A Colour Atlas and Text of DIET-RELATED DISORDERS

Second Edition

Donald S. McLaren
MD, PhD, DTM&H, FRCP(Edin.)
Honorary Fellow, Department of Medicine, University of Edinburgh.
Honorary Head, Nutritional Blindness Prevention Programme, International Centre for Eye Health, University of London.
Formerly Professor of Clinical Nutrition, School of Medicine, American University of Beirut, Beirut, Lebanon.

Wolfe Publishing

First published 1981 by Wolfe Publishing Ltd, now an imprint of
Mosby-Year Book Europe Limited
Second edition published 1992
Printed by BPCC Hazells Ltd, Aylesbury, England
ISBN 0 7234 1800 4

A CIP catalogue record for this book is available from the British Library.

For full details of all Mosby-Year Book Europe Limited titles please write to Mosby-Year Book Europe Limited, Brook House, 2–16 Torrington Place, London WC1E 7LT, England.

Contents

Preface to the Second Edition

Although this is called a second edition it is really a new book because the emphasis, scope and nature have been entirely changed since the *Colour Atlas of Nutritional Disorders* appeared in 1981.

The emphasis then was on nutritional deficiency diseases. These are still among the most important public health problems of developing countries, although some also still arise in societies that are for the most part affluent. Consequently, largely rewritten and expanded sections on these have been included. The change of emphasis has been necessitated by the accumulating evidence, especially in the past decade, that in many, if not most, of the major causes of death and disability in the technologically developed world, diet plays a key role. Included in their number are ischaemic heart disease, hypertension, stroke, diabetes mellitus, obesity, cancer, gallstones, and diverticular disease. These are thoroughly covered as far as their relationship to various dietary factors is concerned.

The expanded scope of the book is evident in several ways. The disease spectrum right around the world now has to be taken into consideration. With this in mind numerous maps have been prepared to help the reader achieve the necessary perspective. The book is also unusual in being all – or at least widely – embracing in the sense that there is hardly a single medical speciality that is not included in some way. Paediatrics, gastro-enterology, dermatology, ophthalmology, cardiology and neurology tend to take the lion's share but others are very well represented. Another reason for the enlarged scope is the increasing number of conditions that respond to intensive care in hospital, and along with other advancing technologies nutritional support provides a greatly improved chance of survival and recovery from advanced states of organ damage and failure that was quite unthinkable only a few years ago. Again, many of the micronutrients, vitamins and essential elements, have recently taken on a new lease of life and interest as it has become evident that states of disturbance from normality, either towards deficiency or excess, bring about changes far beyond those with which they have been traditionally associated for many years. This is especially true of vitamin A, iron, iodine and zinc. All of these trends have been taken into account.

Finally, the nature of the book is very different. This is to some extent reflected in the title but merits some elaboration. The central core of the book remains the profusion of colour plates and their superb reproduction for which Wolfe has long been celebrated. They continue to make their unique contribution to the topics dealt with throughout. There are, however, in medicine increasingly aspects of knowledge that cannot readily be expressed and discussed other than with the aid of graphic and tabular data. These trends have been taken into account and the numerous graphs and tables have been designed to be integral parts of the descriptive text. Where it has been considered that the reader might be most likely to seek a further source of information this has been given.

The final word should, of course, be left with the pictures. They are the products of an extremely wide variety of clinical experience and expertise and could not have been assembled without the greatly appreciated help of the many colleagues gratefully acknowledged. This diversity means that in this field everyone has a great deal to learn from others; among these not least the author. It is his earnest hope and belief that this book will prove to be a good and enjoyable way to do it.

Preface to the First Edition

Although it cannot be stated categorically that all of the essential nutrients for man have been identified it is very unlikely that any of major significance to health remain to be added to the present number of about 50. The latest vitamin, vitamin B_{12}, was discovered more than 30 years ago. During that time many more trace elements have been shown to be essential for animals, and those now number 11 with 4 more of doubtful status. Most of these have been shown, or are suspected, to be essential for man and as food faddism spreads and seriously ill patients are increasingly fed parenterally with specially prepared nutrient mixtures instances of deficiency states have come to the fore. The growth of food processing with risks from contamination have increased the possibility of toxicity from some elements, as well as from other substances in food.

Despite our greatly increased understanding of the nature and extent of malnutrition problems in developing countries, there is little evidence that they are anywhere being brought under control. On the contrary, with the ever increasing world population, especially marked in developing countries, it is clear that more people are suffering from malnutrition today than ever before. The methodology of nutritional assessment has become more sensitive in recent years, particularly with the development of many biochemical tests, but these require sophisticated laboratories and trained personnel, are costly and the results are often difficult to interpret. As in the past, so in the forseeable future, detailed clinical examination for physical signs must be the most practical means of assessing nutritional status of individuals and communities, and of drawing attention to the occurrence and nature of specific nutritional deficiency states.

On the other hand it is only in recent years that recognition has been given to the important role that diet plays in most of the major causes of morbidity and mortality in technologically advanced societies. Although most of these conditions are not directly attributable to an imbalanced diet this does play a part in the aetiology of some and in others dietary measures are an important part of management. It is in these societies also, where advances in diagnosis have made possible the precise identification of the nature of many metabolic derangements, that many more conditions that were previously fatal or untreatable can now be controlled with special diets. Here too the toxic effects of excessive use of vitamins and some trace elements have to be guarded against. Furthermore, it must not be assumed that classic deficiency diseases like rickets, beriberi, scurvy and xerophthalmia need no longer concern the physician practising among over-fed rather than under-fed populations. These and other deficiency states may occur in the presence of an adequate dietary intake from impairment of the utilisation of a nutrient at some stage in the body.

It should also be observed that Nutrition is not only no respecter of persons, but it is also no respecter of systems, organs or tissues. None is exempt from the harmful results of the tipping of the dietary balance beyond the limits of normal that are so difficult to define, or from a failure in utilisation even when those limits are not transgressed.

One final comment may be made. The role of nutrients in the large majority of disorders dealt with in this book is clearly understood and the therapeutic and dietary means to cure or control them are available. That they together account for a high proportion of all illness throughout the world is at least in part due to failure in recognition. It is to be hoped that this atlas, the most comprehensive on the subject as far as it is known, will make a contribution towards remedying the situation.

Acknowledgements

The author and publishers would like to thank the following for provision of the figures listed below.

1 Musée National du Louvre, Paris. 2 & 3 Churchill Livingstone. 5 & 6 T.W. Castonguay, Ph.D. and *Nutrition Reviews*. 8 & 9 Churchill Livingstone. 10 John Wiley and Sons. 11–22 Prof. V. Smil and *Scientific American*. 23 S.J.D. O'Keefe, M.D. and *The Lancet*. 24 Dr R. Passmore and Churchill Livingstone. 26 J. Périssé, Ph.D. and The Food and Agriculture Organization. 27 A. Keys, Ph.D. and The Harvard University Press. 28 H.N. Munro, M.D. and Raven Press. 29 *Medicine Digest*. 30–32 Dr M.G. Dunningham. 36 Royal Botanic Gardens, Kew. 37 Prof. J.R. Anderson and Hodder and Stoughton. 41 & 42 Dr H.M. Gilmour. 43 M.S. Brown, M.D. and J.L. Goldstein, M.D. 44 D. Steinberg, M.D., Ph.D. and American Medical Association. 45–47 Harvard University Press. 48 C.J. Glueck, M.D. and *American Journal of Clinical Nutrition*. 49 Medical Research Council and *British Medical Journal*. 50 D.A. McCarron, M.D. and *The New England Journal of Medicine*. 51 R.L. Weinsier, M.D. and Academic Press. 52 G.L. Montgomery. 53 Dr R.T. Jung. 54 Mr Ching. 55 Dr R. Hall. 56 Dr H.M. Gilmour. 59 Dr R.T. Jung. 60 Dr S. Barclay and Churchill Livingstone. 61 & 62 R.E. Pounder, M.C. Allison and A.P. Dhillon. 63 American Cancer Society. 64 K.K. Carroll, Ph.D. and S. Karger AG, Basel. 67 & 68 Dr H.M. Gilmour. 69 Dr T. Philp. 71 & 72 G.F. Cahill, Jr., M.D. 73 Prof. Dr W. Sandritter. 78–80 J. Murray, M.D., F.R.C.P. 81 & 82 Dr S.P. Allison. 83 & 84 B. Torún, M.D., Ph.D. and Lea and Febiger. 85 & 86 B.R. Bistrian, M.D., Ph.D. and *American Journal of Clinical Nutrition*. 89 M.A. England. 92 Prof. J.D.L. Hansen. 93 World Federation of Public Health Associations. 94 & 95 Dr H. Grossman. 96 & 97 J.E. Rohde, M.D. and *Indian Journal of Paediatrics*. 99 Dr E.M. Widdowson, F.R.S. 100 D.B. Jelliffe, M.D. and Mosby-Yearbook Inc. 101 Prof. L. Mata and *American Journal of Clinical Nutrition*. 102 Prof. R. Hendrickse. 103 Dr R. Cooke. 105 Prof. J.D.L. Hansen and Churchill Livingstone. 106 & 107 Dr S. Lucas. 108 Prof. B. Ochoa. 109 Prof. D. Morley. 112 & 113 *Nutrition*. 114 & 115 Dr I. Maddocks. 116 Prof. D. Morley. 121 Dr H.A.P.C. Oomen. 123–125 Dr F. Mönckeberg. 126 & 127 Dr H. Grossman. 128 Prof. R. Hendricksen. 129–131 Dr H.A.P.C. Oomen. 144 Prof. J.D.L. Hansen. 145 R.B. Bradfield, Ph.D. and *Journal of Pediatrics*. 146 B. Torún, M.D., Ph.D. and Lea and Febiger. 147 D.W. Beaven and S.E. Brooks. 148–151 Dr J. Treasure. 152 A.R. Lucas, M.D., Diane M. Huse, M.S. and Lea and Febiger. 153 Dr Igor de Garine, G.J.A. Koppert and Gordon and Breach Science Publishers. 154 Dr R.T. Jung. 155 & 156 G.A. Bray, M.D. and *The Medical Journal of Australia*. 157 Dr R.T. Jung. 158 & 159 Dr L.J. Taitz (deceased) and Churchill Livingstone. 160 Dr M. Dynski-Klein. 161 & 162 Dr M. Zatouroff. 163–165 Dr M. Dynski-Klein. 166 Dr A.J. Stunkard and *The New England Journal of Medicine*. 168–171 Dr R.T. Jung. 172 Prof. B. Larsson and *British Medical Journal*. 173 Dr M. Krotkiewski and *Journal of Internal Medicine*. 175 MEDDIA, Amsterdam. 177 Dr R. Blomhoff and American Association for the Advancement of Science. 178–180 Upjohn. 181 Medical Research Council. 182–187 A. Sommer, M.D. and *Archives of Ophthalmology*. 188 & 189 Dr J.J.M. Sauter. 190–193 Dr R.R. Pfister. 194 Upjohn. 202–204 Dr J.J.M. Sauter. 214 & 215 Dr J.J.M. Sauter. 216 Dr A. Sommer. 218 Dr H.H.

Sandstead. **221** Upjohn. **222** Dr M.D. Muenter. **223 & 224** Dr H. Grossman. **225–227** Dr I.A. Abrahamson, Snr. **228 & 229** C. Harnois, Ph.D. and American Medical Association. **230 & 231** Dr J. Thomson. **232** E.J. Lammer, M.D. **233** N.R. Belton, Ph.D. and Churchill Livingstone. **234** Dr M. Gebre-Medhin. **235** N.R. Belton, Ph.D. and Churchill Livingstone. **236** Prof. W. Peters and H.M. Gilles. **237** Prof. J.M. Farquhar. **240 & 241** Dr H.M. Gilmour. **243–245** Prof. J.M. Farquhar. **246** Prof. A. Prader. **248** Dr C. Thomas, Jnr. **249** Dame S. Sherlock and J.A. Summerfield, M.R.C.P. **250** Prof. H.R. Wiedemann. **251** Dame S. Sherlock and J.A. Summerfield, M.R.C.P. **252** Dr C. Thomas, Jnr. **253** Dame S. Sherlock. **254–257** Prof. J.O. Forfar. **258** A. Mushin, F.R.C.S., F.C.Ophth. **259 & 260** Dr C.S. Foster. **261** Dr M. Dynski-Klein. **262** Upjohn. **263** Dr M. Dynski-Klein. **264 & 265** Dr M.C. Riella. **267** Dr A. Bryceson. **268 & 269** Dr C. S. Treip. **270** Prof. A.J. Radford. **271** Dame S. Sherlock and J.A. Summerfield, M.R.C.P. **272–274** Upjohn. **283, 284, 290 & 292** Dr H.H. Sandstead. **297–299** Dr M.K. Horwitt. **303 & 304** Upjohn. **305 & 306** Dr R.W. Vilter. **307–309** Dr A.C. Parker. **310** Dr W.R. Tyldesley. **311** D.W. Beaven and S.E. Brooks. **312** Prof. A.V. Hoffbrand. **313** Dr C.S. Treip. **314 & 315** V. Herbert, M.D. and Lea and Febiger. **316 & 317** R.E. Pounder, M.C. Allison and A.P. Dhillon. **318 & 319** Upjohn. **320** Dr M. Zatouroff. **321 & 322** W. Peters and H.M. Gilles. **323** Dr C.S. Treip. **324** Dr W.R. Tyldesley. **325 & 326** D.W. Beaven and S.E. Brooks. **327 & 328** Dr E.J. Watson-Williams. **329–332** Dr C.E. Butterworth, Jnr. **333** H.N. Munro, M.D. and Raven Press. **334–336** D.W. Beaven and S.E. Brooks. **337** M.A. Bedford. **338** Dr C.W. Woodruff. **339** Dr H.E. Sandstead. **340 & 341** Dr C.W. Woodruff. **342** Dr H.M. Gilmour. **343 & 344** Dr R.W. Vilter. **345** Dr C.W. Woodruff. **346–348** Dr R.W. Vilter. **349–351** Upjohn. **352** J. Calder and G. Chessell. **353** Dr R.W. Vilter. **354** Dr H.H. Sandstead. **355 & 356** Dr A. Toft. **358** M.C. Linder, Ph.D. and Elsevier Science Publishers B.V. **359** J.D. Cook, M.D. and *American Journal of Clinical Nutrition*. **360 & 361** Dr A.C. Parker. **362** Dr A.J. Salsbury. **363** Dr M. Zatouroff. **364** D.W. Beaven and S.E. Brooks. **365 & 366** Dr H. Grossman. **367** Upjohn. **368** D.W. Beaven and S.E. Brooks. **369–374** Dr L-G. Larrson. **375** Dr M. Zatouroff. **376** Dr A.C. Parker. **377 & 378** Dr H.M. Gilmour. **379** Dr M. Zatouroff. **380** Dr H.M. Gilmour. **381** M.C. Linder, Ph.D. and Elsevier Science Publishers B.V. **385 & 386** Dr H.M. Gilmour. **388** Dr R. Hall. **389** Dr M. Dynski-Klein. **390** Dr J.T. Dunn. **391** J. Calder and G. Chessell. **393** Upjohn. **394** L.W. Kay. **399 & 400** A.J. Felsenfeld, M.D. and American Medical Association. **402** Dr M. Dynski-Klein. **403–405** Dr L. Finberg. **407** M.C. Linder, Ph.D. and Elsevier Science Publishers B.V. **409 & 410** Dr V. Parsons. **411** M.C. Linder, Ph.D. and Elsevier Science Publishers B.V. **413** I. Murdock, F.R.C.S., F.C.Ophth. **414** E. Randolph Broun, M.D. and American Medical Association. **415** M.C. Linder, Ph.D. and Elsevier Science Publishers B.V. **416** L.W. Young, M.D. and American Medical Association. **417** Dr D.M. Danks. **418 & 419** Dr C.S. Treip. **420** Dame Sheila Sherlock. **421–423** Dr J.M. Walshe. **424 & 425** S. Sherlock and A. Summerfield. **426 & 427** Dr B. Portmann. **428 & 429** Dr A. Kennedy. **430–433** Dr J.F. Sullivan. **434A** G.M. Levene and C.D. Calnan. **434B & C** Profs. Guangqi Yang and Yiming Xia. **436 & 437** Dr M. Zatouroff. **438** S. Sherlock and A. Summerfield. **439** Dr M. Zatouroff. **440** M.A. Bedford. **441–443** Dr S.M. Podos. **444** Prof. H.R. Wiedemann. **445 & 446** Dr R.R. Howell. **447** S. Sherlock and A. Summerfield. **448** Dr S.M. Podos. **449** Prof. K. Weinbren. **450 & 451** S. Sherlock and A. Summerfield. **452** Prof. J.M. Farquhar. **453** Dr von G.-W. Schmidt. **455** Dr R.P. Burns. **456** Dr H. Ghadimi. **457** Prof. H.R. Wiedemann. **458 & 459** Dr S.H. Mudd. **460** R.W. Lloyd-Davies, J.G. Gow and D.R. Davies. **461** Dr S.M. Podos. **462** Dr K. Takki. **463 & 464** Dr L.S. Taitz. **465** S. Sherlock and A. Summerfield. **466 & 467** G.M. Levene and C.D. Calnan. **468** Dr H.M. Gilmour. **469** Dr J.B. Wyngaarden. **470 & 471** Dr H.M. Gilmour. **473** G.M. Levene and C.D. Calnan. **474–479** W.F. Jackson and R. Cerio. **480 & 481** Dr D. Burman and Churchill Livingstone. **482** Dr A. Ferguson. **483 & 484** G.M. Levene and C.D. Calnan. **485** Dr H. Dodd. **486–489** R.E. Pounder, M.C. Allison and A.P. Dhillon. **491–493** Dr H.M. Gilmour. **494 & 495** Dr K.L. Jones. **496** Prof. B. Leiber. **497** S. Sherlock and A. Summerfield. **498 & 499** C. Adams. **500** Dr D.B. Jelliffe. **501** Dr D.O. Gibbons. **502** Prof. J.R. Anderson and Hodder and Stoughton. **504** Dr R. Passmore and Churchill Livingstone. **505** R. Hall and D.C. Evered. **506–508** S. Sherlock and A. Summerfield. **509** Crown copyright © Tropical Products Institute. **510** Dame Sheila Sherlock. **511** Crown copyright © Ministry of Agriculture, Fisheries and Food. **512–515** B.W. Halstead, P.S. Auerbach and D. Campbell. **516** J. Calder and G. Chessell. **517** Federation of American Societies for Experimental Biology. **518–522** Prof. M.M. Meguid. **524** W.R. Beisel, M.D. and *American Journal of Clinical Nutrition*. **525** W. Peters and H.M. Gilles. **526 & 527** Prof. C.M. Anderson. **529** Dr R.V. Heatley. **530 & 531** R.E. Pounder, M.C. Allison and A.P. Dhillon. **532** Dr P. Sweny and Dr Z. Varghese. **533 & 534** S. Sherlock and A. Summerfield. **535** Dr H.M. Gilmour. **536** Dr T. Philp. **537** J. Calder and G. Chessell. **538** Dr J.A. Eisman and *British Medical Journal*. **539–541** R.E. Pounder, M.C. Allison and A.P. Dhillon. **545** Dr A. Bryceson. **546, 547 & 549** W. Peters and H.M. Gilles. **551** G.M. Levene and C.D. Calnan. **552** Prof. M.S.R. Hunt. **555** C. Adams. **556** Dr C.S. Treip. **559** *Journal of Tropical Medicine and Hygiene*. **560** A.C. Boyle. **561** E.E. Kritzinger and B.E. Wright. **Table 13** Dr M.G. Dunningham and Oxford University Press. **Table 18** Dr M.R. Law and *British Medical Journal*. **Table 25** Dr R.T. Jung. **Table 27** Dr R. Peto. **Tables 40 & 41** Dr R.T. Jung. **Tables 42 & 43** World Health Organization. **Table 48** Dr R.T. Jung.

1. Principles of Diet and Nutrition

One of the leading nineteenth century philosophers of materialism, Ludwig Feuerbach (1804–1872), who had the dubious honour of inspiring Marx and Engels, must at least be credited with both a nice play on words and a physiologically sound statement in his well-known dictum 'Der Mensch ist was er isst' – Man is what he eats. Long before this, the sixteenth century artist Guiseppe Arcimboldo produced a series of surrealistic paintings of human figures constructed entirely from everyday items of food; these make the same point in a most striking manner (**1**).

1

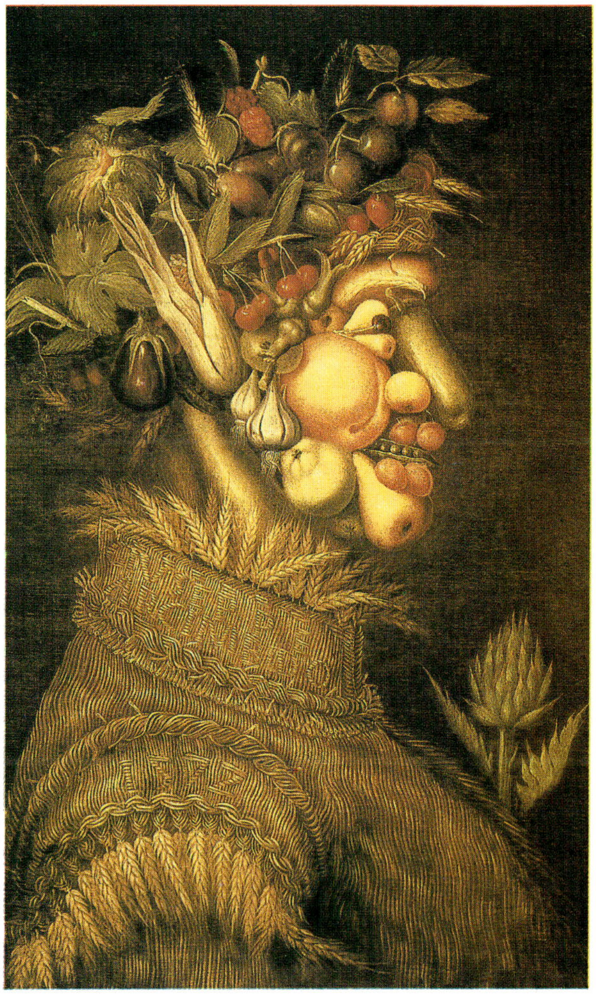

1 Man is what he eats.

The body ingests, rearranges, and utilizes what it consumes for the purposes of maintenance of life, growth, reproduction, functioning of organs, and production of energy. This process is called *nutrition*. Just like some other processes, such as respiration and the functioning of the immune system, it consists of the interaction of the *host* with the *environment* in general and with the relevant *agent* in particular (**2**).

2

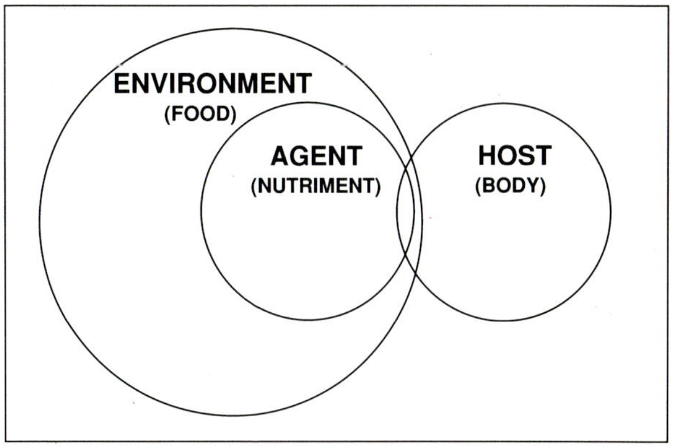

2 Agent–host–environment concept applied to nutrition.

Table 1. Non-nutritional aspects of food.

Dietary fibre	(Chapters 2 and 3)
Food idiosyncrasies	(Chapter 8)
Toxins in food	(Chapter 9)
Food and behaviour	(Chapters 2, 4 and 8)
Analeptic or aesthetic properties	(Chapter 4)

In this case, the relevant part of the environment is that which is ingested, i.e. food, and within that the specific agent is nutriment (or the nutrients). This *agent–host–environment* concept was first developed in epidemiology for application to infectious diseases, but it clearly has wider applications.

Food does more than just provide nutrients; there are a number of other aspects that in various ways have an important bearing on human health and disease (*Table 1*).

3
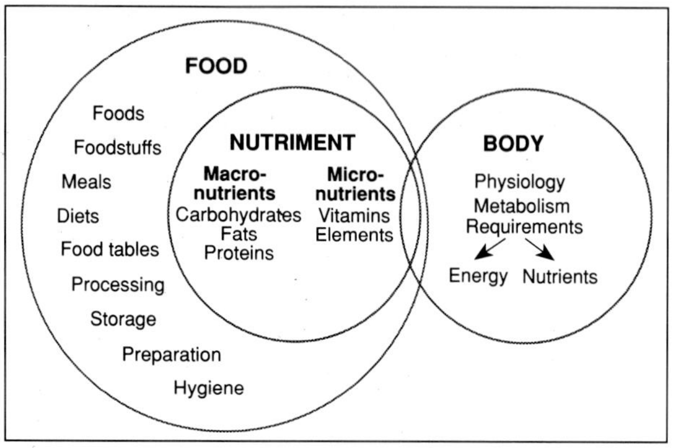

3 Interrelationships of food, nutriment and the body in more detail.

3 is a further elaboration on the same scheme, designed to indicate something of the scope of each of the component parts of the system described here.

Nutrients form a very heterogeneous group of chemical substances, for which the only common feature is the body's need for each to be in the diet, in different amounts, for health to be maintained. This need varies considerably throughout the vegetable and animal kingdoms. In general, the simpler the organism the fewer nutrients it requires. Among higher animals, the need for the approximately 50 known nutrients is allocated in a quite unpredictable fashion. For example, vitamin C (ascorbic acid) is a vitamin only for humans, monkeys, guinea pigs, Indian fruit bats, red-vented bulbuls, and fish, because they possess no L-gulonolactone oxidase, necessary for one of the steps in the pathway for the production of the vitamin.

Nutrients are conveniently divided into *micro-* and *macronutrients* and, as shown in *Table 2*, they have very different characteristics.

The relationship of a nutrient to the body at any particular time is expressed by the term *nutritional status* (or *nutriture*). The nutritional status, like any other status (e.g. financial, social) is the resultant of the opposing forces of supply and demand. In this case it is the resultant of dietary intake of the nutrient in question and utilization of the nutrient by the body. It is now known that for an increasing number of nutrients harm can result not only from a deficiency but also from an excess of nutrient. Recom-

Table 2. Micro- and macronutrients contrasted.

Micronutrients	*Macronutrients*
1. Consumed in small amounts (usually <1 g/day)	Large amounts (many g/day)
2. Absorbed unchanged*	Degraded by digestion
3. Essential, body cannot make them	No single carbohydrate, fat or protein as eaten is essential but products may be (see text)
4. Do not provide energy	Provide energy
5. Major function as coenzymes and catalysts	Enzymes are proteins
6. Structural function limited (calcium, phosphorus mainly)	Protein mainly structural, but also some lipid and carbohydrate

*Exceptions include carotenoids and folates.

mendations that are designed to ensure an adequate intake of nutrients to prevent deficiency among most of the population have been broadened in recent years to include the concept of also setting safe upper limits of intake with a view to preventing toxic effects of excessive consumption in both the long and short term (see Appendix I, Table 7).

4 outlines in principle the concept that for each nutrient and source of energy there is a range of intake that confers optimal biological function. The lower and upper ends of this arbitrarily set range grade into marginal status where structure and function are unimpaired but there are no reserves. Further progress beyond the marginal states leads to uniform evidence of deficiency on the one hand or toxicity on the other.

This spectrum of nutritional status has been most thoroughly explored at its deficiency end in relation to many of the nutrients; *Table 3* relates the progressive stages of depletion to the types of technique used for their assessment, together with specific examples.

4

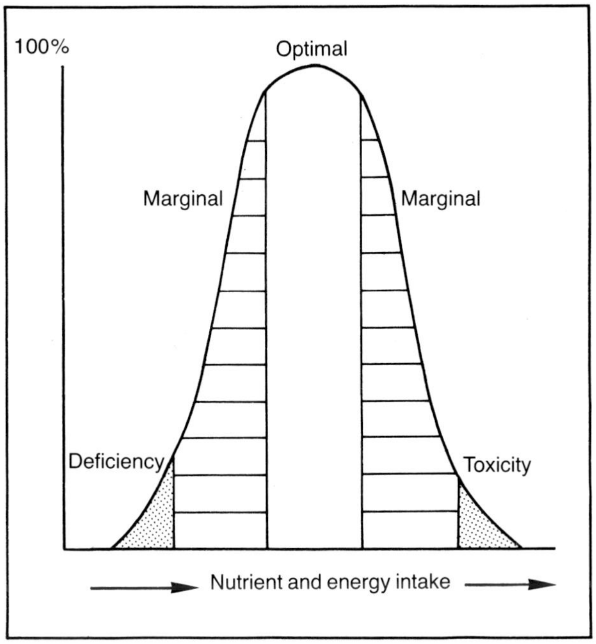

4 'Normal' and 'abnormal' nutrition.

Table 3. Stages in the process of nutritional depletion.

Stage	*Assessment technique*	*Examples of techniques*	*Related deficiency*	*Nutritional status*
Adaptation (physiological)	Biochemical	Urinary urea, Plasma glucose, fatty acids	Protein depletion, Energy lack (temporary)	Well nourished
Reduction in stores	Biochemical, Anthropometric	Autopsy liver sample, Skinfold thickness	Vitamin A, B_{12}, Fe, etc., Starvation, marasmus	↓
Body dimensions	Anthropometric	Weight, height	Protein-energy malnutrition	
Reduction in tissue, blood, urine levels	Biochemical	Plasma retinol, urinary niacin metabolites	Deficiency of vitamin A, niacin	at increasing risk
Biochemical 'lesions'	Enzyme activity	Erythrocyte glutathione reductase activity	Deficiency of riboflavin	
Organ dysfunction/ biophysical defect	Functional	Dark adaptometry (retinal rod function), Hand grip dynamometry	Vitamin A deficiency Protein-energy malnutrition	↓
Early tissue change	Histological	Conjunctival impression cytology	Subclinical vitamin A deficiency	
Clinical symptoms	History	Weakness	Possible anaemia	Actively
Signs	Physical examination	Rickety rosary	Vitamin D deficiency	malnourished

5

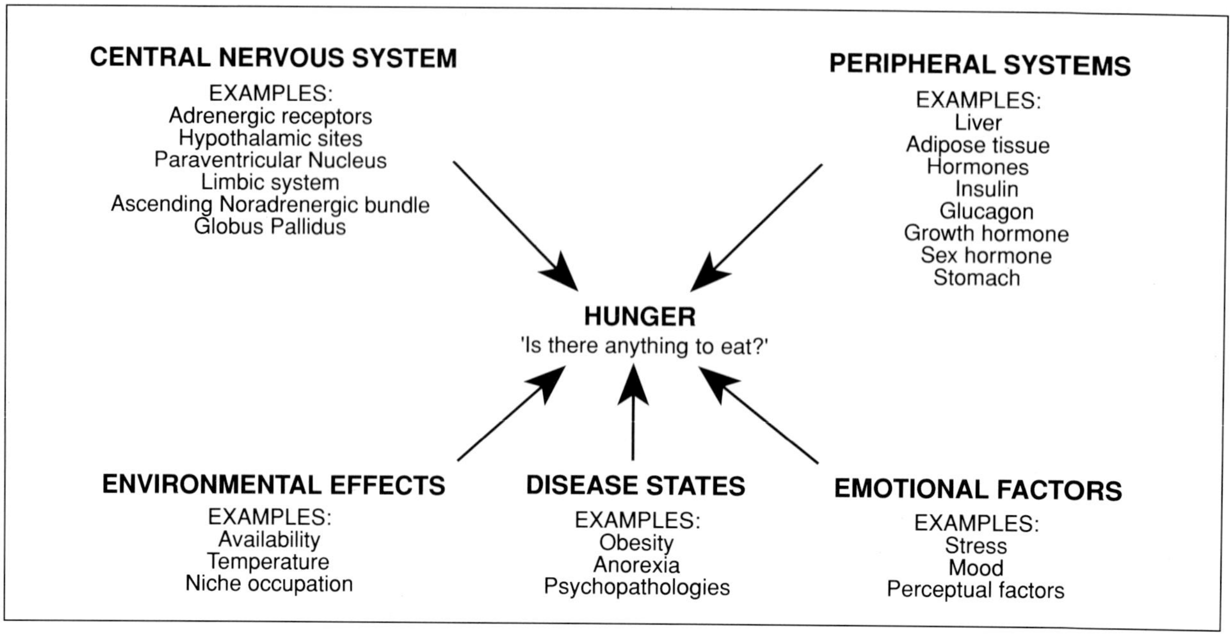

5 A partial listing of the ever-growing number of factors that are known to influence the onset of hunger.

6

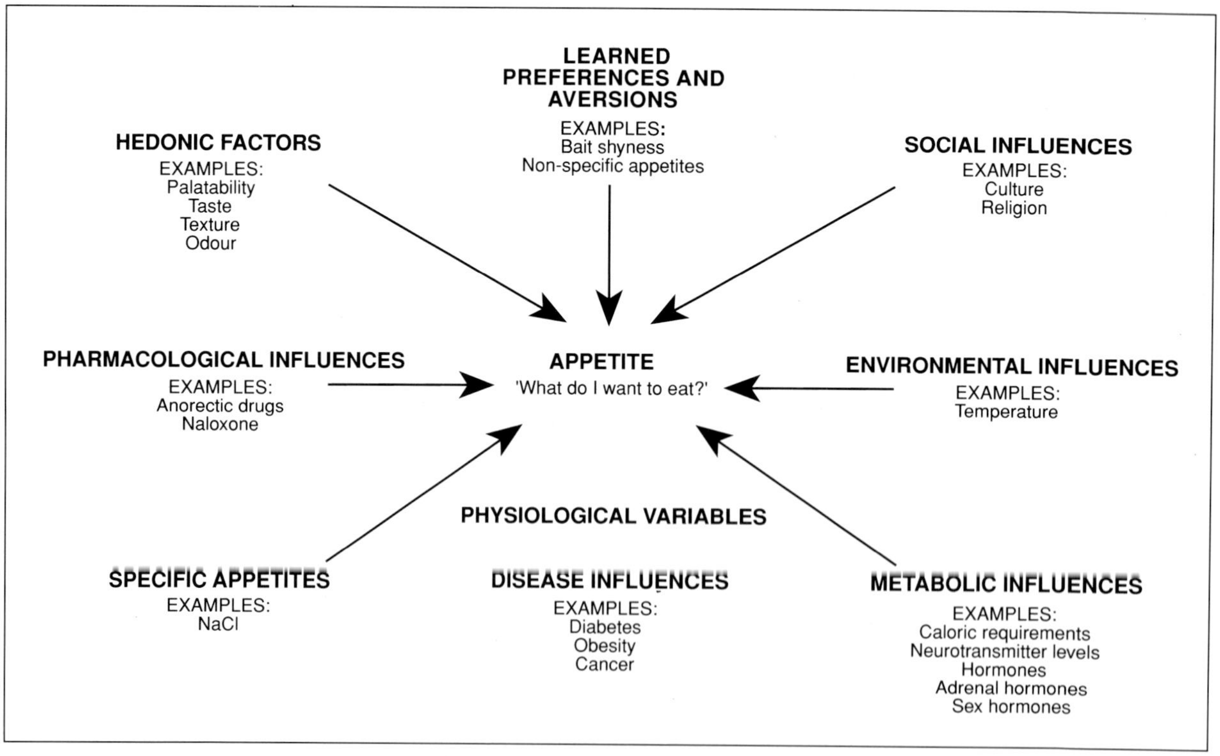

6 Some of the factors that determine appetite.

Determinants of the search for food, i.e. hunger (5) and of appetite (6) are extremely numerous and come both from within the host and also from the environment. The resultant of all these stimuli decides ultimately what food is chosen and how much of it will be consumed. The accompanying figures are by no means exhaustive, but serve to illustrate the complexity of these aspects of dietary intake that are so relevant to health and disease.

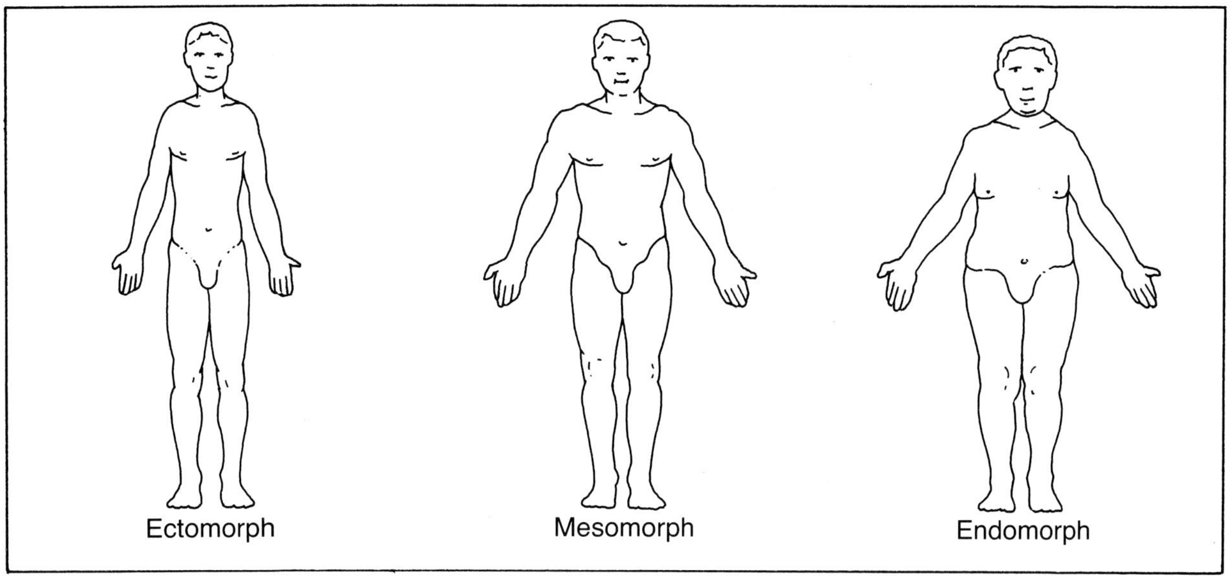

7

7 The three basic contrasting somatotypes; (from left to right) *ectomorph, mesomorph* and *endomorph*. Sheldon described many intermediate stages. In the ectomorph, structures of ectodermal origin in embryology predominate: skin and nervous system. The mesomorph is strong in musculature and this body type predisposes to coronary heart disease, as does the endomorph type if mostly abdominal (see *Table 16* and **167**).

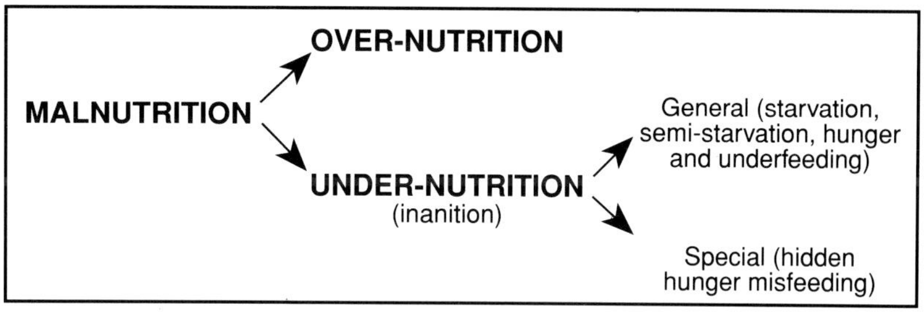

8

8 Types of malnutrition.

An additional complication is provided by the very evident fact that even 'normal' individuals vary greatly in their bodily habitus and therefore in their requirements. There is a vast literature on this subject dating back to the last century and beyond. Of the many classifications devised, Sheldon's[1] (**7**) which consists of the basic somatotypes of *ecto-*, *meso-*, and *endomorph* is one of the best known. Application of this scheme over several decades[2] demonstrated an association between physical type and delinquent behaviour. However, attempts to apply this scheme to various disease states did not meet with similar success. A somewhat different approach was taken by Vague[3], a Marseille physician whose work on the regional distribution of adipose tissue was neglected for many years but which is now seen to be of great importance in unravelling the relationship between obesity and various diseases (see Chapter 4).

Any deviation from 'normal' nutrition may be termed *malnutrition*. The different types of malnutrition are shown in **8**. These are all dealt with in Chapters 4, 5 and 6.

Table 4. Classification of malnutrition.

Cause	primary (exogenous) secondary (endogenous)
Type	excess, toxicity (overnutrition) deficiency (undernutrition)
Nutrient	vitamins, elements, protein, energy sources
Degree	(i) mild–moderate–severe or, alternatively, (ii) depleted stores–biochemical lesion–functional change–structural lesion
Duration	acute, subacute, chronic
Outcome	reversible, irreversible

Table 4 gives a classification of malnutrition which helps to categorize it in different ways.

9

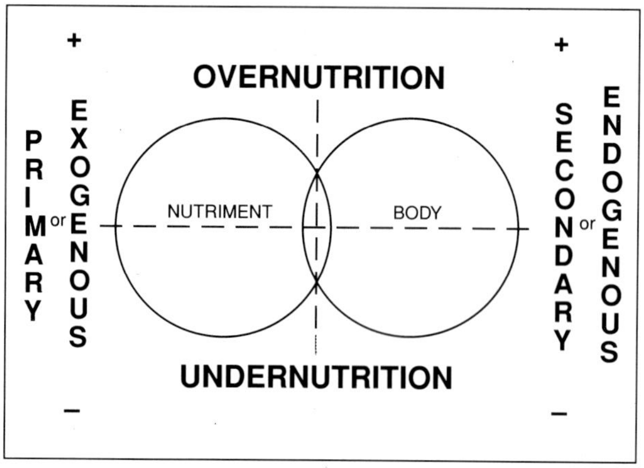

9 Forms of nutritional disorders.

Some of these ideas can be pictured as an interaction between nutriment (the nutrients) and the body (9). In this scheme deviations from normal can originate in nutriment when the abnormality is outside the body (exogenous, primary) or within the body (endogenous, secondary). In either case overnutrition or undernutrition may result. Any combination of nutrients may be affected. In practice it is not uncommon for both exogenous and endogenous factors to be at work and this is well illustrated by protein-energy malnutrition (PEM) (see Chapter 4).

Nutritional deficiency, or impairment of nutritional status, evolves in a steadily progressive way along the lines shown in *Table 3*. Along this way of progression different types of changes occur which may be amenable to investigation by appropriate tests as indicated. Clinical signs which are featured prominently in this Atlas are late manifestations of deficiency. Although much research is being carried out on the development of new tests for the assessment of various aspects of nutritional deficiency in its early stages[4] (see Appendix III, Tables 1 and 2) few are yet available for micronutrient status assessment, and so clinical examination remains of great importance (Appendix IV). In certain fields of hospital practice this is becoming increasingly so as patients with serious organ failure, e.g. liver, kidney, nervous system, and gut survive for long periods and pose problems for nutritional support (see Chapter 10).

Table 5 indicates special groups that are potentially at risk of developing nutritional deficiency and provides additional information on the likely underlying causes and nutritional consequences.

Whenever one of the above groups at risk is involved or if for any reason a nutritional problem is suspected a dietary and nutritional history should be taken using the salient points shown in *Table 6*.

Table 5. Groups at high risk of developing nutritional problems.

Group	*Disabilities*	*Common nutritional consequences*
Infants	low birthweight, birth defects	inadequate stores of nutrients, feeding difficulties
Young children	weaning problems, rapid growth	failure to thrive, poor growth
Adolescents	peer group pressure, growth spurt, anorexia nervosa, bulimia	inadequate energy intake, anaemia
Pregnant and lactating women	increased requirements, pica	iron and folate deficiencies
Elderly	depression, poor dentition, chronic disease, medication	reduced intake and variety, anorexia
Food faddists, obsessive slimmers	unbalanced diets	micronutrient deficiencies
Chronic alcoholics	gastritis, impaired absorption, anorexia, 'empty' calories	thiamin (inadequate for energy intake) deficiency common
Drug addicts	as above, plus chronic infection, especially AIDS, tuberculosis	wasting
Patients of all ages with chronic diseases and/or long-term radio/chemotherapy	anorexia, febrile episodes	weight loss, drug–nutrient antagonism

Table 6. Aspects of personal history that relate to dietary intake.

Recent weight gain or loss
Changes in appetite
Problems with chewing or swallowing
Condition of dentition or dentures
Any changes in sense of taste or smell
Any gastrointestinal symptoms: nausea, heartburn, waterbrash, vomiting, diarrhoea, constipation, blood loss, etc.
Living conditions, including arrangements for meals
Financial circumstances
Any physical or mental handicap
Alcohol consumption
Drugs, prescribed and non-prescribed
Any dietary restriction followed
Use of vitamin or other dietary supplements
Any food allergies
Religious or ethnic beliefs relating to diet

Table 7. Information required for assessment of nutritional status in a community.

Source of information	*Nature of information*	*Nutritional implications*
Anthropometry	Growth, physical development	Indicative of general, rather than specific, undernutrition
Biochemistry	Levels of nutrients, metabolites and other components of body tissues and fluids	Nutrient supplies in the body, impairment of biochemical function
Clinical	Physical signs and symptoms	Deviation from health due to malnutrition
Dietary surveys	Food consumption of different groups	Level of intake of various nutrients
Vital and health statistics	Morbidity and mortality data	Identification of high-risk groups
Background data	Socioeconomic, health, agriculture, cultural, anthropological data, etc.	

Assessment of nutritional status is most appropriately carried out in a community. Reasons for this include, as previously mentioned, the great variability between individuals of nutrient requirements, and therefore the difficulty of applying standards, other than to large groups. Also, while treatment of frank deficiency is a clinical matter, improvement of nutritional status is a public health measure. *Table 7* shows the different methods which have been used to give a direct or indirect assessment of nutritional status. It should be noted that dietary intake, being related only to the input and not to the output side of the status equation (see page 8) does not provide an assessment of nutritional status, although it can be invaluable for planning public health interventions.

2. Diet, Culture and Disease

In Chapter 1, food and the nutrients it contains were considered as that part of the environment which is ingested. In **10** the human environment is pictured at different levels and it is a consequence of resulting interactions that the great diversity of diet-related diseases around the world occurs.

In the agent–host–environment interacting system considered previously, the requirements for nutrients (agent) vary very little and man (host) can undergo physiological adaptation within a certain range of dietary intakes. However, what is considered to be food (the ingested environment) has varied strikingly from culture to culture and throughout the span of human existence. 'One man's meat is another man's poison' had been true long before Lucretius coined the phrase in the first century BC.

There is no such thing as an ideal diet. Each of the great variety of dietaries developed by trial and error throughout human history and under widely differing conditions has proved capable of sustaining normal growth and development and successful continuity of the species, providing it has been available in amounts sufficient to satisfy hunger.

10

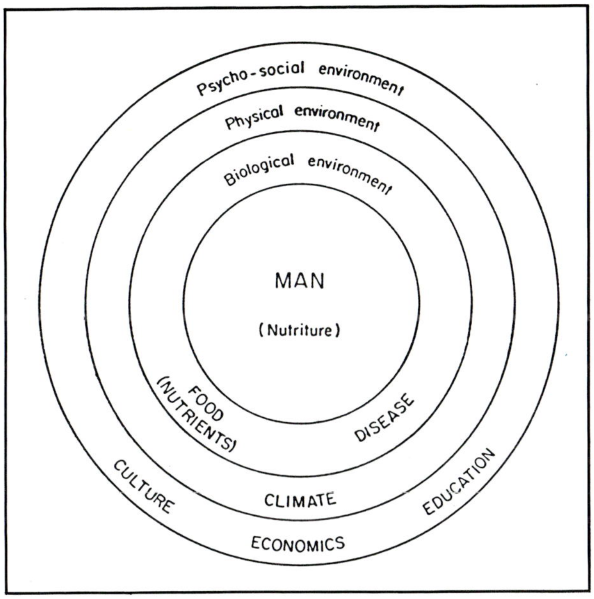

10 Man and his food.

11–22 show the essential foods of the Chinese, most of which will be largely unfamiliar to the non-Oriental. The story could be repeated around the world for other major cultural groups, although increasingly the powerful supermarket culture is breaking barriers down and making the formerly exotic familiar.

11

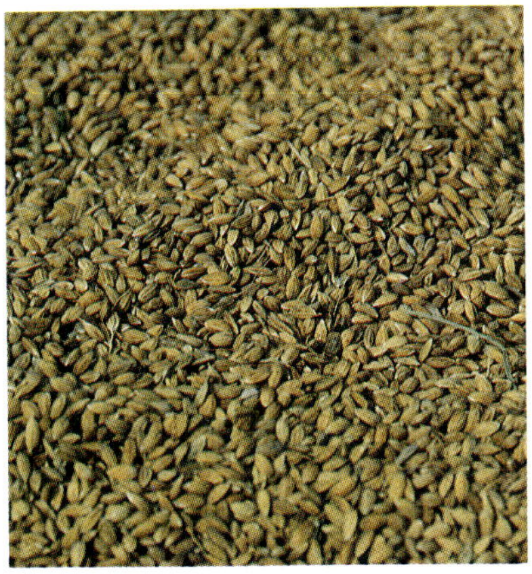

12

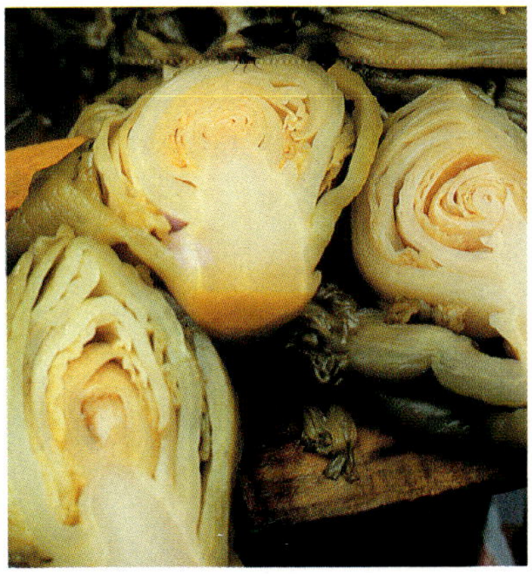

13

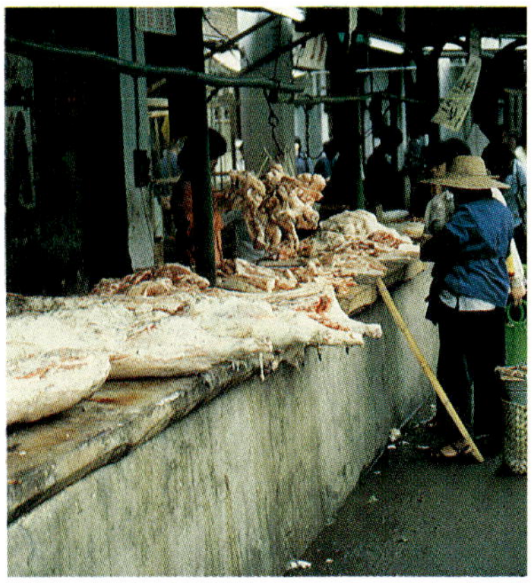

14

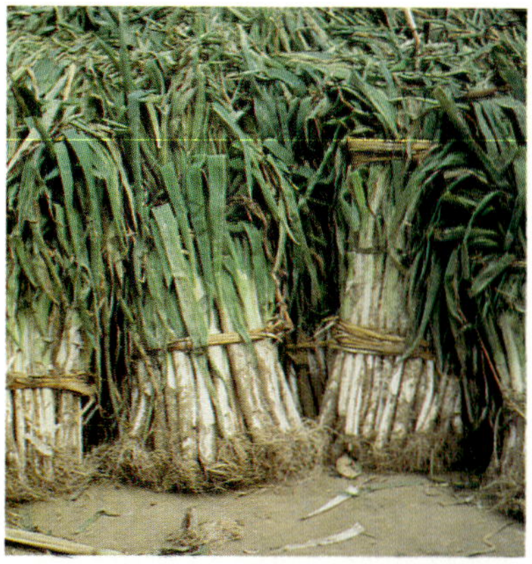

15

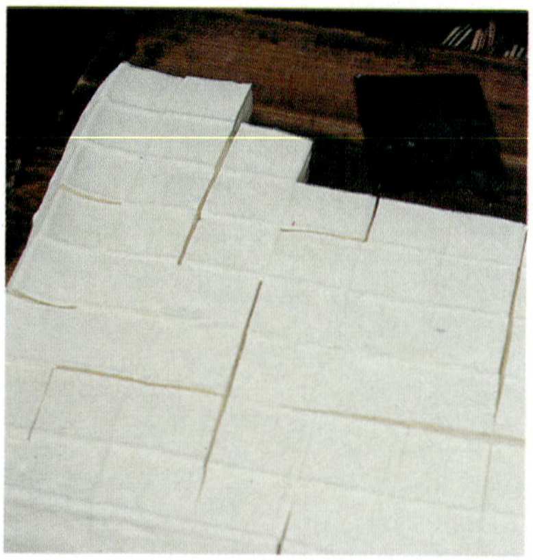

16

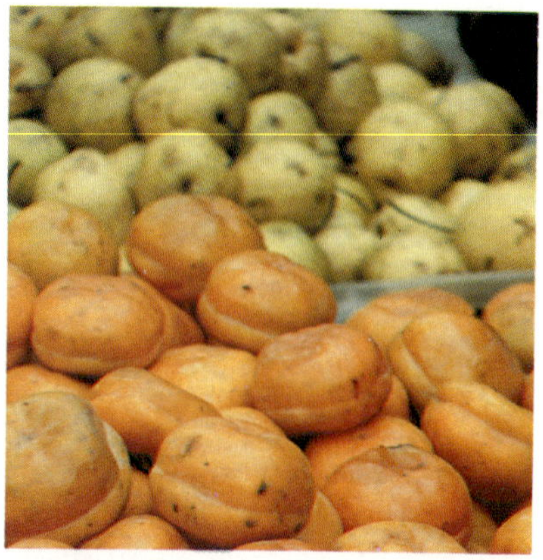

17

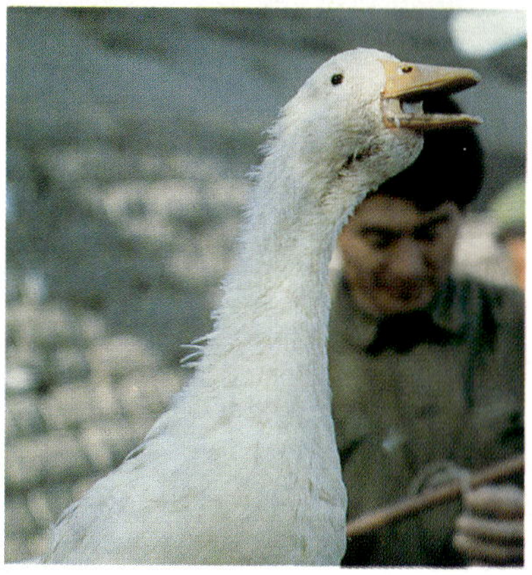

18

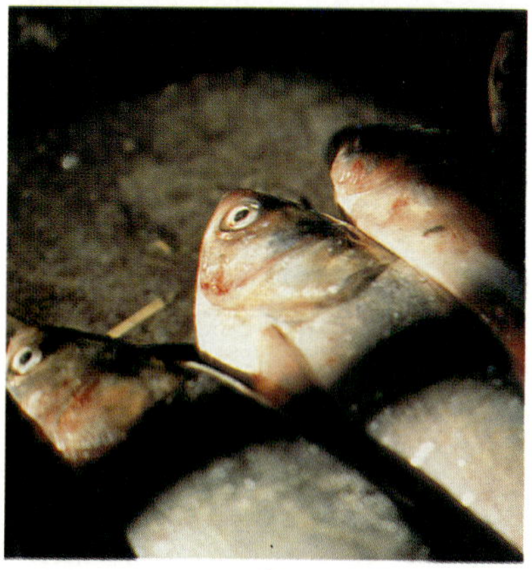

19

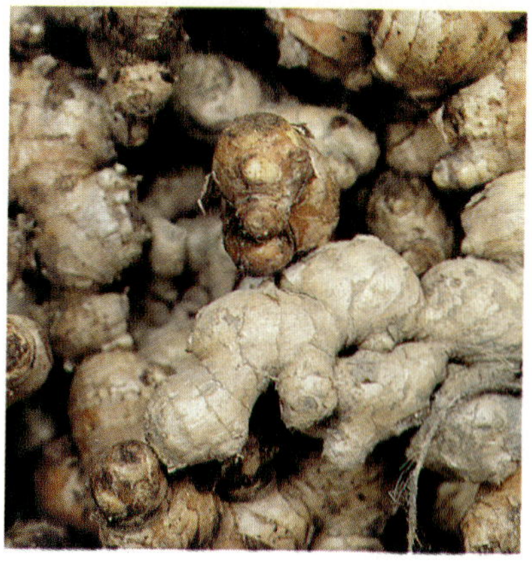

20

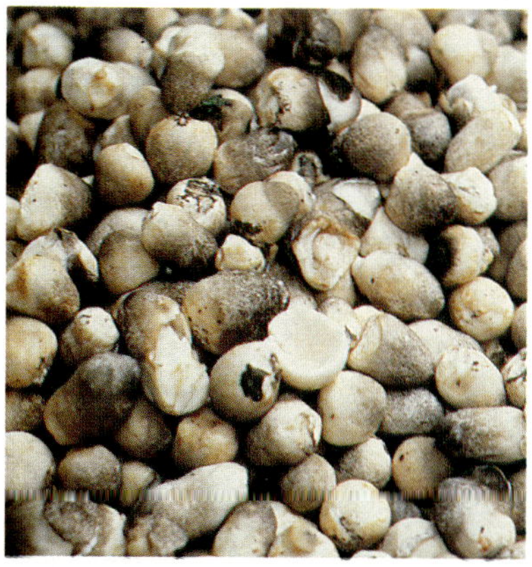

21

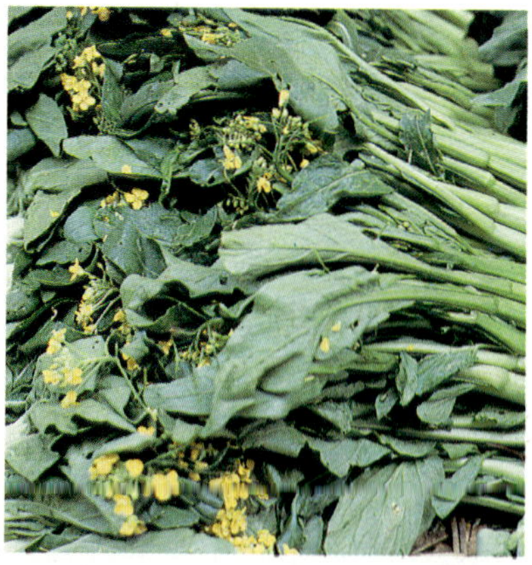

22

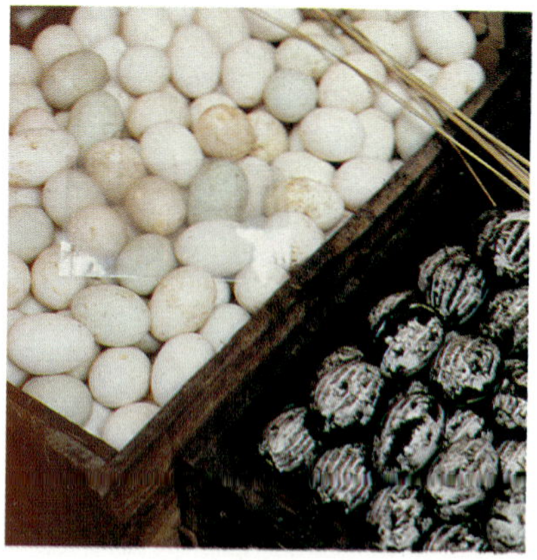

11–22 Essential foods in China are shown here in approximate order of importance. They are: unmilled rice, (**11**); pickled cabbages, (**12**); lardy, nearly meatless pork, (**13**); northern green onions, (**14**); bean-curd cakes, (**15**); pears and persimmons, (**16**); Beijing duck, (**17**); fresh carp, (**18**); ginger root, (**19**); mushroom, (**20**); rape greens, (**21**); and fresh and preserved eggs, (**22**). In the Chinese diet rice is by far the main cereal, cabbage is the main vegetable, pork constitutes 92% of the meat and carp is the main fish. Duck is the most favoured poultry and green onions and ginger are the commonest flavourings in Chinese cooking; mushrooms and persimmons serve widely as delicacies.

Only under conditions of privation is eating dictated by hunger. Habit, custom and social pressure normally determine when and how food is eaten and what is eaten. Religious and other beliefs have a powerful influence over what food is considered permissible and because such beliefs tend to be strict and lasting they have an important influence on nutrition (see page 24).

Paleolithic man was long considered to have been primarily a hunter and therefore to have obtained a high proportion of his diet from meat. This may have been true until the period shortly before the dawn of agriculture about 10,000BC when overhunting, climate changes and population growth brought about a shift to subsistence activities with a way of life not unlike that of the few modern hunter-gatherers who remain relatively untouched.

The dietary intake of some of these societies has been studied in recent years[5] and in general they tend to derive between 50 and 80% by weight of their food from plants. Eskimos and similar people living in the far north are exceptional (see page **25**) in that 10% or less of their food is vegetable in origin. If a conservative estimate of 35% animal and 65% vegetable origin is taken to reflect the late Paleolithic diet then some conjectural comparisons can be made with contemporary western man (*Table 8*).

Hunter-gatherers have tended to merge with pastoral urbanized people around the world with loss of their traditional lifestyle, of which diet is one of the most vulnerable aspects to change. For example the Bushmen of northeast Namibia (**23**) now eat little more than refined maize meal and spend any money earned on alcoholic beverages. In addition to being seriously wasted they show biochemical evidence of protein, vitamins A, C, E and folic acid deficiencies. Eighty-five percent of those hospitalized in one study had tuberculosis.[6]

Table 8. Some broad comparisons of dietary intakes.

Dietary component	*Paleolithic man*	*Current average intake of 'western' man*	*Consensus of recommendations*
Protein (as percentage of energy)	34	16	12
Carbohydrate "	45	45	58
Fat "	21	39	30
P:S* ratio	1.4	0.4	1.0
Cholesterol (mg/day)	590	435	<300
Fibre (g/day)	46	18	25–30
Sodium (mg/day)	690	>3300	1100–3300
Calcium (mg/day)	1580	740	800–1200
Vitamin C (mg/day)	400	88	60

* polyunsaturated : saturated fatty acids

23 Family group of rural Bushmen. Note the difference in stature between Dr O'Keefe (height 1.78m) and Bushmen. Despite the poor living conditions, the large number of children seen is typical of Bushmen settlements.

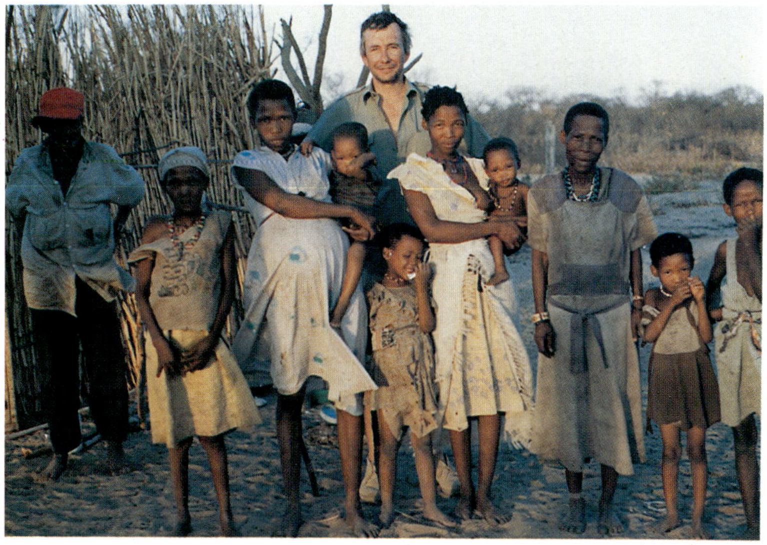

23

24

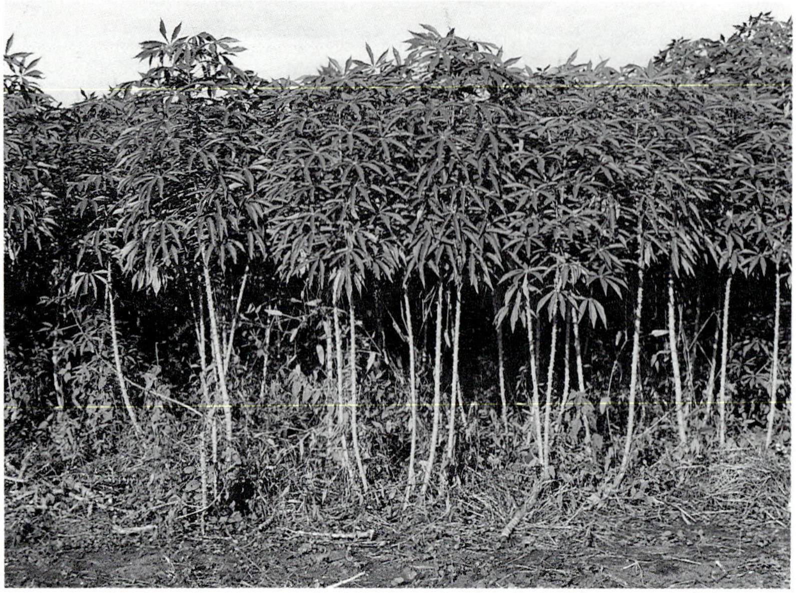

24 Plantation of yuca (**manioc, cassava**) **in Ecuador.** Cultivation is easy, new trees being propagated from stem cuttings. When 2–4 m tall they are dug up and the tubers cooked. The young leaves are rich in carotenoids.

In most of Asia, Africa and Latin America subsistence farming is still the lot of the majority of those who work on the land. In good times they are able to feed their families and have something over to sell, but when hardship strikes in the form of drought, flood or strife they are defenceless. Cereal cultures based on rice, wheat, millet or maize have a sounder nutritional base for a diet with adequate quality and quantity of protein than do those in which the staple is starchy roots such as cassava (**24**). However, social unrest and rapid population growth are contributing to depopulation of the countryside in the less developed countries, with the consequent destruction of the agricultural base, and mushrooming of shanty towns and slums (**25**).

25

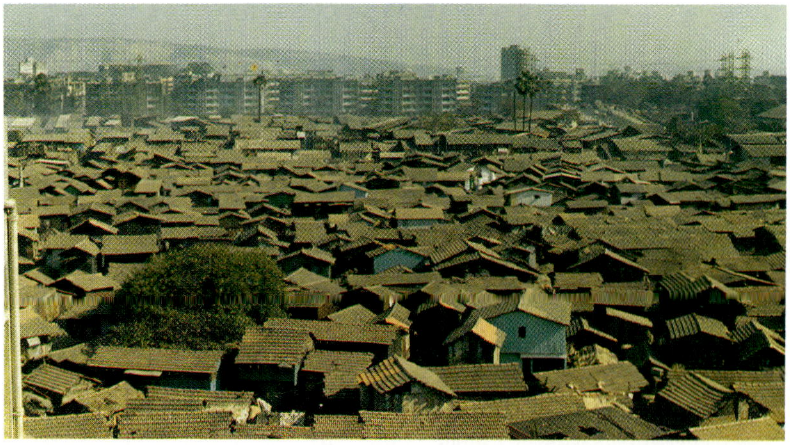

25 Dharavi, covering about 5km^2 in the north west of the Bombay peninsula is notorious as 'the largest slum in Asia'. It houses nearly a million people, migrants from all over India. A typical home is a single room, 3m^2, for three to eight people with no lavatories and communal standpipes providing unsafe water at irregular hours. It is forecast that by the year 2000 nearly half the population of third-world countries will be living in towns and cities and that half of these will be living in slums or shanty towns like those pictured here. The tenements in the background of Dharavi may appear luxurious from a distance by comparison but in reality they are sprawling slums.

Looked at from the perspective of the present situation the world can be divided into two very unequal parts for the occurrence of diet-related disease problems (*Table 9*).

Table 10 shows in more detail the estimated magnitude of the problems of hunger and malnutrition. The contrasting diet-related diseases of the industrialized societies are dealt with in Chapter 3.

Some of the main dietary components require further comment.

Table 9. 'Two halves' of the world.

Factor	*'Westernized' world*	*Rest of the world*
Energy	Deficiency rare, excess considerable	Deficiency widespread (hunger and malnutrition)
Micronutrients	Deficiency rare, excess occasional	Deficiency common
Lack of choice of foods	Rare	Usual; over-reliance on staple
Wrong choice of foods	Considerable (fat, salt, sugar, fibre)	Growing with 'westernization'
Food toxicoses	Little; mostly food technology related	Frequent; mostly natural contaminants

Table 10. Hunger and malnutrition.

Disorder	*Nutrients*	*Precipitating factors*	*Major features*	*Vulnerable groups*	*Geographic distribution*	*Approximate number affected at one time*
Hunger, starvation	All, especially energy sources	Food shortage, poverty	Impaired physical and mental performance	All	Lowest socio-economic group, developing countries	1 billion
Protein energy malnutrition	Protein and energy mainly	Early weaning, infections	Retarded physical, mental development, marasmus, kwashiorkor	Infants and pre-school children	Marasmus throughout developing countries	500 million–mild; 100 million–moderate; 10 million–severe
Xerophthalmia	Vitamin A	Rice staple, infections, early weaning	Night blindness, xerosis, keratomalacia, morbidity, mortality	Young children	S. and E. Asia, parts M. East, Africa and Latin America	250,000–blind/year 10 million–non-corneal/year
Rickets, osteomalacia	Vitamin D	Lack of sunlight, poor diet	Skeletal deformities	Infants, pregnant, aged	Towns, developing countries	Thousands
Beriberi	Thiamin	Non-parboiled rice, alcoholism	Heart failure, nerve and brain damage	Mainly adults	Parts of Asia, cities of Europe, N. America	Thousands
Pellagra	Niacin	Maize diet (not lime treated)	Dermatosis, diarrhoea, dementia	Mainly adults	Parts of Africa, M. East, India	Thousands
Scurvy	Vitamin C	Lack of fruit, over-cooking	Haemorrhages, impaired wound healing	Infants, aged	Mainly famine	Hundreds
Iron deficiency	Iron	Prematurity, milk diet, blood loss	Anaemia, impaired work and learning	Infants, child bearing	Worldwide	Many millions
Iodine deficiency disorders	Iodine	Leached soil, goitrogens	Goitre, cretinism fetal damage	Fetus, young females	Hills of Asia, Africa and L. America	100 million

Energy sources

There is a marked difference between regions in the sources of food energy, as shown in **26**[7]. The proportion of calories from fat rises steeply with income, as the resultant of two opposing phenomena: a rise in the consumption of separated fats (oils, butter, margarine, shortenings and lards) and of unseparated edible animal fats through increased consumption of meat, milk and fish; and a reduction in the consumption of unseparated vegetable fats (in cereals, nuts and oilseeds). On the other hand, the proportion of energy supplied by carbohydrates declines as income rises. This trend conceals two opposing phenomena linked with rise in income: a diminished proportion of starchy staples (e.g. cereals, roots, tubers, plantains) and pulses; and a sharp increase in the consumption of sugar and sugar-sweetened foods.

What **26** does not show is the great disparity between the poor and the better-off within regions. Moreover, it does not take account of the fact that some countries and some communities are in energy deficit and others are in excess of requirements.

26

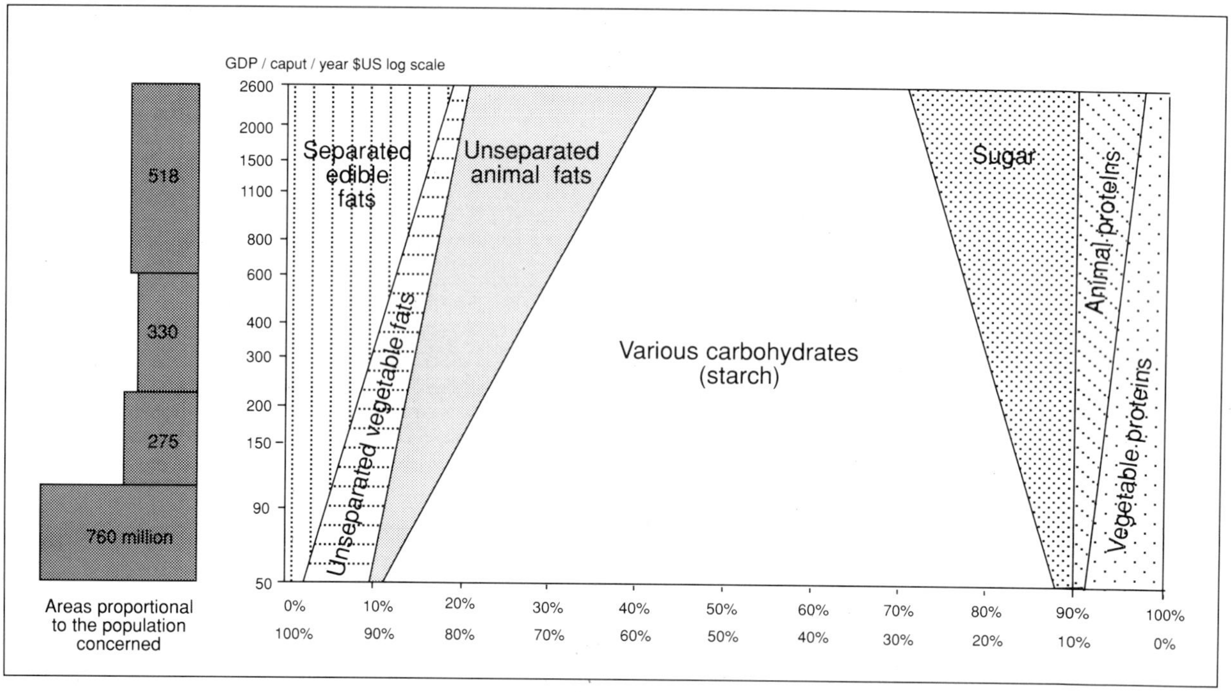

26 Dietary energy derived from fats, carbohydrates and proteins, as a percentage of total energy related to the gross domestic products (GDP) of 85 countries. The figures on the extreme left show the population living in each range of GDP.

Table 11. Changes in energy sources in the United States.

Total calories	*Early 1900s*		*Early 1980s*		
Carbohydrate:		58%		49%	
Polysaccharides	75%		60%		
Mono- and disaccharides	25%		40% (mostly refined)		
Fat:		30%		38%	(42 in 1960s)
Lard and butter	72%		25%		
Margarine	3%		18%		
Shortening	18%		27%		
Salad and cooking oil	7%		30%		
Protein:		12%		12%	
Animal	35%		70%		
Vegetable	65%		30%		
Fibre (g/day)		50	20		

Comparisons over time in the same country can also be informative, although because of the nature of the data these can only be approximations (*Table 11*).

Fat

Few dispute that excess saturated fat is the chief dietary component to have an adverse effect on health in a population and predisposition to hypercholesterolaemia and its consequences[8] in particular (**27**). This relationship has not been found to hold for the individual (see also Chapter 3).

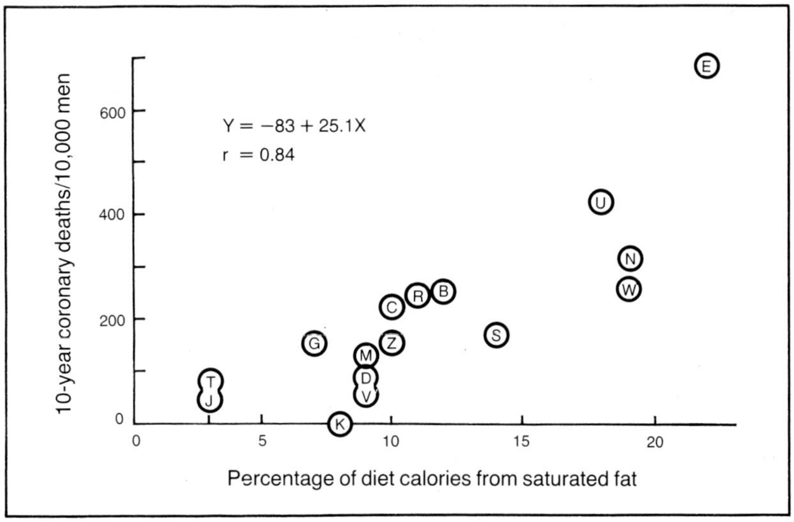

27

27 Ten-year coronary death rates of the cohorts plotted against the percentage of dietary calories supplied by saturated fatty acids. When many more countries are included there are notable exceptions to the general trend. It has also not been explained why in industrialized countries with very similar life expectancy, IHD mortality may differ by as much as threefold (circles represent people in 16 different cohorts in 7 countries).

Protein

28

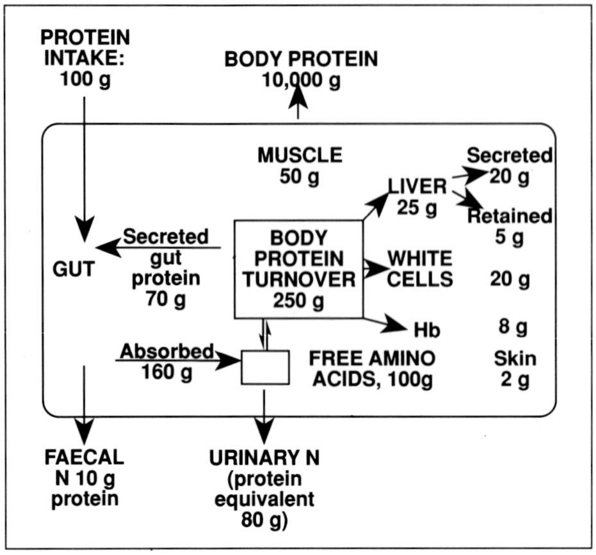

28 **Estimated daily turnover of protein** in the whole body and some organs of a 70kg man. The total quantity of plasma proteins secreted daily by the liver (20g) has been estimated for albumin (12g), gammaglobulins (3g), fibrinogen (2.5g), transferrin (1g), and caeruloplasmin (0.2g), the balance (1.3g) allowing for the turnover of other plasma proteins.

In any diet providing adequate nourishment the proportion of energy provided by protein is about 12%, which contrasts with that from various sources of both fat and carbohydrate (see above). With increasing income the proportion supplied by animal protein increases steadily (see **26**). The daily turnover of body protein (**28**) is about 2.5 times that of the intake.[9] For protein requirements (see Appendix I, Table 3) to be met, not only must the total amount of protein be adequate but the balance of essential amino acids must be correct (see Appendix II, Table 1). If deficiency occurs adaptive changes take place to allow body reserves to be drawn upon (see **70–72**) and when these are exhausted frank malnutrition results (see page 54).

Salt

Salt intake is coming to be increasingly recognized as a major influence on blood pressure (see Chapter 3).

Sugar

Average sugar intake in the West has increased several-fold during the century up until about 1960 when a decline set in. Most of this can be accounted for by the refining of sucrose from cane and later beet, thus converting a luxury food into one of everyday consumption. A recent report[10] examined the evidence for adverse effects on health from this level of consumption. It was exonerated in the cases of IHD, diabetes, gallstones, cancer, renal stones and any effect in obesity apart from contributing to overall energy intake. Non-milk extrinsic sugars, mainly sucrose, were implicated as the most important dietary factor in the development of dental caries (see Chapter 6).

Dietary fibre

This is the most important non-nutritional component of the diet. It has been defined as a large group of substances present in the plant foods of man which are not digested by human gut enzymes. The principle members of this group are cellulose, hemicelluloses, and pectic substances – all polysaccharides; and lignin, a noncarbohydrate (see **29**).

Different forms of dietary fibre have very different effects on the body (*Table 12*). The distinction is sometimes made between soluble fibres that dissolve in water to form a gel and insoluble fibres. Guar gum and pectin are soluble fibres and lower serum cholesterol but have little effect on bowel function. Cellulose and the arabinoxylans of bran fail to affect serum cholesterol but are good laxatives (see Chapter 3). However, it is not possible to classify dietary fibre according to function in any rigid way.

The average western diet of today is low in all kinds of fibre in comparison with that of a century ago and diets in third-world countries, as well as what we know of the diet of early man (see *Table 8*). Many of the diseases associated with a western lifestyle (Chapter 3) can be attributed in part to lack of fibre in the diet.

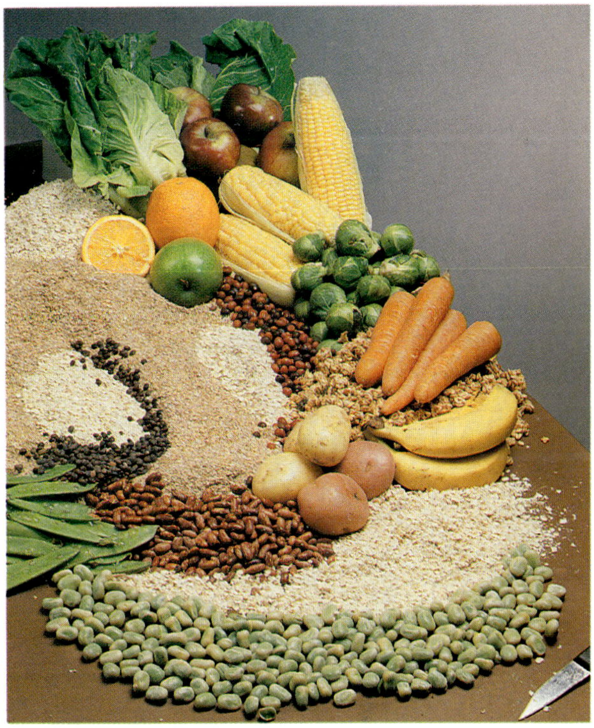

29

29 Cereal, vegetable and fruit sources of dietary fibre in the British diet.

Table 12. Properties of different types of dietary fibre.

Type of fibre	*Physico-chemical property*	*Physiological effects*	*Clinical applications*
Wheat bran	Particle formation and water-holding capacity	Increased gastric emptying and Increased faecal bulk Decreased transit time Decreased colonic pressure	Peptic ulcer Constipation Diverticular disease
Gums, mucilages	Viscosity	Decreased gastric emptying Decreased absorption in small intestine	Dumping syndrome Diabetes, hypercholesterolaemia
Lignin	Adsorption	Increased steroids output Decreased faecal fat losses	Hypercholesterolaemia Cholelithiasis
	Antioxidant	Decreased free radicals	?Anticarcinogenesis
Acidic polysaccharides	Cation exchange	Increased intestinal losses of elements	Negative mineral balance

Vegetarianism

An adequate supply of all nutrients can readily be obtained from a varied selection of foodstuffs from which the flesh of animals and fish has been excluded, but containing milk and eggs. This is the most common form of vegetarianism and is known as ovo-lactovegetarianism. Only iron may be in short supply. If all animal products are excluded – veganism – vitamin B_{12} will be deficient (see Chapter 5) and calcium, iron and zinc supply may be marginal. Infants may be especially vulnerable in a new community following vegan principles[11] and may suffer from multiple deficiencies including PEM, rickets, osteoporosis and vitamin B_{12} deficiency.

Dunnigan and his colleagues in Glasgow[12] have shown the important part that varying degrees of vegetarianism play in the development of osteomalacia among Asian women living there (*Table 13* and 30–32). Lactovegetarians who consume no meat, fish or egg had a significantly higher risk than ovo-lactovegetarians, the vitamin D in eggs apparently making the difference.

30

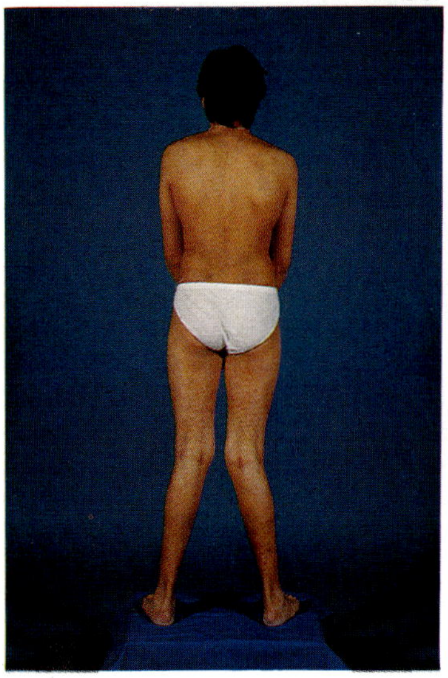

31

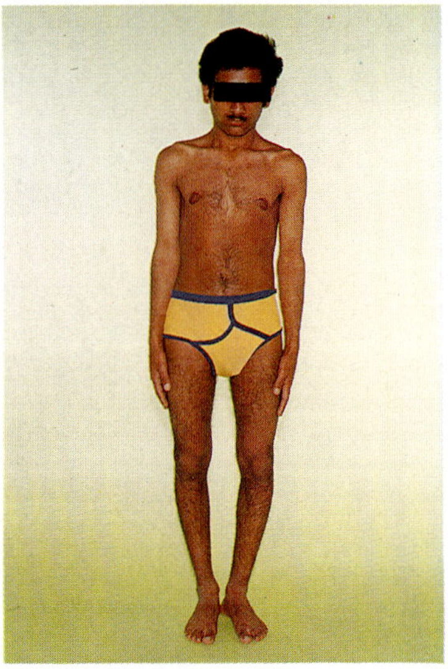

32

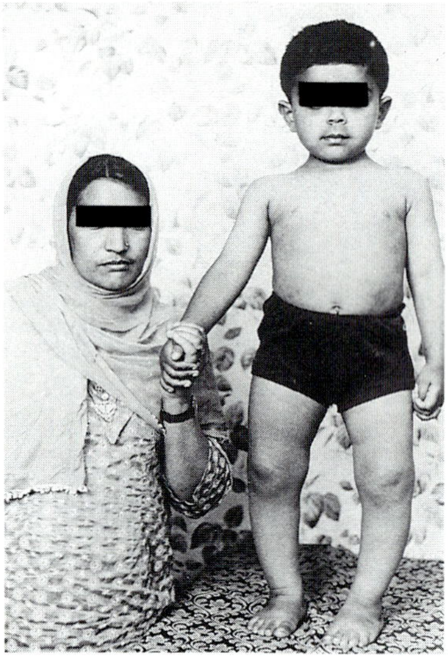

30 This adolescent Asian boy required an osteotomy for severe genu valgum. He had adopted 'junk vegetarianism' after leaving school. He managed an uncle's shop and subsisted on a diet of chappati, dal and a variety of sweets, lemonade and crisps.

31 This Muslim Asian non-vegetarian adolescent has severe tibial deformity, an unusual deformity in late rickets. He had very high intakes of chappati with a high fibre and phytate content. His meat intake was in the normal range.

32 Classical toddler rickets in an Asian child in Bradford. The usual history in such a case is prolonged breast feeding, supplementation with vegetarian foods containing no vitamin D, failure to utilize welfare vitamin D supplements, and marginal exposure to ultraviolet light.

Table 13. Vegetarianism and osteomalacia in Asian women.

	Osteomalacia		*Normal*	*Osteomalacia: Normal*
	X ray +ve	*X ray −ve*		*p**
Lactovegetarian	10	4	1	<0.001
Ovolactovegetarian	2	2	5	<0.04
Non-vegetarian	0	9	71	<0.001

* χ^2 test

Case studies

In a work of this kind it is only possible to hint at some of the salient features of the subject of this chapter and it seems fitting to select some illustrative stories to round off this account. The hunt for the cause of a new disease demands scientific detective work, objective assessment of the evidence, and great patience. Bradford Hill proposed the application of six criteria, or canons as he called them, to test a hypothesis: the correlation of the proposed cause with the diseases should–

- be biologically plausible;
- be strong;
- reflect a biological gradient;
- be found consistently;
- hold true over time; and
- be confirmed by experiment.

Only in the first of the following accounts do all of these apply.

Eskimos and EPA

The diet of the Eskimo peoples of the North has long been of interest. Traditionally it has mainly been animal, including seal, whale and fatty fish. The rarity of ischaemic heart disease (IHD) and atherosclerosis among them was repeatedly noted and blood cholesterol was found to be low. In the 1970s several expeditions were made to study Eskimos on the coast of northwest Greenland and to compare them with those living in Denmark (**33**).[13,14] Dietary analyses showed differences in polyunsaturated fatty acids (PUFA) (*Table 14*) (**34**).

33

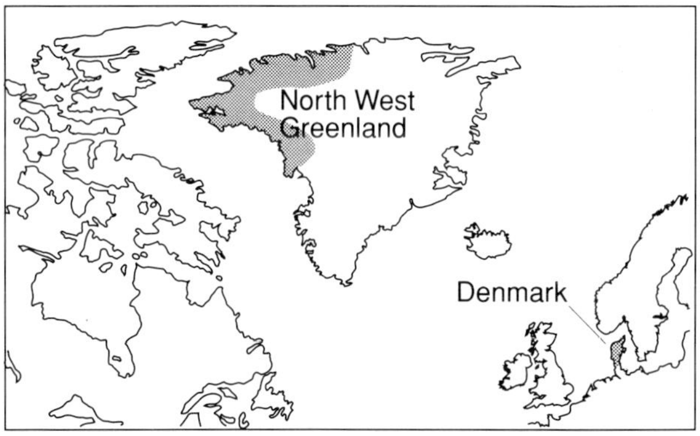

33 Eskimos and EPA.

34

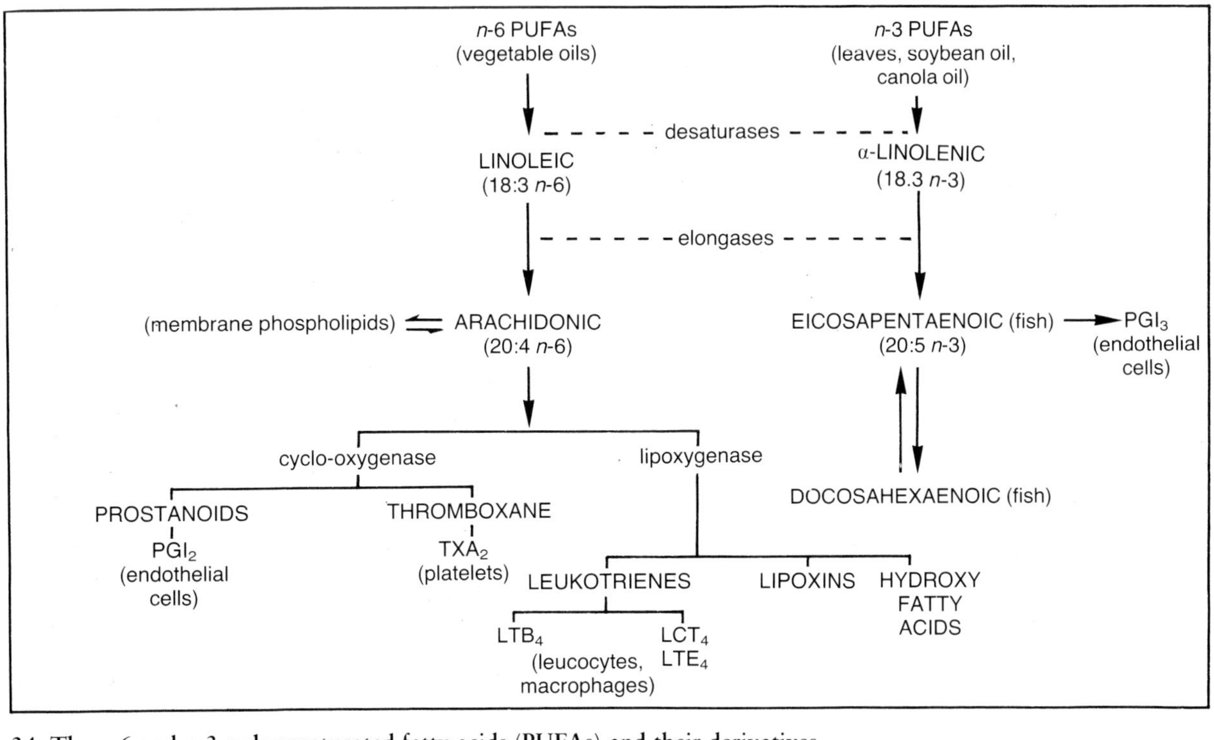

34 The *n*-6 and *n*-3 polyunsaturated fatty acids (PUFAs) and their derivatives.

Two fatty acids of the n-3 series, eicosapentaenoic acid (EPA) and docosahexaenoic acid (DHA) were high in blood samples as was HDL, but LDL was low and VLDL very low in Greenland Eskimos. Bleeding time was prolonged, platelet count low and platelet aggregation less than normal. All these findings are consistent with a low incidence of IHD. Similar results have been obtained in fishing communities in Japan and elsewhere. Feeding studies in animals and man of these n-3 fatty acids provide confirmatory evidence.

n-3 PUFAs appear to have their anticoronary effect by several mechanisms[15]. They depress plasma lipids and in phospholipid pools arachidonic acid is replaced by EPA and DHA which, when released, inhibit enzymes responsible for the synthesis by platelets and macrophages of some eicosanoids, especially thromboxane (TXA_2) and leukotriene B_4(LBT_4) resulting in lessened thrombotic activity of platelets. n-3 PUFAs also depress eicosanoid metabolism and in this way may retard the progress of atherogenesis.

In the form of Maxepa these marine fatty acids are now available on prescription for treatment of hypertriglyceridaemia and prevention of IHD and pancreatitis.

Table 14. Comparison of dietary fat consumed by Eskimos in Greenland and Denmark.

	Greenland	*Denmark*
Total energy from fat (%)	39	49
n-3 PUFAs (g/day)	14	3
n-6 PUFAs (g/day)	5	10
Cholesterol (g/day)	0.7	0.42
Fatty acids (dietary fat %)		
Saturated	23	53
Monounsaturated	58	34
Polyunsaturated	19	13

Motor neuron disease and cycads

The Chamorro people, the original inhabitants of Guam and other Mariana Islands in the northern Pacific between the Philippines and Japan, commonly develop damage to the nervous system that has been attributed to the consumption of cycad seeds (**35**).

The cycad (**36**) is a palm-like tree, the false sago palm, *Cycas circinalis* and a number of other species, that survives well in drought and has provided an emergency source of food.

35

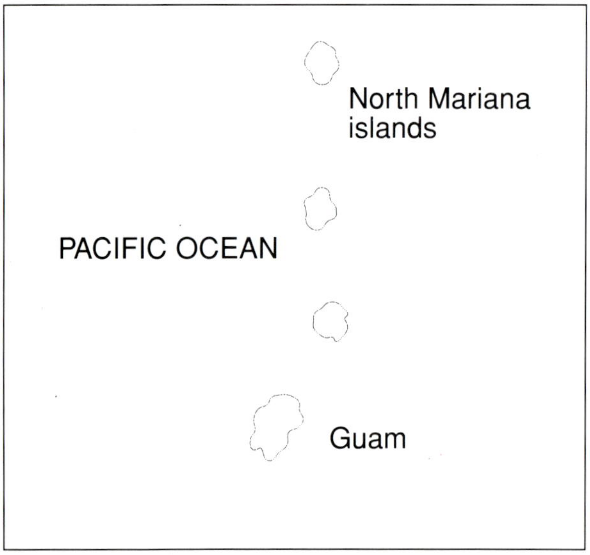

35 Motor neuron disease and cycads.

36

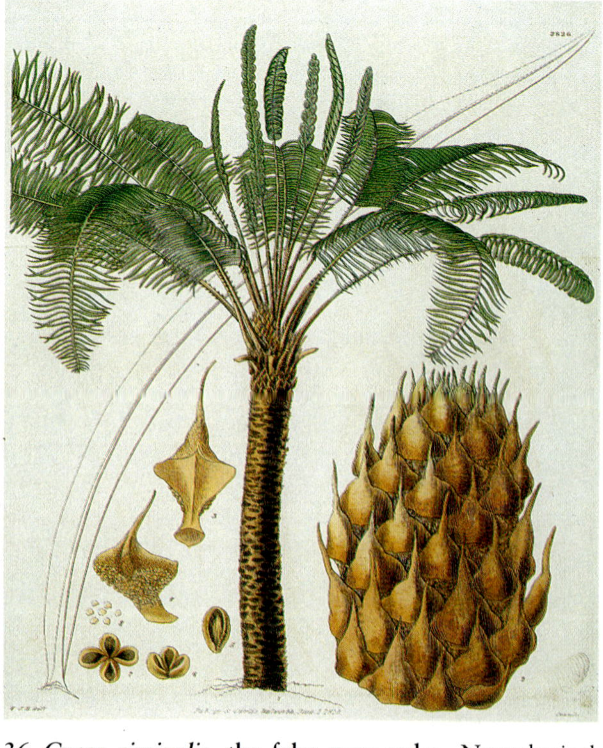

36 *Cycas circinalis*, the false sago palm. Neurological disease has been attributed to consumption of the seeds.

Amyotrophic lateral sclerosis (ALS) is about one hundred times more common among the Chamorro than elsewhere and a parkinsonism–dementia complex is also often found (**37**). Neurofibrillary tangles in neurons of the cerebral cortex, basal ganglia and brain stem have been reported in these patients but these lesions are common even among healthy Guamanians and their significance is uncertain.

A toxin, cycasin, has been isolated from cycad seeds but it has been found in experimental animals that it causes cancer and does not bring about changes in the nervous system. A preliminary report claiming that degenerative changes in the motor system of monkeys were produced by another toxin from cycad has not been confirmed.

With recent diversification of the diet and infrequent consumption of cycad seeds the diseases are said to be waning and they may disappear before their aetiology is proved (see also Chapter 9).

37

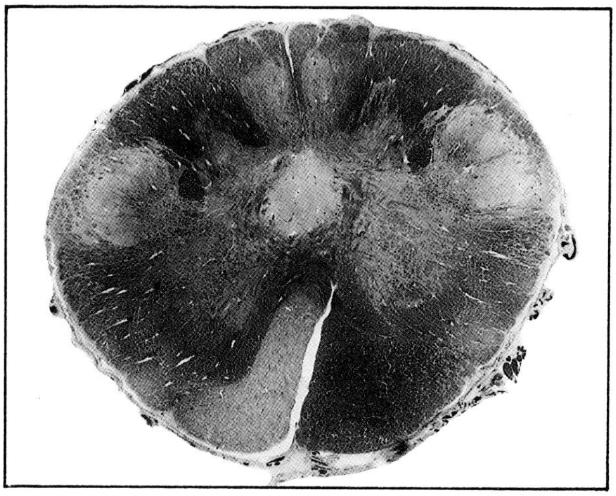

37 **Degenerative changes** are present in both anterior horn cells, producing a lower motor neuron lesion, and of the long motor tracts causing an upper motor neuron lesion. The pyramidal tracts are maximally involved, but the anterior and lateral white columns are degenerate, and the posterior columns are spared.

Balkan endemic nephropathy

After the second world war evidence began to emerge from Yugoslavia, Bulgaria and Romania that renal failure was a common cause of death. At autopsy the kidneys were wasted, with large tumours affecting the tubules often present. A considerable proportion of the population from scores of villages along the banks of the river Danube and its tributaries in these countries was affected (**38**). Investigation of the disease was largely confined to two centres in Yugoslavia (Croatia and Serbia) and one in Bulgaria. Facilities were limited and there was rivalry rather than cooperation. Many theories were put forward including that it was hereditary, or was due to lead poisoning from water mills.

The discovery in Copenhagen, Denmark in 1972 that pigs fed mouldy barley developed kidney damage led to the identification of ochrotoxin as the cause. This is produced by the mould *Aspergillus ochraceus*. In Croatia this mould was found in food stored in cellars and in attics. It was also present in human blood but its occurrence did not coincide well with the endemic area.

38

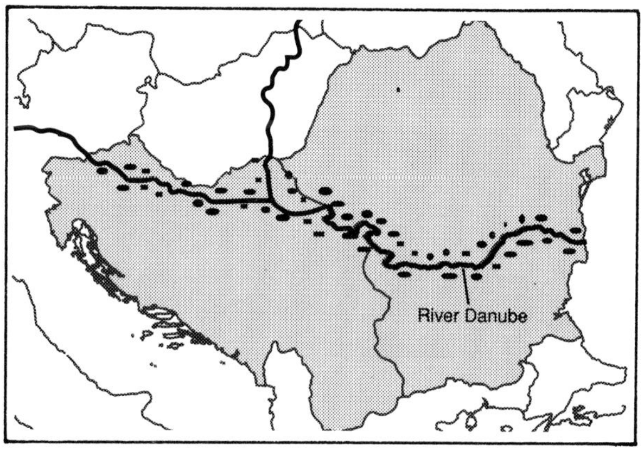

38 **Balkan endemic nephropathy.**

In Bulgaria ochrotoxin was found in food and blood at much higher levels in areas with the nephropathy. Animal experiments in the United States showed that ochrotoxin could cause renal tumours. Ochrotoxicosis seems to be the most likely explanation.

Sudden cardiac death (SCD)

39

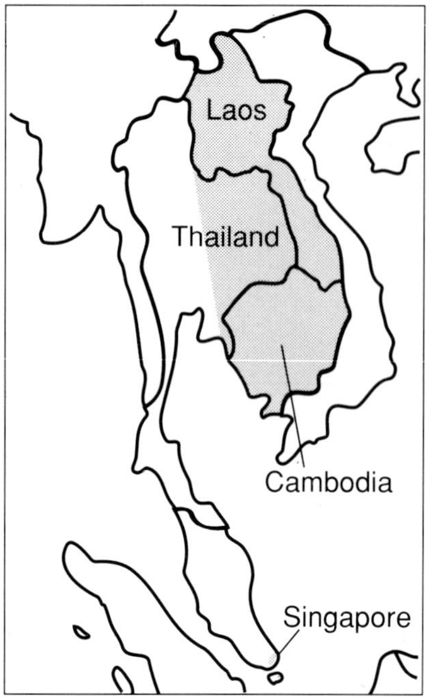

39 Sudden cardiac death.

Much of the building construction in Singapore is carried out by poorly paid immigrant labourers from northeast Thailand. More than 200 sudden cardiac deaths have occurred among these young men in the past six years or so. Autopsy reveals only subendocardial haemorrhage, indicative of terminal hypoxia, with normal coronary arteries. Similar reports have come from Mong people (a hill tribe from Laos) based in refugee camps in Thailand, from the Khmer in Cambodia, and among rural Thai themselves (**39**).

In the West most SCD is due to IHD but about 10% have normal vessels and the rapidly fatal ventricular fibrillation is attributed to electrical instability. This may result from excess sympathetic stimulation. A long QT interval on the ECG, signifying delay in transmission between atria and ventricles, suggests impending sudden death.

It has been suggested that thiamin deficiency (see Chapter 5) might underlie SCD in Asia. Dietary surveys have shown the thiamin intake to be less than half of the required amount and the highly polished rice eaten as staple contains hardly any. Sudden deaths from cardiac arrest occurred in Japanese prisoners of war; human deprivation studies involving thiamin deficiency after the second world war reported lengthening of the QT interval. SCD is likely to be of multifactorial aetiology, but where diet is severely restricted beriberi is likely to be causal.[16]

'Toxic oil syndrome'

This is the name approved by WHO for the largest outbreak of food poisoning in Europe in recent times, which affected about 25,000 people and caused at least 700 deaths. The cause has never been satisfactorily determined and it has been called an 'unresolved scientific and criminal mystery'.

The outbreak began suddenly in May 1981 in the poorer suburbs of Madrid and spread rapidly throughout northern and western Spain (**40**). The earliest symptoms were breathing difficulties and intense muscle pain. By about the sixth week it had been concluded that contaminated cooking oil was responsible. It was alleged that rapeseed oil, suitable only for industrial use, had been retailed cheaply on the streets. It was traced to two refineries, and 38 merchants were arrested. Years later only two had received prison sentences, which brought violent protests from the relatives of the many victims who by then had died or been crippled. However, samples of the cooking oil did not reproduce the disease when fed to animals and a toxin has never been identified.

Suspicion fell later on salad items and in particular tomatoes which were traced to one area in the south of the country. Horticulture had begun there recently with intensive use of fertilizers and pesticides by illiterate farm workers. The symptomatology would fit with organophosphate poisoning. Until today the Ministry of Health has refused to revise its view that cooking oil was responsible or to consider other evidence offered.

40

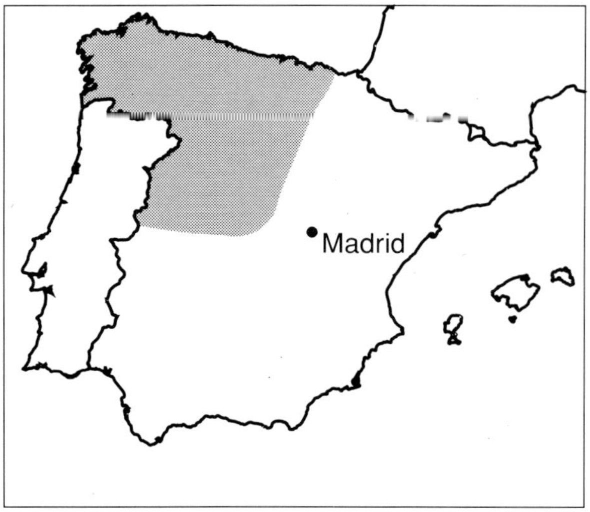

40 'Toxic oil syndrome'.

3. Western lifestyle-related diseases

In Chapter 2 evidence was presented for the concept that diet as an integral part of human culture plays a major determining role in the epidemiological pattern of non-infectious disease around the world. This relationship is explored in more detail below as it concerns the major causes of morbidity and mortality in the West[17] (*Table 15*).

Table 15. Estimated total deaths and percentage of total deaths for the ten leading causes of death in the United States, 1987.

Rank	*Cause of death*	*Number*	*Deaths (%)*
1 *	Heart diseases	759,400	35.7
	(Coronary heart disease)	(511,700)	(24.1)
	(Other heart disease)	(247,700)	(11.6)
2 *	Cancers	476,700	22.4
3 *	Strokes	148,700	7.0
4 **	Unintentional injuries	92,500	4.4
	(Motor vehicle)	(46,800)	(2.2)
	(All others)	(45,700)	(2.2)
5	Chronic obstructive lung diseases	78,000	3.7
6	Pneumonia and influenza	68,600	3.2
7 *	Diabetes mellitus	37,800	1.8
8 **	Suicide	29,600	1.4
9 **	Chronic liver disease and cirrhosis	26,000	1.2
10 *	Atherosclerosis	23,100	1.1
	Subtotal	1,740,000	81.9
	All causes	2,125,100	100.0

* Causes of death in which diet plays a part.
** Causes of death in which excessive alcohol consumption plays a part.

Ischaemic heart disease (IHD)

It is generally agreed that this archetypal 'western' disease emerged in Europe and North America in the early part of the present century, to reach epidemic proportions by the 1960s. Since then there has been a dramatic decline in some countries, notably the United States, but not in others for reasons that are not fully understood. As a western lifestyle has been increasingly adopted in the urbanized areas of the rest of the world coronary heart disease has emerged where previously it was unknown (**41** and **42**).

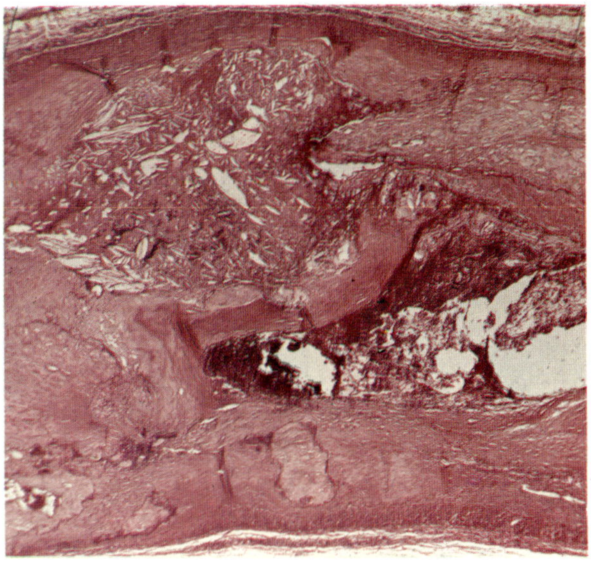

41

41 Coronary artery thrombosis. Fatty streaks evolve into raised subintimal plaques which encroach on the vascular lumen. Superimposed thrombosis occurs on fissured, or more often ulcerated lesions, as shown here.

42

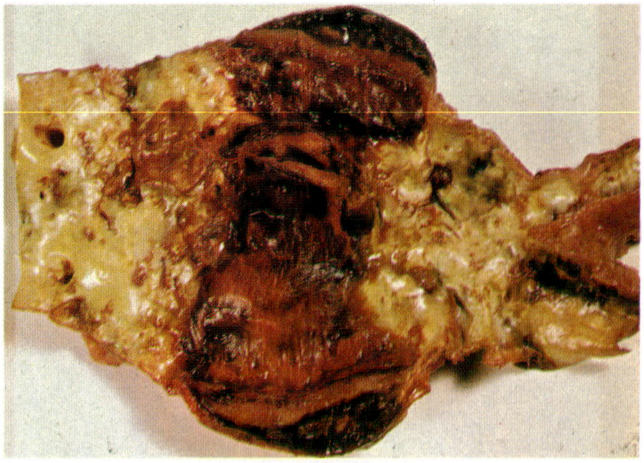

42 Atheromatous aortic aneurysm. There is gross atheromatous plaque formation, and weakening of the wall has resulted in aneurysm formation.

Despite recent improvements IHD remains the most common cause of death in western countries, partly because other major causes like cancer and stroke are also declining. The risk factors that are known to be most closely associated with death from IHD are cigarette smoking, raised blood pressure and raised serum cholesterol. Measures to control these factors have formed the basis of most community intervention trials. More than 250 associated factors have been reported and yet it is generally recognized that about 50% of the variance in causation remains unaccounted for (*Table 16*).

There is still incomplete understanding of the nature of the pathological processes that underly the

Table 16. Factors associated with ischaemic heart disease.

Some associated characteristics
Maleness
Increasing age
Family history of premature vascular disease
Mesomorph body build
Certain personality traits

Primary risk factors
Smoking (1 or more packs of cigarettes/day)
Blood pressure (diastolic > 90 mmHg; systolic > 140 mmHg)
Elevated plasma cholesterol (> 250 mg/dl or 6.50 mmol/l)

Secondary risk factors
Elevated plasma triglycerides
Obesity (especially abdominal)
Diabetes mellitus
Chronic stress
Oral contraceptives
Vasectomy
Hyperuricaemia and gout

Correlation of mortality with intake of certain nutrients *

Positive correlations ($p < 0.05$; correlation coefficient in brackets)	*Negative correlations*
Animal protein (0.782)	Starch (–0.464)
Cholesterol (0.762)	Vegetable protein (–0.403)
Meat (0.697)	
Total fat (0.676)	
Eggs (0.666)	*No correlations*
Sugar (0.638)	Plant sterols, fish, vegetable fat,
Total calories (0.633)	vegetables
Animal fat (0.632)	

* Men 55–59 years of age

changes which result in IHD. Most research has centred on the changes in arterial walls that take place in atheromatosis and the accompanying changes in blood lipoproteins. Brown and Goldstein[18] received the Nobel prize for identifying the single gene defect involving the low-density lipoprotein (LDL) receptor in patients with familial hypercholesterolaemia. The lipoproteins themselves are also involved[19] (see also Chapter 7) (**43** and **44**).

Genetic defects of cholesterol metabolism occur in about 0.2% of the population and account for about 50% of deaths from IHD before the age of 55 years.

Of the many dietary factors that have been studied for their effect on blood cholesterol the strongest and most consistent evidence relates to fat, both amount and nature. Excess fat, especially saturated and usually from animal sources, is strongly associated with hypercholesterolaemia (see **27**).

43

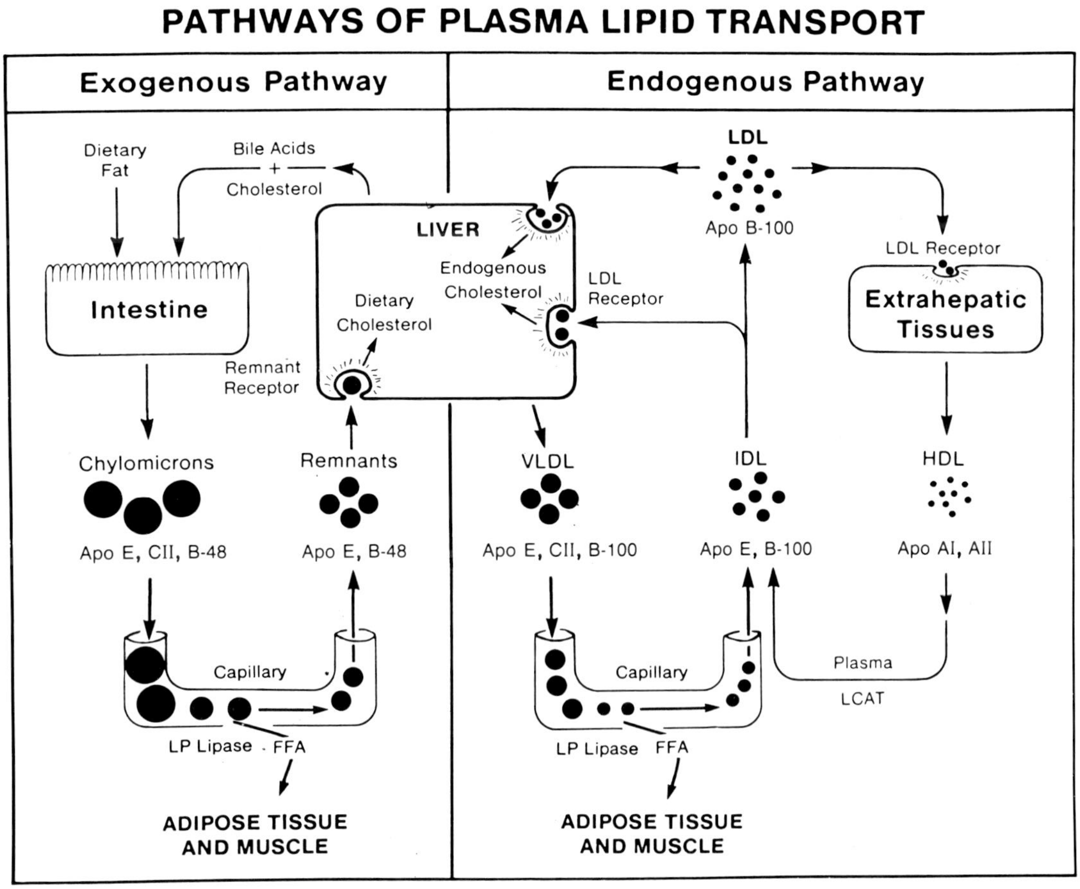

43 The plasma lipoproteins in man.[18]

44

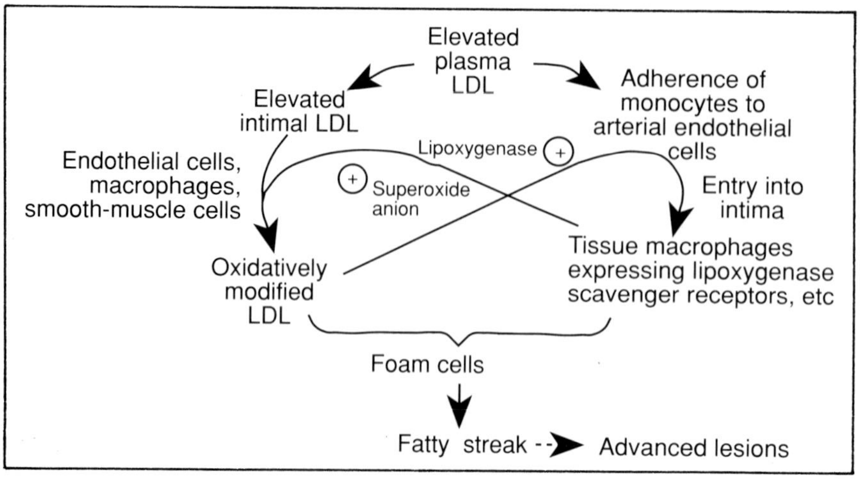

44 Some of the essential processes believed to be involved in the generation of the fatty streak lesion of atherosclerosis. Briefly, hypercholesterolaemia induces adherence of monocytes to the endothelium, after which these monocytes penetrate, alter their phenotypic expression, and become tissue macrophages. They express scavenger receptors that can rapidly take up oxidatively modified LDL and become foam cells. All three of the major cell types in the intima can contribute to oxidation of LDL, including the macrophage. Oxidatively modified LDL is chemotactic and could play a role in recruiting more monocytes into the lesion area. Thus the stage could be set for an almost 'autocatalytic' expansion of a lesion once initiated.

Data from the Framingham study[20] and other sources show a close relationship between each of blood cholesterol, blood pressure, and diabetes mellitus with death from IHD (**45–47**).

Polyunsaturated fatty acids tend to lower blood cholesterol and recent evidence[21] suggests that olive oil, which is monounsaturated, works equally well and appears not to have some of the possible adverse effects of PUFAs, i.e. predisposition to gallstones, cancer, autoxidation, immune suppression and lowering of serum HDL cholesterol (which is known to be protective). Saturated fat may act by reducing the expression of receptors for LDL in the liver, thus decreasing the clearance of LDL cholesterol from the circulation.

45

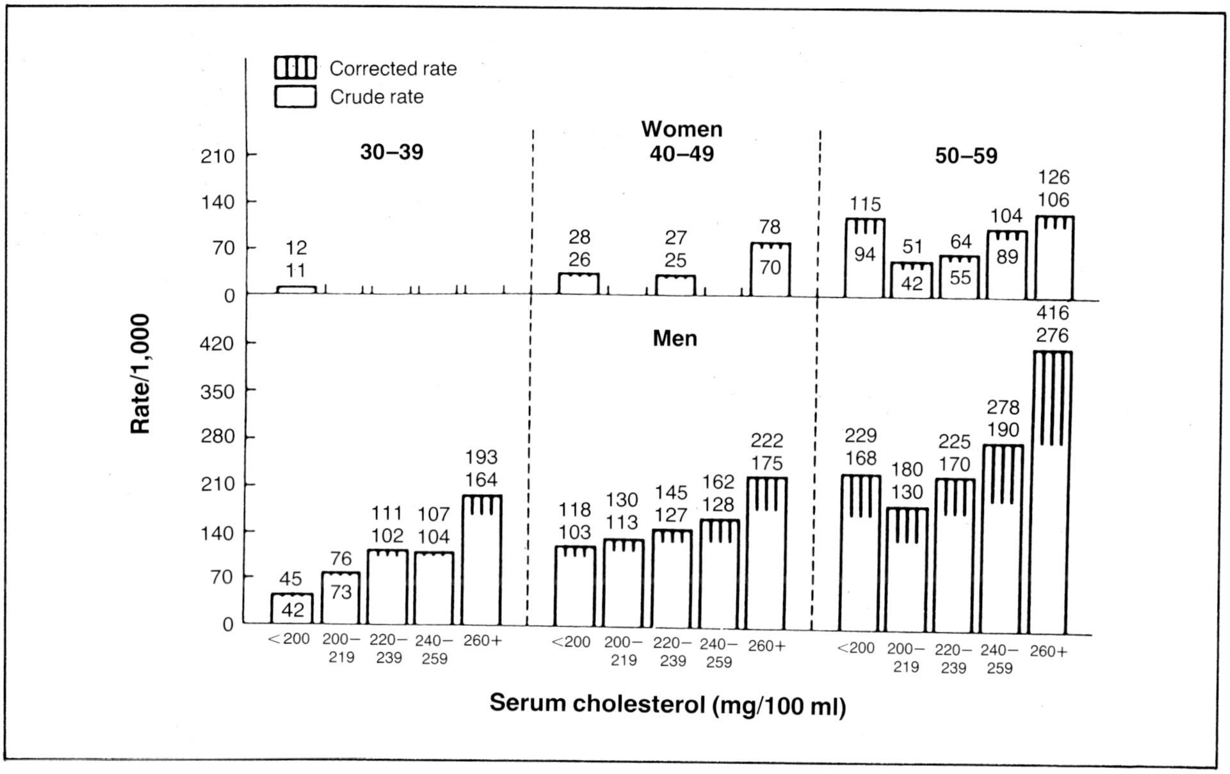

45 Twenty-four-year incidence of myocardial infarction, by serum cholesterol levels in the Framingham study.

46

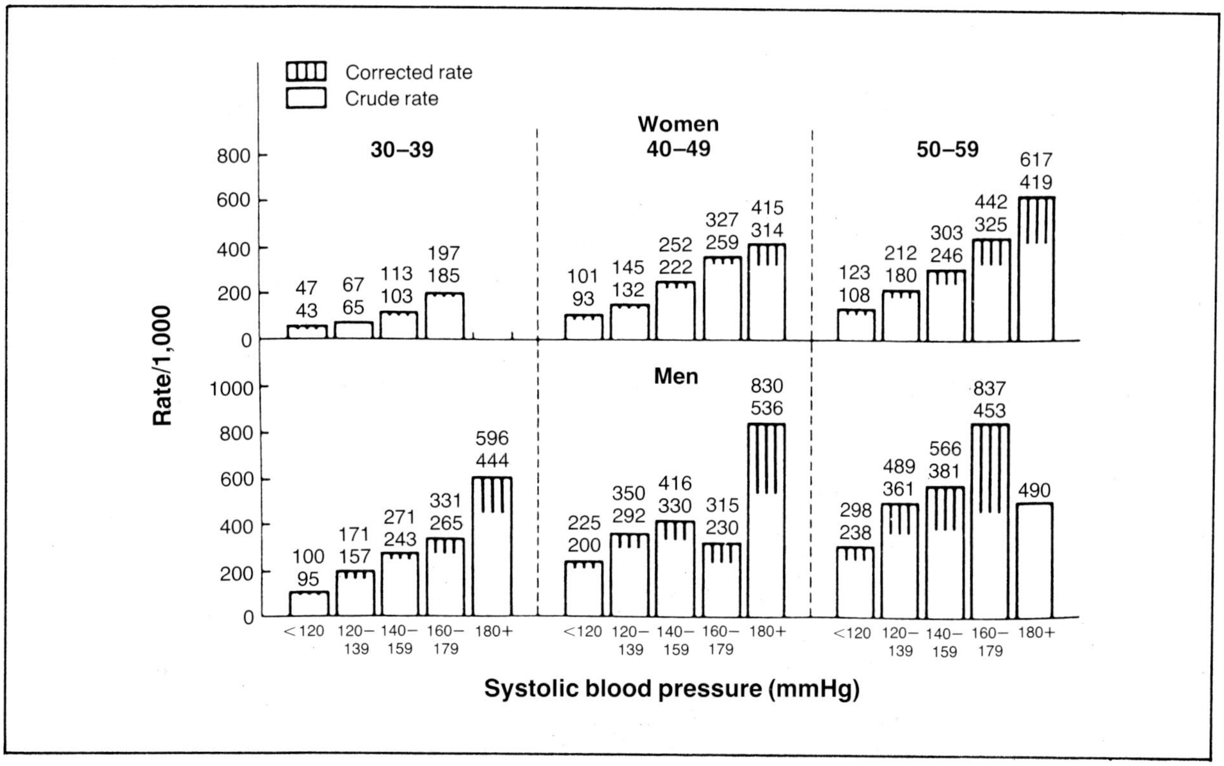

46 Twenty-four-year incidence of coronary heart disease, by systolic blood pressure in the Framingham study.

47

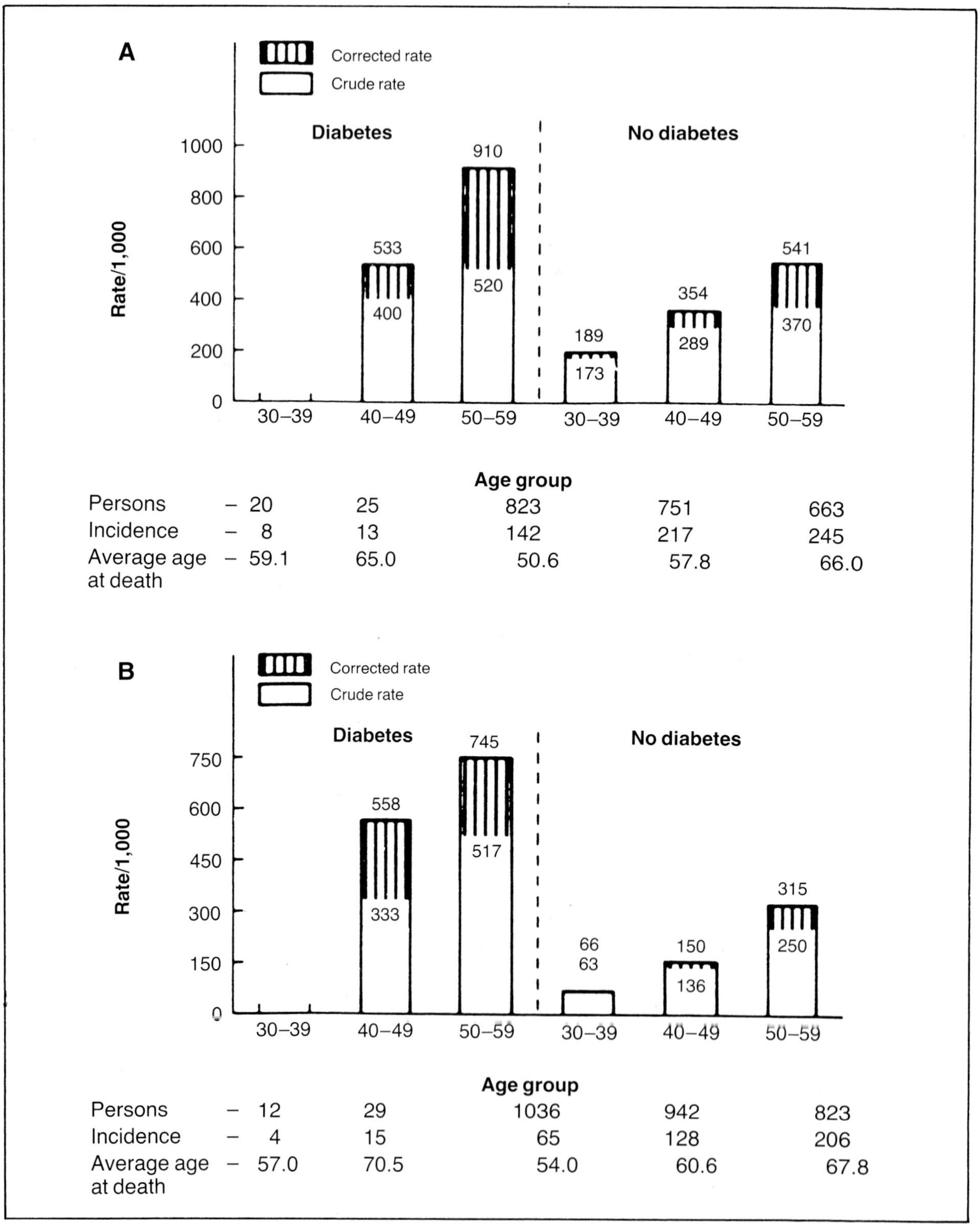

47 Twenty-four-year incidence of coronary heart disease in subjects with diabetes mellitus, aged 30–59 at entry: **A**, men; **B**, women.

48 The effects of different intakes of dietary cholesterol levels in humans. The baseline data in all instances were virtually cholesterol-free.

48

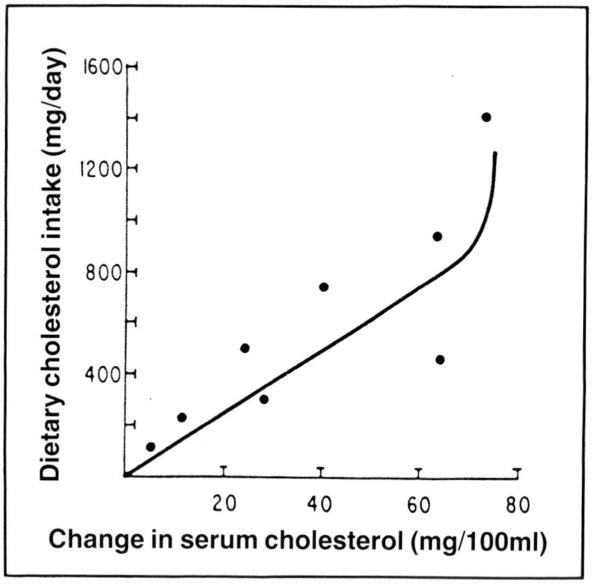

Other dietary factors seem to be much less important. An association with high sugar consumption is now discounted, but dietary fibre has been shown to be hypocholesterolaemic (see Chapter 2). Obesity of the abdominal type predisposes to IHD as well as to other western diseases (see Chapter 4). Chronic alcoholism is associated with IHD but moderate intake (one drink more than once per month but less than one per day) has been reported to be associated with reduced risk.[22] Dietary cholesterol at customary levels of intake has little effect.[23] (**48**)

Evidence is accumulating that garlic reduces cardiovascular risk factors through effects on serum lipids, blood pressure, coagulation, platelet aggregation and vasodilatation.

Thrombus formation is an integral part of IHD and factors that are responsible for it are not necessarily the same as those associated with atheromatosis. *Table 17* presents a summary of results which show that abnormalities in clotting factors are good indicators of risk of developing IHD, but they do not appear to provide new leads to the control of the problem. Dietary fat affects plasma factor VII coagulant activity,[24] as well as influencing plasma cholesterol. Saturated fat tends to induce arterial thrombosis and platelet aggregation, as well as raising plasma cholesterol.[25]

Until fairly recently research on the effects of PUFAs was confined to the fatty acids of the omega-6 series (see Chapter 6). Since the discovery of the low incidence of IHD in Greenland Eskimos and their thrombotic tendency attention has been focused on those of the omega-3 series (see Chapter 2).

Table 17. Clotting factors as cardiovascular risk factors.

Factor	*Normal values*	*Under what conditions found raised*
Fibrin-related antigen	48–184 ng/ml	Acute myocardial infarction and unstable angina; normal in chronic stable angina*
D dimer (principal breakdown product of fibrin)	40–50 ng/ml	
Fibrin monomer (intermediate product of fibrin formation)	15–20 ng/ml	
Factor VII coagulant activity		In smokers and those with other socioeconomic risk factors **
Plasma fibrinogen	3 g/l	
Enlarged platelet size		

* Ref.[25]
** Ref.[24]

Hypertension

High blood pressure is usually defined in terms of diastolic pressure (90–104 mmHg, mild hypertension; 105–114 moderate; and greater than 115 severe). Occasionally diastolic pressure may be normal (less than 90 mmHg) and systolic pressure raised (greater than 140 mmHg) when isolated systolic hypertension is recognized. It can be seen from recent studies that about 58 million people in the United States either have a blood pressure of greater than 140/90 mmHg or are receiving antihypertensive treatment. The prevalence increases with age (but see below) and is higher in blacks (38%) than whites (29%).

Blood pressure control in both the short and long term is under a complex array of haemodynamic, nervous, hormonal and other factors. In more than 95% of people with high blood pressure the specific cause is unclear and the condition is known as primary or essential hypertension. It is this disease that is considered here in relation to diet, although

49

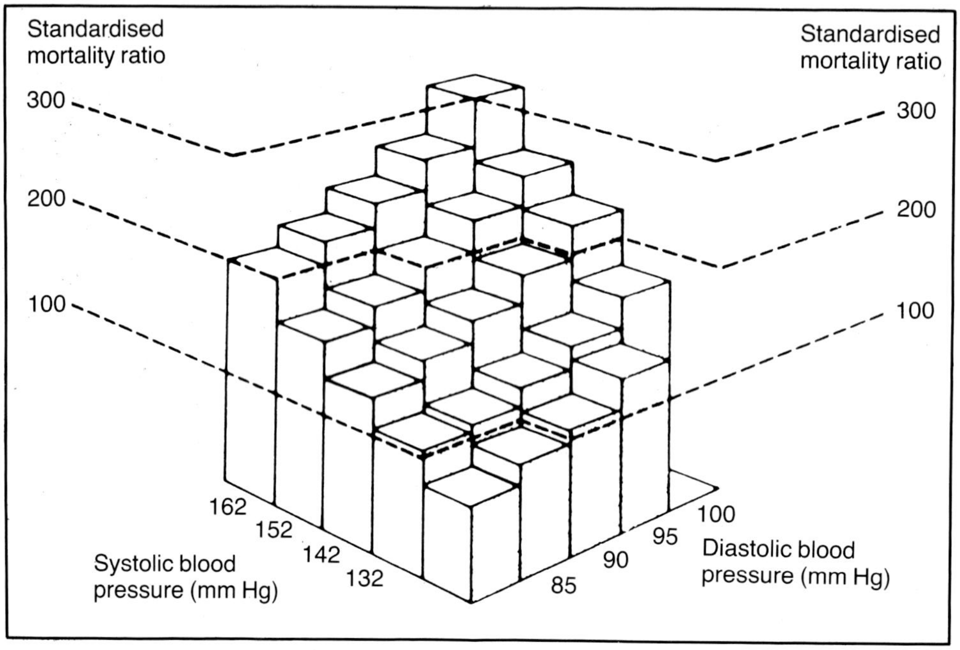

49 Life insurance data linking risk and levels of arterial pressure, standardized to average risk (= 100).

Table 18. Estimated mean blood pressure at zero sodium intake for economically developed communities* according to age.

Age (years)	*Systolic*	*Diastolic*
15–19	113.4	67.3
20–29	117.0	69.4
30–39	119.0	73.8
40–49	121.3	76.1
50–59	125.3	77.0
60–69	133.9	78.9

* For economically underdeveloped communities mean blood pressure was 109.9 systolic and 71.8 diastolic at all ages.

salt restriction is part of the management of all forms of established hypertension (**49**).[26]

The steady rise of blood pressure with age observed in the West is now considered not to be physiological[27] (*Table 18*).

There are many non-nutritional as well as nutritional factors that might be contributing to the general rise in blood pressure in industrialized societies. Stress might be expected to be prominent among the former. Nutritional factors might either ameliorate or potentiate a rise in blood pressure and those for which the evidence is best substantiated are shown in *Table 19*.

Abnormalities in handling of both extracellular and intracellular calcium in hypertension lend importance to the possible role of this essential element (**50**).[28]

It is often difficult to translate these findings into dietary recommendations; fortunately, foods low in sodium tend to be high in potassium and vice versa.

A family history of hypertension predisposes an individual child to develop hypertension in later life but the association weakens as other influences, including diet, become stronger. The high correlation between dietary sodium intake and blood pressure in different populations (**51**) does not hold true within populations.[29]

The physiological mechanisms capable of maintaining sodium homeostasis in the face of widely differing sodium dietary intakes (*Table 20*) complicate the interpretation of the significance of the different intakes.

Table 19. Dietary factors and their possible influence on blood pressure.

Reduce	*Increase*
Potassium	Total energy
Calcium	Sodium
Magnesium	Alcohol
Fibre	Chloride
	Sucrose
Less well substantiated	
Linoleic acid	Cadmium
Omega-3-fatty acids	Lead
Oleic acid	Caffeine (temporary)
Protein	
Taurine	

50

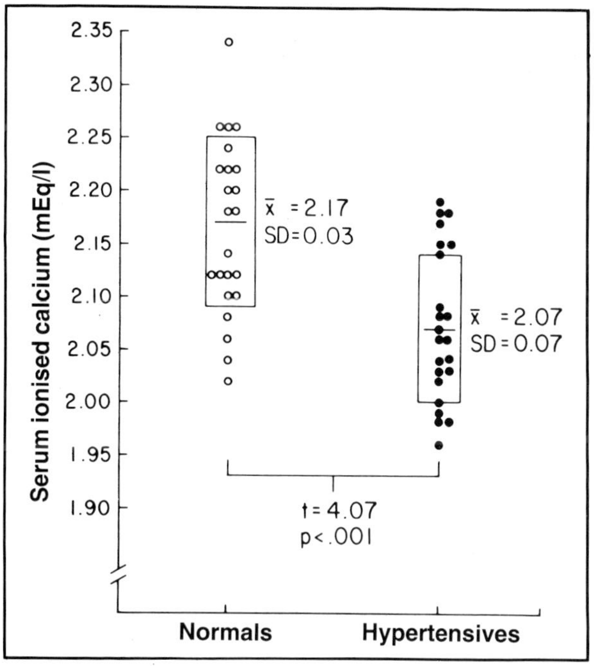

50 Serum concentrations of ionized calcium in 23 normotensive and 23 hypertensive subjects (means ± SD).

51

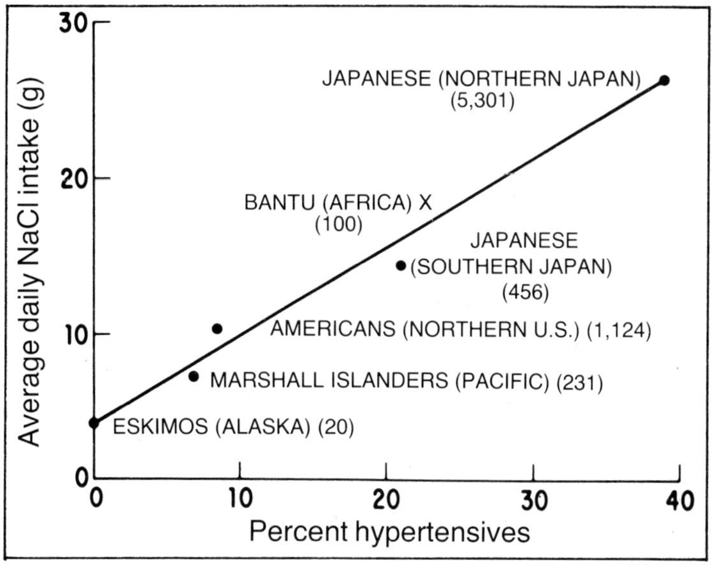

51 Comparison of the prevalence of hypertension among various populations according to their average salt (NaCl) intake. (Number of persons studied given in parentheses.)

Table 20. The range of sodium status in human health and disease.

Daily sodium intake	*Sodium balance*	*Plasma aldosterone*	*Examples*
+ 500–600 mmol	Positive	Very low	Population of Northern Japan
+ 50–400 mmol	Positive	7ng/100ml ('normal')	Westernized societies
+ 2–10 mmol	Positive	28ng/100ml	New Guinea highlanders Patients on low sodium diet
	Neutral (input = output)		
– 100 mmol	Negative	Very high	Low sodium vegetarian diet, mild sweating
– 300 mmol	Negative	Very high	Low sodium diet with mild diarrhoea
– 500 mmol	Negative	Very high	Cholera, dysentery, severe sweating

Cerebrovascular disease (stroke)

Cerebrovascular disease that leads to sudden loss of brain function, results usually from one of four vascular events in a cerebral artery: thrombosis, embolism, stenosis (which often causes transient ischaemic attack (TIA)), or haemorrhage.

Blood pressure in individuals as well as in communities is highly correlated with risk of stroke regardless of age and sex: this appears to be true for salt intake as well (52). Fibrinogen, total cholesterol and high density lipoprotein cholesterol are risk factors for minor strokes, which in this resemble IHD (see page 30).

Reduction in the risk of stroke developing has been claimed on the basis of carefully conducted trials involving individually the following measures: moderate sodium restriction, alcohol restriction, high potassium intake, vegetarian diet, calcium supplementation, and weight reduction. Sodium restriction and weight reduction appear to be the most effective.[30]

Complications of stroke (*Table 21*) are widespread and very disabling, underlining the importance of early recognition of the risk factors and institution of corrective measures, including diet modification.

Table 21. Complications of stroke.

Respiratory
Pneumonia, inhalation, pulmonary embolism

Cardiovascular
Myocardial infarction, cardiac failure, cardiac arrhythmias

Infections
Pneumonia, urinary, skin, septicaemia

Metabolic
Dehydration, acid–base imbalance, hyperglycaemia, renal failure

Mechanical
Spasticity, contractures, subluxation or 'frozen' shoulder, falls and fractures

Others
Pressure sores, deep vein thrombosis, dependent oedema, acute peptic ulceration, incontinence of urine and/or faeces, pressure palsies of peripheral nerves

52 **Massive intracerebral haemorrhage.**

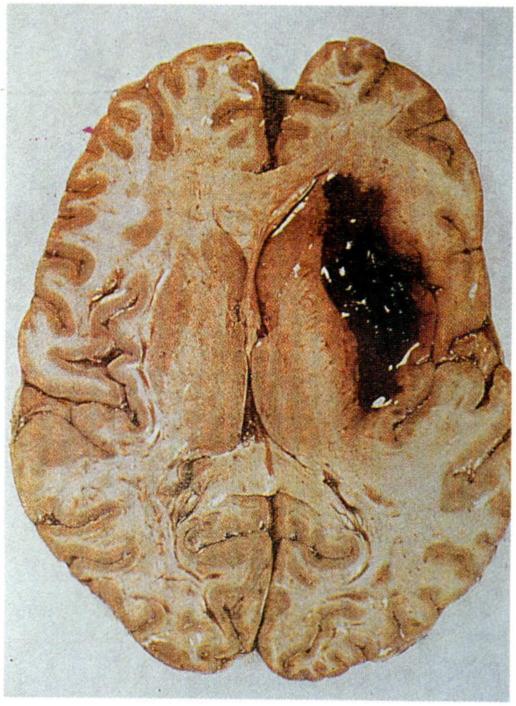

52

Diabetes mellitus

Diabetes mellitus is characterized by abnormal insulin secretion, elevated blood glucose and various end-organ complications. Hereditary and environmental factors interact in ways that are incompletely understood at present.

In broad terms diabetes mellitus is manifest in two very different forms (Type I and Type II or insulin-dependent and non-insulin-dependent diabetes mellitus, respectively (IDDM and NIDDM)) (*Table 22*).

Table 22. Characteristics of Type I and Type II diabetes mellitus.

Characteristics	*Type I Insulin-dependent*	*Type II Non-insulin-dependent*
Age of onset	Often < 30	Often > 30
Body build	Usually lean	90% are overweight
Histocompatibility antigens (HLA DR3/DR4)	Present	Decreased with different distribution
Family history	Minor (10% in parent or sibling)	Marked
Twin concordance	Low	High
Islet cell morphology	Loss of B cells	Hyperplasia
Symptoms	Polydipsia, polyphagia, polyuria	Often asymptomatic
Plasma insulin	Low to absent	Normal to high
Acute complication	Ketoacidosis	
Vascular disease predominating	Microangiopathy	Atherosclerosis
Diet therapy	Maintaining ideal weight Maintaining good glycaemia control Prevention of hyperlipidaemia	Weight reduction Maintaining ideal weight Prevention of hyperlipidaemia
Insulin therapy	Essential	Often not required

Of particular relevance in the present context is the occurrence in various parts of the world of forms of diabetes that appear to be closely related to malnutrition which also affects other aspects of pancreatic function (*Table 23*).

Table 23. Features of malnutrition-related diabetes mellitus.

Alternative names
- Tropical diabetes
- J type diabetes (Jamaica)
- K type (Kerela, south India)
- Z type (Zuidema – a Dutch researcher in the 1950s)

Aetiological factors
- Alcohol may be important
- Malnutrition (PEM) and cassava consumption also implicated

Clinical characteristics
- Often underweight with history of malnutrition
- Mostly restricted to tropical countries and non-Caucasians
- May have severe insulin resistance
- Frequently associated with exocrine pancreatic malfunction, pancreatic fibrosis and calculi
- Endogenous insulin secretion intermediate between Type I and Type II

53 demonstrates the consistent rise in incidence of diabetes mellitus with age, and even more strikingly with increasing adiposity.

53

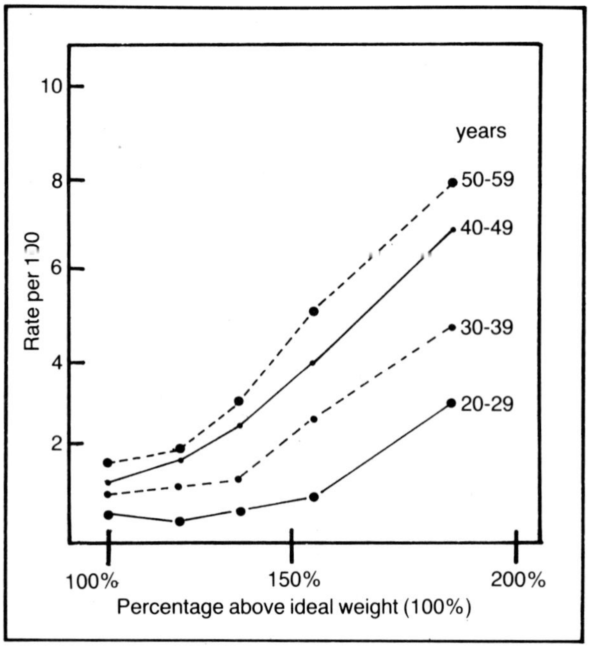

53 Diabetes mellitus incidence increases both with the degree of obesity and with age.

As will be discussed in Chapter 4 the distribution of body fat has an even greater influence in predisposing to diabetes than does overall increase in weight. It is probably as a result of inbreeding that among some isolated populations, such as the Pima Indians in North America and the Micronesian islanders, the incidence of diabetes may be as high as 50% by middle age with a strong association with abdominal obesity. Impairment of insulin response to glucose loading is associated with a rise in blood pressure.[31] Black Americans and Pima Indians appear to be particularly susceptible.[32]

The rise in blood glucose following ingestion of a food has been used to calculate a glycaemic index for use in planning diet therapy.[33] However, the glycaemic response is influenced by many factors (*Table 24*) and its use is not recommended at present.

The importance of trying to maintain glycaemic control throughout life would seem to be borne out by the seriousness of the complications of diabetes (*Table 25*) (**54, 55**). Although prevention of hypoglycaemia will protect the nervous system and good control will improve the outcome of pregnancy it has not yet been established that any of the long-term complications can be influenced.[34]

Table 24. Factors affecting the glycaemic response to food.

Rate of digestion	Hormone response
Pre-stomach hydrolysis	Pancreatic
Stomach hydrolysis	Gut
Gastric emptying rate	Colon effects
Intestinal hydrolysis and absorption	
Food form	
Starch characteristics	
Fibre content	
Food ingredients	
Intestinal response	

Table 25. Complications of diabetes mellitus.

Skin	— Stiff hand syndrome Necrobiosis lipoidica Dermopathy	**Neuropathy**	— Polyneuropathy Mononeuritis Autonomic abnormalities Neuropathic ulceration Charcot joint
Eye	— Maculopathy Retinopathy Vitreous haemorrhage Retinal detachment Rubeosis of iris Cataracts	**Infections**	— Bacterial e.g. osteomyelitis Boils Fungal Tuberculosis
Kidney	— Microalbuminuria Proteinuria Nephrotic syndrome Renal failure	**Impotence**	—
		Coma	— Hypoglycaemia Ketoacidosis Hyperosmolar Lactic acidosis
Vascular	— Peripheral vascular disease Cerebrovascular disease Coronary artery disease Ischaemic ulcers		

54

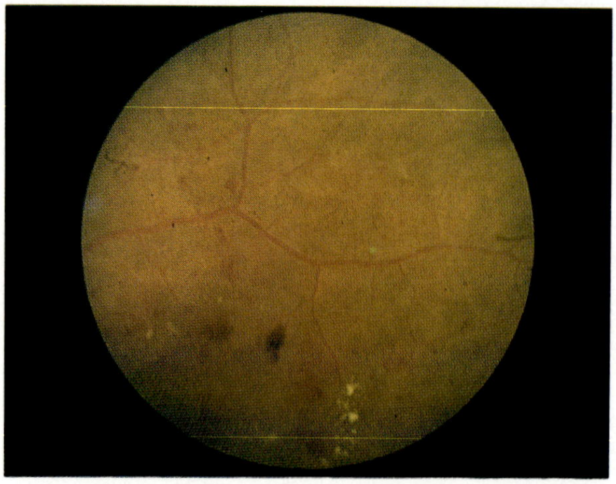

54 Diabetic retinopathy. Note the vascular changes, predominantly at the posterior pole of the eye, with 'dot and blot' haemorrhages and hard exudates arranged side by side. There are minimal arterio-venous changes. Microaneurysms are a characteristic feature. Iridopathy leading to glaucoma and vitreous haemorrhages also occur.

5.

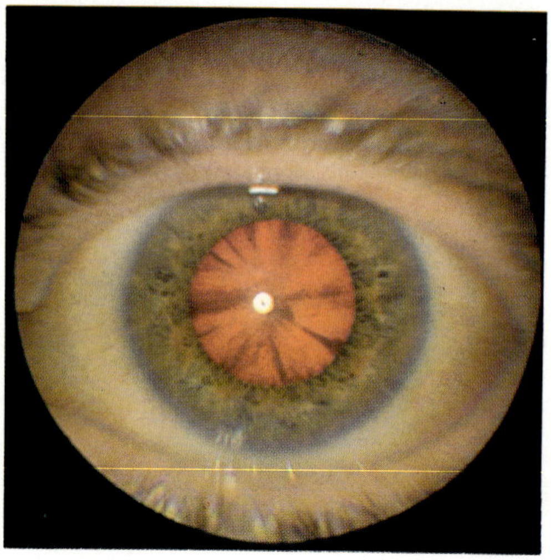

55 Diabetic cataract. The most common type of true diabetic cataract, shown here, consists of posterior subcapsular opacity with radial striae extending into it from the equatorial zone. Less frequently numerous white flaky opacities in the cortex give a snowstorm appearance. In more advanced cases lens fibres become distorted with intervening vacuoles.

'Senile' cataract, distinguished by the uniform opacification, occurs more frequently and at an earlier age in diabetics.

There is much current interest in the amount and type of carbohydrate and fibre that should be recommended in diabetes.[35] Carbohydrate should not be restricted as it was in the past, and a high proportion of this should be complex rather than sugar. Different forms of dietary fibre vary in their physiological effects (see Chapter 2) and it is the water-soluble fibres – pectins, gums, storage polysaccharides and a few hemicelluloses – that reduce serum levels of glucose and insulin. In other dietary aspects advice for diabetics is no different from that for the general population (see Appendix V, Table 1): weight control is of primary importance in NIDDM.

Gallstones

These frequently fail to produce significant symptoms and may remain undetected during life. They are more common in women than men. Cholesterol gallstones predominate in western societies and the diet-related risk factors are very similar to those for IHD – diabetes, obesity, excess energy and fat intake.[36] Reports in the relevant literature indicate that gallstones are more likely to occur in people following a western lifestyle (**56, 57**).

Several factors have been implicated in the degree of readiness with which cholesterol may be held as a micellar liquid in bile. A further array of influences is shown in *Table 26*.

The elegant studies of Small[37] and subsequently of

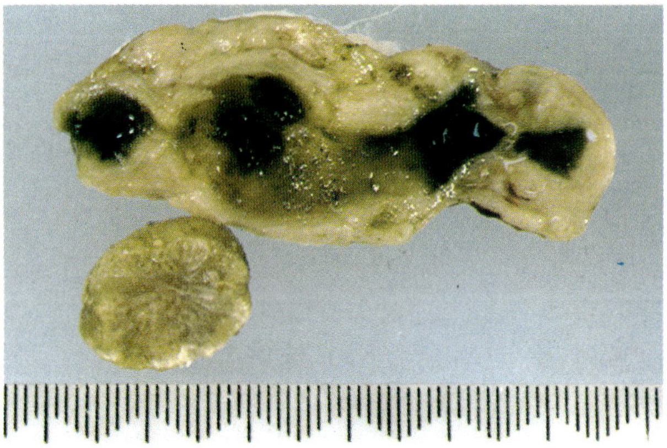

56

56 Cholelithiasis. A cholesterol stone is shown, against a centimetre scale, and chronic cholecystitis is present in the gallbladder.

57

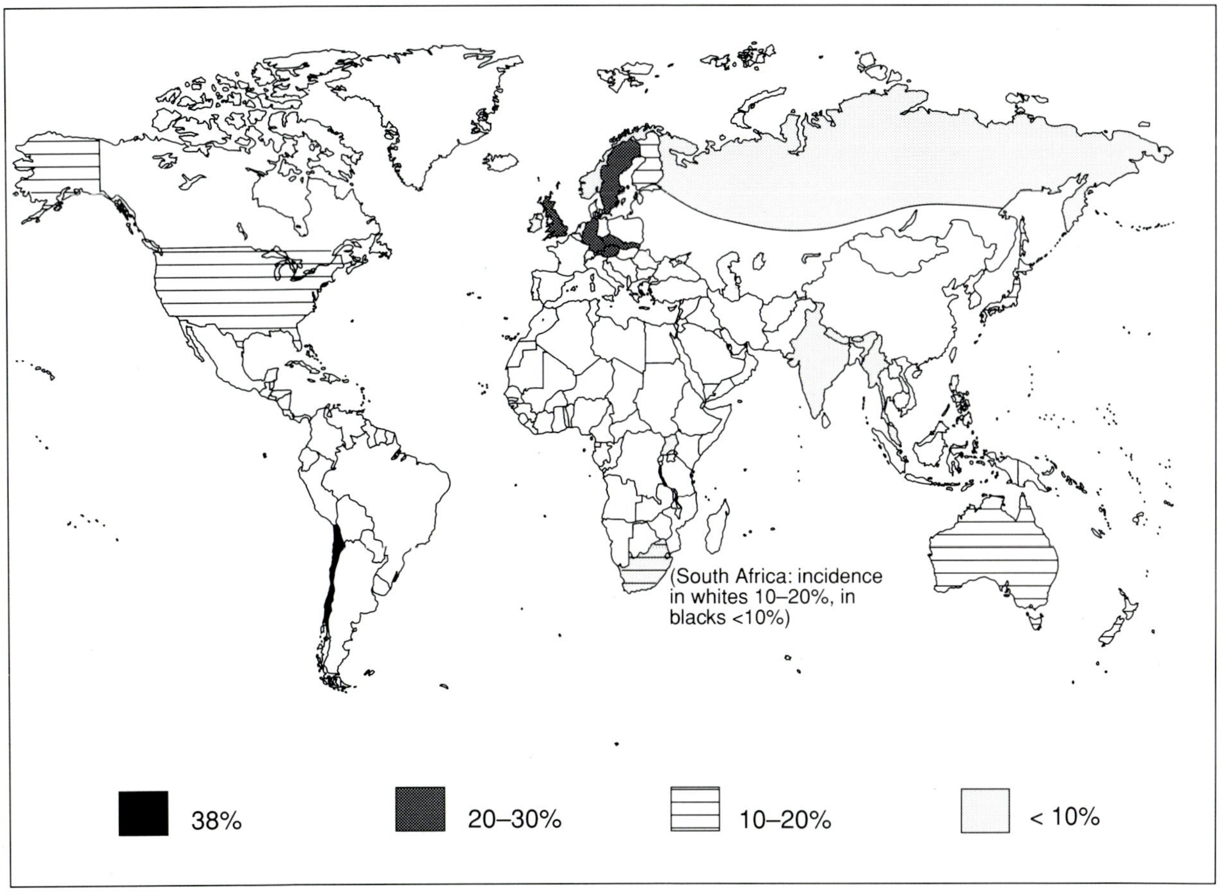

57 Incidence of gallstones at autopsy in females (age is standardized, male incidence about half that of females).

Table 26. Factors in cholesterol gallstone formation.

Factor	*Influences*
Supersaturation of bile	Age – increases with age Sex – ratio of females to males, 2:1 Genetics – certain families Obesity – especially in females < 50 years Drugs – increased by contraceptive pill, oestrogens post-menopausal Diet – lack of fibre predisposes Liver disease – increased
Cholesterol nucleating factors (nucleation of cholesterol monohydrate crystals is the crucial first step)	Infection, glycoprotein, mucus, bile protein and ? others
Gallbladder contraction	Decrease in cholecystokinin receptors
Enterohepatic circulation of bile salts	Interrupted in: biliary fistula, ileal resection, and cholestyramine
Nidus formation	Calcium bilirubinate, biliary protein

58

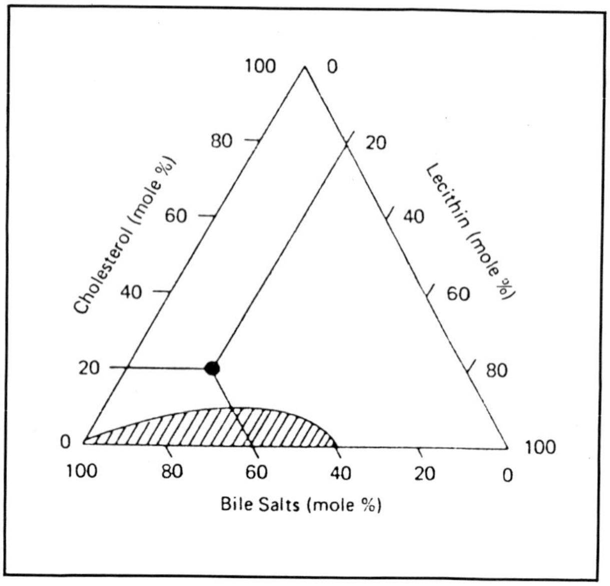

58 Solubility of cholesterol in bile. Cholesterol is present as a micellar liquid when in the presence of high concentrations of bile salts and lecithin (shaded area).

59

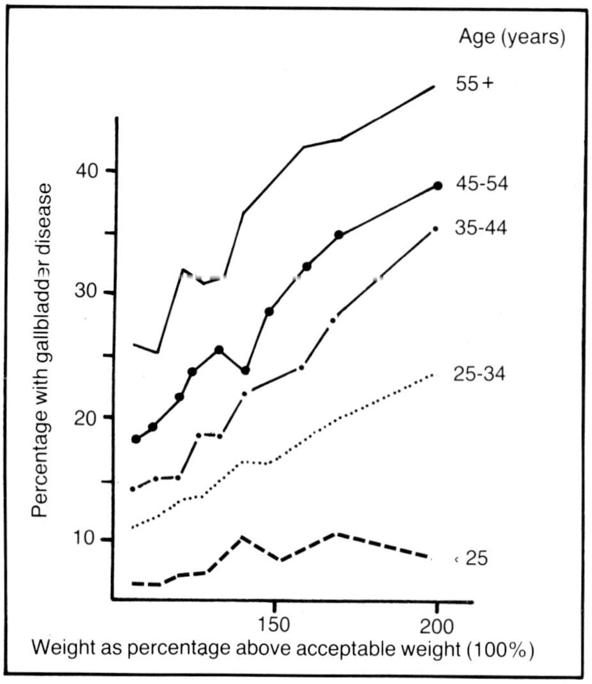

59 Relationship of gallbladder disease to weight and age in adult women in the USA. Note the rising incidence with age and obesity.

Montgomery *et al.*[38] illustrated in **58** have quantified the dynamics between cholesterol, lecithin and bile salts.

59 shows the increasing incidence of gallbladder disease with both age and weight in women – certain similarities with diabetes can be seen (see **53**).

Dietary factors that predispose to gallstone formation include excessive energy intake, especially as saturated fat, and a lack of soluble components of dietary fibre (**60**) but they probably play only a minor role, as large segments of western society consume such a diet without forming gallstones.

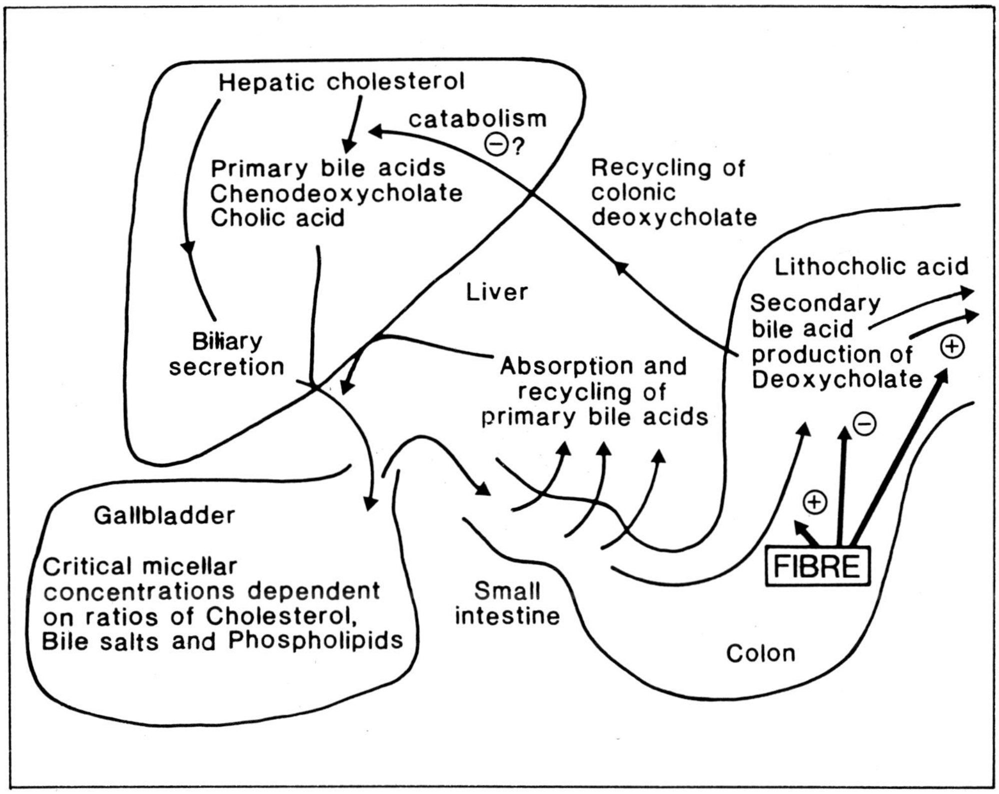

60 The positive and negative effects that dietary fibre is believed to have on different aspects of the recycling of bile salts.

Diet and cancer

Most cancers in western countries have been attributed to various environmental factors[39] (*Table 27*). Among these it is considered that nearly 40% are related to diet. The leading form of cancer in western society (which is also likely to assume a similar position in developing countries in coming decades) is *bronchogenic carcinoma*. Although in the large majority of cases cigarette smoking is responsible, a

Table 27. Proportions of cancer deaths attributed to various factors*.

Factor or class of factors	*Percentage of all cancer deaths* *Best estimate*	*Range of acceptable estimates*
Tobacco	30	25–40
Alcohol	3	2–4
Diet	35	10–70
Food additives	1	(–5**)–2
Reproductive and sexual behaviour	7	1–13
Occupation	4	2–8
Pollution	2	1–5
Industrial products	1	1–2
Medicines and medical procedures	1	0.5–3
Geophysical factors	3	2–4
Infection	10?	1–?
Unknown	?	?

* It should be understood that these figures are speculative, and there is considerable uncertainty associated with them.
** Some factors (e.g. food fortification) may be protective.

61

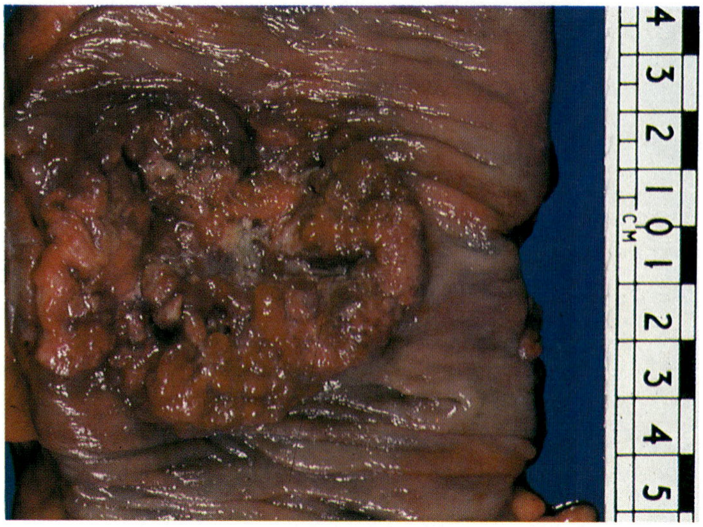

61 Colorectal carcinoma. A colonic resection specimen from a patient with a polypoid ulcerating colonic carcinoma 6cm in diameter.

strong negative association has been observed with some micronutrients, especially vitamin C and B-carotene (**61, 62** and *Table 28*).

It is instructive to consider the evidence for the association of diet with the major forms of cancer affecting different sites.

Review of the literature to date suggests that the strength of the association and also whether this is positive or negative varies as indicated for both nutrients (*Table 28*) and non-nutrients (*Table 29*).

The evidence has been obtained using different methodologies, such as epidemiological, ecological, case–control, cohort, clinical intervention and animal studies.[40] In all of these it is virtually impossible to distinguish between statistical association and causation. Not surprisingly, as more investigations are being carried out, so more associations are discovered.

62

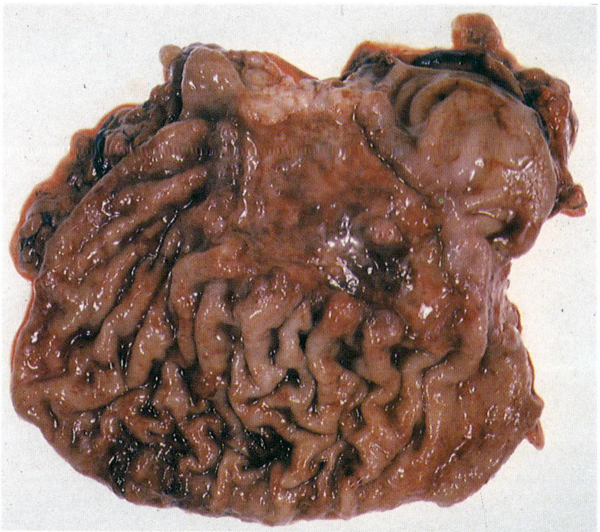

62 Gastric carcinoma. This surgical resection specimen demonstrates a large, malignant gastric ulcer with irregular surrounding folds and rolled edges. Blood clot is visible from recent haemorrhage from this ulcer.

Table 28. Nutritional factors in human cancer.

Cancer site	*Positive energy intake and overweight*	*Fat (especially saturated)*	*Protein*	*'Carotene' (vitamin A)*	*Vitamin C*	*Salt*	*Selenium*
Nasopharynx*						+	
Oesophagus				(−)	(−)	(+)	
Stomach			(+)	(−)	(−)	+	
Colon	(+)	+	(+)				
Pancreas		(+)					
Gallbladder	(+)						
Lung				−			
Kidney	(+)						
Breast	+	(+)		(−)			
Endometrium	+						
Ovary		(+)					
Prostate	(+)	(+)					(−)

\+ = good evidence for a positive relation
− = good evidence for a negative relation
* = salted fish as prepared in parts of the Orient
(+) = suggestive evidence only
(−) = suggestive evidence only

Table 29. Non-nutrient dietary constituents and human cancer.

Cancer site	*Vegetables and fruits*	*Other fibre, starch, cereals*	*Alcohol*	*Aflatoxin*	*Soya products (contain oestrogens)*
Oesophagus	−		+		
Mouth			+		
Tongue			+		
Pharynx			+		
Larynx			+		
Stomach	−	(+)			
Colon	−	(−)			
Liver			+	+	
Pancreas	(−)				
Lung	(−)				
Breast	(−)		(+)		−
Ovary	(−)				
Prostate	(−)				−

\+ = good evidence for a positive relation
− = good evidence for a negative relation
(+) = suggestive evidence only
(−) = suggestive evidence only

63

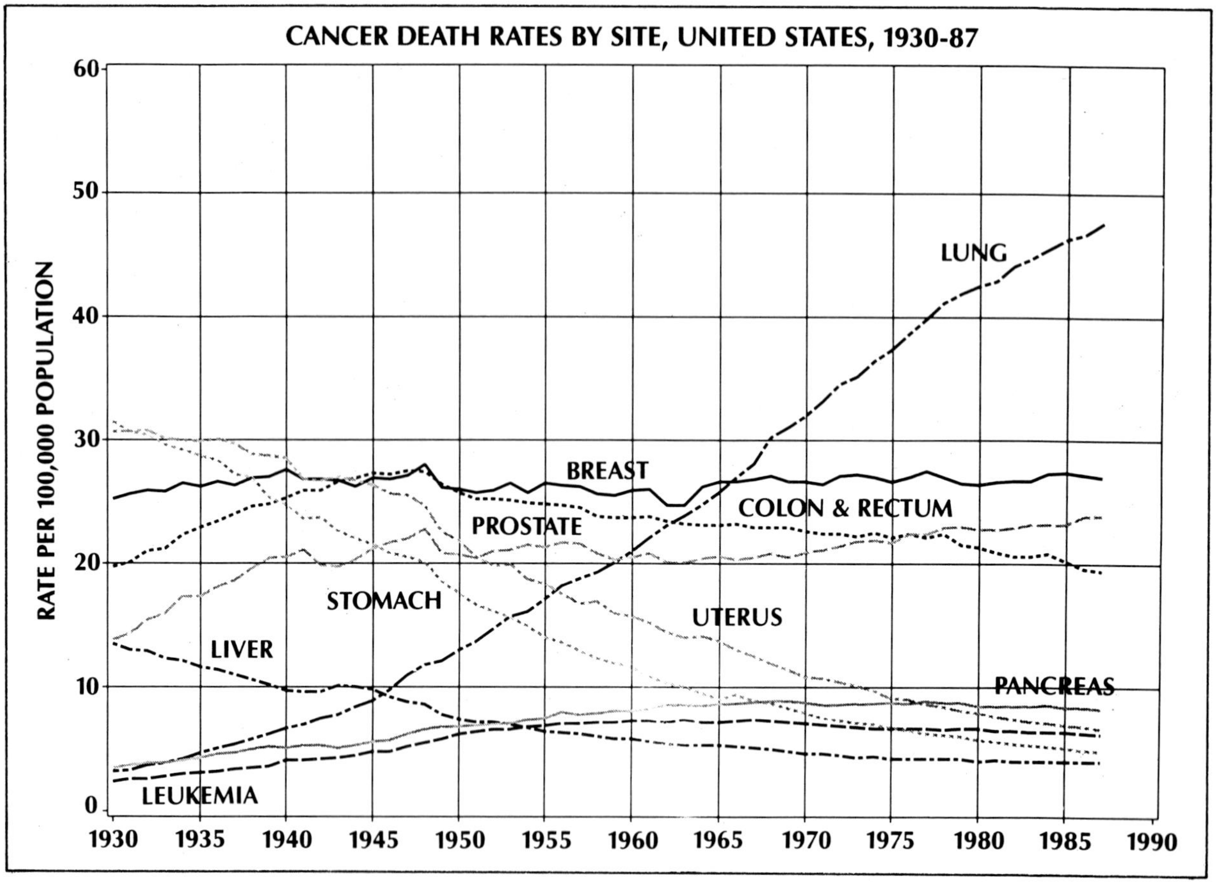

63 Cancer death rates by site, United States, 1930–1987. (Note: rates are for both sexes combined except breast and uterus (female population only) and prostate (male population only).

63 indicates the trends in cancer death rates over the past years in the United States which are in general typical of western societies.[41] It is immediately evident that the only instance of steady and striking increase throughout the period is cancer of the lung. Although this is largely related to the popularity of cigarette smoking, it is likely that a decade or two previously the dietary factors shown in *Tables 28, 29* also played a minor part. Most other major cancers have been declining in recent decades and some of this effect must be attributed to better diagnosis and treatment.

Ecological studies in which cancer rates are related to certain aspects of diet in particular countries are chiefly of value in generating hypotheses rather than providing precise explanations. The data from both cancer registries and food consumption surveys nationwide are quite crude and subject to many kinds of error. Nevertheless the close correlation for example between breast cancer mortality and daily fat intake is very striking (**64**).[42]

That environmental, including dietary, factors are involved in tumourigenesis in some way is also suggested by the marked difference in incidence figures for a given cancer between countries (**65**).

In this case chronic alcohol consumption may be partly responsible through its known association with cirrhosis[43] in which a certain proportion progress to malignant change. In some areas aflatoxin may play a part (see Chapter 9) and hepatitis B virus carrier state is associated with a several hundred-fold increased risk of hepatocellular carcinoma. A combination of these and possibly other factors makes this the most common form of internal cancer in parts of Africa and southeast Asia.

In the high incidence areas shown in **66** squamous cell carcinoma predominates and seems to relate to high alcohol, tobacco or opium consumption and poor nutrition. In most of Europe there is a considerable increase in adenocarcinoma at present although the squamous type still accounts for about 70%.

64

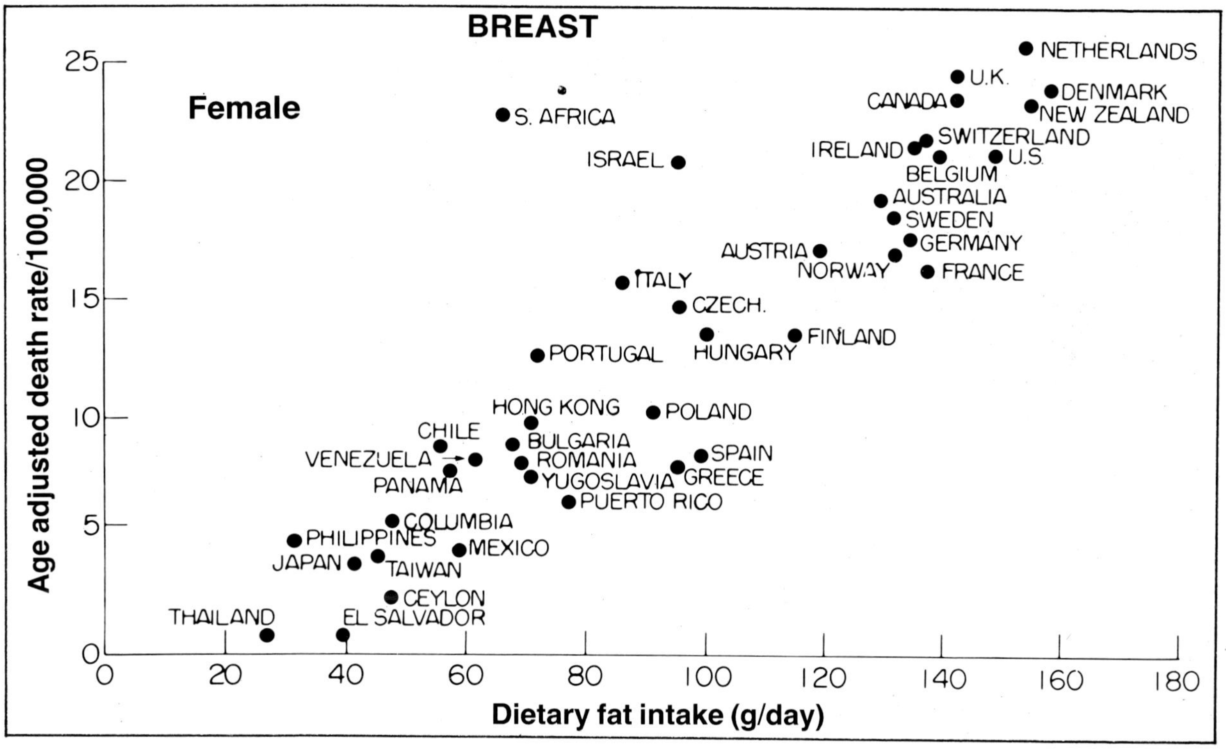

64 Dietary fat intake in relation to breast cancer-related death rate.

65

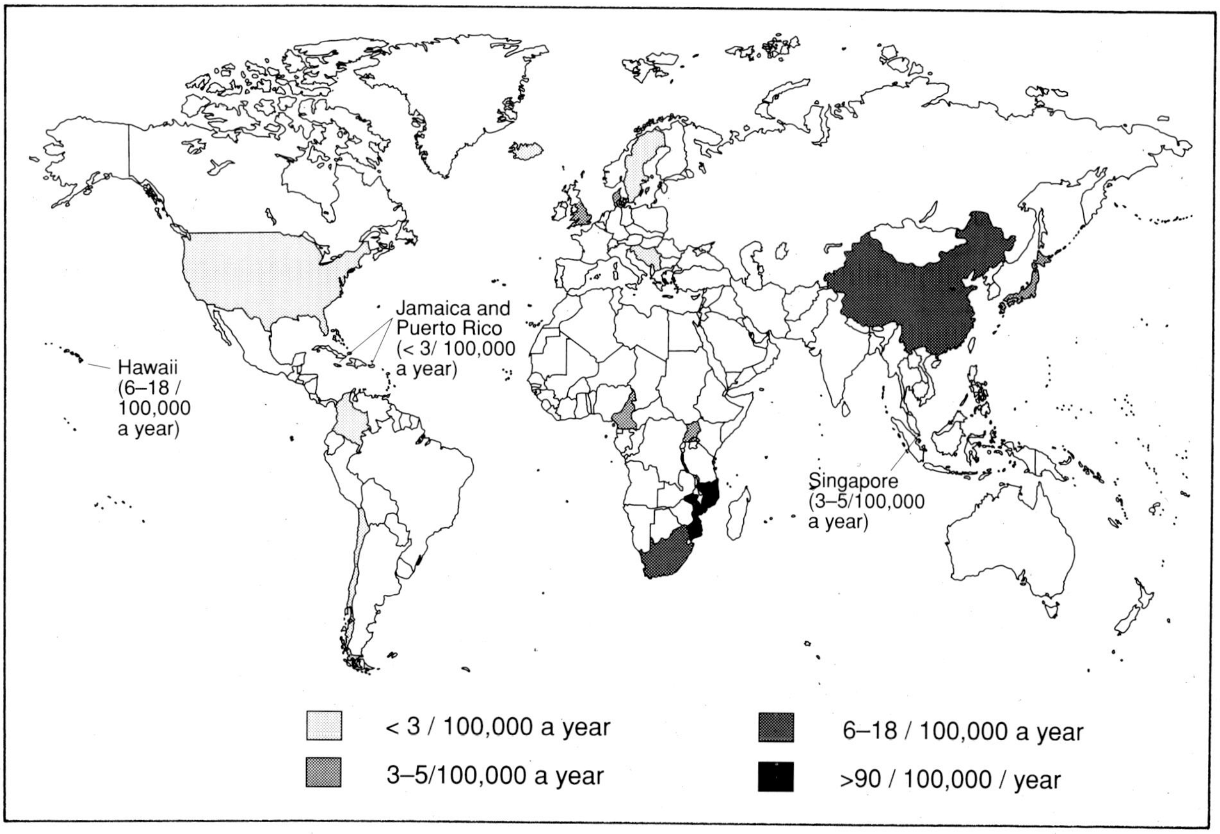

65 Prevalence of hepatoma in cancer registries.

66

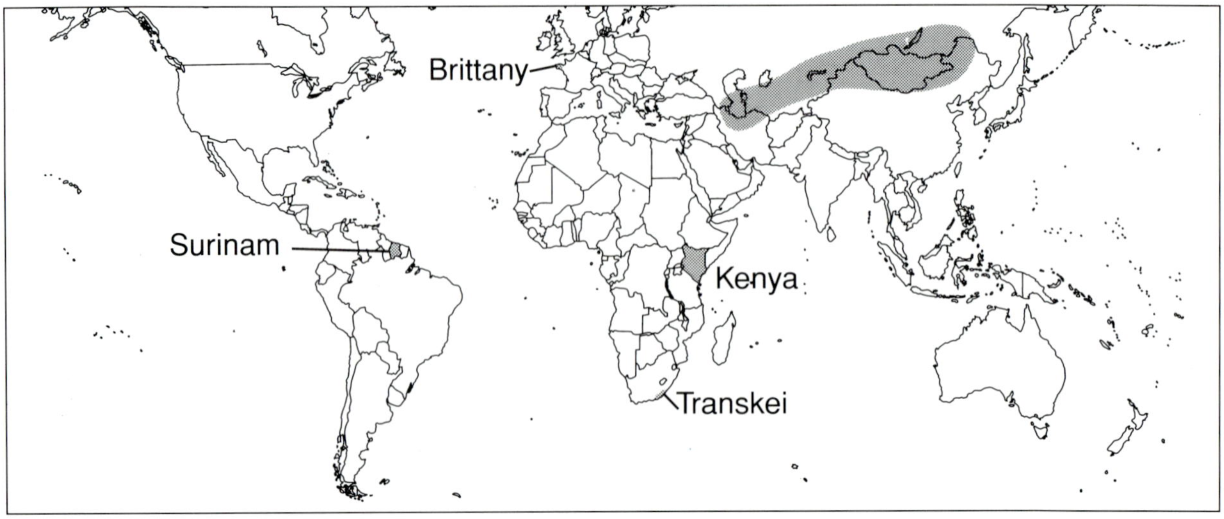

66 Areas of high prevalence of carcinoma of the oesophagus.

Diverticulosis and related diseases

Chronic constipation and its consequences (diverticular disease, varicose veins and haemorrhoids) are especially characteristic of a western lifestyle (**67–69**) (see also Chapter 2). The association with a fibre-depleted diet is strong and increasing dietary fibre, particularly from cereals such as coarse wheat bran, usually relieves constipation although advanced changes are irreversible.

Carcinoma of the colon is the second most common form of cancer in western communities and in many studies has been strongly associated with a diet low in fibre (see *Table 29*). Several theories have been advanced for the possible mechanism and the subject has been reviewed recently.[44]

67

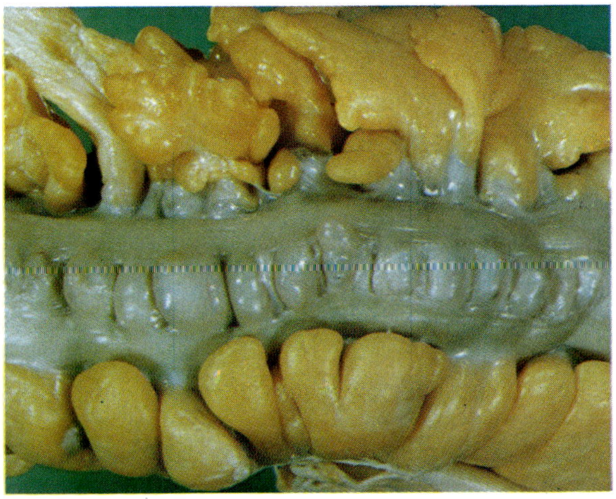

67 Diverticular disease. External appearance shows marked hypertrophy of the muscularis.

68

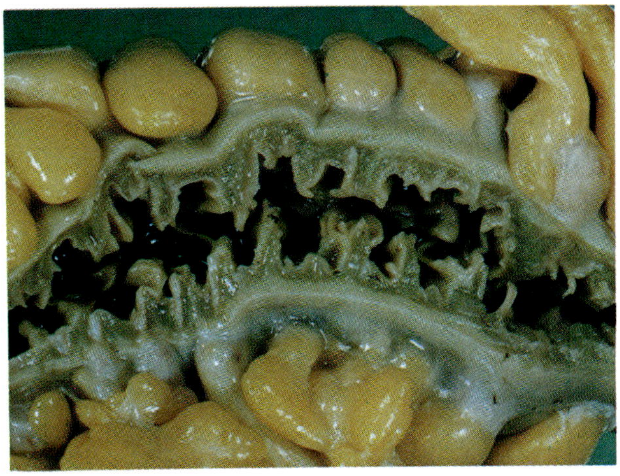

68 Diverticular disease. Viewed from the serosal surface there are numerous outpouchings aligned along one margin of the taenia coli. The sigmoid colon is most commonly and seriously affected. About 10% of all people in the West over the age of 40 are affected, rising to about 65% in old age. Many are asymptomatic. Diverticulitis causes left lower quadrant pain and repeated attacks result in fibrotic colonic narrowing.

Communities consuming a diet high in fibre content rarely have diverticular disease or other conditions associated with constipation and increased intraluminal colonic tension, such as haemorrhoids, varicose veins, pelvic vein thrombosis and appendicitis. Wholemeal bread and vegetables are good sources of fibre.

69

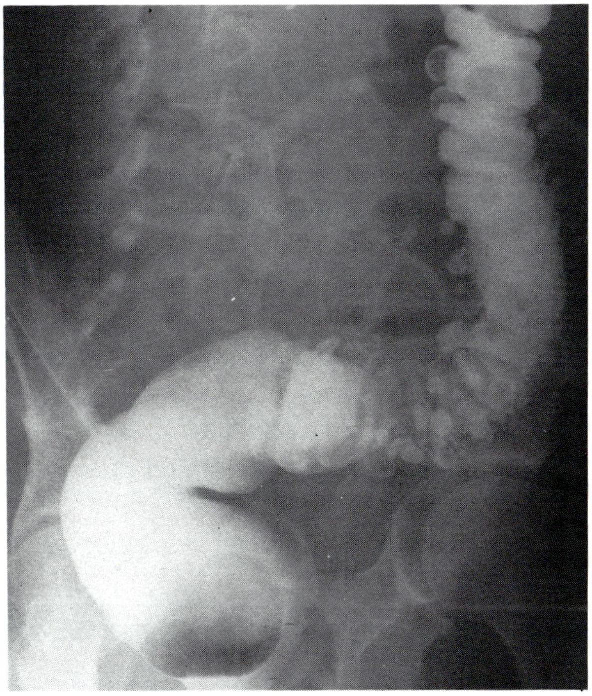

69 Diverticular disease. X-ray appearance of the most commonly affected sigmoid colon showing barium-filled diverticulae.

4. Disorders of Energy Metabolism

The conditions dealt with here might all be considered to be examples of what may be termed *macronutrient malnutrition* (in contrast to the *micronutrient malnutrition* disorders in Chapters 5 and 6). In clinical practice features of the two groups overlap considerably. All of the present disorders relate to deficient, or in the single case of obesity excessive, consumption of food in general and not to any particular nutrient. The deficiency states are therefore instances of general inanition.

The main energy sources involved are, of course, carbohydrate and fat, but part of protein intake provides energy and the complex of disease states seen in what is generally called protein-energy malnutrition (PEM), for want of a better term, is also best considered here. At the kwashiorkor end of the spectrum of severe PEM where protein deficiency is prominent, there is good evidence that excessive energy intake in the form of starch is also important (see page 76).

A qualitative deficiency of protein consists of a deficiency of specific essential amino acids. Although such states have been induced experimentally in animals the only counterpart in man is the aminoacidopathies of genetic origin described in Chapter 7 (see also Appendix II).

Normal nutrition which, as pointed out in Chapter 1, eludes precise definition, is a matter of balance. Energy balance is the best example of the phenomenon and provides the most varied and important examples of the ways in which it can be disturbed and give rise to disease.

Thus general inanition has differing causes but presents with certain common features in whatever circumstances it occurs. Starvation as caused by famine at the community level affects all members, but those with the greatest nutritional requirements – infants and young children, pregnant and lactating women – will suffer most and die first. Inanition also operates on a long-term basis in the community when inadequate feeding practices target the young child, giving rise initially to failure to thrive and going on to marasmus; or the pregnant woman, resulting in fetal malnutrition and low birthweight newborn. Malnutrition in the hospitalized patient also takes the form of general inanition with many underlying pathological processes giving rise to the same end result – negative energy balance. Anorexia nervosa illustrates the importance of psychological influences in feeding and how vulnerable it is to distortion, especially in adolescence. Finally, energy balance may equally readily be tipped towards the positive side, leading to overweight and obesity. The causes are very complex and still imperfectly understood and it is now evident that there are different forms of obesity with very different consequences for health.

Starvation

Like any other machine the body cannot continue to function without an adequate supply of energy. Unlike ordinary machines, when energy intake is restricted it can begin to catabolize its own tissues.

70 shows the average amounts of the various energy sources in the body and how they may be assessed. The ways in which energy is provided from tissues when intake is reduced were the subject of now classical studies by Cahill and his associates. They were able to carry out these studies by treating obese patients with diets consisting of only water, vitamins and minerals over periods of a number of weeks. **71** and **72** show the differences occurring after only 24 hours of fast (**71**) compared with 5–6 weeks later (**72**). In **71** the small glycogen reserves are used up and amino acids derived from protein of skeletal muscle become a major source of gluconeogenesis. Adipose tissue triglyceride gives rise to both fatty acids and ketones. As fasting continues several adaptive mechanisms come into operation designed to preserve life as far as possible, although eventually extreme wasting will lead to death. Ketone production is boosted to offset a reduction in glucose formation from muscle protein breakdown. Nervous tissue, including the brain, and other tissues now use ketones instead of glucose. The consequent reduction in protein catabolism causes a fall in urinary nitrogen excretion and ammonia formed in the kidney from glutamine now predominates over urea in the urine. This has the advantage of serving to maintain acid–base balance. A further adaptation is the reduction in energy requirements resulting from loss of body mass. Physical activity is also reduced and in the young child growth ceases.

70

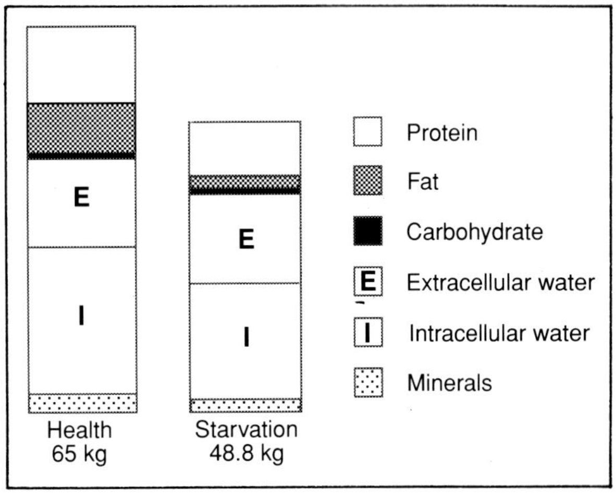

70 Body composition changes in starvation. These amount to about a 25% reduction in body weight and the release of about 70,000 kcal (293.3 MJ) of energy. This is made up of over 80% from 6.5kg of fat, 17% from 3kg of protein, almost all from skeletal muscle, and only about 1% from 200g of carbohydrate. Energy expenditure is reduced to about 1600kcal (6.70MJ) per day and the reserves would last about 50 days.

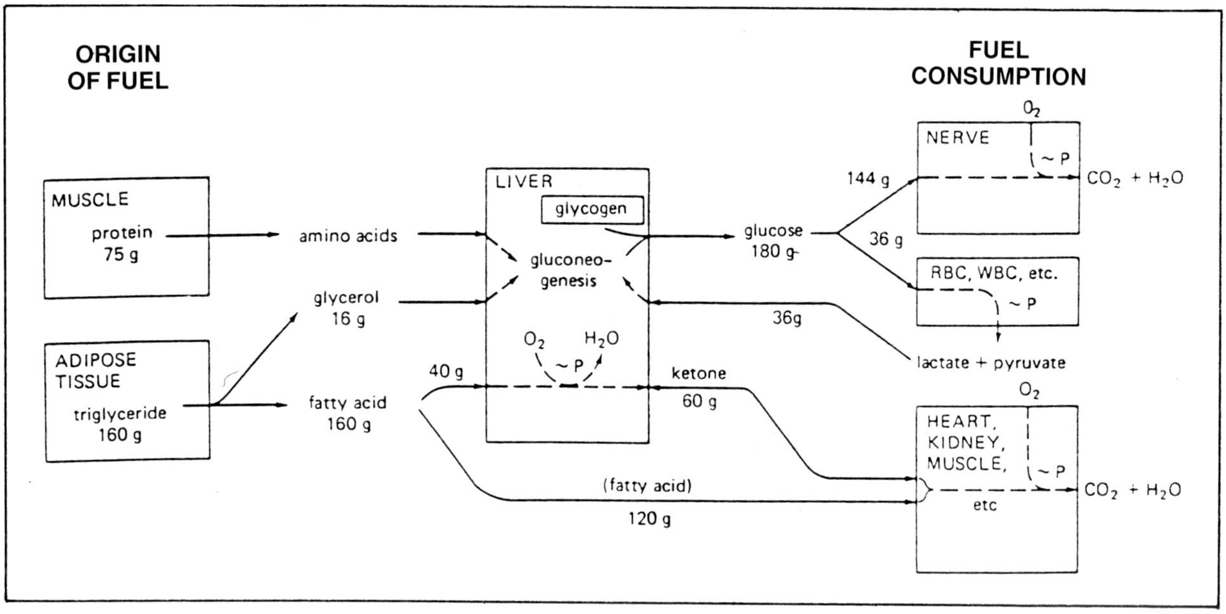

71

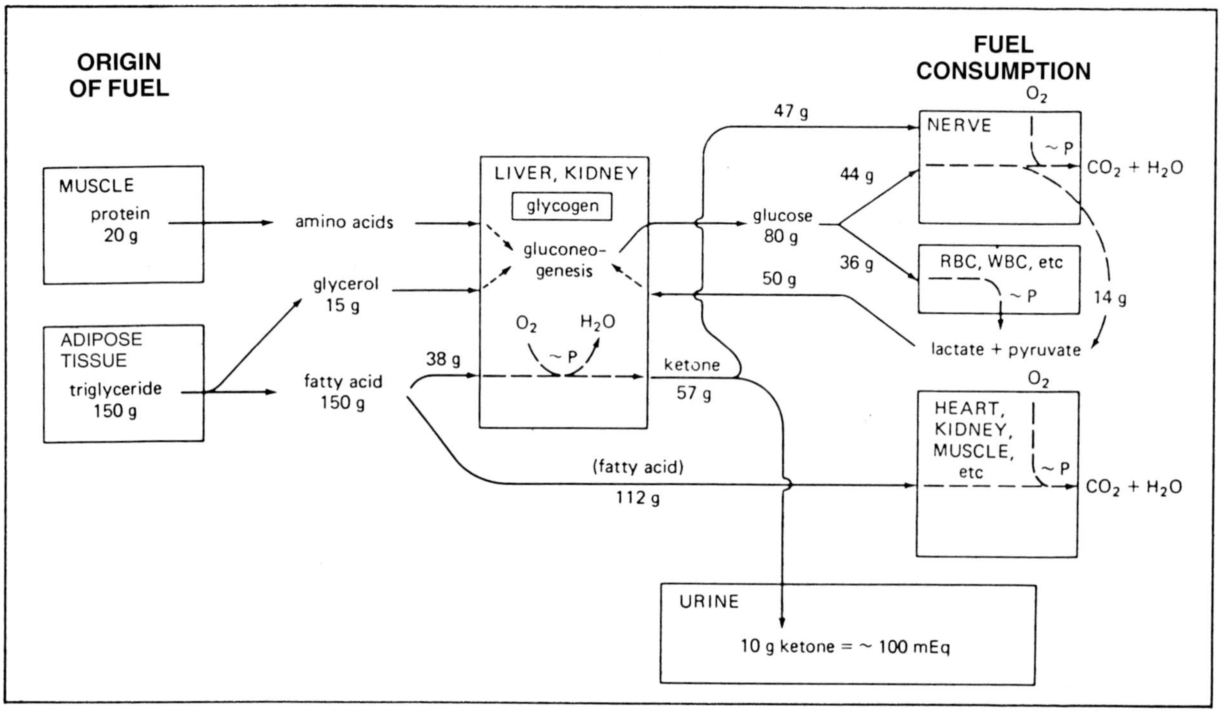

72

71, 72 Fuel utilization and gluconeogenesis from muscle protein in early and prolonged fasting or starvation. 71, Adult man after a 24-hour fast (24-hour basal: 1800 cal). 72, Adult man after 5–6 weeks of fasting (24-hour basal: 1500 cal). Data show loss of muscle protein and adipose tissue triglyceride (main sources of fuel), their use in production of glucose and ketone bodies by the liver, and uptake of glucose, ketones, and fatty acids by organs requiring fuel for energy. Values given are g/day, based on studies of numerous obese individuals fasting for various periods of time.

The general appearance in starvation is all too familiar (73). The skin undergoes several characteristic changes (**74–76**) and no system is spared (77).

73

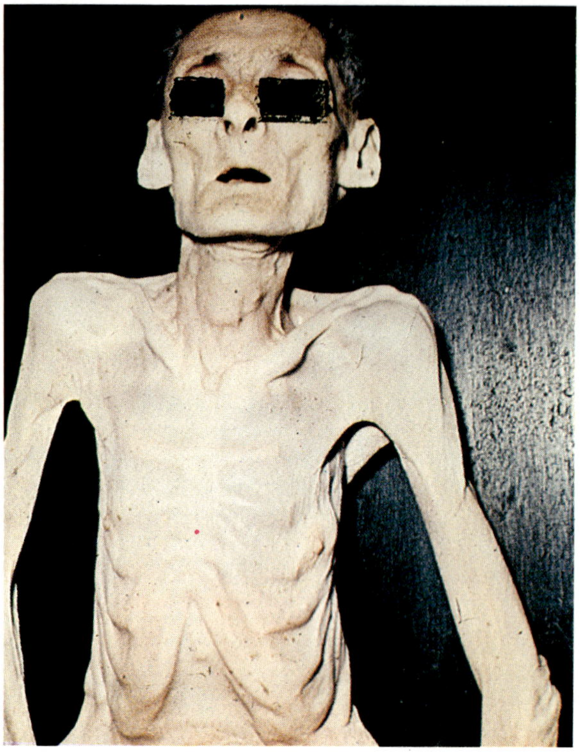

73 **Cachexia.** An extreme example of the loss of muscular and adipose tissue in terminal illness.

7

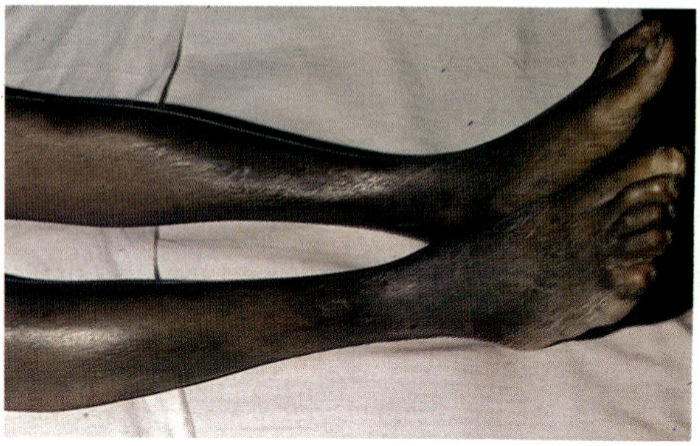

74 **Xerotic skin.** In chronic undernutrition in adults the skin of the extremities is frequently abnormally dry and superficially fissured. The skin over most of the body is thinned, wrinkled and has lost its usual elasticity, amounting to premature ageing.

75

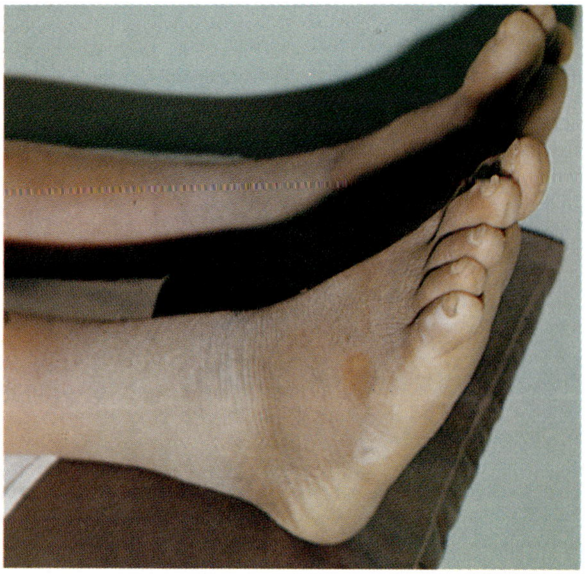

75 **Hyperkeratosis.** The skin over parts of the body is thickened, dry and wrinkled. The perifollicular areas are sometimes affected, with heaping up of hyperkeratotic material, but this appearance is more especially associated with vitamin A deficiency (see **218, 219**).

76

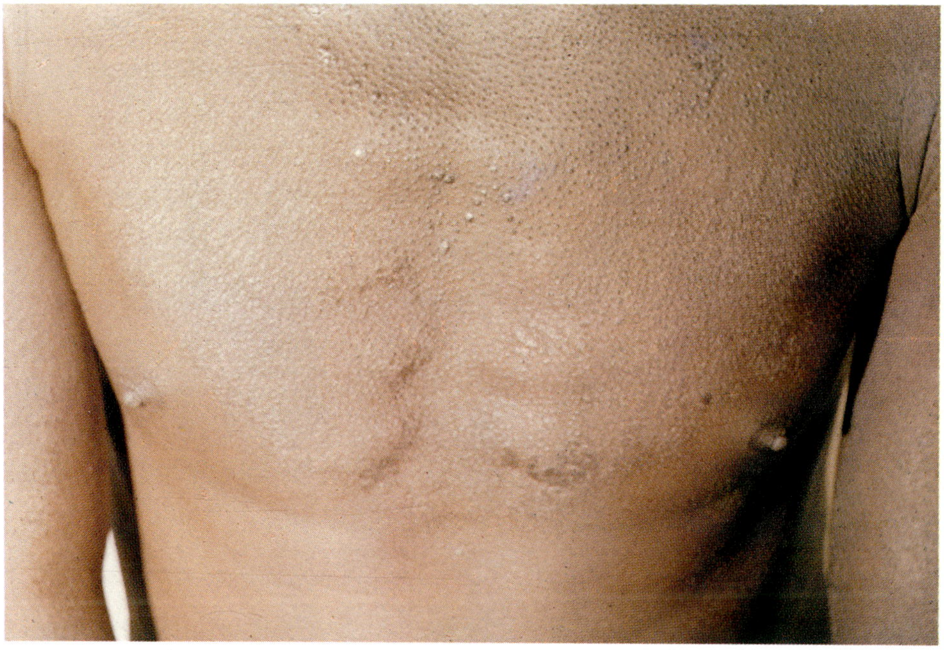

76 **'Permanent goose flesh.'** This term was given to a condition of the skin commonly seen in chronically undernourished adults by B.S. Platt. It superficially resembles cutis anserina, with prominence of the pilosebaceous follicles but they are not frankly keratotic, as in perifollicular hyperkeratosis (see **218, 219**). Its significance remains uncertain.

77

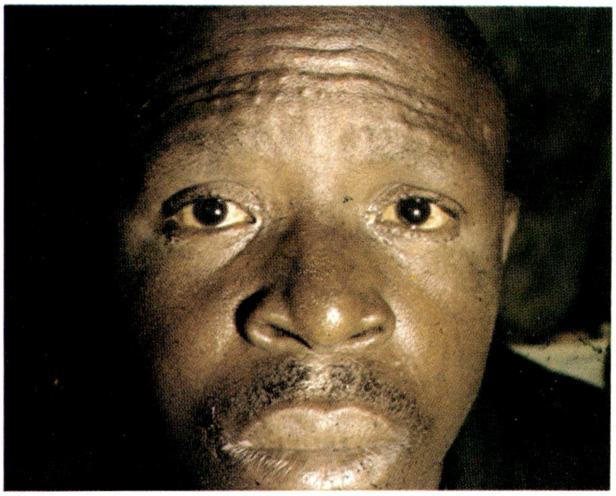

77 **Parotid enlargement.** There is bilateral, chronic, non-inflammatory swelling of the parotid glands, with no change in the overlying skin. It is usually seen in older children and adults and is an indication of prolonged undernutrition. It has also been reported to occur in chronically starved subjects during refeeding (see also **149**).

Refeeding of famine victims has brought its own problems. In prisoner-of-war camps overloading of the enfeebled digestive system with amino acid infusions hastened death and there is evidence[45] that it has caused resurgence of infections previously quiescent (78–80).

78

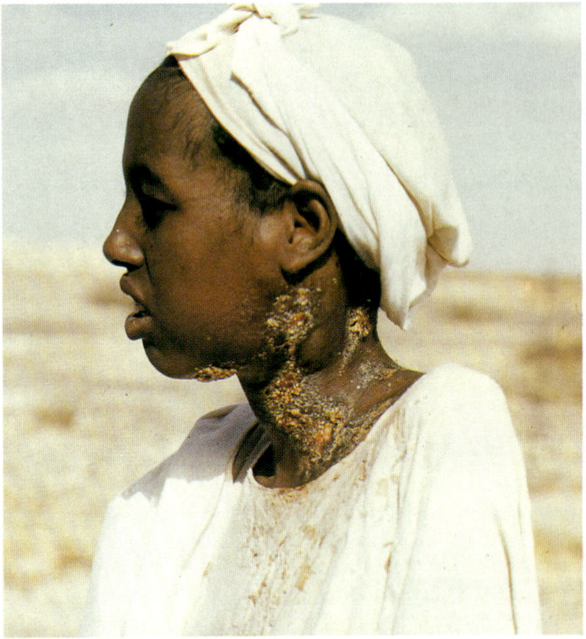

78 **Breakdown of tuberculous adenitis** (scrofula) after 1 month refeeding and a gain of 7kg in a Somali woman.

79

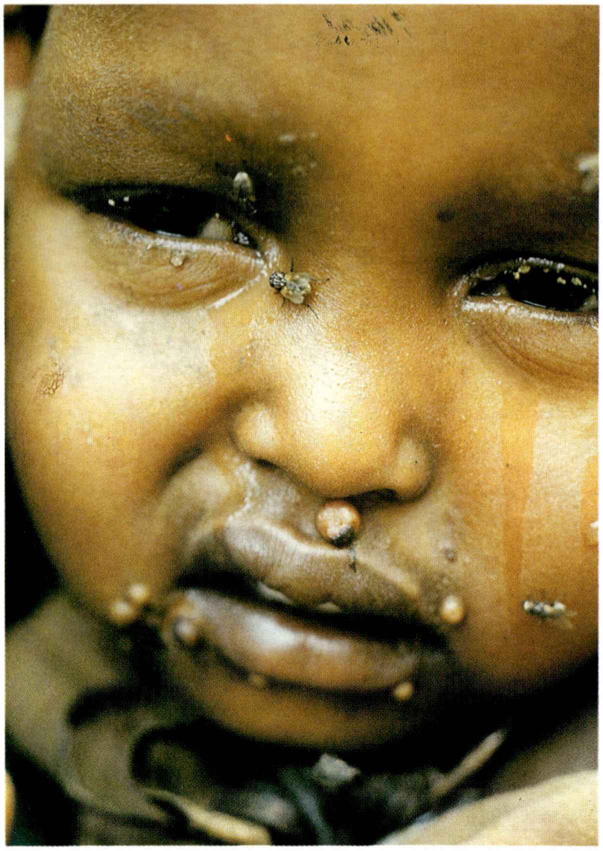

79 **Molluscum contagiosum** in a Maasai child during an epidemic following refeeding after famine.

80

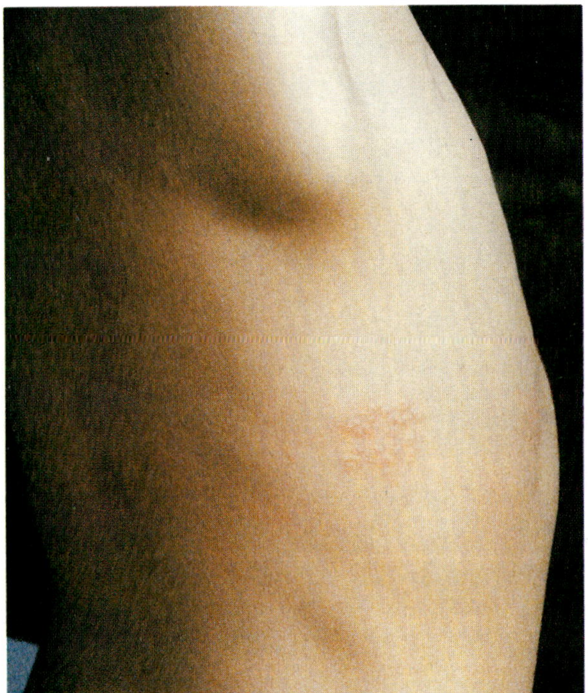

80 **Herpes zoster** in a Vietnamese 'boat' child following refeeding on arrival in Hong Kong.

Hospital malnutrition

Despite pioneering studies by Moore in the United States[46] and Cuthbertson in the United Kingdom[47] on the nutritional and metabolic consequences of illness and injury it has only been in the past two decades that much attention has been paid to malnutrition occurring in patients in hospital, at least some of which is iatrogenic. Part of the problem has been, and remains, how to assess nutritional status that falls short of the frank deficiency states that can be readily recognized by clinical signs. Even so a powerful clinical subspeciality called Nutritional Support has been developed and is now available in most medical centres. Its primary aim is to restore or maintain normal nutrition in a wide variety of medical and surgical diseases affecting patients of all ages and in this way to assist the natural processes of the body concerned with such functions as wound healing and response to infections, drugs, radiotherapy, etc. The subject is explored further in Chapter 10.

Hospital malnutrition is almost always of the general inanition, marasmic type whether in children or adults (**81, 82**).

81

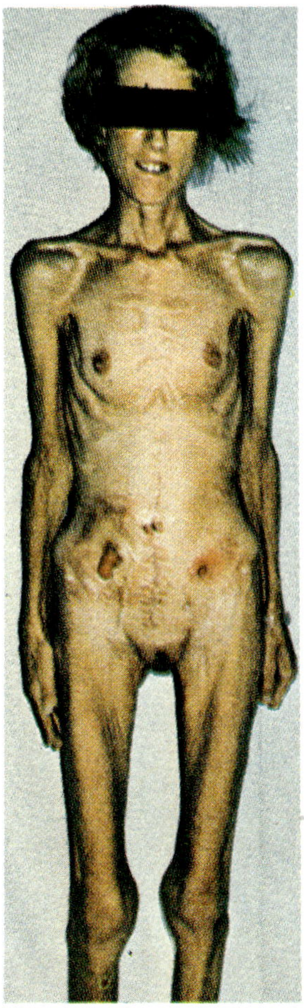

82

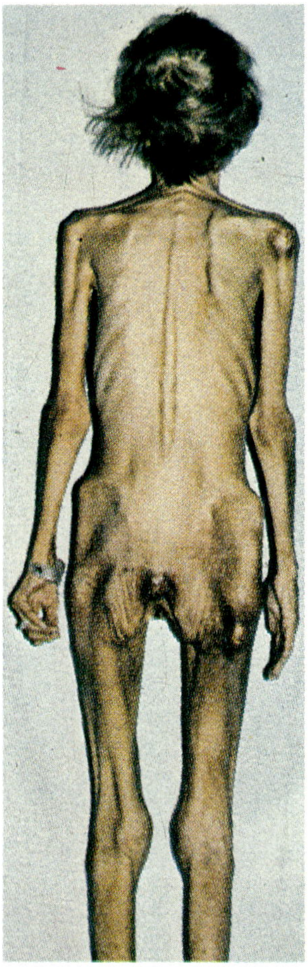

81 Hypercatabolic disease. This occurs in acute illness or injury usually associated with sepsis in which there is an increase in metabolic rate and of net protein catabolism of 25% or more. This 27-year-old patient with ulcerative colitis required an emergency colectomy after losing weight from 44 to 25kg. After operation the weight continued to fall to 22kg and normal weight was only regained after 3 months in hospital.

82 Hypercatabolic disease. Posterior view of the same patient.

True kwashiorkor with skin changes, oedema, fatty liver and hypoalbuminaemia is hardly ever seen under these circumstances and it is preferable to use the term hypoalbuminaemic malnutrition[48] and reserve kwashiorkor for the full syndrome (**83–86**).

83

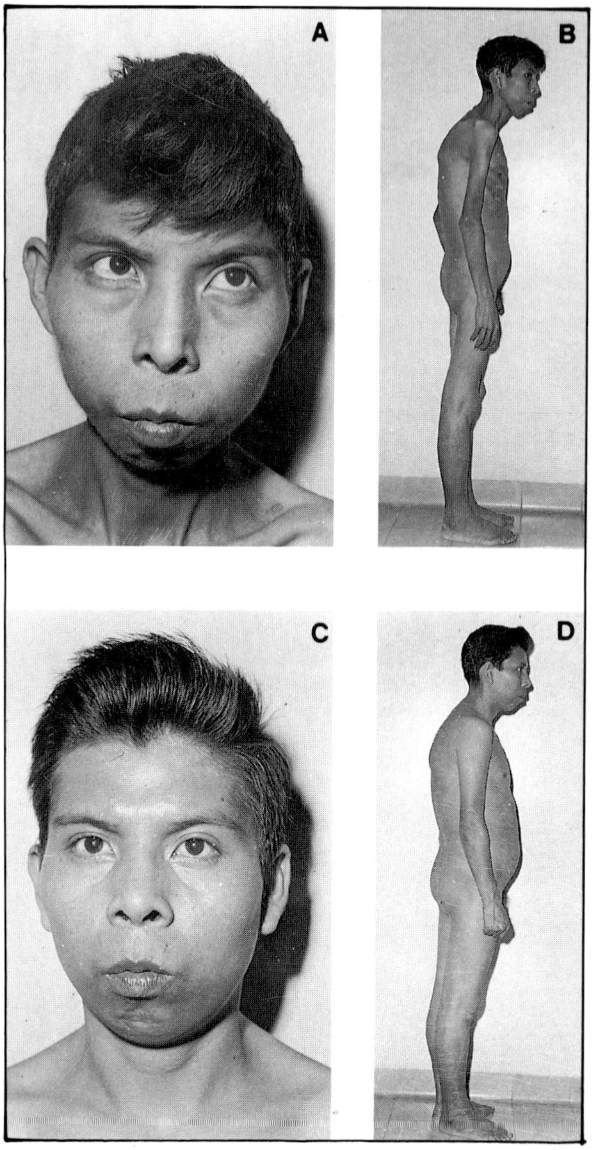

83 Marasmic protein-energy-malnutrition in a 29-year-old man, A and B; patient after three months of treatment, C and D.

84

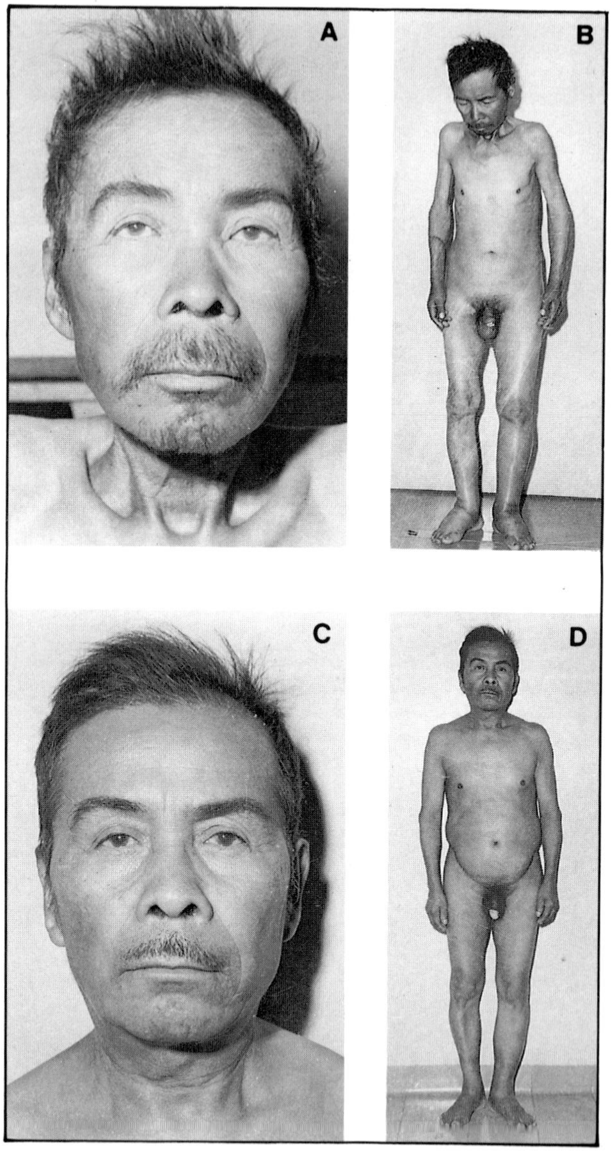

84 Oedematous protein-energy-malnutrition in a 46-year-old man, A and B; patient after three months of treatment, C and D.

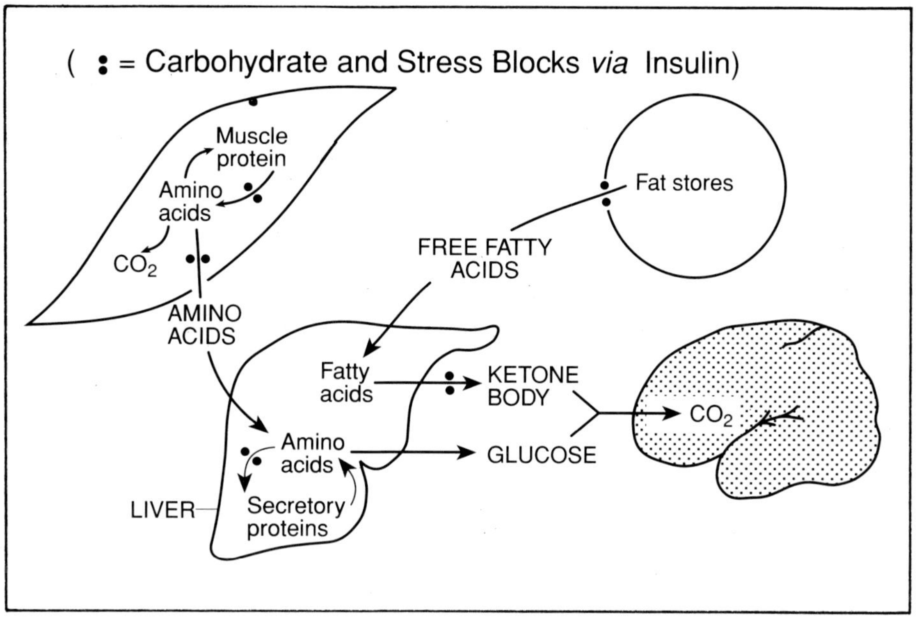

85 Aetiology of adult kwashiorkor-like syndrome. The combined effect of stress and carbohydrate to produce hyperinsulinaemia impair the metabolic response to infectious stress. Amino acid and free fatty acid mobilization from the periphery are curtailed while visceral protein synthesis is reduced through diminished substrate availability.

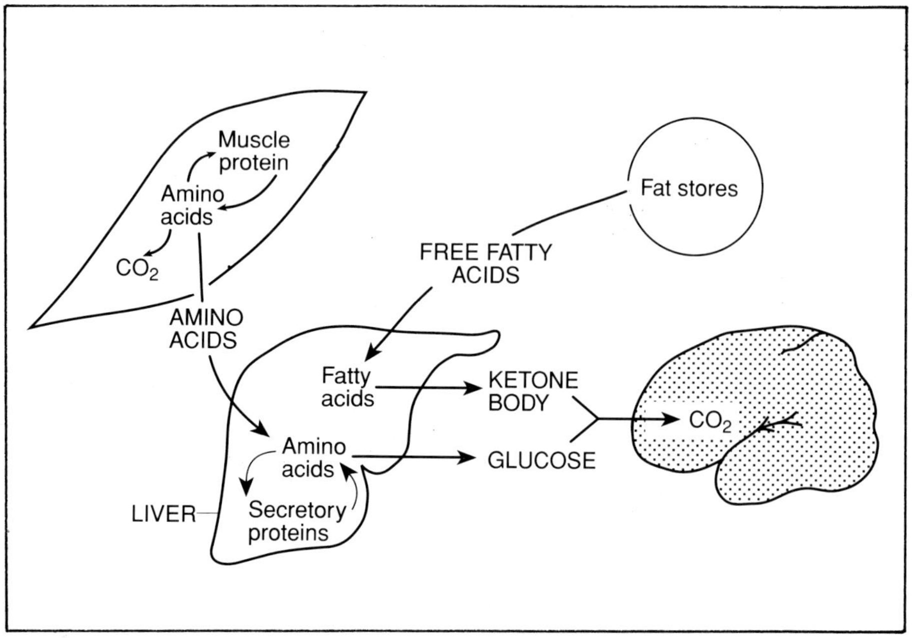

86 Why plasma amino acid levels are low in adult marasmus. A deficient supply of amino acids from depleted body protein stores is compounded by inadequate dietary protein such that protein synthesis is impaired. This is shown here schematically by the relatively smaller fat and skeletal muscle compartments.

This condition can be attributed largely to acute phase response (APR) in trauma and infection (87).

There are a number of reasons why serum albumin or other transport proteins such as retinol-binding protein (RBP), prealbumin, or transferrin are unreliable for assessment of protein status in many hospitalized patients (*Table 30*).

87

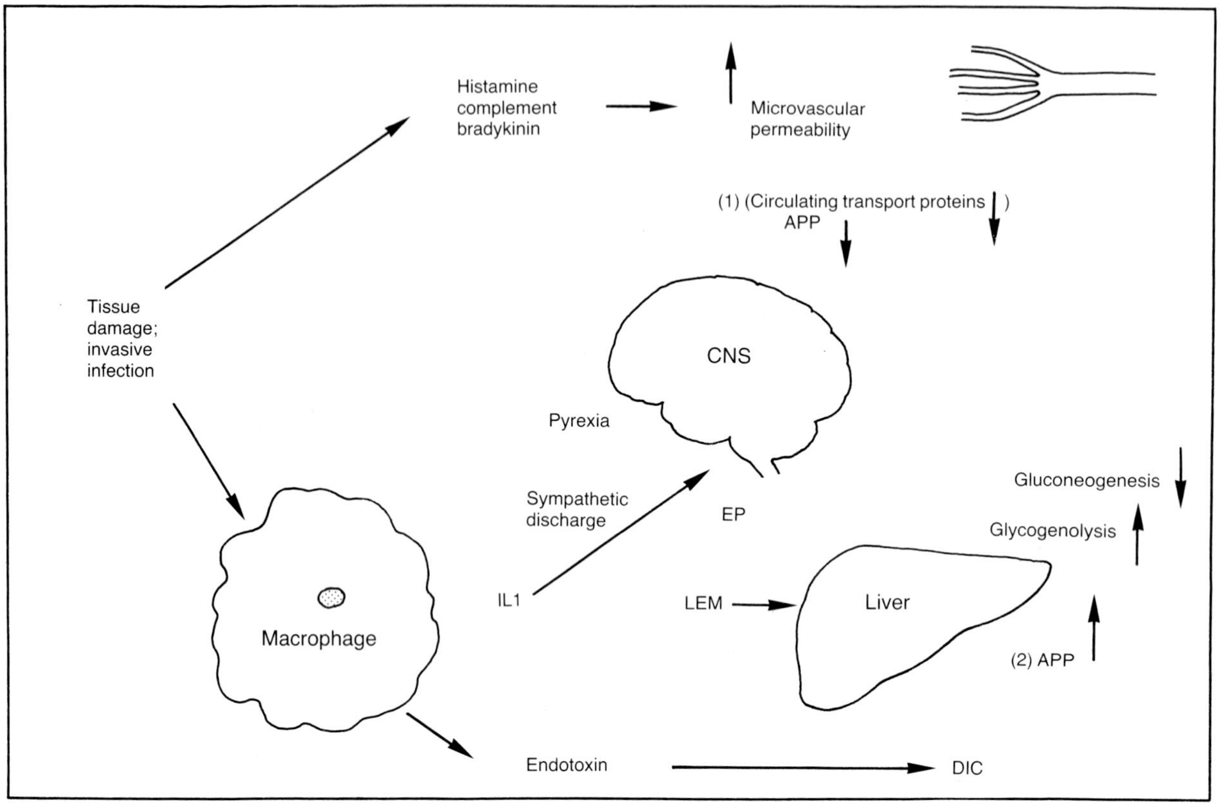

87 Some metabolic and nutritional consequences of tissue damage and invasive infection. (**Key:** IL1, Interleukin 1; EP, Endogenous pyrogen; LEM Leucocytic endogenous mediators; DIC, Diffuse intravascular coagulation; APP, Acute phase proteins; (1), First or second day; (2), Third to fifth day).

Table 30. Non-nutritional causes of depression of serum albumin and other transport proteins.

Mechanism	*Disease*
Diminished synthesis	Liver disease, chronic infections and malignancy
Normal synthesis but release from liver impaired	Acute infections
Reduced efficiency of reutilization of amino acids	Trauma, surgery
Translocation of serum proteins to interstitial space	Trauma, acute infections, cancer, radiation and chemotherapy, ascites
Loss from the body	Nephrotic syndrome, protein-losing enteropathy, burns, pressure sores

Cardiac cachexia

Wasting has long been noted to be common in chronic heart disease, especially in right-sided failure with tricuspid regurgitation. The mechanisms have not been understood until recently. Whole-body protein synthesis is depressed while breakdown of myofibrillar protein is increased. In other forms of cachexia there is also a fall in protein synthesis but protein breakdown is normal or even depressed. Postulated mechanisms are shown in *Table 31*.

Numerous attempts have been made to try to relate nutritional status to outcome in hospital, especially in surgical patients. One of the more widely used is the prognostic nutrition index (PNI)[49] (*Table 32*). It relies heavily on transport protein assessment (criticized above) and uses triceps skinfold which is generally regarded as insensitive. Correlation with outcome in practice is, however, good and this suggests that it relates more to APR and other factors than to nutritional status *per se*.

Table 31. Postulated mechanisms for cardiac cachexia.

Reduced blood flow to limbs
Immobility leading to disuse atrophy
Anorexia from hepatic congestion, hypoxia or drug toxicity
Protein-losing enteropathy, steatorrhoea
Energy requirements increased, resulting in increased myocardial oxygen consumption and increased metabolic cost of breathing
Secretion of catecholamines and corticosteroids accelerates muscle protein breakdown
Cellular hypoxia causes decreased ATP production necessary for protein synthesis
Cachetin (tumour necrosis factor) and interleukin are raised

Table 32. Assessment of nutritional status of the hospitalized patient.

Signs indicative of a significant degree of protein-energy malnutrition	
Recent weight loss $> 10\%$	
Serum albumin < 35g/l	
Serum transferrin < 2g/l	
Triceps skinfold thickness	< 10mm males < 13mm females
Upper arm circumference	< 23cm males < 22cm females
Lymphopenia $< 1.2 \times 10^9$/l	
Skin anergy to a battery of antigens: candida, mumps, streptokinase, streptodornase, dermatophytin, PPD	

Prognostic Nutritional Index (PNI) uses four of these indicators in a linear predictive model of increased morbidity and mortality following surgery, according to the following formula:
PNI % (chance of complications) $= 158 - 16.6(A) - 0.78(TSF) - 0.2(TFN) - 5.8(DH)$ where A = serum albumin; TSF = Triceps skinfold thickness; TFN = serum transferrin; and DH = delayed hypersensitivity response.

Low birthweight

Babies of low birthweight may be of normal gestational age but have failed to grow at the usual rate ('small-for-dates' or small for gestational age) or may have grown normally but have been born prematurely. It is important to distinguish between the two types of low birthweight, as those small for gestational age have a higher mortality and morbidity; this type falls below the tenth centile of weight for age and may not have had a pre-term delivery (less than 37 weeks). The old criterion for low birthweight of 2.5 kg should be abandoned.

It is estimated that about 22 million low birthweight babies are born every year, about 90% in developing countries where in turn 80% are 'small-for-dates'.[50] It is these latter babies who are especially likely to have suffered *in utero* from fetal malnutrition as a consequence of maternal malnutrition (88).

All of the factors shown in this figure in some way or another interfere with fetal nutrition and lead to growth retardation. In particular deficiency of energy, iron, iodine, zinc and folic acid has been implicated in developing countries. Ultrasound is being used increasingly in prenatal care and can assist in the diagnosis of fetal growth retardation (**89**).

All except very low birthweight infants (between 0.8 and 1.5kg and less than 32 weeks gestation) usually gain weight well after birth, undergo catch-up growth (**90**) and suffer no permanent ill effects.

It has been claimed in a series of studies[51] that adverse social circumstances in very early life, including those *in utero*, predispose to death from degenerative disease in later life. The claim has been contested on the grounds that such conditions tend to persist and that the influences later on in life are responsible.[52]

88

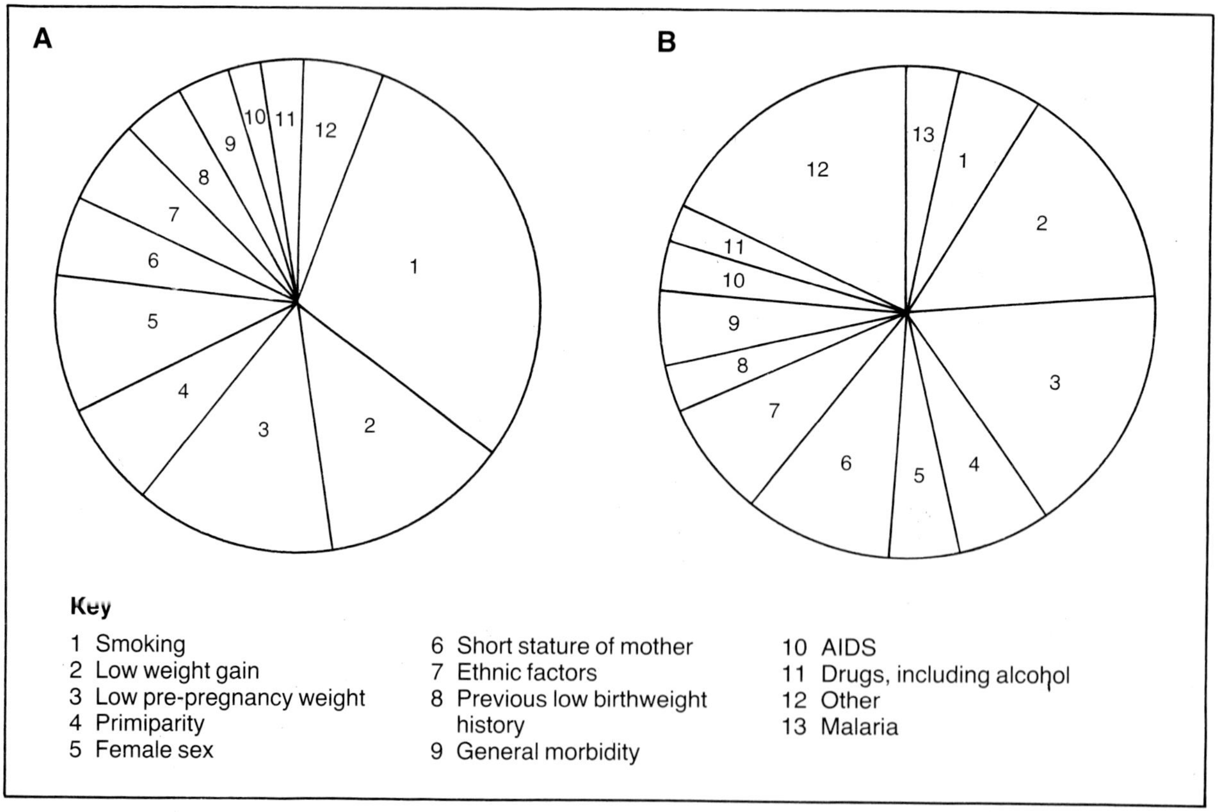

88 Relative importance of factors associated with low birthweight in industrialized (A) and developing (B) countries.

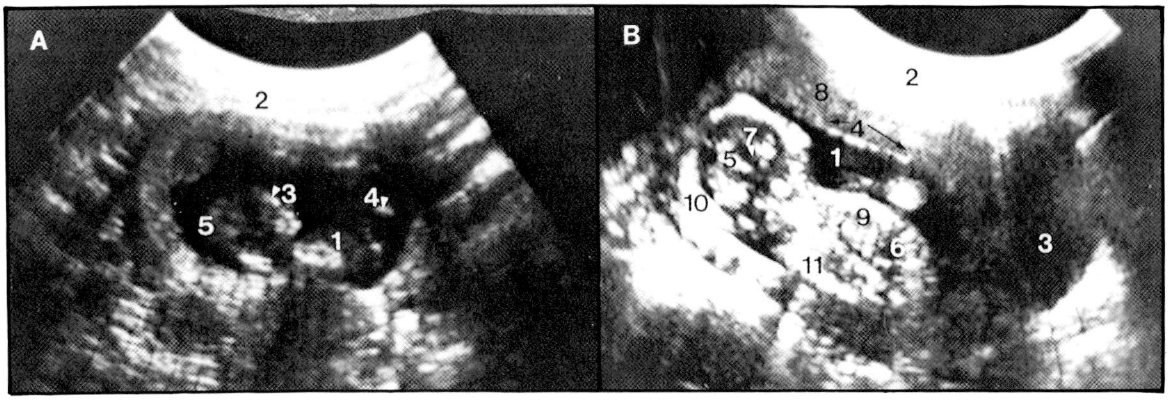

89 **Ultrasound method** used to assess very accurately development *in utero* by scanning the maternal abdomen. Measurements of the biparietal diameter and femur are used for dating gestational age, and thus for detecting growth failure. Growth is best assessed by serial circumference measurements of the fetal head and abdomen. In late pregnancy fetal weight is estimated by using in addition abdominal circumference, crown–rump length and amniotic fluid volume. (**Key:** A, longitudinal scan of a 12 week fetus: 1, abdomen; 2, anterior abdominal wall (maternal); 3, face; 4, limb; 5, skull. B, longitudinal scan of a 15.5 week fetus: 1, amniotic fluid; 2, anterior abdominal wall; 3, bladder (maternal); 4, chorionic plate; 5, falx cerebri; 6, fundus of the stomach; 7, lateral ventricle; 8, placenta; 9, rib; 10, skull, 11; spine).

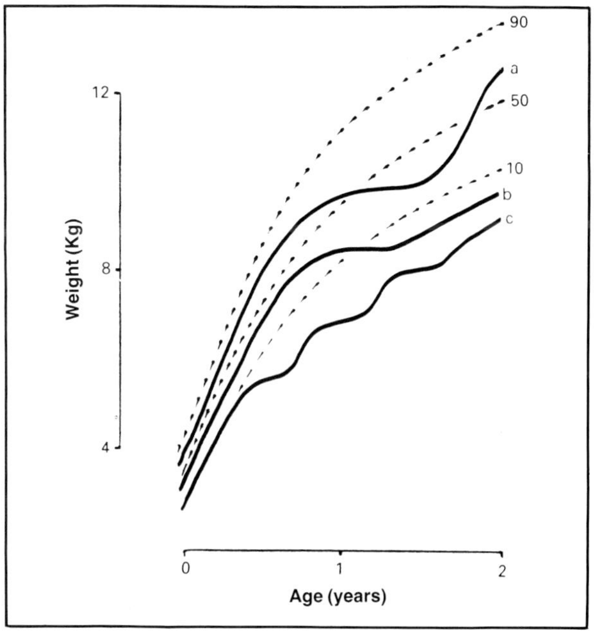

90 **Weight curves of children failing to thrive** plotted against the 10th, 50th and 90th weight centiles. Showing: a, complete catch-up growth; b, incomplete catch-up growth; and c, recurrent growth faltering and incomplete catch-up.

Failure to thrive (FTT)

This is failure to gain in height and weight at the expected rate (**91, 92**) and therefore refers to growth speed and not to absolute size.

Immediate causes of FTT consist of one or any combination of the following: inadequate intake, failure to absorb, failure to utilize, increased losses, increased requirements. Conditioning factors are often of a more social, cultural, economic and environmental nature (**93**).

Infections are prominent under the above conditions and may induce FTT in various ways (*Table 33*).

91

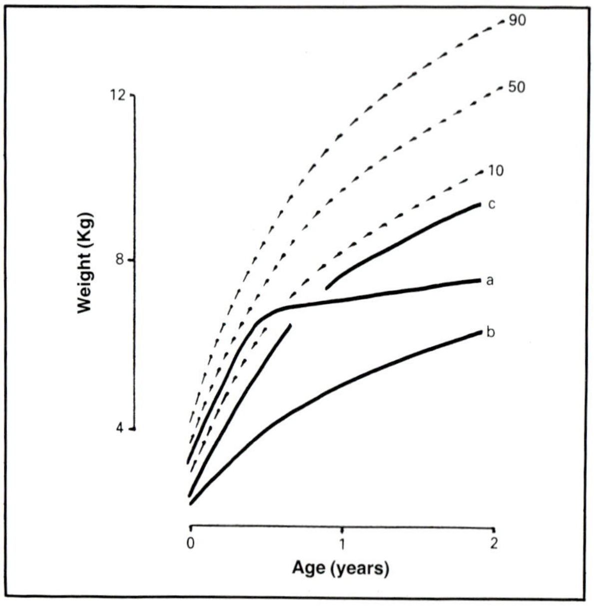

91 Weight charts of children failing to thrive (a and b), and small normal child (c) plotted against the 10th, 50th and 90th weight centiles.

92

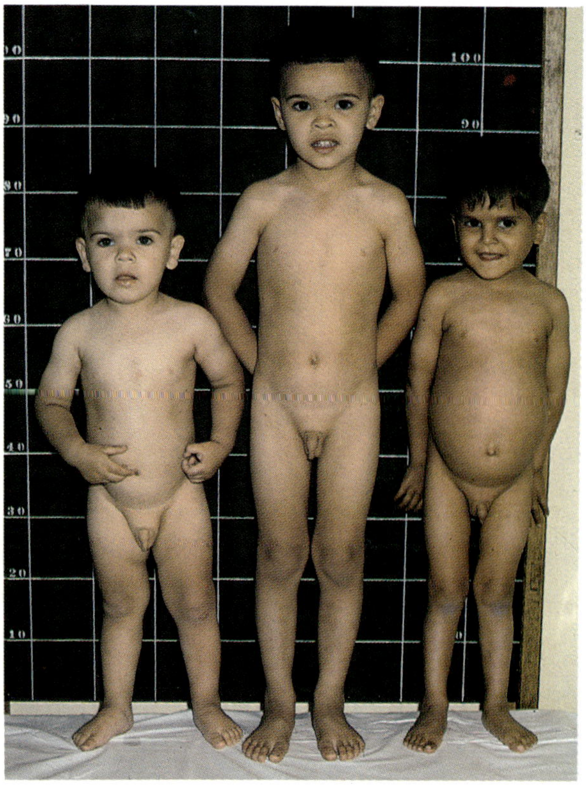

92 Growth failure. The children in this picture were aged 2, 4.5 and 5.5 years from left to right. The first two are normal but the last is grossly retarded in growth although the weight:height ratio is normal and there is no evidence of clinical malnutrition. Stunting is the commonest evidence of chronic, mild PEM.

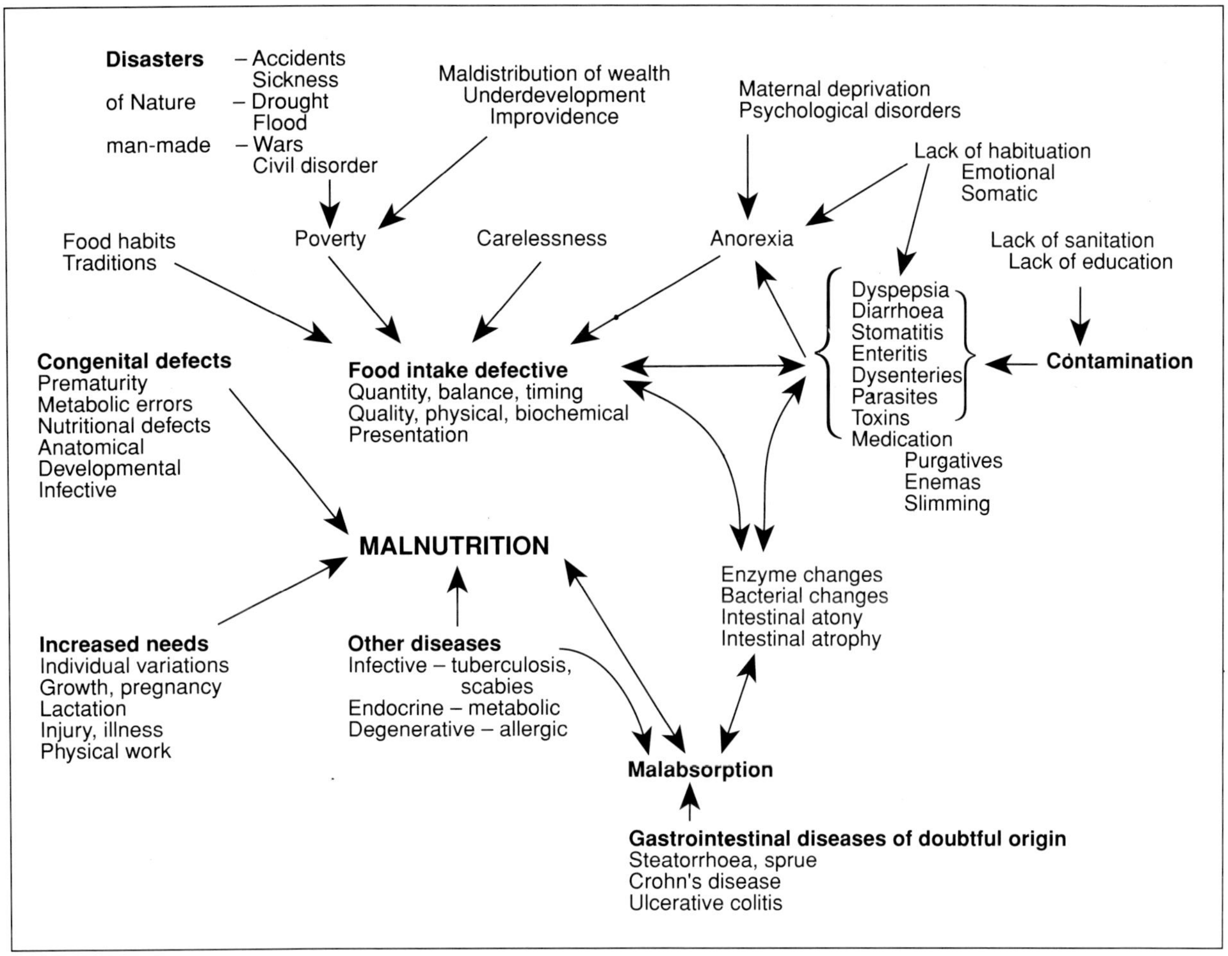

93 General scheme of causes of malnutrition. This was devised by Dr Cicely Williams who identified kwashiorkor in Ghana in the early 1930s as a disease due mainly to protein deficiency. Strangely, the 'deposed child situation' which she showed was the main predisposing condition in kwashiorkor, and recognized as such by the local people in naming the disease, does not appear. In very different circumstances in tribal India the author found the same main cause underlying the occurrence of keratomalacia in one group and not in another. **110** shows how markedly different the underlying causes of kwashiorkor and marasmus tend to be.

Table 33. Ways in which infections affect nutritional status.

Appetite is reduced and nutrient intakes become inadequate.
Gut infestations, such as giardiasis and ascariasis, lead to mucosal damage, malabsorption (particularly for disaccharides), or secondary nutrient losses.
Pyrexia increases energy requirements: a 1°C rise in body temperature causes a 13% increase in basal metabolic rate.
Pyrexia inhibits gastrointestinal absorption of iron and, possibly, other elements.
Infection may also lead to failure in nutrient utilization through as yet ill-defined toxic effects at the cellular level.

94

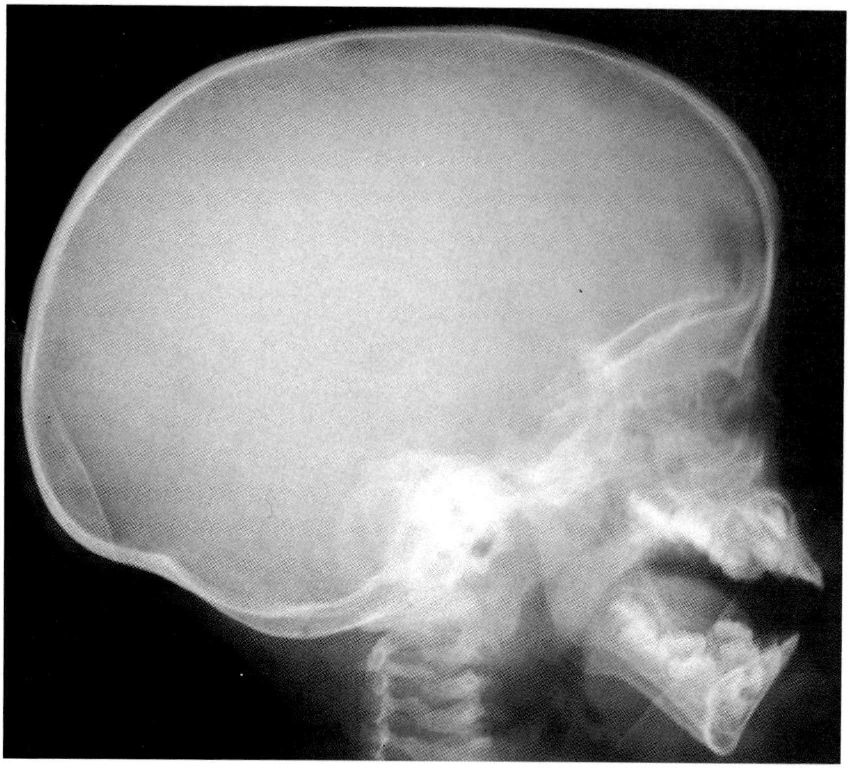

94 Skull in failure to thrive. A 30-month-old male hospitalized for FTT; the lateral skull X-ray at time of admission is normal.

95

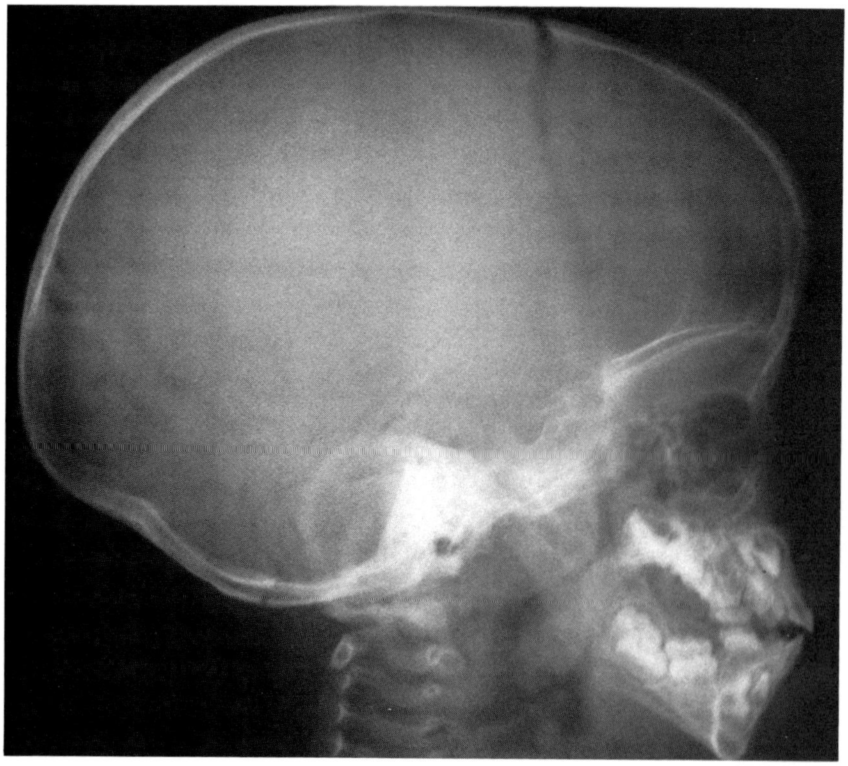

95 FTT. Two months later, when the child had gained weight and was well, the lateral X-ray demonstrates wide coronal and lambdoid sutures indicating growth of the brain. The increased head circumference and separation of the cranial sutures are caused by cellular growth of the brain when nutrition is improved in previously malnourished young children. Although the sutural diastasis simulates increased intracranial pressure, there are no abnormal neurological signs or symptoms, and intracranial pressure is not increased.

Table 34. Features of FTT attributable to neurological and psychological problems.

Emotionally and/or physically depriving environment
Often good or excessive appetite; may be bizarre appetite and food stealing
Developmental delay, especially in psychological skills
Disturbed affect with passivity and lack of interest; alternatively, attention seeking behaviour
Short stature
Retarded bone age
Underweight for height, as well as age
Infantile proportions to body
Distended abdomen
Acrocyanosis of hands and feet
'Radar gaze' or 'frozen watchfulness'
Acceleration in growth, and developmental and emotional progress, on change of environment only

FTT is just another name for mild or 1st degree PEM (see page 71) at which stage clinical signs and biochemical derangements are absent and retarded growth is reflected in substandard somatic measurements. There is, however, a small group of children in whom neurological and psychological factors predominate and some of the clinical features are specific to this form of FTT (*Table 34* and **94**, **95**). This form is suggestive of an infantile version of anorexia nervosa (see 89).

Data from a number of countries in the third world show a rather consistent pattern, with the prevalence of FTT (less than 80% weight for age in this study) increasing steadily up to about 5 years of age (**96**).

96

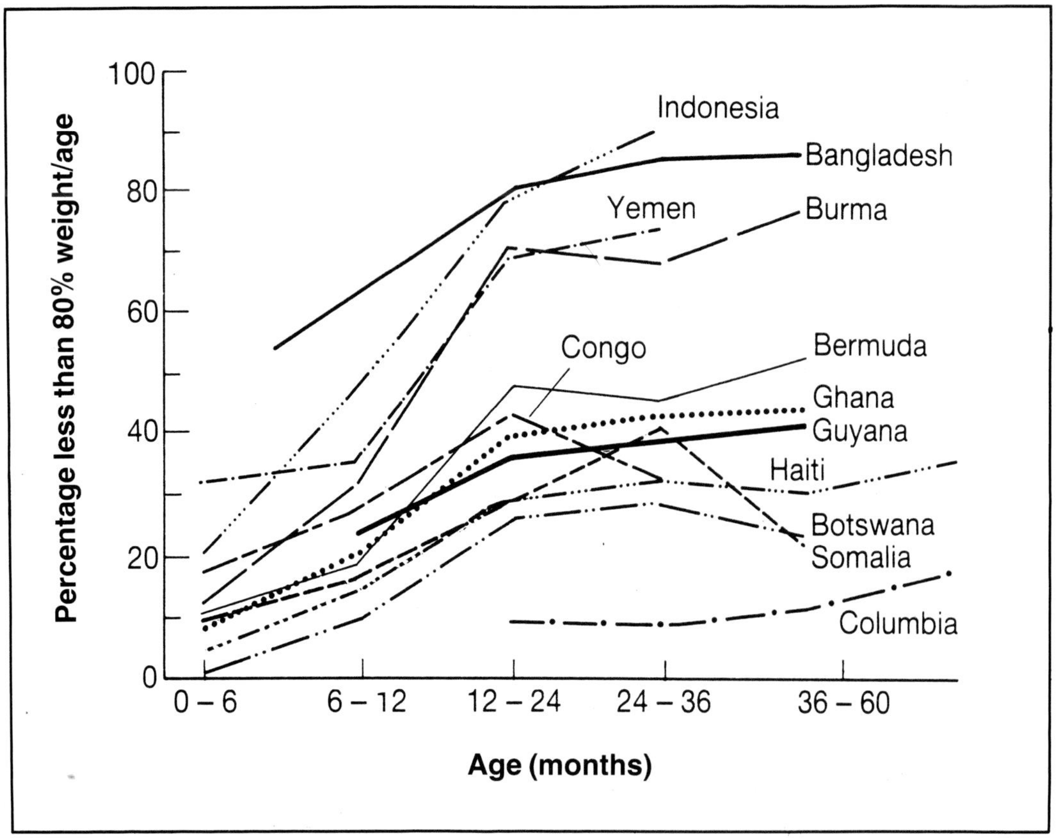

96 Prevalence of malnutrition (less than 80% weight for age) at different ages in various countries. It is maximum in the age group 2–4 years.

97

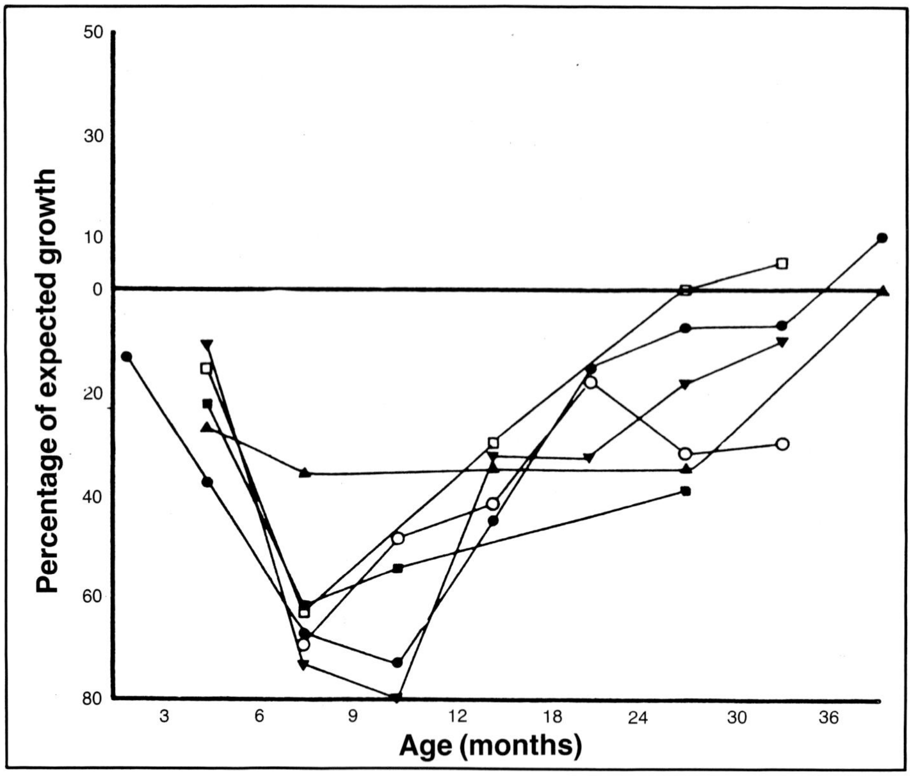

97 Growth faltering in early infancy (data drawn from same study as 96).

98

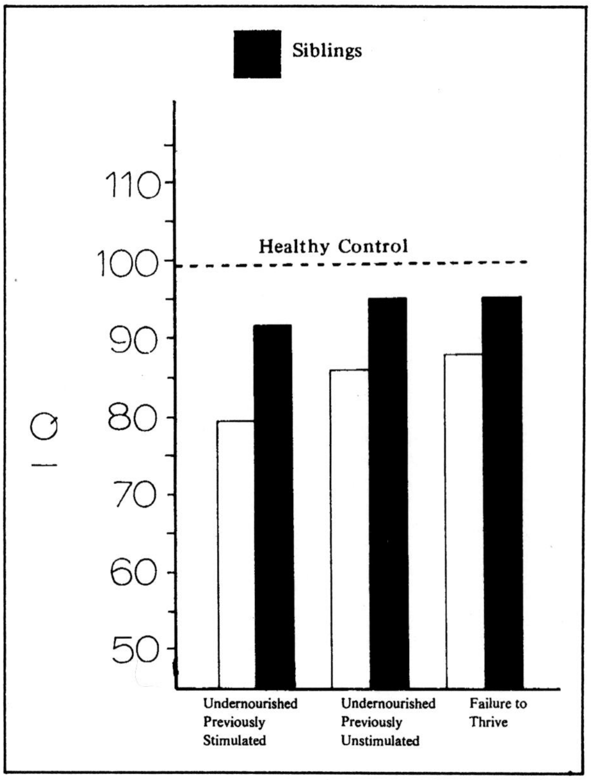

However, the same data looked at in terms of growth-rate faltering reveals that the average deficit is maximum at a much earlier stage in all cases, i.e. during the second half of infancy (97); if preventive measures are to be effective they should be instituted at this age.

Also very impressive is the degree of catch-up growth that occurs in some countries, but the probable impairment of mental development should not be ignored[53] (98, 99).

98 Undernutrition and mental development. This diagram shows seven groups of Lebanese pre-school age children matched for age and sex. There were 15 in each group. The mean IQ measured by the Stanford-Binet test is shown for each. The healthy controls from a middle-class group score almost 100. Three groups of undernourished children all scored significantly less than the controls. They also scored less than their 'healthy' but socially deprived siblings. The previous state of the malnourished children did not influence the tests; one group had been stimulated during rehabilitation; another had not; and a third had never been severely malnourished but had failed to thrive. These results suggest that both undernutrition and social deprivation can adversely affect mental development of the young child.

99 **Quality of care and growth.** Changes in the weight of children from two German orphanages during 1948. Both groups were given the same diet up to week 26 after which those in orphanage A received supplements of unlimited bread, jam, and orange juice. At the same time a cruel and unpopular sister-in-charge was transferred from orphanage B to orphanage A. The growth curves follow the presence or absence of the sister, not the diet. However, eight children who were favourites of the sister and were transferred with her did benefit from the supplemented diet.

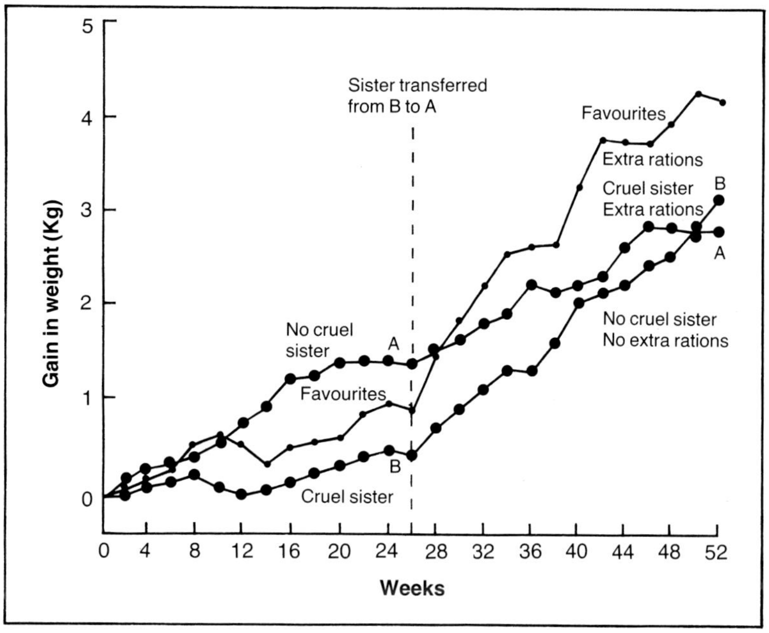

99

Protein-energy malnutrition

After more than 30 years the nutritional pyramid of Jelliffe[54] (**100**) is still the best visual representation of the degrees of PEM (1st, 2nd, 3rd) and the types of severe PEM.

Infections and infestations play a constant part (**101–109**) (see Chapter 10).

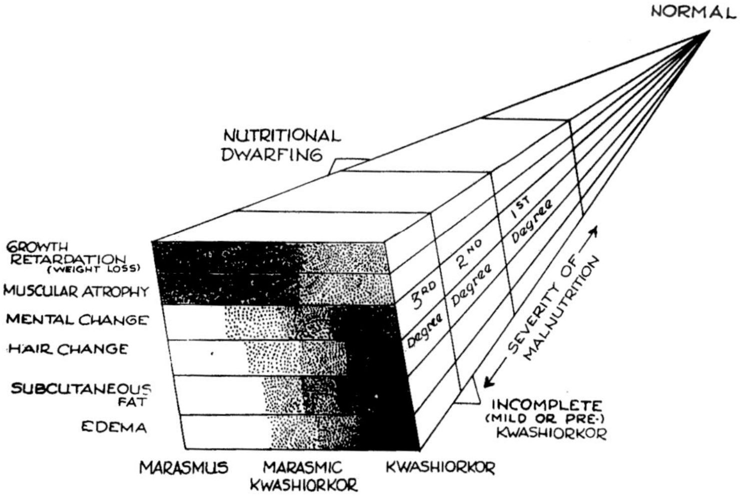

100

100 Nutritional pyramid. This shows interrelationships between various forms of protein-energy malnutrition in tropical pre-school children. Base shows usual gradation of *main* features of kwashiorkor (probably due to a low-protein, high-calorie diet) → marasmic kwashiorkor → nutritional marasmus (probably due to a low-protein, low-calorie diet). Interrelationships between classifications employed in some different countries can be identified on the pyramid: *Jamaica* — kwashiorkor, marasmic kwashiorkor, nutritional marasmus; *Haiti* — kwashiorkor, incomplete kwashiorkor, nutritional marasmus, nutritional dwarfing; *Mexico* — first-, second-, and third-degree malnutrition.

101

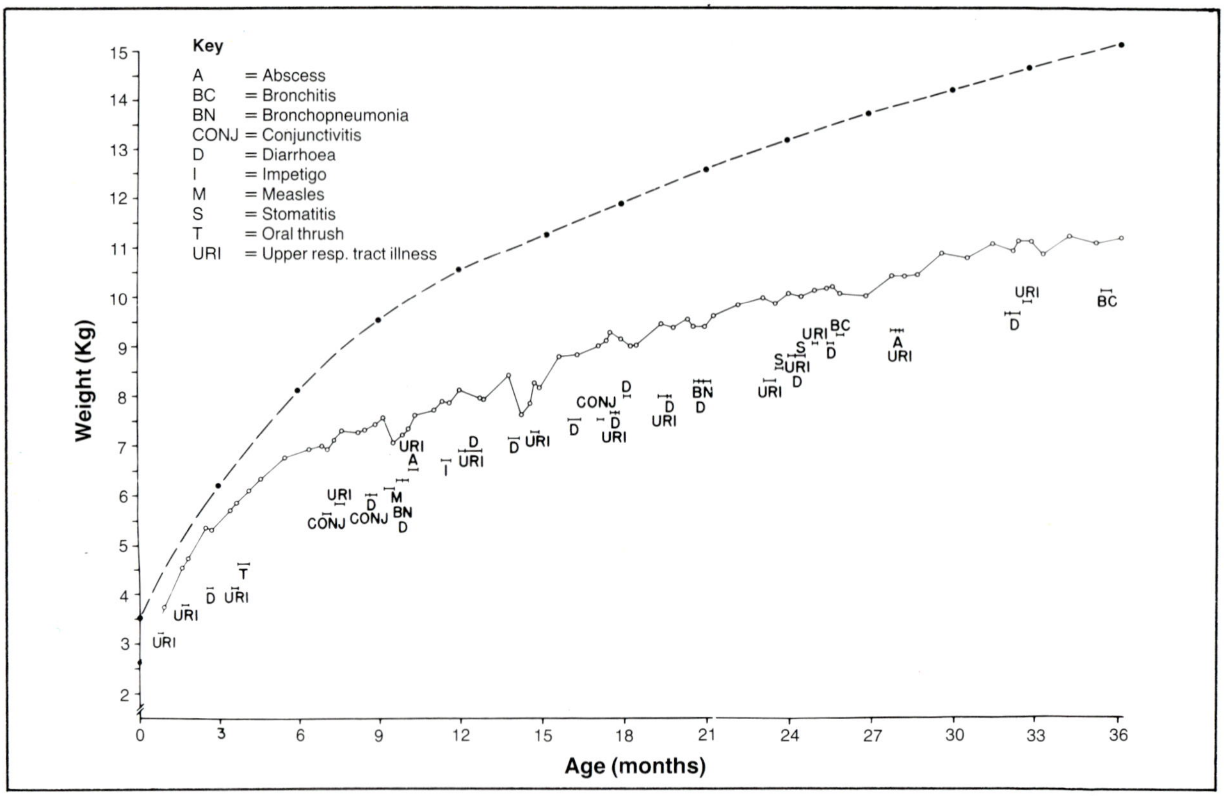

101 Multiple infection and growth. This remarkable and oft-cited chart was recorded by Professor Leonardo Mata from Guatemala. Although, no doubt, it was chosen for the multiplicity of the infections and the very close monitoring of both occurrence of disease and weight it does illustrate graphically the serious impact that chronic infection has on nutrition and growth in early life.

102

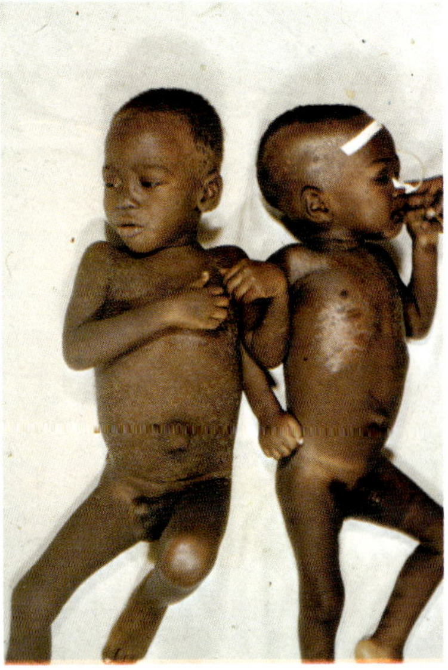

10

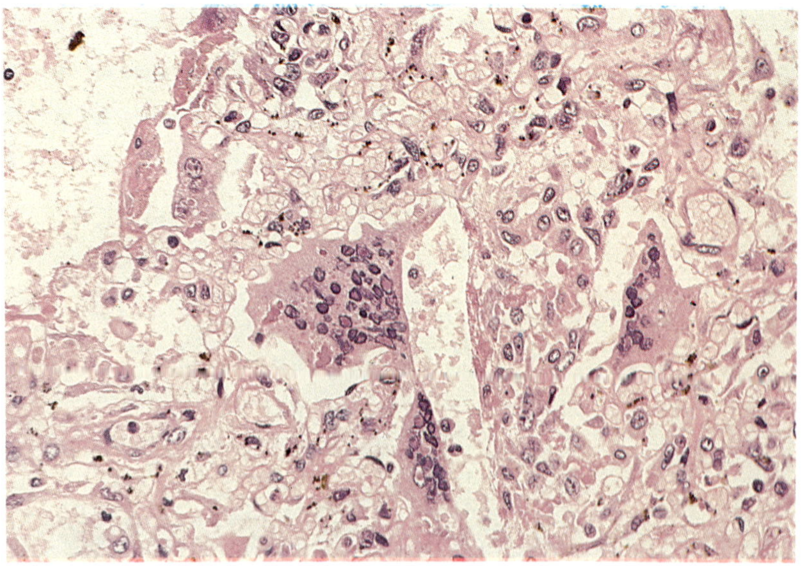

102 Measles in twins. Measles is one of the most important causes of childhood mortality in the tropics. The twin on the left shows typical post-measles desquamation but is otherwise recovering. The other twin has post-measles encephalitis.

103 Lung in giant cell pneumonia. Mortality is commonly associated with giant cell pneumonia during the prodromal stage. This section was from a 10-year-old girl who contracted measles while receiving steroid therapy for treatment of her nephrotic syndrome. (*H&E*, × 500)

104 Measles in the undernourished child is always a serious disease. The rash often assumes a florid form as in this Guatemalan child. It frequently precipitates overt kwashiorkor (see **128–143**) with a marked fall in serum albumin, and xerophthalmia (see **195–216**). Cell-mediated immunity is markedly impaired.

104

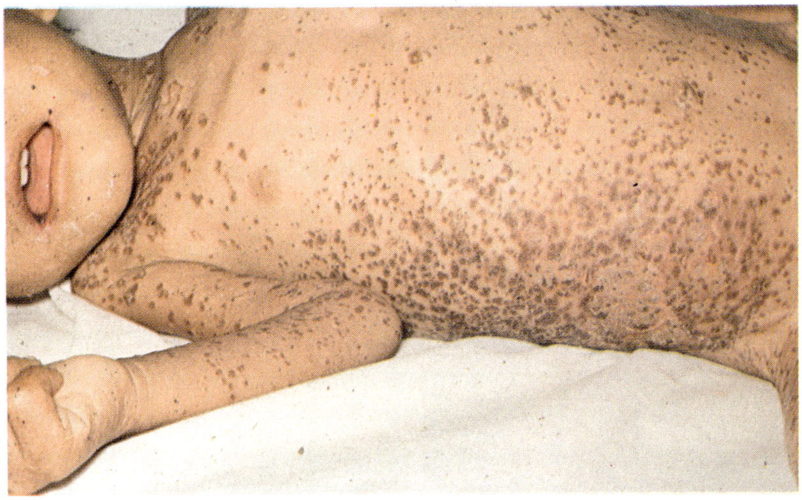

105 The liver in generalized herpes simplex infection. The prognosis is extremely poor (see *Table 37*).

105

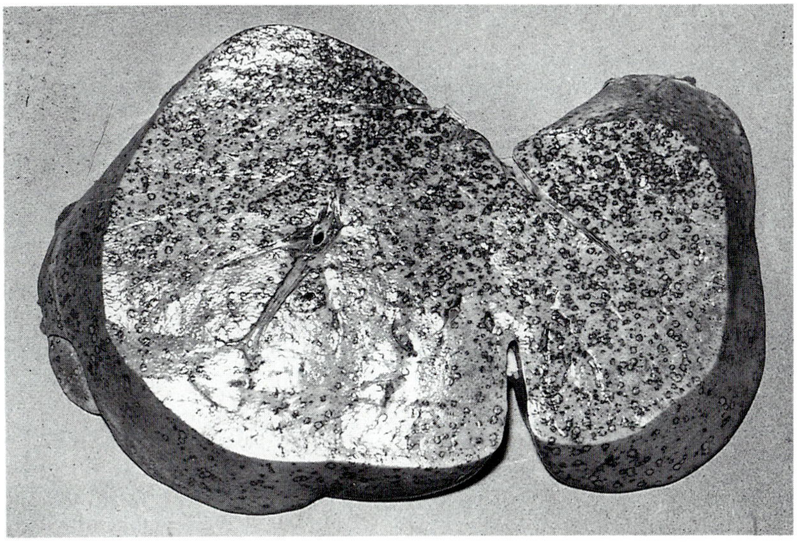

106, 107 Jejunal epithelium. Severe infection with *G. lamblia* can result in partial villous atrophy of the duodenum or jejunum, with resulting flattening of the villi (**107**) compared with the normal pattern (**106**). Although the organism is commensal in many individuals, it is considered particularly pathogenic in children in the New World, and is a common cause of diarrhoea and a malabsorption syndrome characterized by steatorrhoea in travellers. (*H&E*, × 40)

106

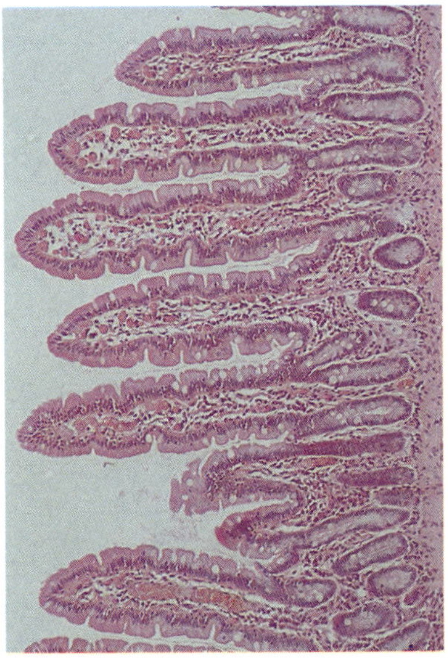

107

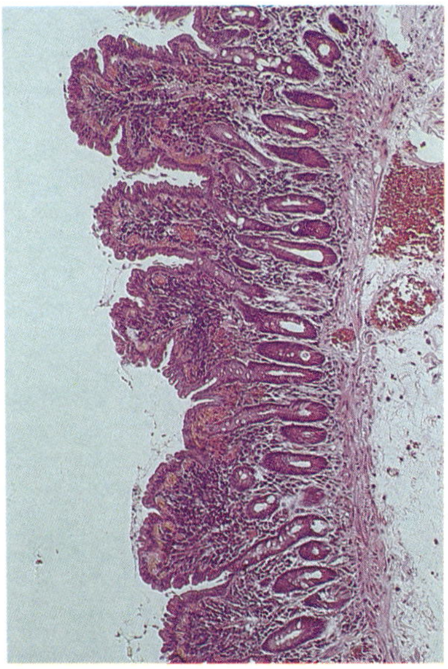

108

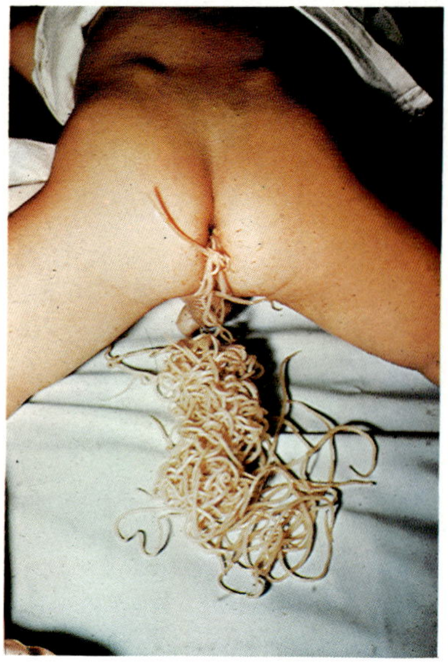

108 Massive *Ascaris* infection in child. A large bolus of roundworms was expelled following anthelminthic treatment. Malabsorption of nutrients may be severe.

109

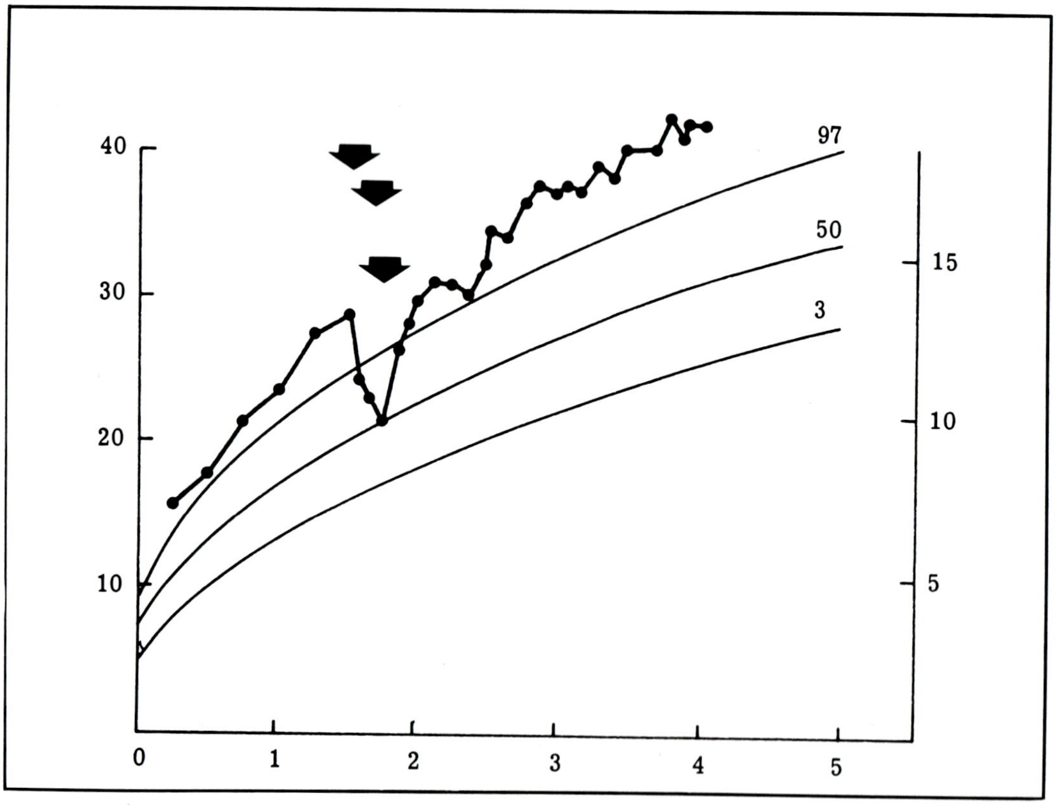

109 Growth chart in mild PEM. Supervision and weighing at regular intervals form a useful means of monitoring progress. In this case weaning from the breast was followed by a dramatic fall in weight and frank kwashiorkor was precipitated by an attack of measles, but a good recovery was made. An apparently satisfactory weight gain may mask a change in body composition towards extracellular fluid retention preceding kwashiorkor, and weight should be related to height. In severe PEM X-rays show transverse lines of bone growth retardation with thinning of bone texture.

Social and cultural factors tend to vary considerably in their occurrence and determine to a large extent the type of PEM that prevails in a particular place[55] (**110, 111**).

110

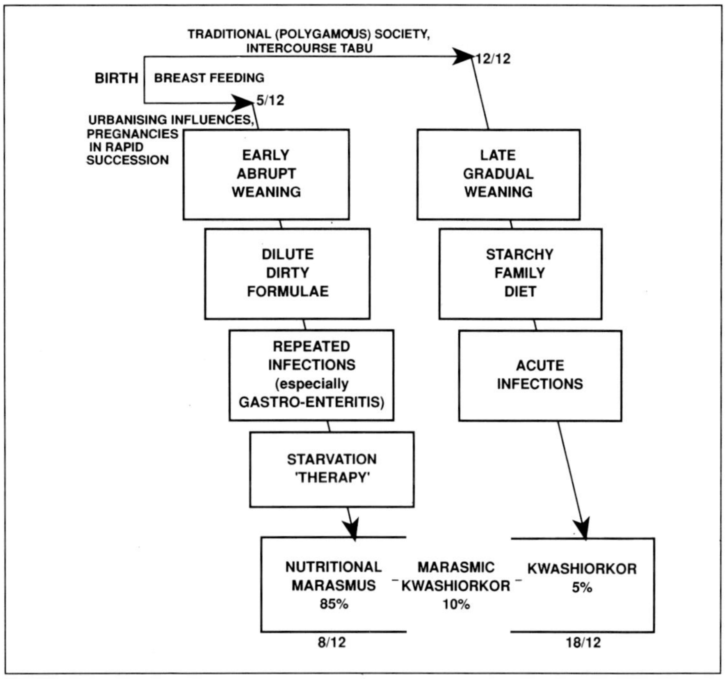

110 Pathogenesis of marasmus and kwashiorkor.[55] This flow diagram is based on a study of approximately 200 cases in Jordan. The percentage figures indicate the type of severe PEM in the study, with marasmus predominating as it does in most situations. The other numbers indicate months; mean of 5 months weaning for marasmus contrasted with 12 months for kwashiorkor; mean age on admission, 8 months marasmus 18 months kwashiorkor. The other elements show the very different aetiological factors found for the two conditions.

111

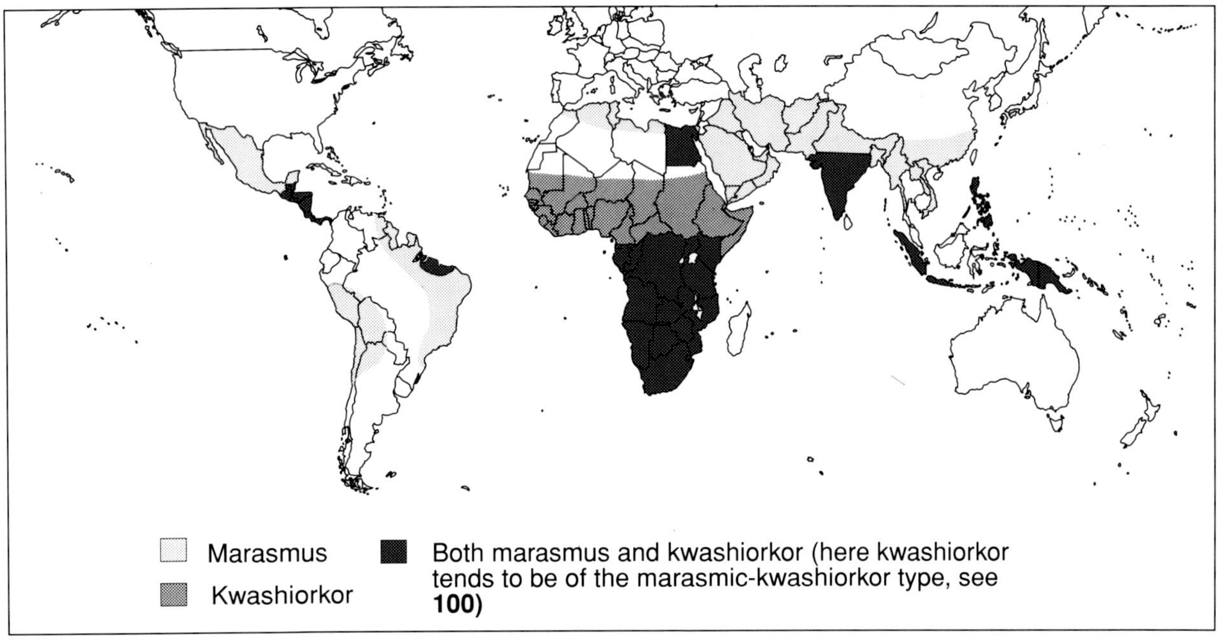

111 Global distribution of the different forms of severe PEM.

General inanition in marasmus (**112**) and protein lack, starch excess and infections in kwashiorkor (**113**) can be related to the observed biochemical disturbances.[56]

Typical marasmus and kwashiorkor differ in many points (*Table 35*).

Many of these contrasting features are illustrated in **114–147** and *Table 36*.

112

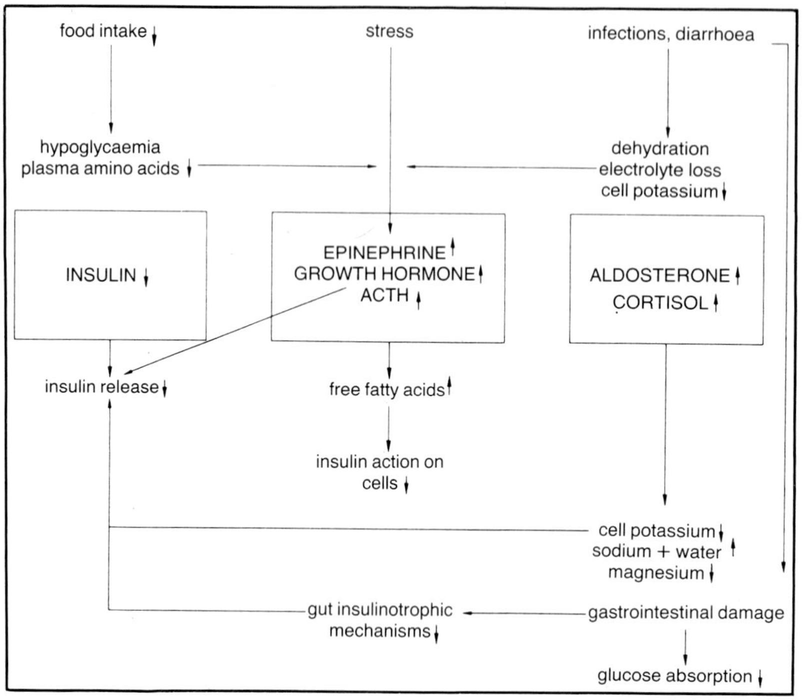

112 Adaptive mechanisms in marasmus.

113

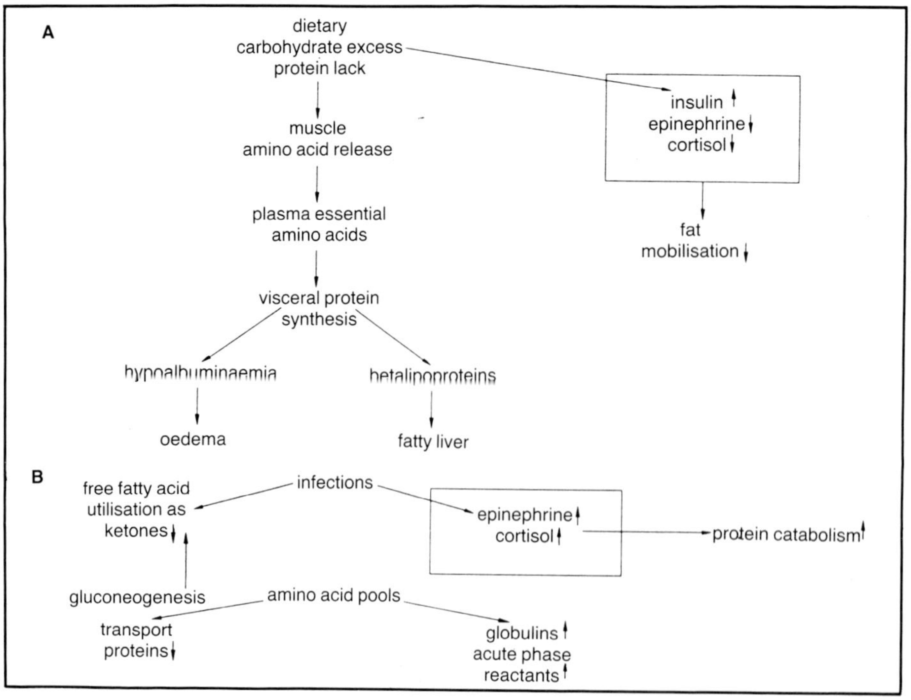

113 Kwashiorkor. Either carbohydrate excess (A) or infections (B) or both abolish the adaptive changes to starvation.

Table 35. Some features of marasmus and kwashiorkor compared and contrasted.

	Marasmus	*Kwashiorkor*
General features		
Occurrence	Throughout the third world	Limited, mainly Africa
Usual age	Infancy	Second and third years
Response to treatment		
immediate	Poor	Good (occasional sudden death)
ultimate	Fair	Good
Long-term effects		
mental	Can be severe	Rare
physical	Stunting	Mild or none
liver damage	Nil	Nil
Clinical signs		
Oedema	Absent	Present
Dermatosis	Rare, mild	Common
Hair changes	Common	Very common
Hepatomegaly	Rare	Very common
Psychomotor change	Alert, hungry	Miserable
Wasting of fat and muscle	Severe	Mild
Anaemia	Common	Very common
Vitamin deficiencies	Uncommon	Common
Laboratory tests		
General		
Total body water	High	High
Extracellular water	Some increase	More increase
Body potassium	Some depletion	Much depletion
Renal function	Impaired	Impaired
Glucose tolerance	Normal	Impaired
Response to adrenaline	Exaggerated	Lowered
Serum		
Albumin, transferrin, etc.	Slightly low	Very low
Trace elements	Normal	Low
Non-essential/essential amino acids	Normal	High
Non-esterified fatty acids	Normal	High
Glucose	Low	Very low
Insulin	Low	High
Urine		
Urea/total N	Above 65%	Below 50%
3 methyl histidine	Very high	High
Hydroxyproline index	Low	Low
Liver		
Urea cycle enzymes	Low	Low
Amino acid-synthesizing enzymes	High	High

114

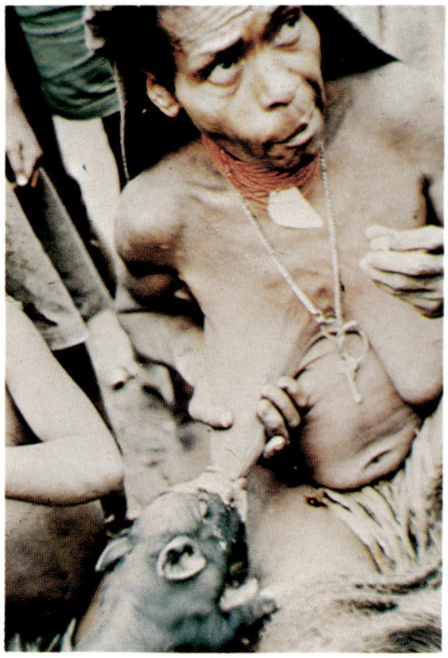

114 Enteritis necroticans (pigbel). Old woman feeding her pig. In the highlands of New Guinea, enteritis necroticans is related to pig feasting which is an integral and complex part of the indigenous culture of the highland tribes. The feeding of infant pigs may even take priority over the feeding of human infants. An interesting, if rare, example of how the 'deposed child' situation can lead to malnutrition.

115

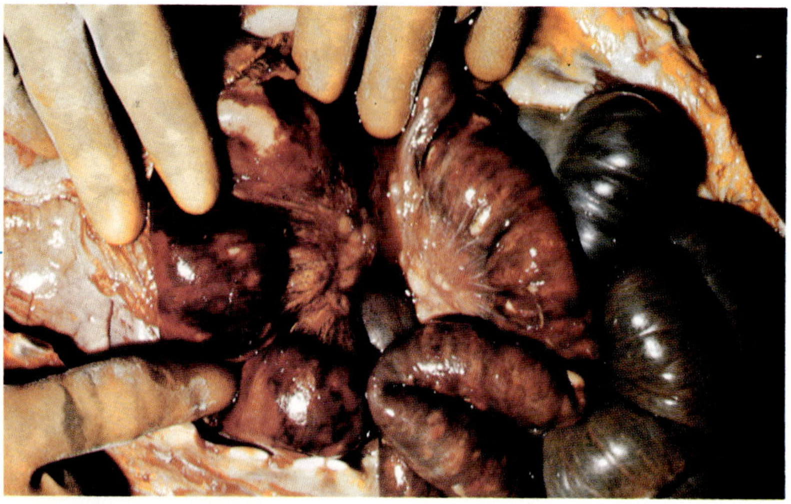

115 Pigbel. Appearance of intestine at operation. Extensive sloughing and necrosis of the large bowel occur in this condition which is endemic in the highlands of Papua New Guinea. It is associated with the B toxin of *Clostridium perfringens* type C (which can be found in the faeces of 70% of highland villagers) and the intermittent consumption of inadequately cooked pork with baked sweet potatoes, especially in children whose normal diet is protein deficient. Vaccination with *C. perfringens* type C B toxoid gives protection lasting a few years.

116

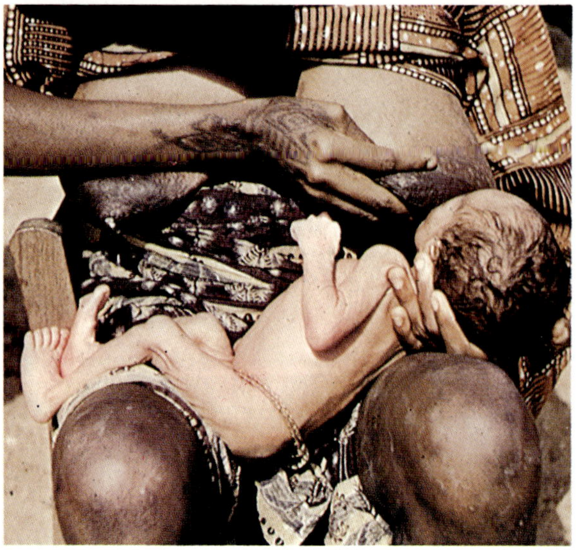

116 Inanition despite adequate lactation. The breasts are engorged and the flattened nipples make sucking difficult. The 6-week-old baby is wasted, weighing only 2.25 kg.

117 Extreme wasting in marasmus. This affects all body tissues and the marked loss of subcutaneous fat and skeletal muscle results in a 'skin and bone' appearance. Body weight may be reduced to only 40% or so of the normal mean for age. The prognosis is especially grave in those cases with 50% or more loss of body weight.

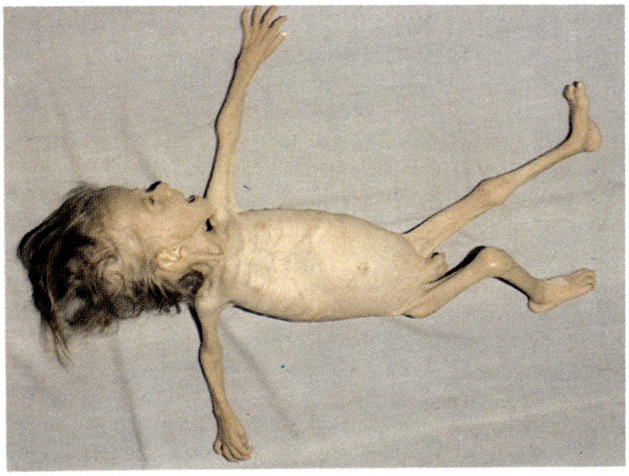

117

118 'Monkey' facies. The wizened, 'old man' appearance of the face with sunken, wrinkled cheeks, is characteristic of prolonged and severe marasmus. In milder cases the normally large buccal fat pads are preserved long after wasting of deeper fat elsewhere.

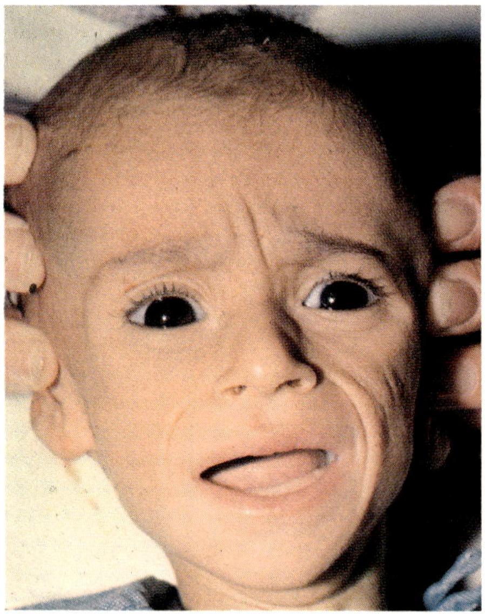

118

119

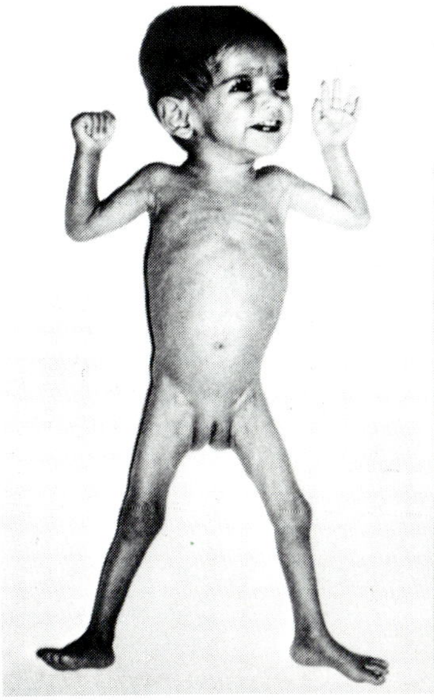

120

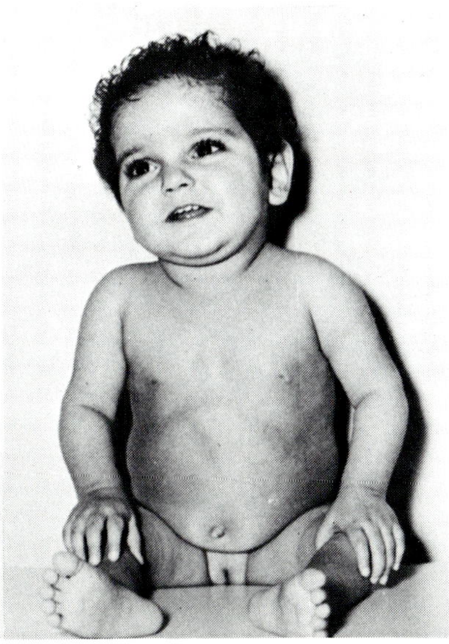

119 **Severe marasmus before treatment.** There is generalized wasting and, in contrast to kwashiorkor, these infants are extremely hungry.

120 **Severe marasmus.** The same patient after 3 months of treatment. A modified cow's milk formula with added arachis or other oil provides a concentrated source of energy. The diet should be introduced stepwise to provide eventually about 200kcal and 3–5kg protein/kg/day. Catch-up growth is usually slow during the first month but rapid thereafter.

121

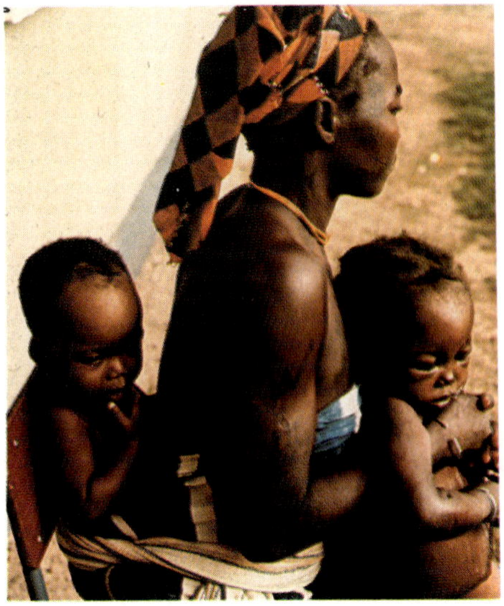

121 **Identical twins.** Twins constitute a serious feeding problem in poor communities. They are usually given a special significance, being regarded as lucky by some and unlucky by others. The twin in front of the mother has kwashiorkor.

12

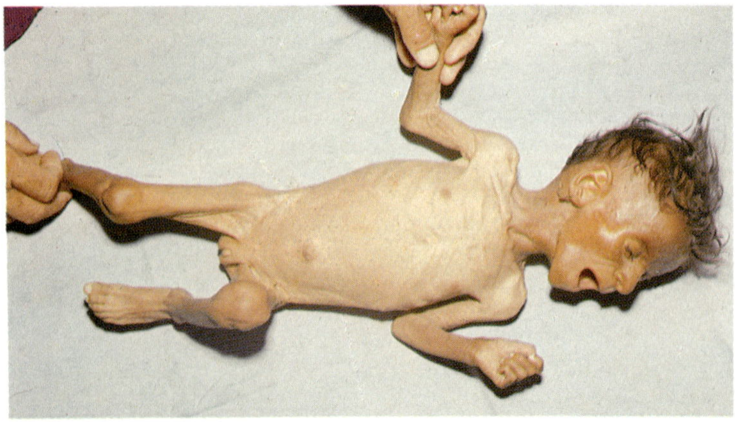

122 **False appearance of 'enlarged joints'.** Marked muscle wasting, as in this 5-month-old infant, may mislead the physician into believing that the limb joints are swollen (see also **221**).

123

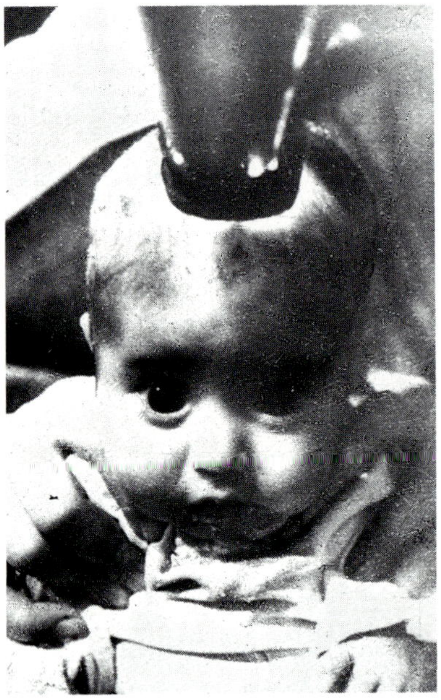

124

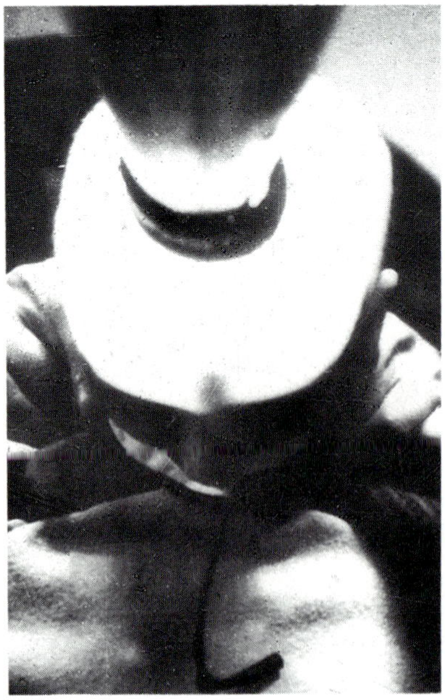

125

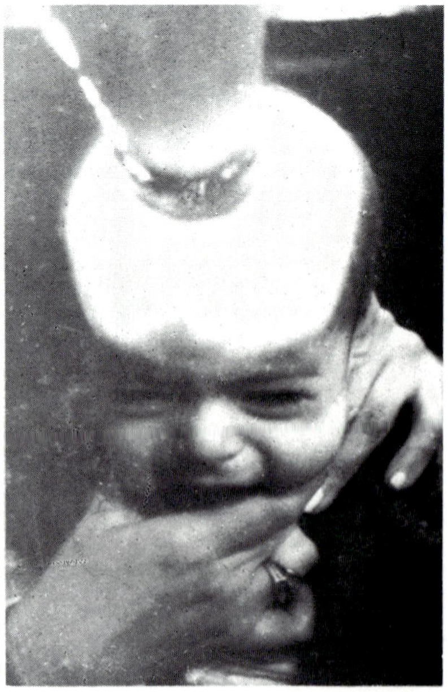

123 **Cranial transillumination.** Appearance of the skull of a normal child.

124, 125 **Cranial transillumination.** The appearance of this child with severe marasmus and of that in the next picture with kwashiorkor both contrast markedly with the normal. The brain substance fills the cranium less completely and the skull table is less well outlined. With experience this can form a simple non-invasive test.

126 Gastrointestinal tract in marasmus. Gastrointestinal series 2 weeks after admission demonstrates a large stomach and separate loops of small intestine with thickened valvulae conniventes.

126

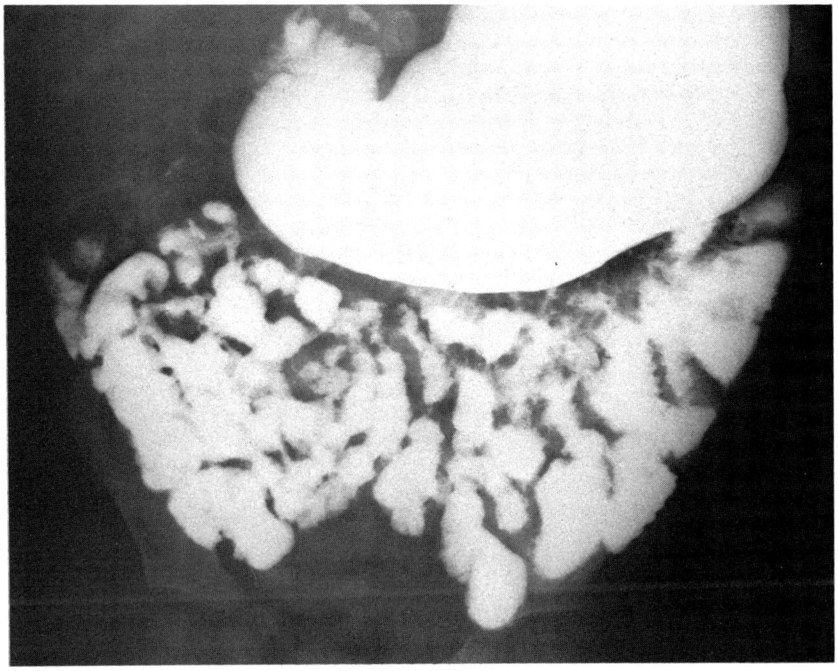

127 Gastrointestinal tract in marasmus. Four weeks after the original study when the patient was well, a repeat intestinal series shows the small intestine to be normal.

127

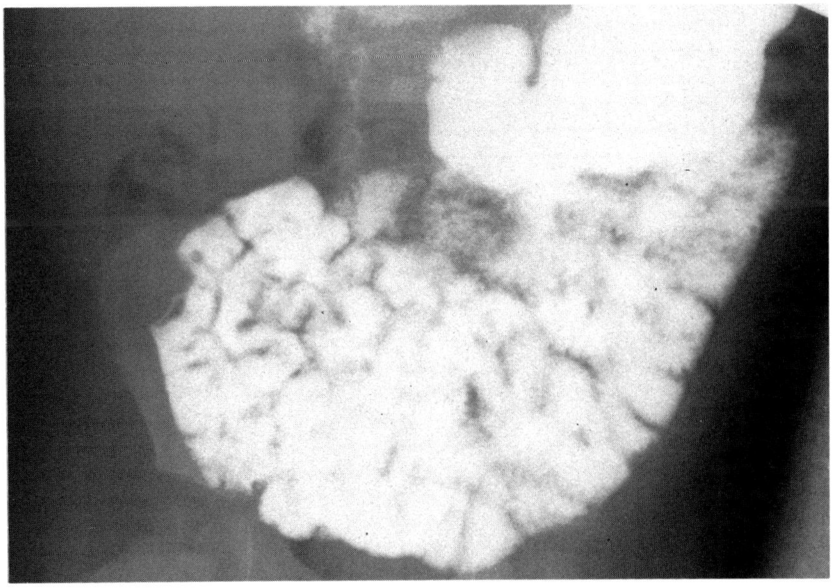

Table 36. Gastrointestinal changes in PEM.

Stomach Chronic atrophic gastritis, hypochlorhydria	**Bile acid metabolism** Impaired micelle solubilization
Pancreas Acinar cell atrophy; perilobular fibrosis; reduced enzyme secretion	**Small bowel contamination** Bile acid deconjugation, defective absorption of water and nutrients
Small intestine Mucosal thinning; villous atrophy; reduced disaccharidase activities; greater susceptibility to injury	**Immune function** Reduced secretory IgA; increased macromolecular uptake

128

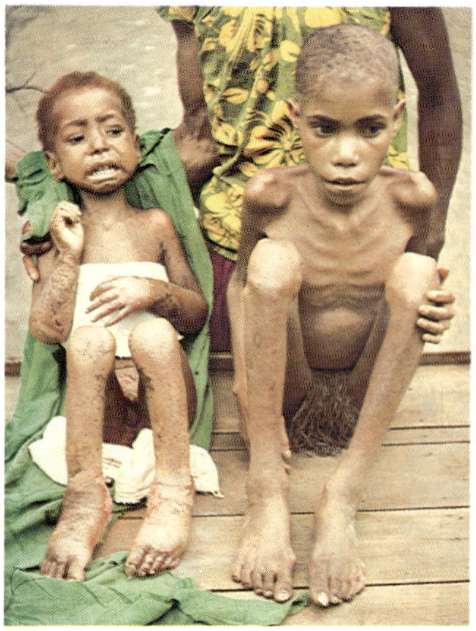

128 Kwashiorkor and marasmus in brothers. Compare the miserable expression, pale hair, generalized oedema and skin changes in the child on the left with the marasmic wasting of his older brother. Kwashiorkor frequently follows acute infection and/or diarrhoea in a child during the weaning period. Some have speculated that this might occur because of genetic differences, involving in particular the endocrine system. It seems more reasonable to suppose that, just as the same child may go through various phases and forms of malnutrition, so siblings might be exposed to somewhat different diets and other predisposing factors within the family, which is itself a constantly changing microenvironment.

129

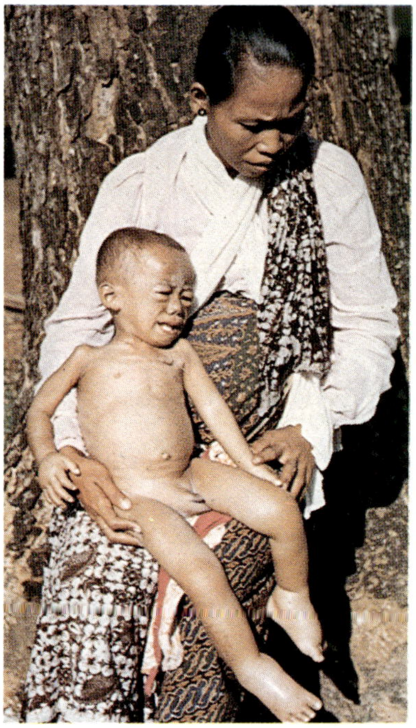

129 Typical kwashiorkor. This Indonesian child shows marked oedema, mental changes and sparse, light-coloured hair, which contrasts with that of his mother.

13

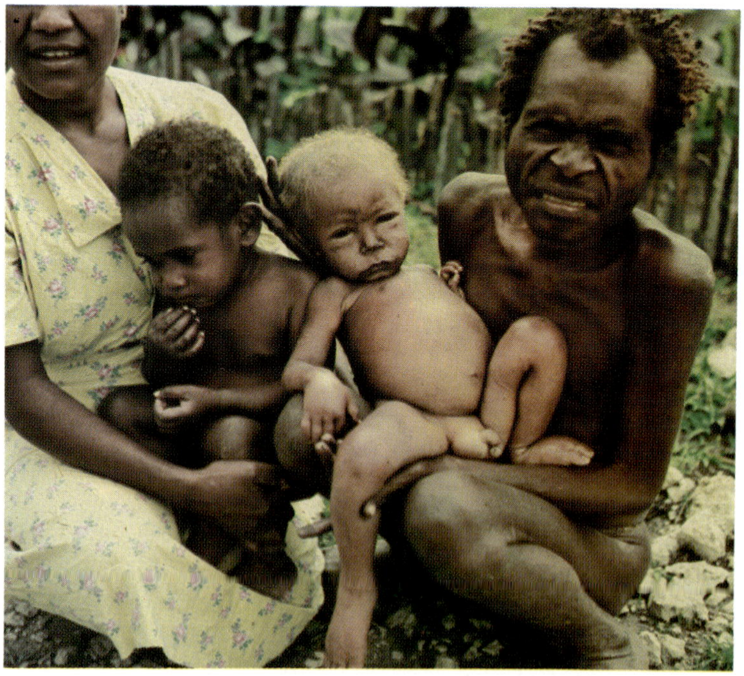

130 Depigmentation in kwashiorkor. The contrast with the normal child is striking (a tribe in New Guinea).

131

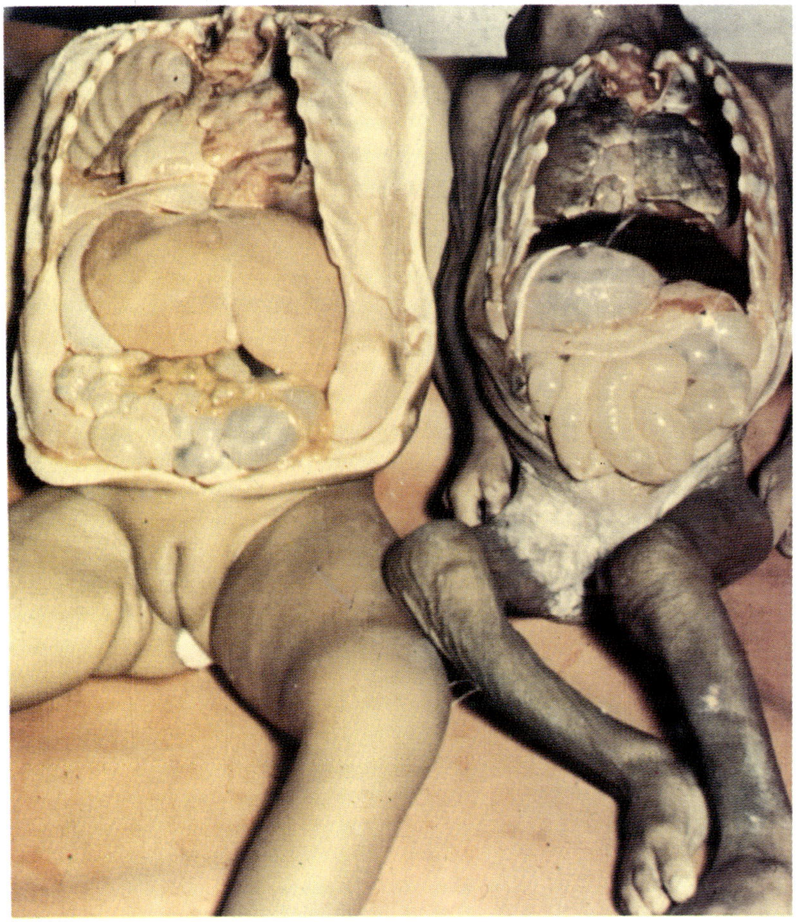

131 Kwashiorkor and marasmus. Contrasted appearance at post-mortem. The child on the left with kwashiorkor has generalized oedema, preservation of subcutaneous fat and gross enlargement of the liver with fatty infiltration. In marasmus (right) there is no oedema, muscle and fat are wasted, and the liver is shrunken.

132

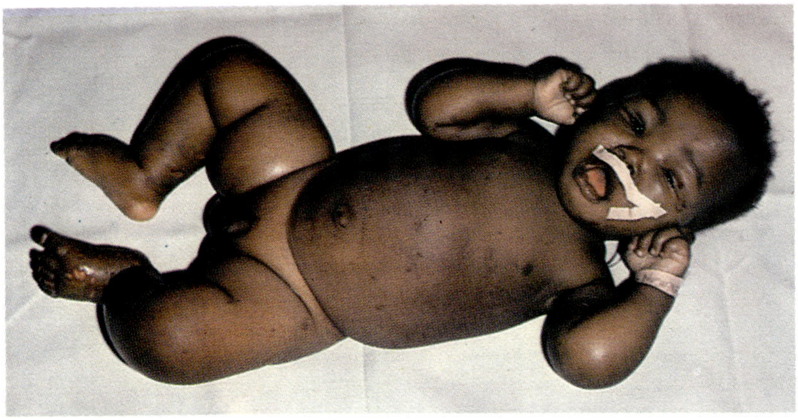

132 'Sugar baby'. This term was first used for the severe form of kwashiorkor commonly seen in Jamaica and attributed to a high sugar, and consequently very low protein, diet. Marked oedema, fatty liver and low serum albumin are the main features and skin changes are absent or minimal. This is a Bantu baby in Johannesburg.

133

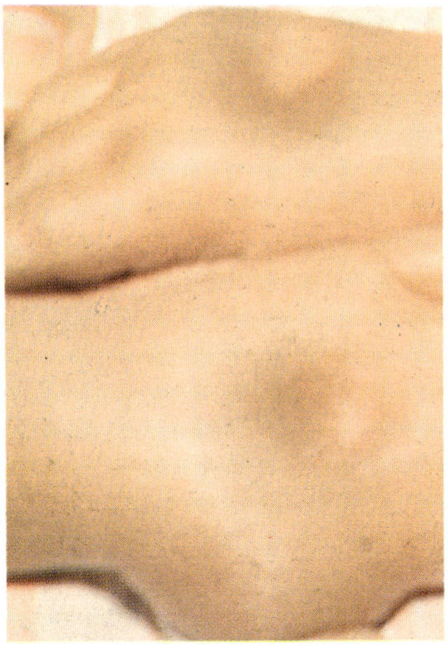

133 Oedema of the hands in kwashiorkor. The occurrence of oedema is related to hypoalbuminaemia and impaired renal function leading to increased sodium retention.

134 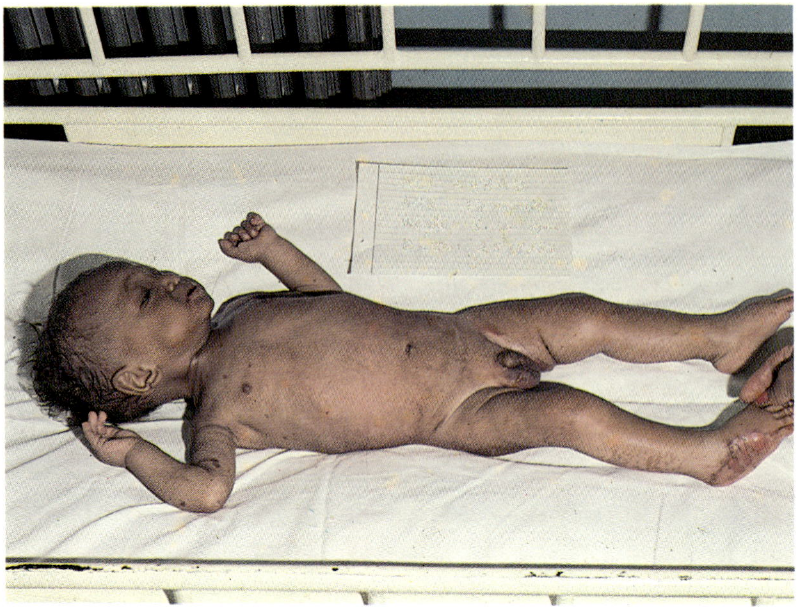

134 Dermatosis of kwashiorkor. This is one of the most characteristic features and is absent in marasmus. There is a generalized increase in pigmentation with a tendency to desquamation (less noticeable in dark-skinned people) with desquamation leading to patchy depigmented areas. Confluent areas have been termed 'flaky-paint' or 'crazy-paving' dermatosis, and small lesions 'enamel spots'. The skin on most parts of the body may be involved, especially the buttocks, inner thighs and perineum, but the photosensitive areas affected in pellagra (275–279) are spared. Although characteristic of kwashiorkor the lesion has been wrongly attributed to burns or scalds. A careful history and general examination will readily lead to a correct diagnosis.

135 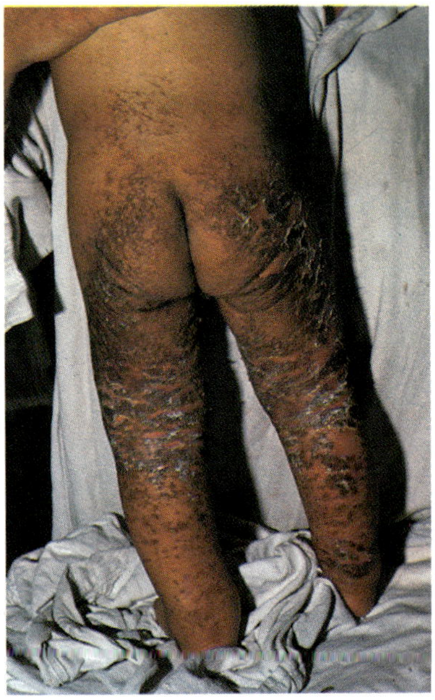

136 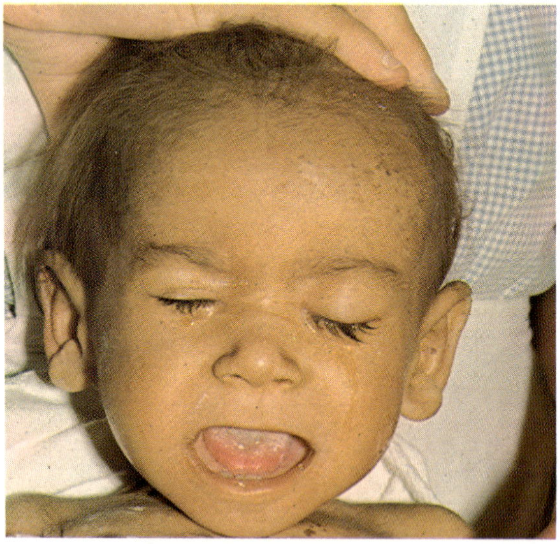

135 Kwashiorkor dermatosis. The skin in the flexures of the legs is especially liable to become dirty, soggy and devitalized and so subject to peeling.

136 Hyperpigmentation in a fair skin. In contrast to the frequent patchy desquamation depigmentation in the dark-skinned, kwashiorkor skin changes are less marked in those with a fair skin in whom hyperpigmentation may predominate. This characteristically occurs on the forehead as in this Jordanian child.

137 Marasmic-kwashiorkor. Many children with PEM, as this Jordanian child, show features of marasmus (emaciation) and of kwashiorkor (oedema of the hands and legs).

137

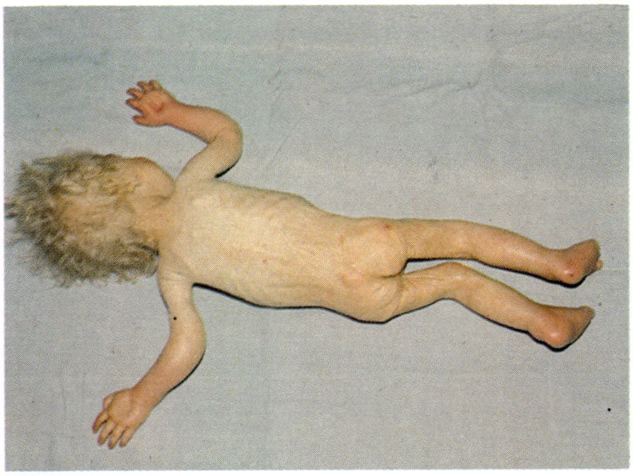

138 Marasmic-kwashiorkor. In many areas this is the most common form of kwashiorkor and tends to have a better prognosis than the full-blown form.

138

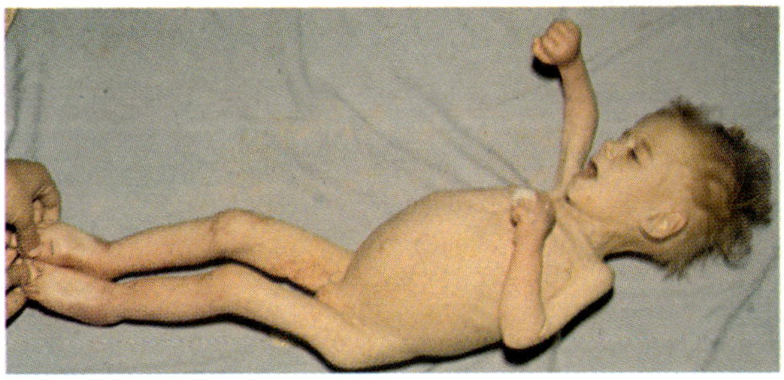

139 Noma in kwashiorkor. This severely malnourished young Egyptian child has the uncommon complication to kwashiorkor of noma (cancrum oris) (see **553**, **554**). Keratomalacia was also present in both eyes (one is shown in **208**).

139

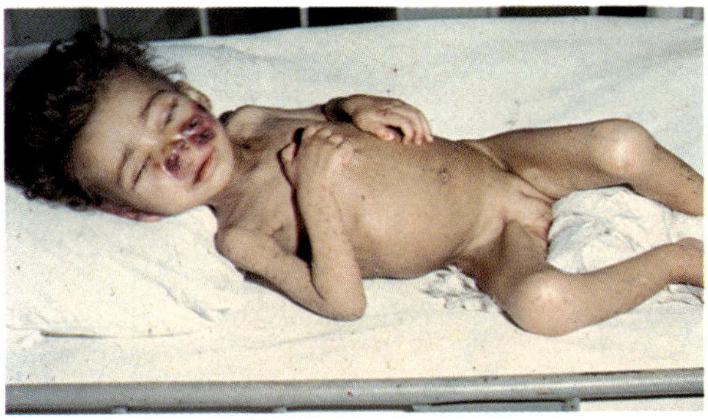

140 Moon face. This is seen usually in those cases of kwashiorkor with marked oedema of the extremities and lumbar region. It subsides rapidly with treatment. The emaciated, 'monkey' facies of marasmus (**118**) should be contrasted with it. Moon face is also seen in chronic ankylostomiasis with severe anaemia; it is rare in pre-school children. Unlike the moon face of obesity (**162**) it is not due to excess deposition of fat. In hypercorticalism there is often erythema.

140

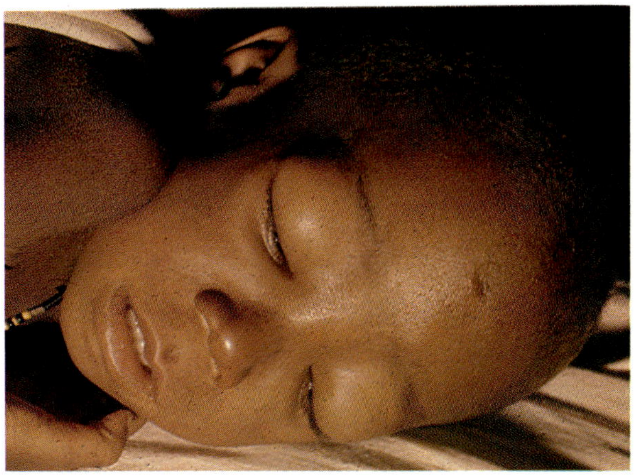

141

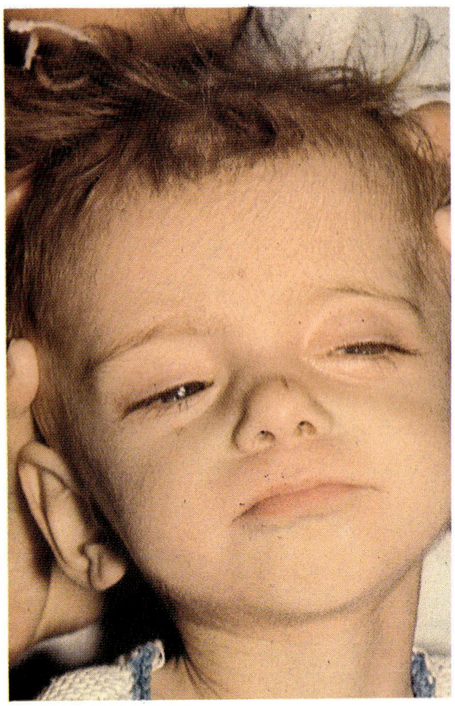

141 **Hair changes.** These are a constant feature of kwashiorkor but may also be seen in marasmus. The hair is dull and dry and lacks its normal lustre. It is finer and more silky in texture than normal, and sparse – covering the scalp less abundantly and with wider spaces between hairs. Naturally long hair is unusually straight, untidy and 'staring'. In black children the thick, tight, short curls become unruly and straightened. Hairs become loose and are readily plucked out. Normally black hair becomes greyish or reddish in colour – dyschromotrichia; but local factors such as dyeing, the effect of sunshine, salt-spray and dust should be taken into account.

142

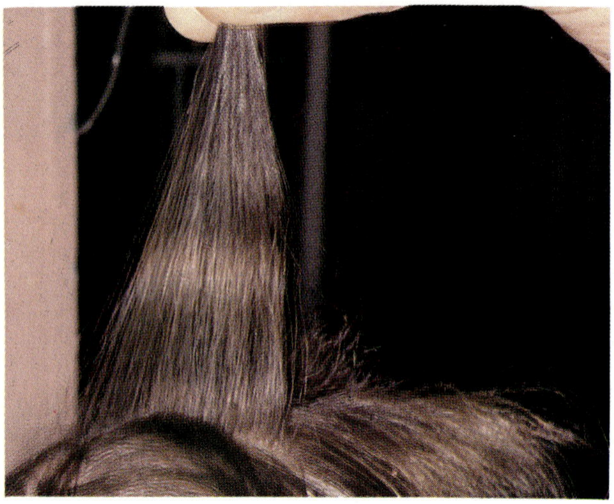

142 **The 'flag-sign' or signa de bandera.** This was first described from Costa Rica. When the hair is long and naturally dark, as in this child in El Salvador, it may show alternating darker and lighter bands when held up, corresponding respectively to periods of better and poorer nutrition.

143

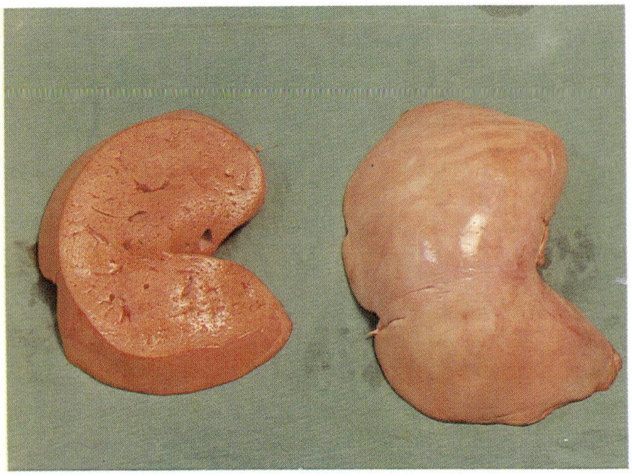

143 **Fatty liver of kwashiorkor.** Infiltration of fat as yellowish areas is evident on the uncut surface. The cut surface is much more greasy than normal.

144

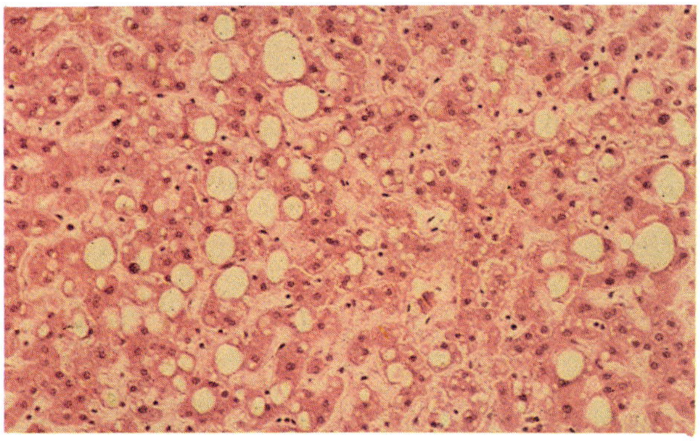

144 Fatty liver in kwashiorkor. This is not seen in marasmus, in which the liver is shrunken. Fat droplets appear first in the periphery and spread progressively to the central vein area. With treatment the fat disappears in the reverse order. Cirrhosis does not result, in contrast to the fatty liver in alcoholism (see **491–493**).

145

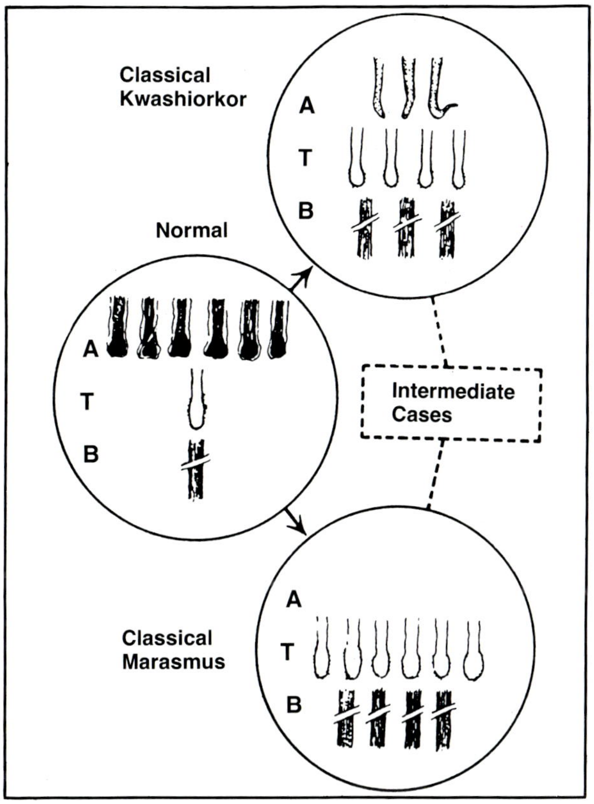

145 Simulated microscope view of normal hair and the alterations which occur in the two classical forms of protein-energy malnutrition. (*A*, anagen or growing phase; *T*, telogen or resting phase; *B*, broken hairs). Note that in kwashiorkor the number of growing hairs is reduced and those that are found are atrophied. The number of resting bulbs increases as does the number of broken hairs. In marasmus essentially all bulbs are found in the resting phase.

146

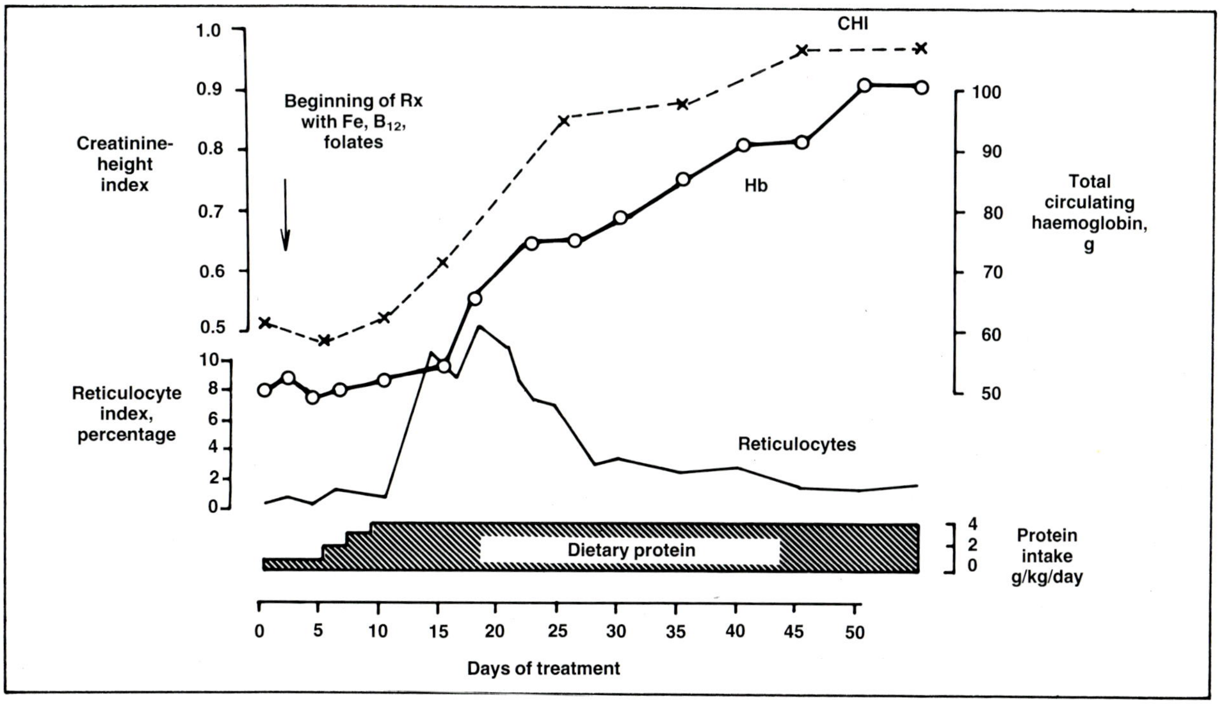

146 Haematological response of a child with severe PEM. Treatment with iron, folic acid, and vitamin B_{12} began on day 2; dietary energy and proteins were increased gradually to 150kcal and 4g protein/kg/day on day 9. There was no reticulocyte or haemoglobin response until lean body mass, assessed by the creatinine/height index, began increasing, suggesting the importance of adequate protein and energy intake for a full haematological response under these circumstances.

147

Koilonychia

(1) Iron deficiency
(2) Sulphur-containing amino-acids ↓
(3) ♂ Diabetics 15 to 20 years disease
(4) Raynaud's disease (uncommon)
(5) Developmental abnormality

147 Koilonychia. Table to show conditions which may give rise to koilonychia. Sulphur-containing amino acids require growth hormone and insulin to be used in cells of nail bed, and metallo-enzymes containing iron are rate-limiting in this step. Hence, severe protein-energy malnutrition or iron deficiency will produce koilonychia as also will long-term insulin deficiency.

Certain clinical signs have been found to carry a poor prognosis (*Table 37*).

Table 37. Features suggesting a poor prognosis in severe PEM.

Male, about twice mortality of female
Age less than 6 months
Deficit in weight for height greater than 30% or weight for age greater than 40%
Stupor or coma
Infections especially measles, herpes simplex, pneumonia, HIV
Purpura, often associated with septicaemia
Jaundice, suggesting liver failure
Deficiencies of vitamin A, potassium
Tachycardia, suggesting heart failure
Severe anaemia with hypoxia
Noma (cancrum oris)
Hypoglycaemia
Hypothermia

Anorexia nervosa and bulimia

These two conditions are frequently associated and both might be classified with other disorders of eating behaviour (see Chapter 8) but, in contrast to them, energy balance is so disturbed, with marked wasting and intermittently in bulimia obesity, that they are best considered here.

Table 38 lists the generally accepted diagnostic criteria for the two conditions. **148–151** show some characteristic clinical appearances.

The term anorexia is applied inappropriately as there is no loss of appetite until an advanced stage of cachexia has been reached. The condition is a serious one with overall rates of mortality as high as 20%. There are many theories as to the aetiology of anorexia nervosa, falling into categories of organic, psychodynamic, familial and sociocultural. Each has its advocates but none is generally accepted.

Table 38. Features of anorexia nervosa and bulimia.

Anorexia nervosa
- Inability to maintain body weight above a minimum for age and height that is 15% below that expected
- Intense fear of gaining weight, even though underweight
- Distortion of experience of weight, size or shape
- In females, absence of at least three consecutive menstrual cycles when otherwise expected to occur
- No other explanation for the clinical symptoms and signs.

Bulimia
- Recurrent episodes of binge eating – at least 2 episodes/week for 3 months
- Lack of control over eating behaviour
- Engaging regularly in either self-induced vomiting, laxative use or diuretics; strict dieting or fasting or vigorous exercise to prevent weight gain
- Persistent overconcern with body shape and weight

No other explanation for the clinical symptoms and signs (applies to both conditions).

148

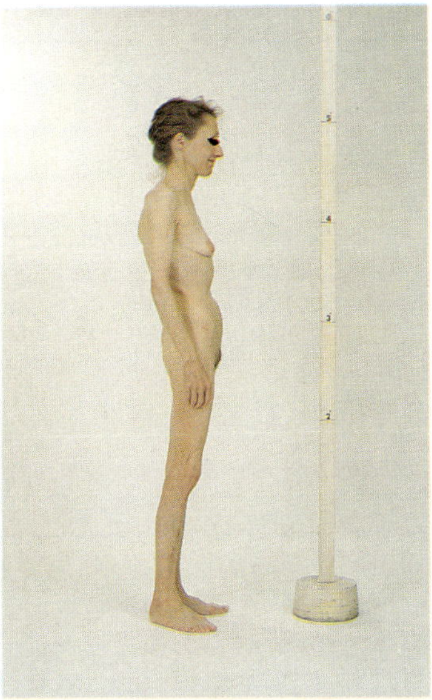

149

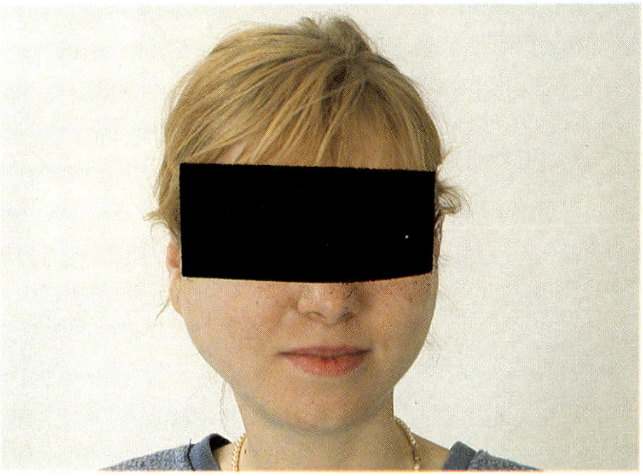

148 Anorexia nervosa. A 40-year-old lady who has had anorexia for 20 years. She has a dorsal kyphosis as a result of wedge fractures of several of her thoracic vertebrae.

149 Bulimia nervosa. A 20-year-old girl with asymmetrical parotid hypertrophy. Bulimia nervosa developed at the age of 17. She was vomiting four times each day.

150

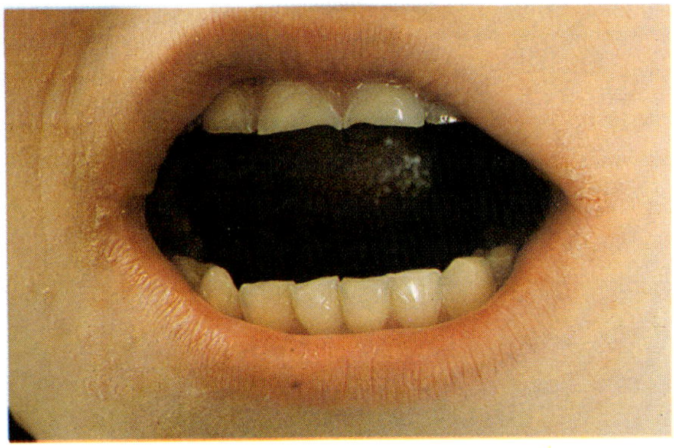

151

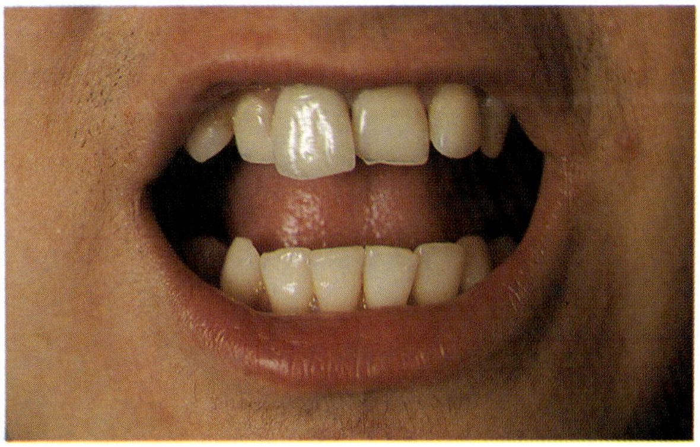

150 Bulimia nervosa. This 18-year-old girl had been vomiting to control her weight from the age of 15. Her top incisors have been gradually eroded.

151 Bulimia nervosa. This 22-year-old woman had an incisor capped because of dental caries. She continued to vomit and the surrounding teeth have diminished in size, whereas the dental prosthesis remains unchanged.

Table 39. Laboratory findings in anorexia nervosa.

Erythrocyte sedimentation rate	Raised
Blood white cells	Leukopenia with relative lymphocytosis
Red cells	Acanthocytosis common
Plasma albumin	Normal
oestradiol	Low
LH (luteinizing hormone)	Low in day, high at night (reverse of normal)
potassium	May be very low, suggesting purgation or bulimia
cholesterol	High in one third
carotenoids	High, reason unknown
growth hormone	Increased
cortisol	Increased
thyroid hormone	Low
catecholamines	Increased
insulin	Decreased

The profound psychological changes are associated with biochemical disturbances, some of the most consistent of which are given in *Table 39*.

They are more profound than those seen in marasmus (see *Table 35*). Bulimia is present in about half of patients with anorexia nervosa, is relatively uncommon in the obese, and occasionally occurs even in patients of normal weight. Depression is prominent in bulimia, suggesting that it is a variant of mood disorder, and behavioural therapy has given encouraging results.

152 illustrates a concept of eating disorders that attempts to relate them in a continuum.

152 Continuum of eating disorders.

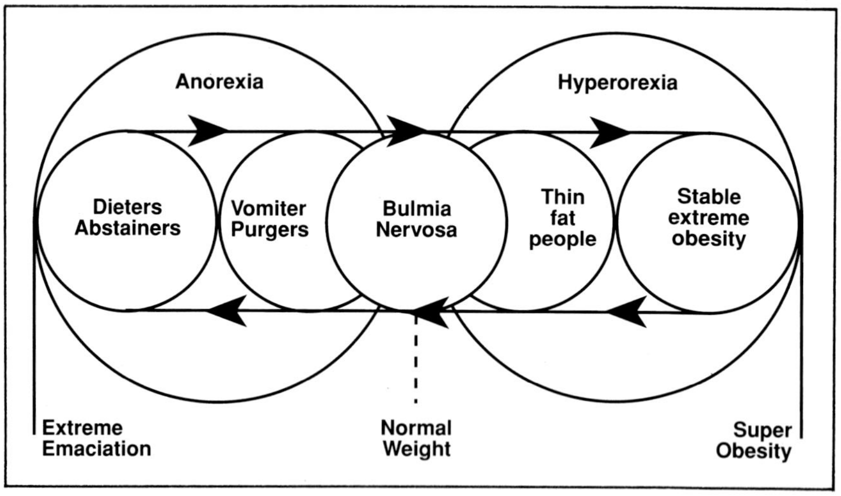

15

Obesity

Obesity can be defined as an excess of adipose tissue, but where the line should be drawn has to be somewhat arbitrary, although an increased mortality risk seems to be a good indicator (see **156**).

It is customary to include a category of overweight between normal and obesity. Women have almost twice as much fat (about 25% of body weight) as men (about 14%) and any standard should therefore take this sex difference into account.

De Garine and Koppert[57] have recently reviewed the value placed on fatness by different societies; it is a phenomenon which is much less commonly seen among males. They studied *guru* fattening sessions, which may be either individual or collective, among men aged 15–25 years of the Massa of Northern Cameroon and Chad (**153**).

The techniques for assessing degrees of adiposity are fully discussed in Jung's *Colour Atlas of Obesity*.[58] Among these are skinfold calipers (**154**) and weight adjusted in some way for height. A popular method at present is the Quetelet or Body Mass Index (BMI) (**155**).

153

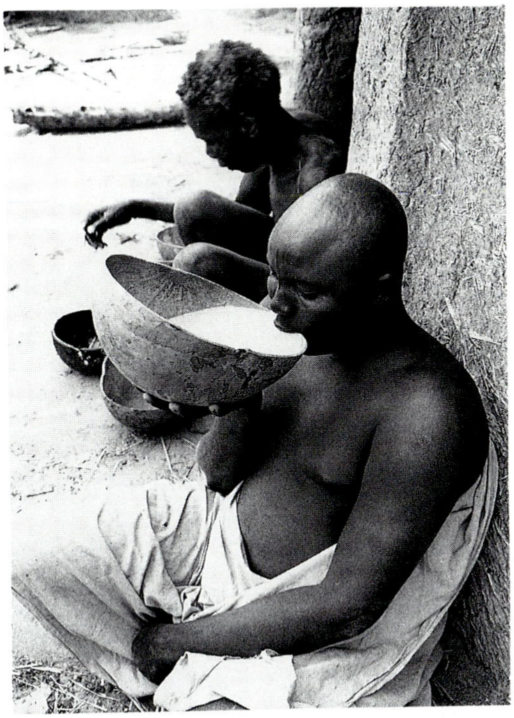

154

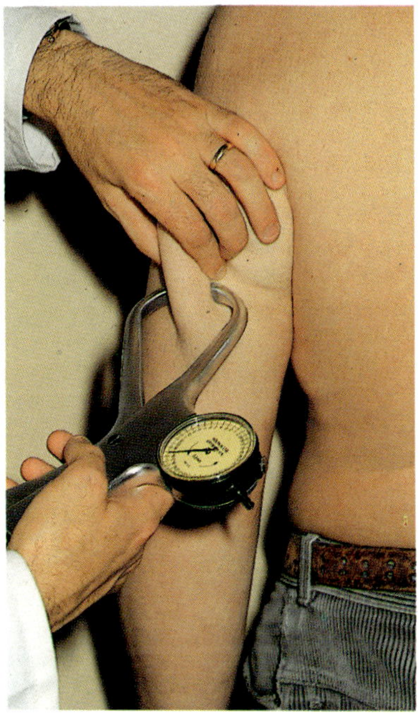

155

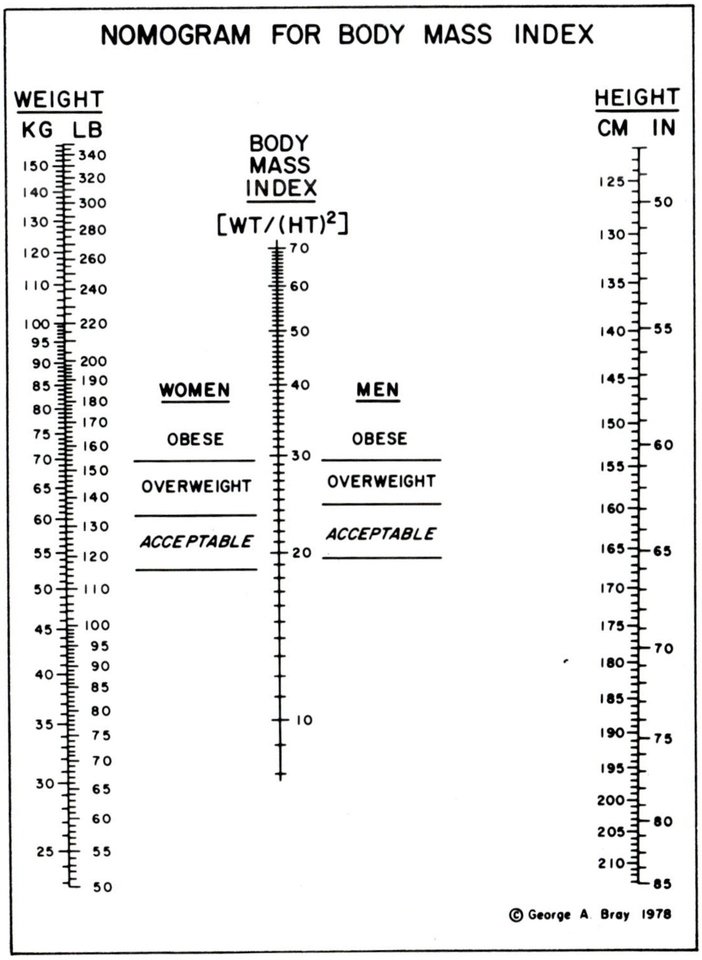

153 *Guru* **fattening.** Gorging on milk at the end of the fattening season. This 18-year-old male consumed during one week of a 2-month session an average of 16,823kcal/day provided mainly by 3136g sorghum flour and 3255g of milk.

154 **Skinfold thickness** measured by Harpenden callipers can be used to measure body fat. The best established system is to measure the skinfold thickness of four sites. Triceps skinfold is measured half-way between the acromial and olecranon processes. A fold of skin and subcutaneous tissue is pinched between the operator's thumb and forefinger. The grip is maintained with the left hand while the right hand relaxes the pressure of the callipers.

155 **Nomogram for Body Mass Index.** To use this nomogram place a straight edge between the two outer columns at the points indicating the patient's weight and height respectively. Where the straight edge intersects the centre line is the appropriate body mass index (BMI). The horizontal lines show the diagnoses are slightly different for men and women (nb. the asymmetric position of the BMI scale is correct).

156

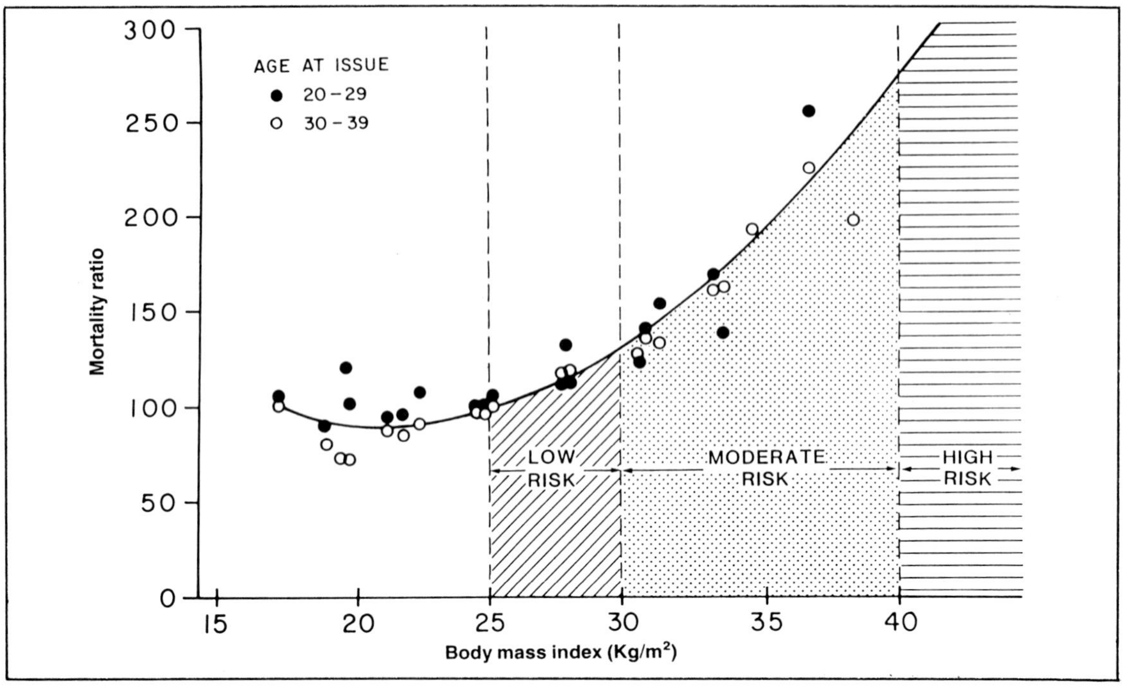

156 Body Mass Index (kg/m^2) and mortality. Above the acceptable range (see **155**) of about 20–25 there is a steady rise. Below this range there is a suggestion that mortality risk also rises as a state of wasting occurs.

Table 40. Morbidity in obesity.

Cardiovascular
- Hypertension
- Coronary artery disease
- Cerebrovascular disease
- Peripheral vascular disease
- Varicose veins
- Varicose ulcers
- Ankle swelling
- Deep venous thrombosis
- Pulmonary embolism

Respiratory
- Breathless
- Pickwickian syndrome
- Cor pulmonale
- Sleep apnoea

Gastrointestinal
- Hiatus hernia
- Gallstones and cholelithiasis
- Gallbladder and biliary cancers
- Fatty liver
- Constipation
- Haemorrhoids
- Herniae
- Cancer of the colon and rectum

Metabolic
- Hyperlipidaemia
- Diabetes mellitus
- Polycystic ovarian syndrome
- Acanthosis nigricans
- Hirsutism
- Menstrual irregularities and menorrhagia

Neurology
- Nerve entrapment (e.g. neuralgia paraesthetica)

Renal
- Proteinuria

Breast
- Gynaecomastia in males
- Breast cancer

Uterus
- Endometrial cancer
- Cervical cancer

Urological
- Prostate cancer

Skin
- Sweat rashes
- Fungal infections
- Striae
- Lymphoedema
- Dry ulcers
- Cellulitis

Operations
- Respiratory risk
- Poor wound healing
- Ventral herniae
- Postoperative infections

Orthopaedic
- Spinal disc problems
- Osteoarthritis
- Exacerbates effect of all arthritides
- Gout
- Baker's cyst rupture

Psychological disturbances

Pregnancy

The close association between increasing weight and mortality is shown clearly in **156**.[59]

Much of this association can be explained by the predisposition to many other disorders that excessive weight brings (*Table 40*).

The public health magnitude of the problem of obesity in western societies in particular is indicated by the data shown in **157**. **158–165** illustrate various clinical aspects of obesity.

157

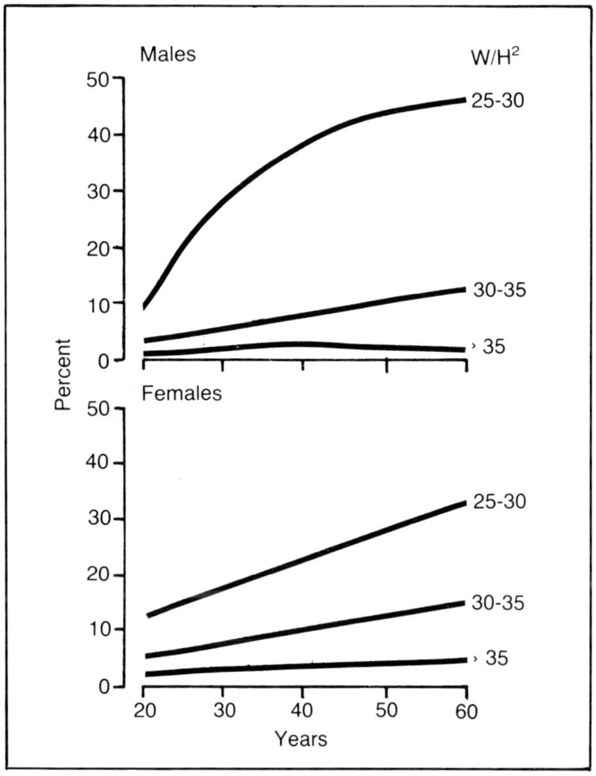

157 Prevalence of obesity. In a sample of 10,021 adults representing the distribution of social class and living style in the UK, 40% of men and 32% of women were overweight or obese. The percentage of those overweight and obese increases with age in both males and females. The corresponding figures for the US are 43% of males and 36% of females and for Australia, 41% of males and 31% of females are overweight or obese.

158 **159**

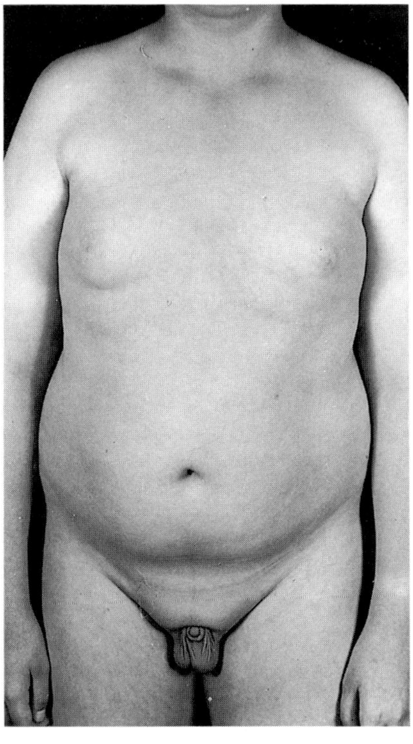

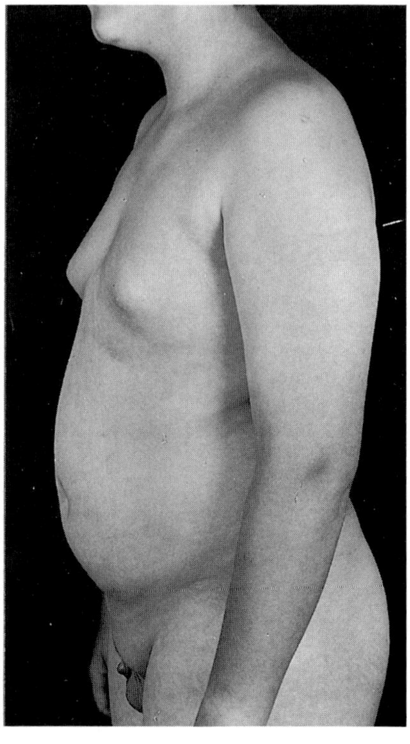

158, 159 Normal genitalia in a pre-pubertal boy buried by pubic fat. It is doubtful whether obesity associated with hypogenitalism in the male is a genuine entity apart from that associated with Prader-Willi syndrome.

160

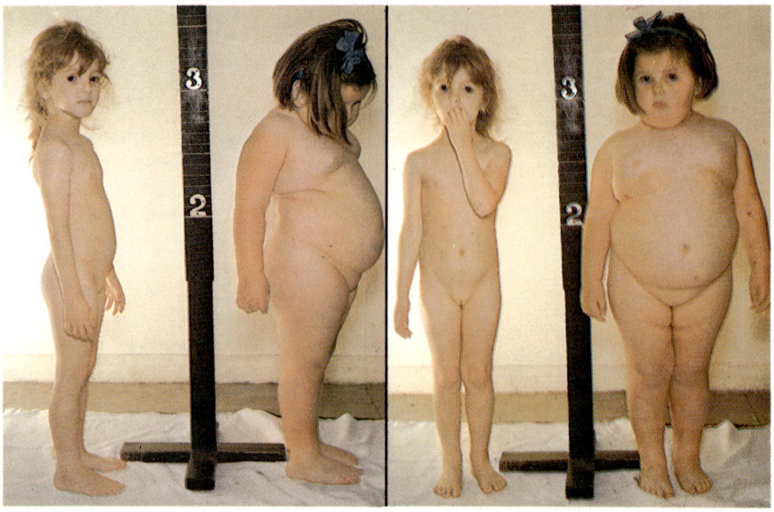

160 Obese girl and normal child of the same age. Weight difference was 15.25kg. Note the difference in height.

161

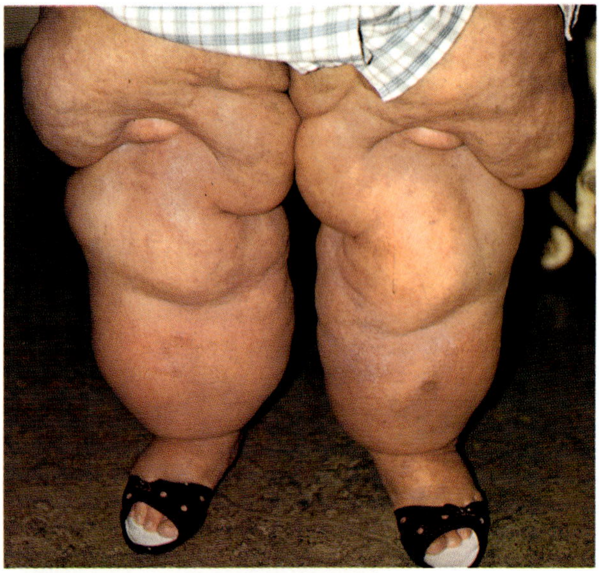

161 Obesity, adipose dimpling and oedema. No pitting. There may be oedema as a secondary effect due to the sheer physical weight obstructing the venous and lymphatic return, as can be seen in the feet. This oedema will pit.

162

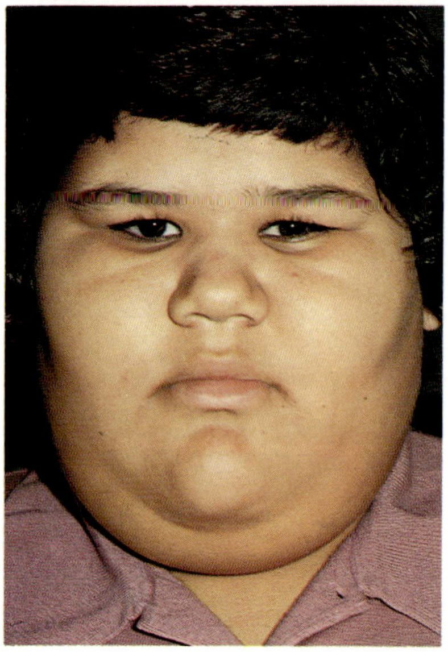

162 Obesity. The roundness and fatness of the face in obesity must be differentiated from the appearance of hyperadrenocorticalism. In the latter there is oedema of the facial tissues and frequently erythema.

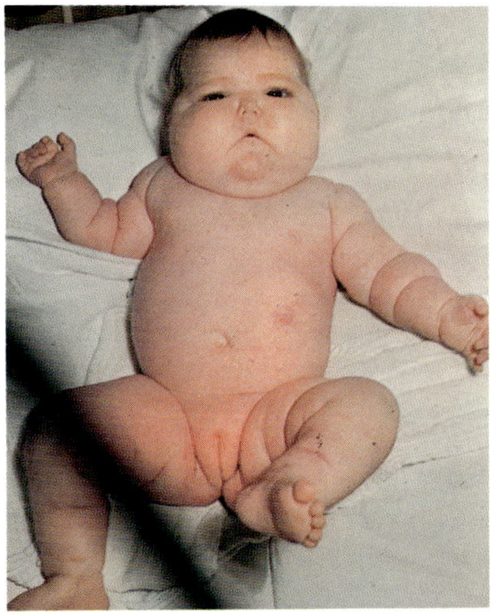

163

163 Calorie excess. Girl of 4 months, weight 9070g (75th centile for 9 months). Birthweight was 3850g. Overfeeding was the only cause of the excess deposition of adipose tissue on the face, buttocks and limbs, and the cushingoid appearance.

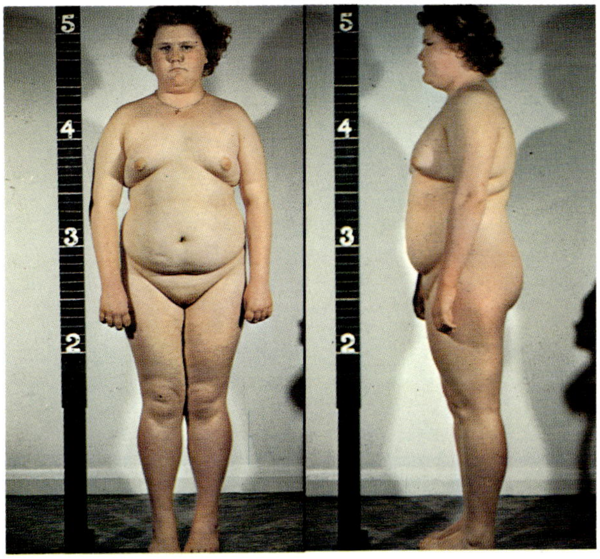

164

164 Precocious development. Girl aged 10 years. Weight 65kg, height 165cm corresponding to the 75th centile for 15 years. The distribution of fat tissue on the breasts and abdomen with relatively slim limbs is of adult type. The girl was a compulsive eater (hyperphagia).

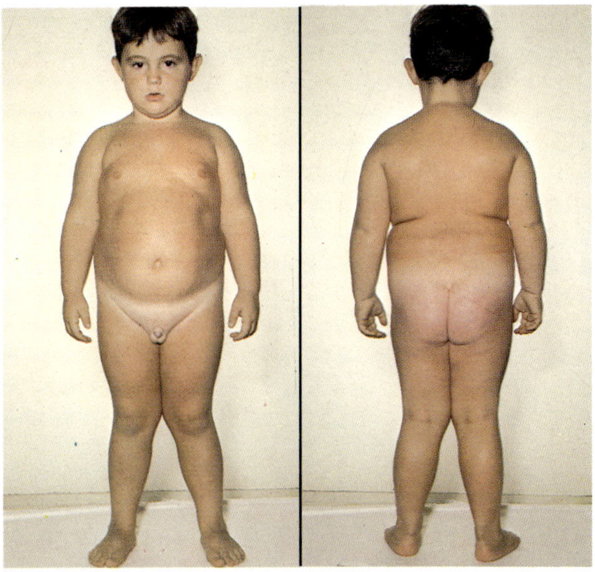

165

165 Postural defects in obesity. The 3-year-old boy shows valgus deformity of the legs and lordosis, which may persist throughout life.

Table 41. Causes of obesity

Essential (simple or idiopathic)		
	Multifactorial, inheritance, racial	
Genetic		
	Prader–Willi	
	Laurence–Moon–Biedl	
	Alström	
	Morgagni–Stewart–Morel	
	DIDMOAD (diabetes insipidus, diabetes mellitus, optic atrophy, deafness syndrome)	
	Carpenter's syndrome	
	Cohen's syndrome	
Mental retardation		
	e.g. Down's	
	Hurler's	
Physical Disability		
	e.g. Spina bifida	
	Paraplegic	
Hypothalamic		
	Trauma	
	Inflammation	– meningitis
		encephalitis
		tuberculosis
		syphilis
	Infiltration	– sarcoidosis
		histiocytosis X
	Tumours	– craniopharyngioma
		astrocytoma
	Leukaemic leucodystrophy	
Endocrine		
	Hypothalamus and pituitary	– **growth hormone failure**
		Laron dwarf
		hypogonadotrophic hypogonadism (Kallman)
		hyperprolactinaemia
		Cushing's disease
		hypopituitarism
	Thyroid	– cretinism
		primary and secondary hypothyroidism
		rarely thyrotoxicosis
Endocrine cont.		
	Parathyroid	– pseudohypoparathyroidism
		pseudo-pseudo hypoparathyroidism
	Adrenal	– Cushing's syndrome
	Ovaries	– polycystic ovarian syndrome
		postmenopausal
		Turner's syndrome
	Testes	– primary hypogonadal
		Klinefelter's syndrome
		Sertoli cell only syndrome
		Noonan's syndrome
Metabolic		
	Diabetes mellitus therapy	
	Nesidioblastoma	
	Insulinoma	
	Beckwith–Wiedemann syndrome	
	Hyperlipidaemia III and IV	
Drugs		
	Sulphonylurea	
	Insulin	
	Oestrogen	
	Contraceptive pill	
	Alcohol	
	Corticosteroids	
	Cyproheptadine	
	Sodium valproate	
	Non-selective B adrenergic blockade	
	Phenothiazines	
	Tricyclic antidepressants	
Abnormal fat distribution		
	Multiple lipomatosis	
	Partial lipodystrophy	
Painful fat		
	Dercum's disease	

Table 41 is a reminder of the extremely wide variety of possible causes of obesity. It is estimated that 99% of all cases are idiopathic or 'essential' in nature and it is this form that will be discussed almost exclusively here.

Idiopathic obesity does not always take the same form, as will be seen later, and while energy intake always exceeds energy requirement and the first law of thermodynamics is not contravened this does not mean that overeating is inevitably to blame. It is becoming increasingly well recognized that genetic and family environmental influences are of great importance (**166**).[60]

Psychological factors play a part and to a certain extent obesity is a disorder of eating behaviour (see **152**).

Only in recent years has the concept that there are different kinds of obesity become generally accepted. For many years the Marseille physician Vague[3] had divided his patients into a more typical female (gynoid) distribution of fat mainly on hips and thighs ('pears') and male (android) with abdominal distribution ('apples') (**167**).

166 Genetic and family environmental influences investigated by Stunkard and his colleagues in 540 adult Danish adoptees where information was available on both the biological and the adopted parents. The adoptees were divided into four groups depending on whether they were thin, average, overweight or obese, each group being then compared with the body mass index of the biological and adoptive parents. Note the close association of the weight of the adoptees with their biological parents: the heavier the parents, the heavier the adoptee. For biological mothers the association was highly significant ($p < 0.0001$) but less so for biological fathers ($p > 0.02$). In contrast, there was no apparent relation between the body mass index of the adoptive parents and the weight of the adoptees. The conclusion was that genetic influences are important in determining body fatness and that childhood family environment alone has little effect in this Danish society where food was in abundance. The latter is important since environmental factors do influence genetic expression where food availability may alter dependency on the family's attitude, finances and education.

166

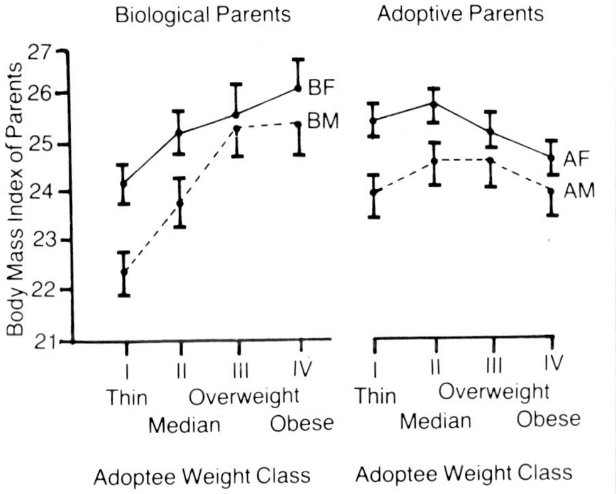

BF denotes biologic fathers, BM biologic mothers, AF adoptive fathers, and AM adoptive mothers.

167

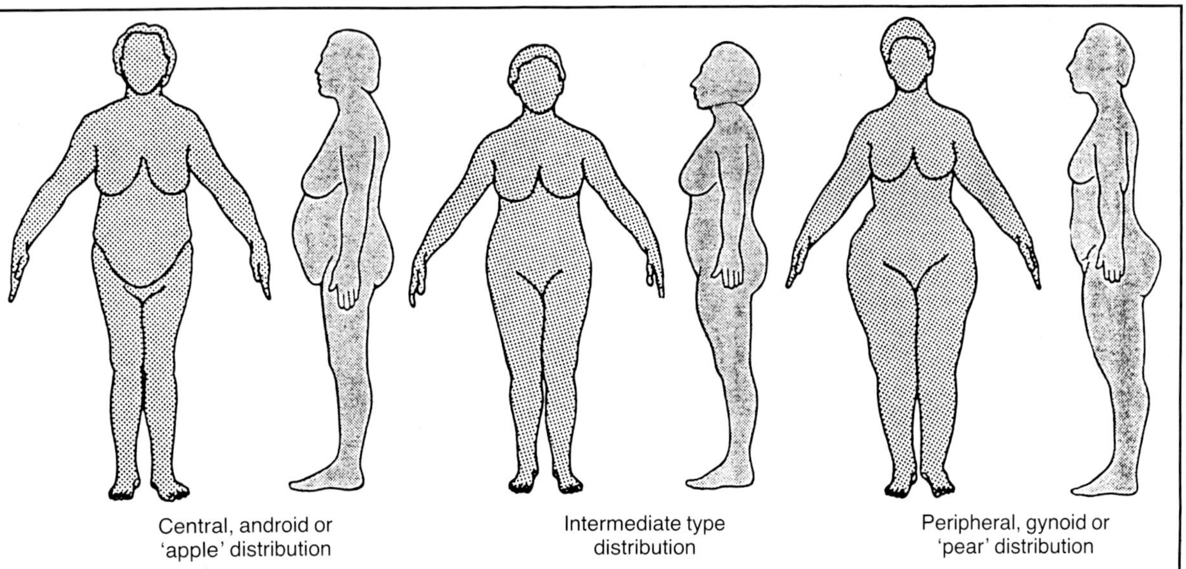

167 Fat distribution. Outline of three obese women with approximately the same Quetelet's index, but differing in pattern of fat distribution.

168

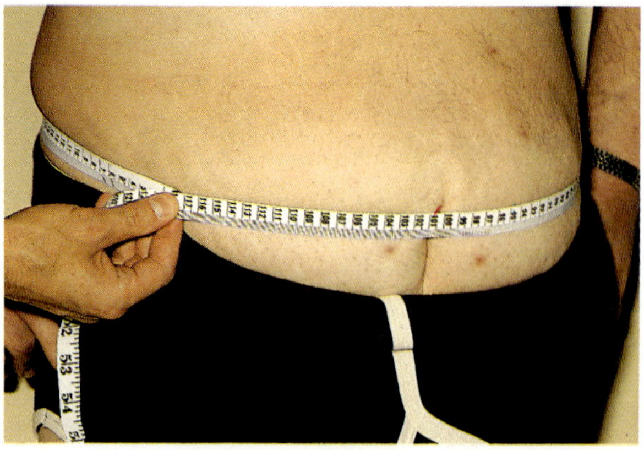

16

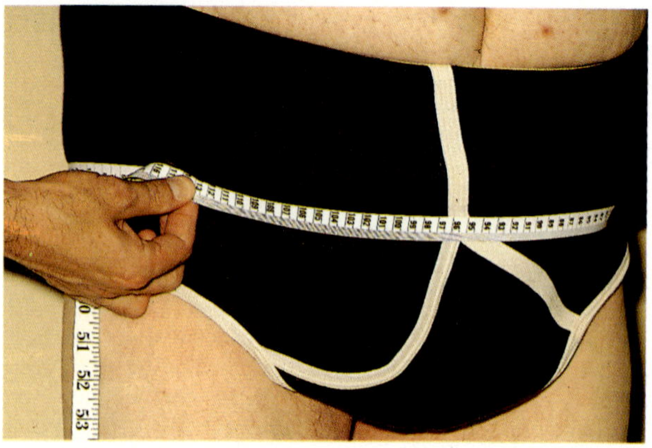

168, 169 Regional fat distribution. Comparison of the circumference of waist and hip is often measured. The circumference is measured around the waist in the erect position. Some measure at the umbilicus (**168**), others at a point one-third the distance between the xiphoid process and umbilicus. This measurement can be difficult in the very obese with large abdominal obesity. The hip circumference (**169**) is measured 4cm below the anterior superior iliac spine (without pants). Others advocate measuring the hip at a point one-third of the distance between the anterior superior iliac spine and the patella. The importance of these measurements appears to be that those who deposit their fat abdominally rather than on their hips are particularly susceptible to cardiovascular disease and diabetes mellitus. In this respect a ratio of abdominal to hip girth of over 0.8 is considered hazardous.

170

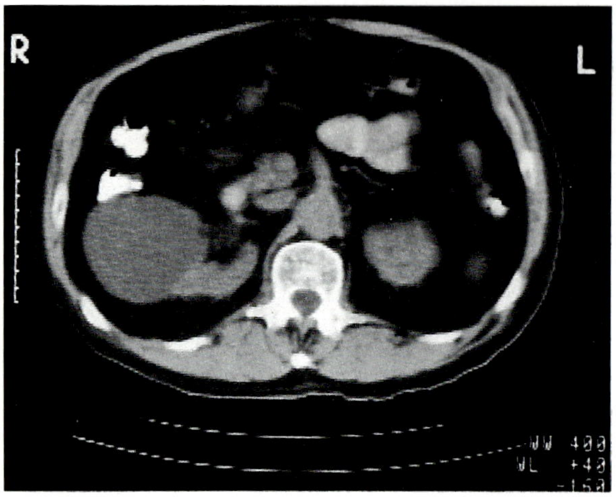

170 Computer assisted tomography (CAT) of a typical obese male patient shows that much fat is contained within the abdomen.

171

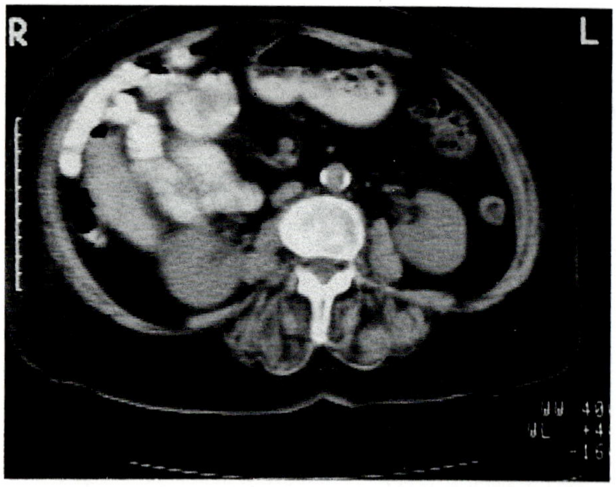

171 CAT of a typical obese female shows that fat is mainly subcutaneous with little intra-abdominal fat.

Vague noted that various metabolic disorders such as diabetes, hyperlipidaemia, hyperuricaemia, hypertension and atherosclerosis were common in abdominal obesity (**168**) and much less so in gluteal obesity (**169**).

During the past decade or so many studies have been undertaken using more simple methods of characterizing fat distribution, among which the waist to hip ratio for application to large numbers of subjects has been most used. For more precise location of fat deposits, including importantly those that are intra-abdominal, CT scan has been employed (**170, 171**).

Disease association with abdominal obesity is most impressive (**172**).[61]

It has become evident that location of fat is much more important than amount of fat in relation to disease susceptibility. This is a weakness of weight to height measures like the BMI.

At present it is unclear why central or abdominal obesity carries much greater health risks. There are several theories and one of these[62] is illustrated in **173**.

Fat patterning appears to be under strong genetic predisposition, according to the results of sibling studies.[63]

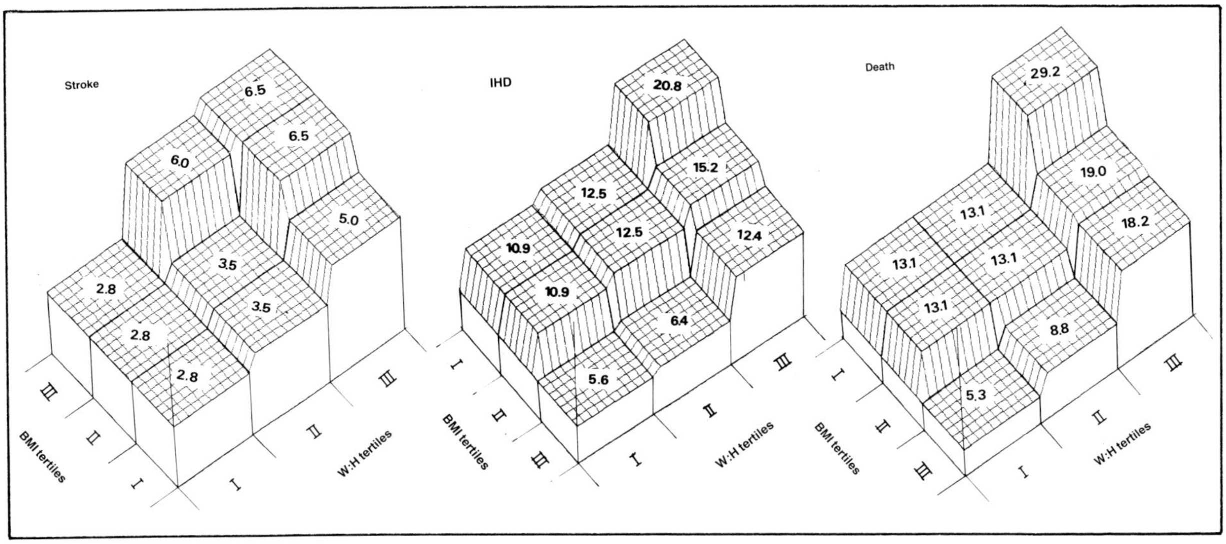

172 **Fat distribution and disease and death.** Percentage probabilities of stroke, ischaemic heart disease (IHD) and death from all causes in relation to tertiles of BMI and waist:hip circumference (W:H) ratio. (BMI axes reversed for death and IHD). Although associations with the W:H ratio were not significant in multivariate analysis when blood pressure and serum cholesterol concentration were taken into account, the ratio was more closely associated with the risk of cardiovascular disease than were other indices of obesity such as BMI.

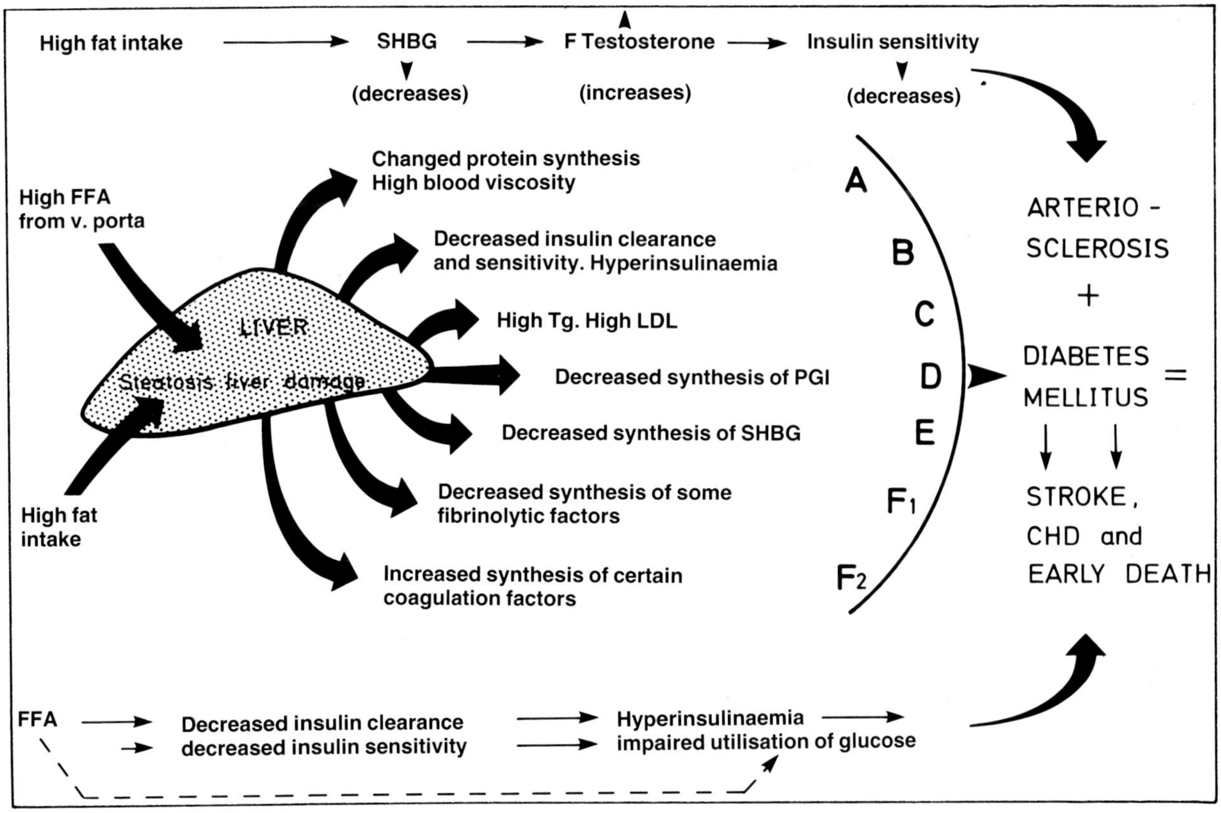

173 **How liver steotosis in android obesity can contribute to *higher* cardiovascular morbidity.** A hypothetical chain of events to explain the acceleration of the development of diabetes and arteriosclerosis in android obesity. A high intake of fat and a high concentration of FFA in the portal circulation both contribute to impairment of the liver function with subsequent decreases in SHBG (serum hormone binding globulin) synthesis and fibrinolytic activity and impaired insulin clearance.

5. Vitamins in Medicine

Vitamins are non-energy producing organic compounds occurring naturally in food and which are necessary for health. Depending upon their isolation during the first half of this century from either fat- or water-soluble fractions of foodstuff extracts, they have come to be classified into *fat-soluble vitamins* (A, D, E, K) and *water-soluble vitamins* (thiamin, niacin, riboflavin, pyridoxine, folic acid, vitamin B_{12}, biotin, and vitamin C). In itself this would hardly be sufficient reason to retain this division, but the members of the two groups tend to have rather different characteristics. Fat-soluble vitamins (and the essential fatty acids which are usually considered in this context) are stored in the body, whereas the water-soluble vitamins, with the notable exception of vitamin B_{12}, are not to any extent. Water-soluble vitamins function mainly as coenzymes, assisting enzymes in many important metabolic processes. None of the fat-soluble vitamins has coenzyme function and their roles in the body are diverse and incompletely understood. Vitamin A is involved in vision, fertility and epithelial cell differentiation; vitamin D has hormone-like actions in calcium homeostasis; vitamin E is an antioxidant; vitamin K is required for blood coagulation factor formation; and essential fatty acids are precursors of prostaglandins and other compounds.

Until recently most attention has been focused on deficiency states of vitamins which still predominate in most parts of the developing world. However, in the West, abuse of vitamin supplements has led to the recognition of toxicity for an increasing number of vitamins. Some forms of hypervitaminosis may be very difficult to distinguish from other diseases unless the possibility of their occurrence is continually borne in mind.

Finally, there is a group of rare disorders in which shortly after birth some form of genetic defect which involves an error in the interaction between a vitamin coenzyme and its apoenzyme becomes manifest. This state is known as *vitamin dependency* and can usually be overcome by routine massive dosing with the appropriate vitamin (see *Table 81*). The clinical picture produced in no way resembles that due to the deficiency state.

Vitamin A (retinol)

This alcohol ($C_{20}H_{30}O$) is derived in the mucosa of the upper small intestine by biodegradation of a relatively small fraction of the large class of coloured compounds, carotenoids of which B-carotene is the most important. Dark green leafy vegetables (**174**) such as spinach, turnip tops and parsley are rich sources of the provitamin, as are carrots (**175**) and yellow fruits like papaya and mango. Red palm oil (**176**), the traditional cooking oil in much of west and central Africa, is so rich (about 33,000µg provitamin A activity/100g oil) that prolonged use induces hypercarotenosis (see also **225–227**).

174

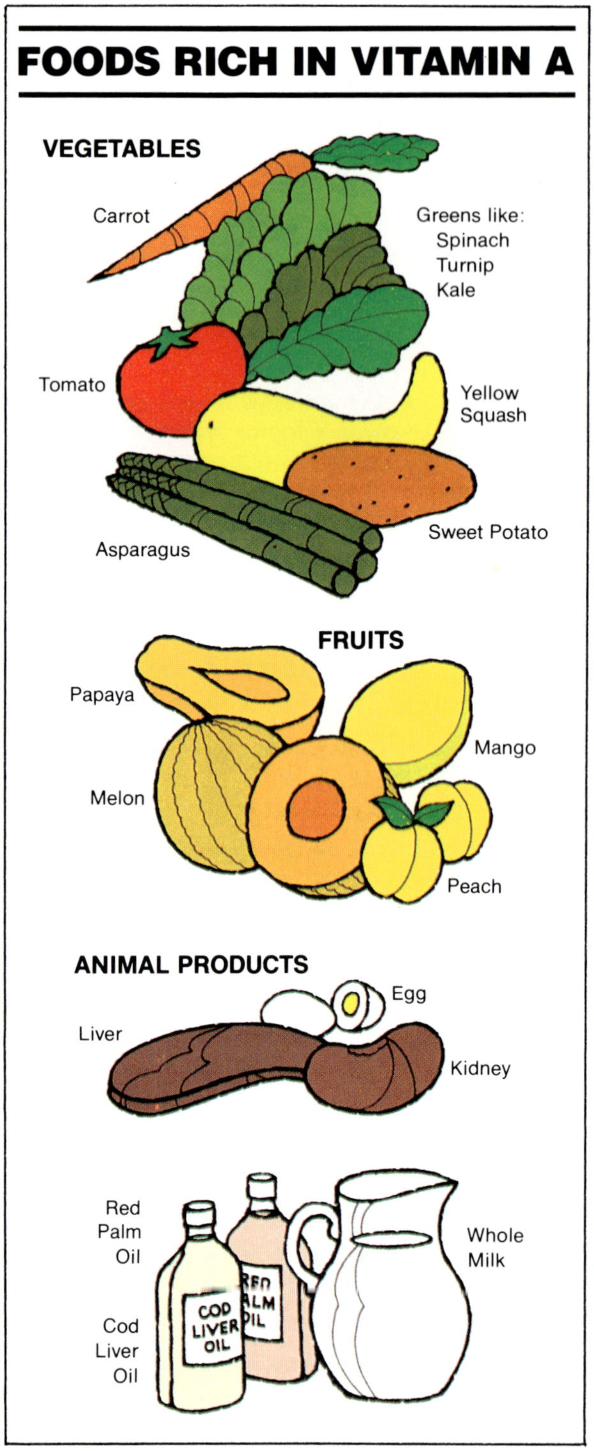

174 Vitamin A poster. Example of a poster used for health and nutrition education for combating vitamin A deficiency and xerophthalmia.

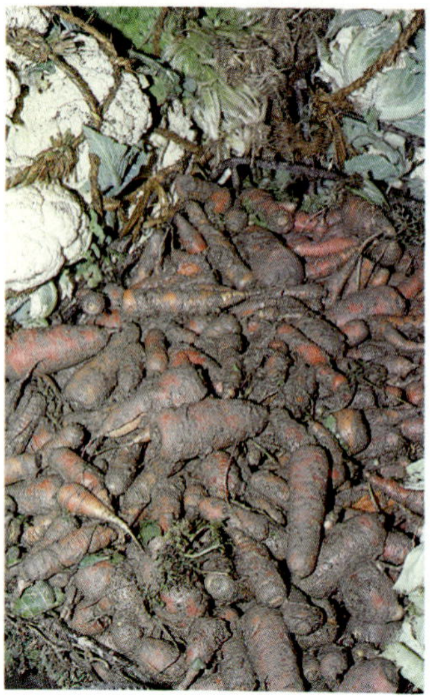

175 Vegetables in an Eastern market. These carrots are likely to be heavily contaminated with helminth eggs, as well as protozoal cysts, but the parasites will be destroyed when the vegetables are cooked.

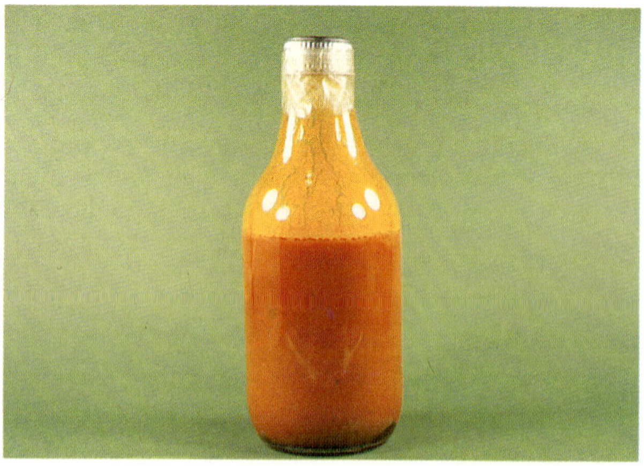

176 A sample of red palm oil, extracted from the fruit coat of *Elaeis guineensis*, the traditional cooking oil in much of west and central Africa. It contains as much as 100,000 IU (33,000 μg) of provitamin A activity per 100g oil.

The physiology of vitamin A is outlined in **177**.[64]

The best understood function of vitamin A is its role in vision. An early sign of vitamin A deficiency is night blindness (see page 105), resulting from impairment of retinal rod function in dark adaptation. Vitamin A plays a key role in the normal differentiation of epithelial cells all over the body. Xerosis, loss of goblet cells and keratinization occur in deficiency and these changes form the basis of cytological assessment of vitamin A status[65] and also of the clinical eye signs (see **182–215**).

Vitamin A is also necessary for normal growth, fetal development, fertility, haemopoiesis and the immune response. The increased mortality associated with even mild vitamin A deficiency may be related to increased susceptibility to common infections such as diarrhoeal and respiratory diseases.

The daily requirement for vitamin A may be met from animal or plant sources or more usually a combination of both. Preformed vitamin A is much more efficiently used than provitamin carotenoid and allowance is made for this in determining the RDA (Recommended Dietary Allowance) expressed in RE (retinol equivalents) (see Appendix I, Table 4). It is set at approximately 750μg for an adult. Normal blood levels are shown in Appendix III, Table 1.

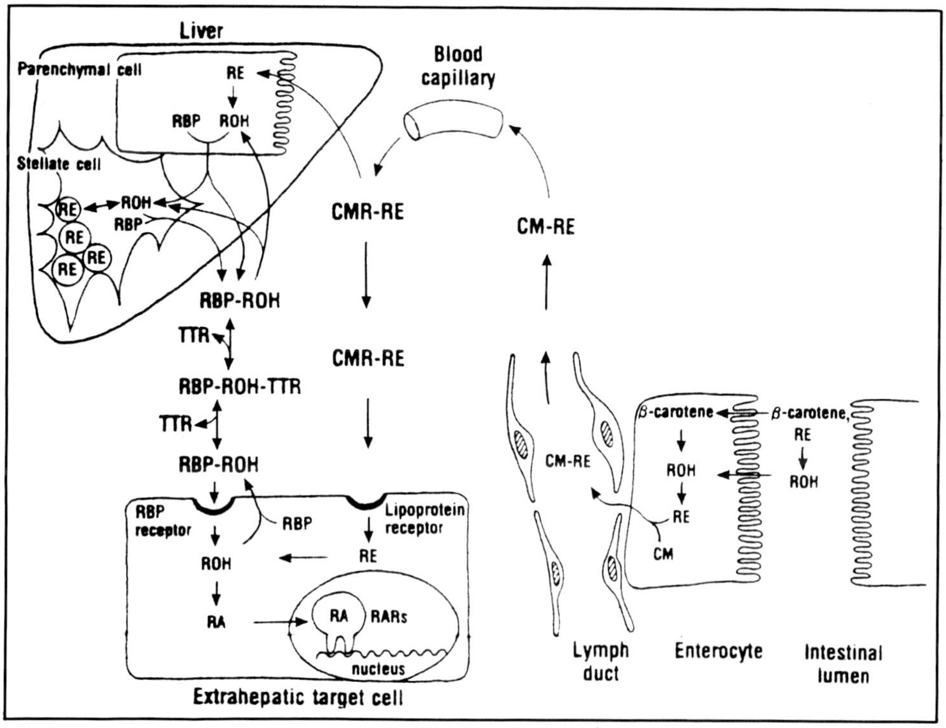

177

177 Major pathways for retinoid transport in the body. Dietary retinyl esters (REs) are hydrolysed to retinol (ROH) in the intestinal lumen before absorption by enterocytes, and carotenoids are absorbed and then partially converted to retinol in the enterocytes. In the enterocytes, retinol reacts with fatty acids to form esters before incorporation into chylomicrons (CMs). Chylomicron remnants, which contain almost all the absorbed retinol, are mainly cleared by the liver parenchymal cells and to some extent also by cells in other organs. In liver parenchymal cells, retinyl esters are rapidly hydrolysed to retinol, which then binds to RBP (retinol-binding protein). Retinol-RBP is secreted and transported to hepatic stellate cells. Stellate cells may then secrete retinol-RBP directly into plasma. Most retinol-RBP in plasma is reversibly complexed with TTR (transthyretin). The uncomplexed retinol-RBP is presumably taken up in a variety of cells by cell surface receptors specific for RBP. Most of the retinol taken up will then recycle to plasma, either on the 'old' RBP or bound to a newly synthesized RBP. (RA, retinoic acid; RAR, retinoic acid receptor.)

Vitamin A deficiency (xerophthalmia)

Characteristic clinical signs occur in the eye and the World Health Organization (WHO) has introduced a classification shown in *Table 42*.

Early among these to appear is impairment of dark adaptation which is recognized subjectively as night blindness (**178–181**). About the same time and preceding clinically-evident structural changes, the bulbar conjunctiva undergoes early changes of xerosis consisting of disappearance of goblet cells and mucin lakes and enlargement and distortion of epithelial cells. These changes can be readily documented by taking superficial conjunctival impressions obtained by application of a cellulose acetate strip followed by fixation and appropriate staining (**182–187**).

178

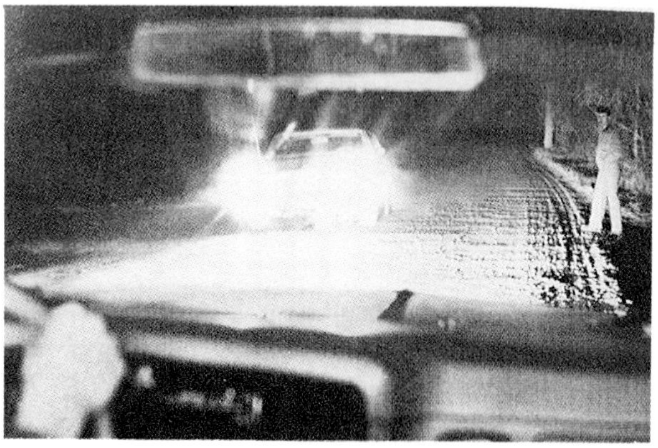

Table 42. Xerophthalmia classification by ocular signs.

Night blindness (XN)
Conjunctival xerosis (X1A)
Bitot's spot (X1B)
Corneal xerosis (X2)
Corneal ulceration/keratomalacia < ⅓ corneal surface (X3A)
Corneal ulceration/keratomalacia ≥ ⅓ corneal surface (X3B)
Corneal scar (XS)
Xerophthalmic fundus (XF)

179

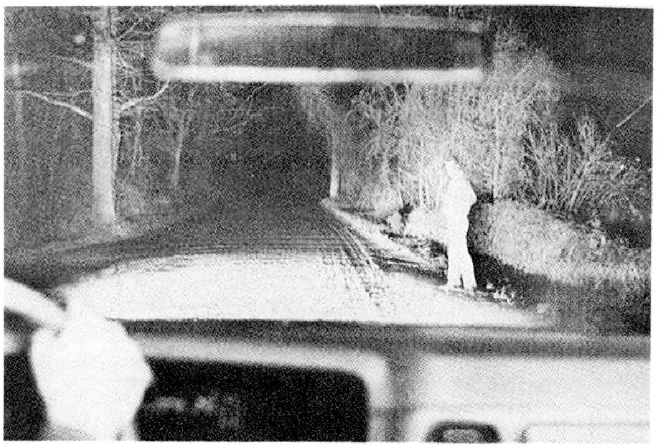

180

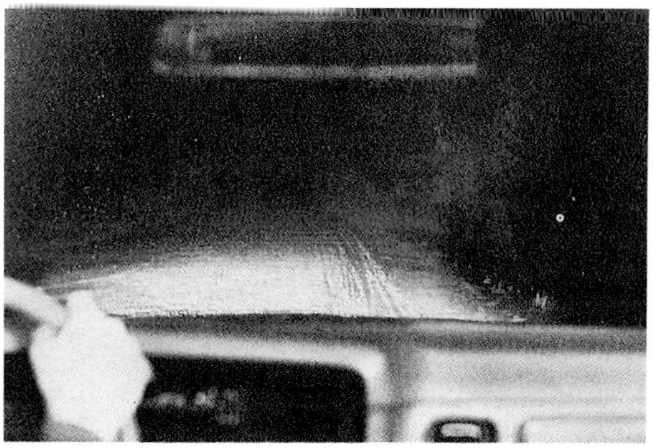

178 **Night blindness.** Both the normal person and the vitamin A-deficient patient see the headlights of an approaching car, as shown.

179 **Night blindness.** After the car has passed, the normal person sees a wide stretch of road.

180 Night blindness. The vitamin A-deficient patient can barely see a few feet ahead and cannot see the pedestrian at all.

181 **Curves of dark adaptation** for a subject deprived of vitamin A. The final rod threshold is at the right-hand side of the figure. It was tested on five occasions (the dates are indicated in day, month and year) and in general there is a rise with time in the threshold which indicates a progressive deterioration in the ability of the rods of the retina to respond to a standard low level of illumination.

181

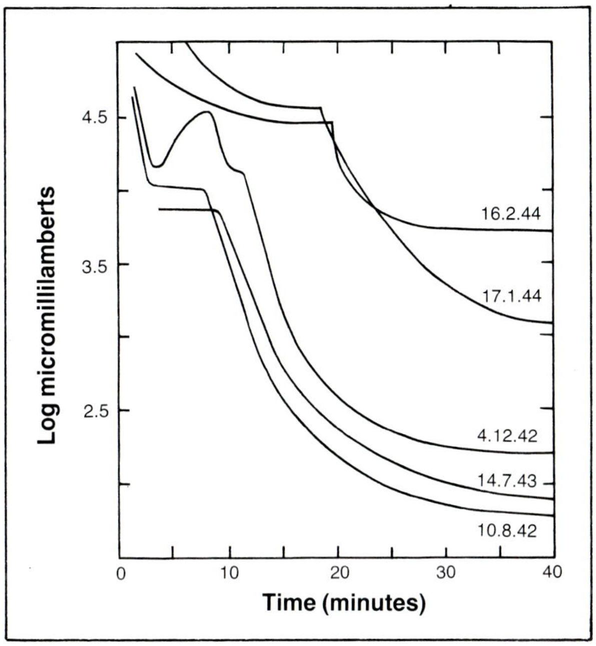

2

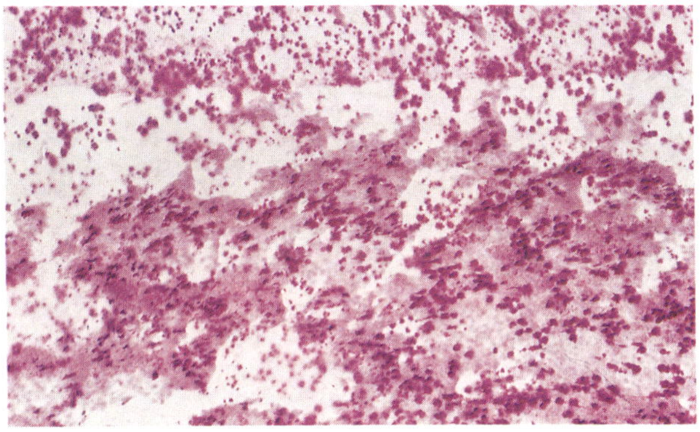

183

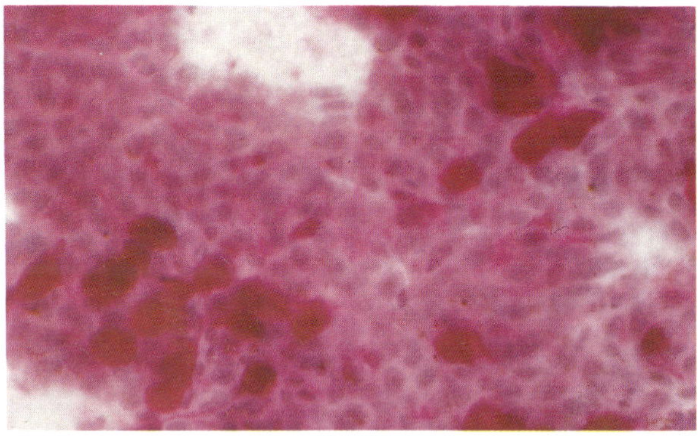

182 **Normal conjunctival impression** with abundant goblet cells, sheets of small epithelial cells, and mucin spots (periodic-acid Schiff (PAS) and Harris' haematoxylin, × 160).

183 **Higher power of normal conjunctiva,** showing contrast between PAS-positive goblet cells and epithelial cells (PAS and Harris' haematoxylin, × 400).

4

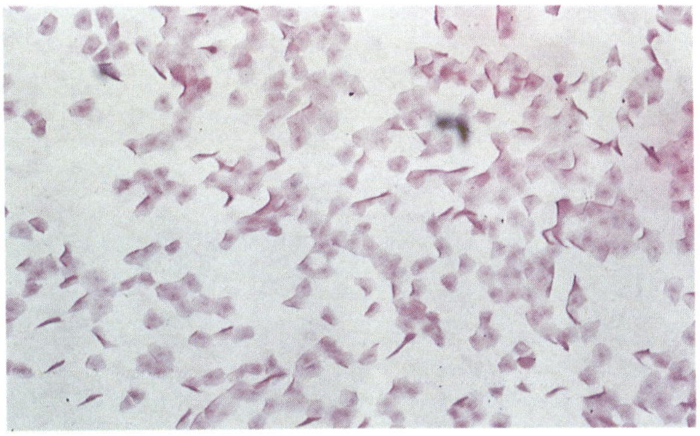

185

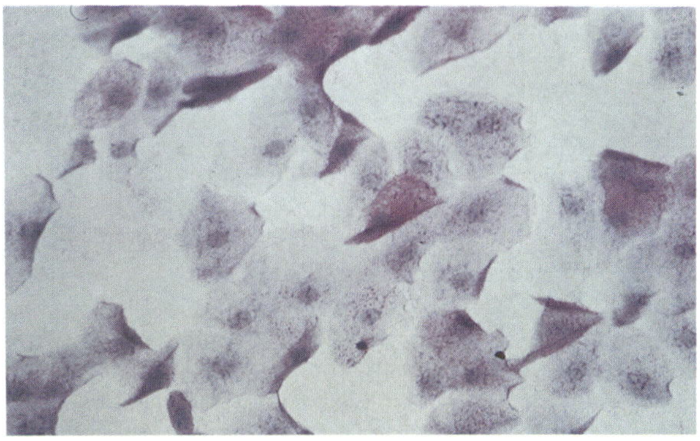

184 **Abnormal conjunctival impression** with complete loss of goblet cells and mucin spots, along with appearance of enlarged epithelial cells (PAS and Harris' haematoxylin, × 100).

185 **Higher power of abnormal, enlarged conjunctival cells** (PAS and Harris' haematoxylin, × 400).

186

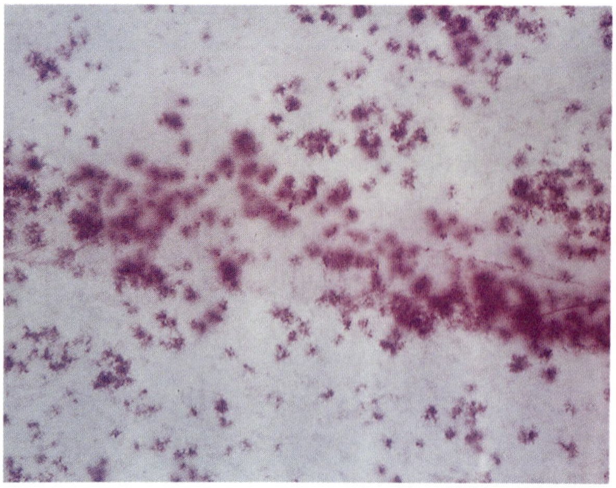

186 PAS-positive mucin spots representing 'impressions' of goblet cells on conjunctival surface (PAS and Harris' haematoxylin, × 400).

18

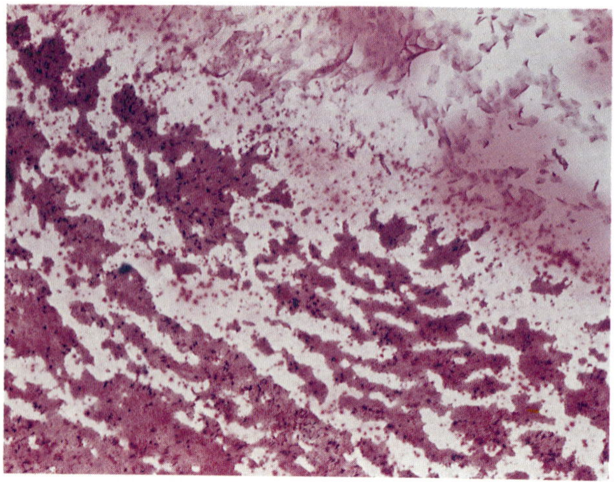

187 Impression cytology from normal child showing transition from abundant normal epithelium (lower left) to abnormal epithelium (upper right). Specimen was graded as normal (PAS and Harris' haematoxylin, × 100).

The progressive histological changes in conjunctiva and cornea are illustrated in **188–193**. Similar changes affect most other epithelial tissues in experimental animals; the few human post-mortem studies carried out also show keratinization (**194**). Early xerosis, as shown by conjunctival impression cytology above, is thought to be the basis for increased morbidity and mortality from infections in mildly vitamin A deficient young children.

188

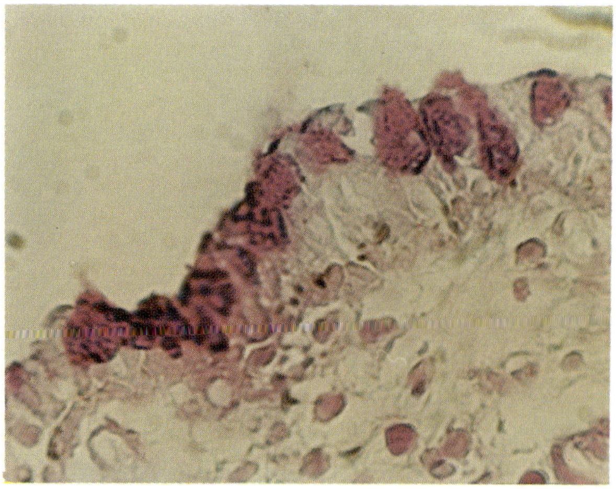

188 Conjunctival histology in xerophthalmia. The very thin epithelium is desquamating and consists of keratinized cell layers with flattened nuclei. The basal cell layer retains the ability to regenerate normal epithelium once vitamin A is supplied, (*H&E*, × 100).

18

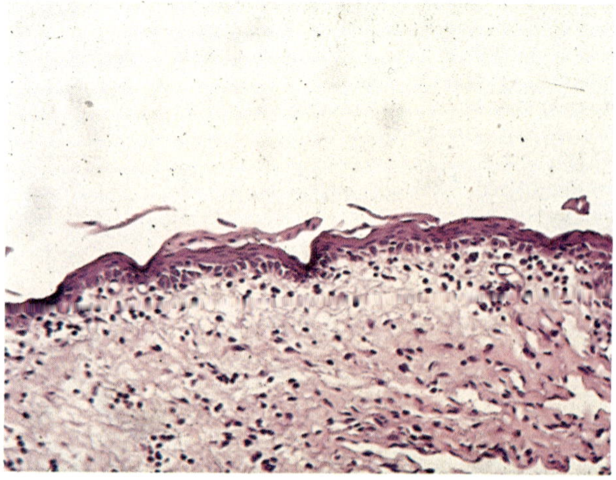

189 Conjunctival histology of healing xerophthalmia. The epithelium is still only one or two cells thick. There are now numerous mucus-secreting goblet cells. (PAS & AB, × 400)

90

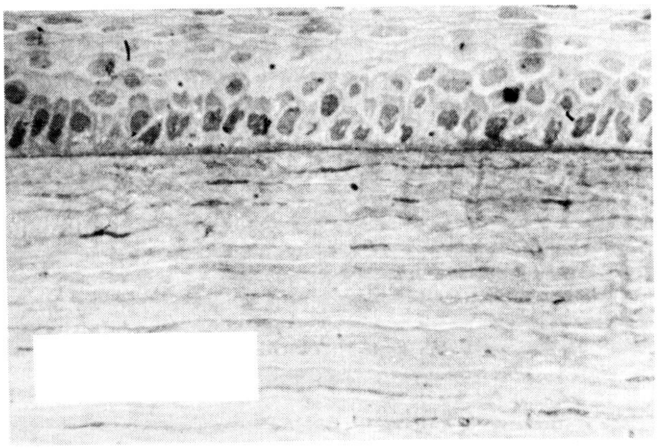

190 Normal cornea. This section shows the normal appearance of basal, wing and squamous epithelial cells. Many keratocytes are found in the anterior stroma. (× 500)

191

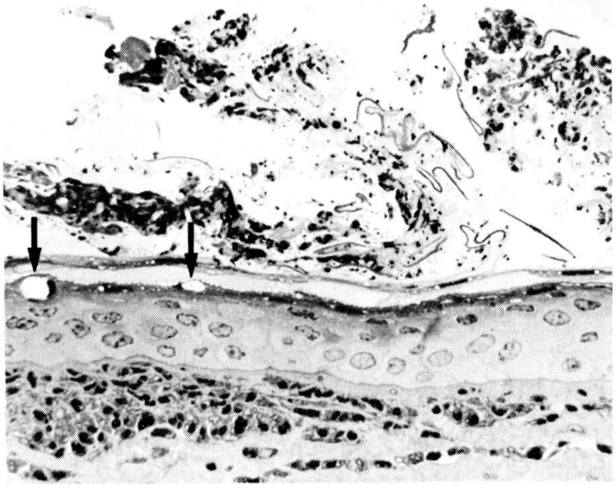

191 Vitamin A deficient cornea. After 6 weeks of experimental deficiency in the rat the columnar appearance of the basal epithelium is lost, with keratinizing epithelium at the surface. There is accumulation of keratin, inflammatory cells, and amorphous cellular debris. Two cysts (*arrowed*) are located in the superficial epithelial layers. (× 500)

92

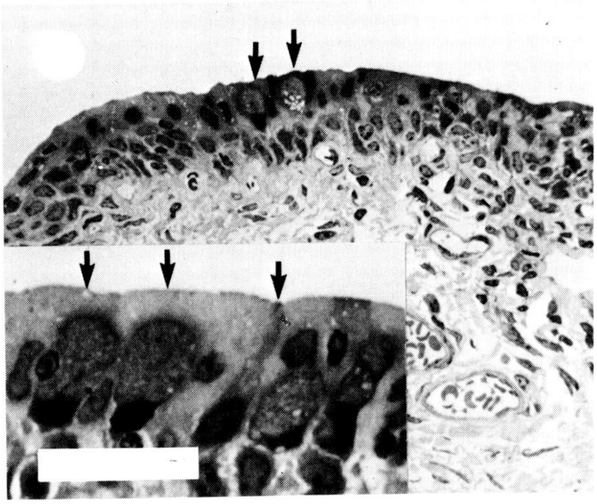

192 Normal conjunctiva. The epithelium shows three or four layers of cells with goblet cells (*arrowed*) interspersed. (× 500, inset × 1000)

193

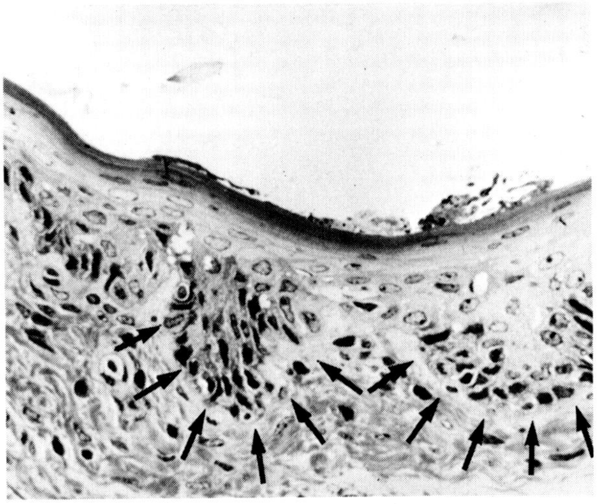

193 Vitamin A deficient conjunctiva. There is superficial keratinization of the epithelium, loss of goblet cells, and rete peg formation (*arrowed*) where the thickness is twice normal. (× 500)

194

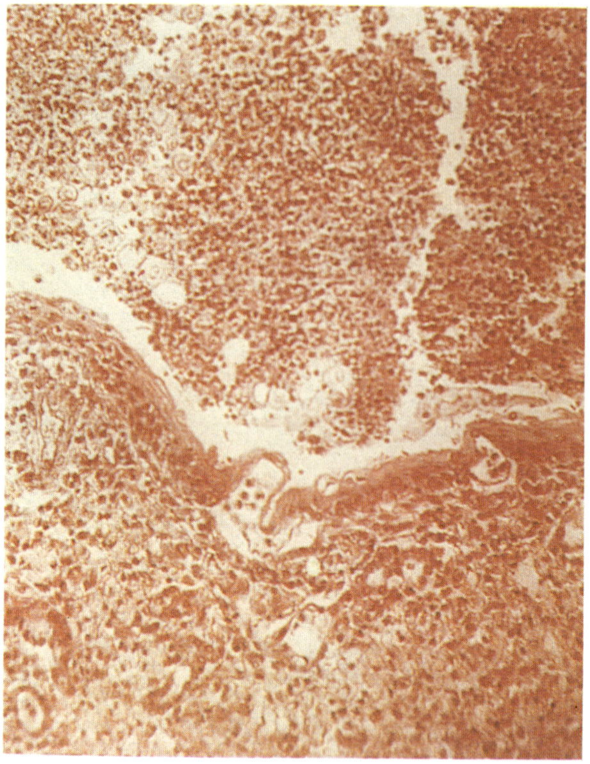

194 Section of lung in vitamin A deficiency. The bronchial epithelium, running transversely across the middle of the section, has undergone keratanizing metaplasia.

Examples of the ocular manifestations of vitamin A deficiency illustrating progressive stages which lead eventually to irreversible blindness are shown in **195–216**. To assist in the recognition of a problem of xerophthalmia of public health magnitude in a community (**217**) WHO has published criteria that are applied to selected signs as shown in *Table 43*.

195

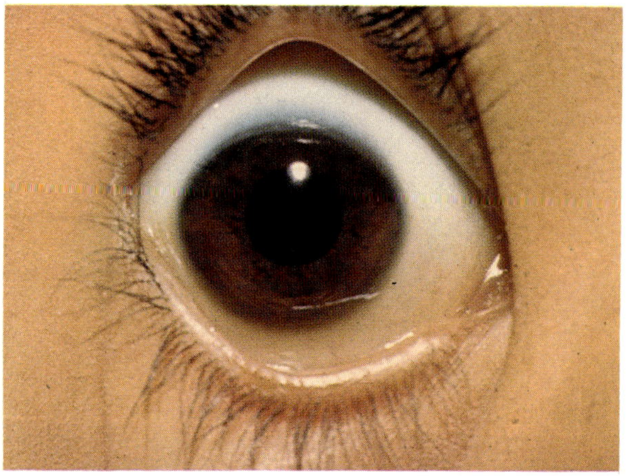

195 Early conjunctival xerosis (**X1A**). Dryness and unwettability of the conjunctival surface are characteristic of this early stage of vitamin A deficiency. Wrinkling and increased pigmentation may also be present, as in this case, but are not on their own an indication of vitamin A deficiency. Plasma vitamin A was 9 μg/100ml (normal 20–50 μg/100ml). Evidence of night blindness can be elicited by careful history taking and observation of the behaviour of the young child at dusk even at this early stage.

196 **Bitot's spots (X1B).** These are single or, as in this case, multiple areas of desquamated, keratinized conjunctival cells together with lipid material from the Meibomian glands. They are not pathognomonic of vitamin A deficiency, as sometimes supposed, but only of nutritional aetiology if accompanied by conjunctival xerosis, as here.

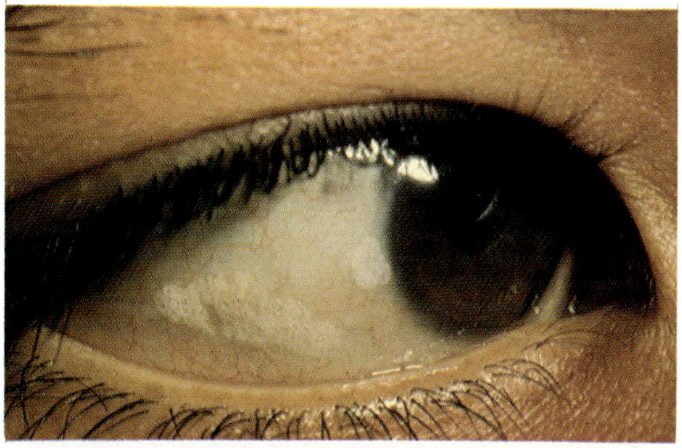

196

197 **A large, diffuse, foamy Bitot's spot.** Bitot's original description in 1868 mentioned 'Particles arranged in a series of wavy parallel lines, which give the lesion the appearance of an undulating and rippled surface'. *Corynebacterium xerosis* can usually be grown from these lesions and it has been suggested that this gas-forming organism is responsible for the bubbles that give the foamy appearance.

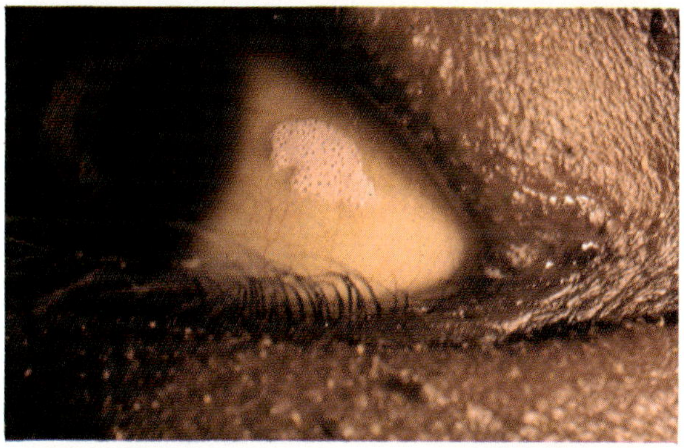

197

198 **A large, compact Bitot's spot.** This is a less common appearance than the foamy lesion (**196, 197**), in which the desquamated epithelial material is more dense and has a 'cheesy' appearance. The 'cheesy' lesion appears to be more chronic than the 'foamy' and those that occur in older children are often of this kind and may be stigmata of previous vitamin A deficiency. Under these circumstances they do not respond to vitamin A treatment.

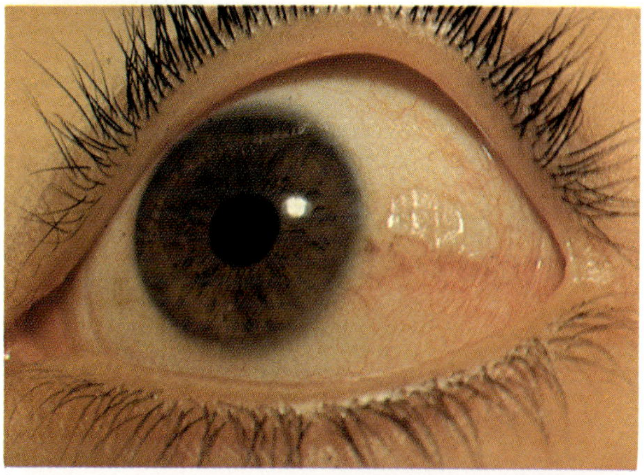

198

199 **Nasally situated Bitot's spot.** This is rare compared with the temporal position. The reason is unclear. It has been suggested that exposure, a factor thought to play a part in the accumulation of Bitot's spot material, is less on the nasal side. Another theory is that the lids are less closely applied on the nasal side and therefore less likely to mould desquamating epithelial cells into a spot.

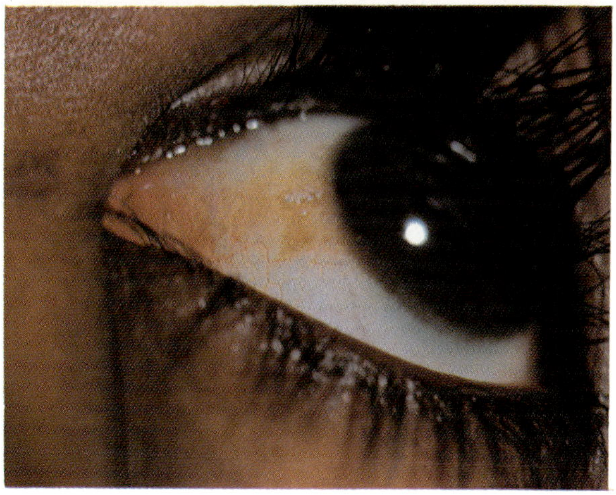

199

200

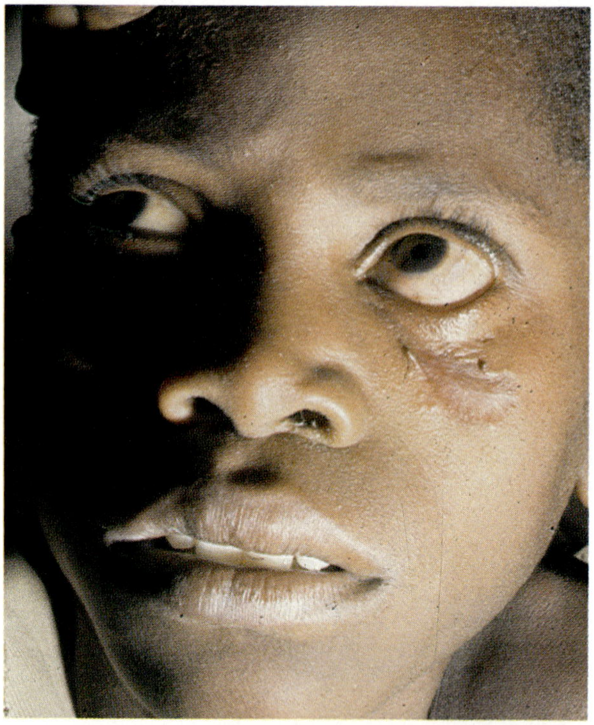

200 Bitot's spot related to ectropion. Light is thrown on the aetiology of Bitot's spot by this and other rare instances in the literature of material accumulating on part of the conjunctiva not normally exposed to the atmosphere. That exposure does play a part, possibly by creating instability of the tear film covering the conjunctiva, is also borne out by the fact that Bitot's spots are often confined to the normally exposed interpalpebral area of the conjunctiva, or if more extensive most of the material accumulates there.

201

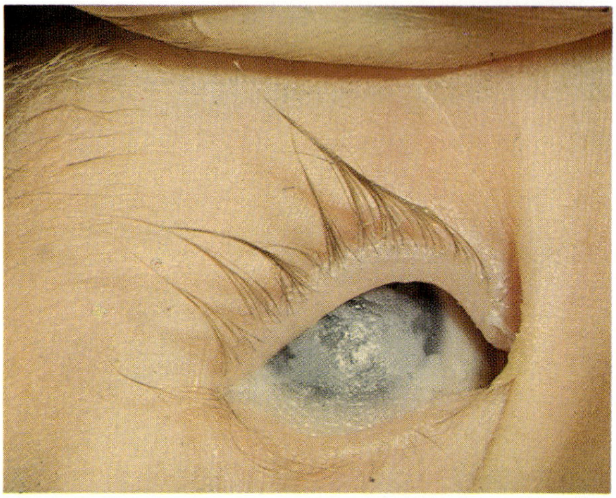

201 Extensive Bitot's spot material involving cornea and conjunctiva. Bitot's spots are usually confined to the conjunctiva even when quite extensive. Rarely xerosis and desquamation also affect the cornea, especially if the process is very low-grade and chronic, as in this Jordanian child. There was no corneal ulceration or keratomalacia and complete clearing occurred with vitamin A therapy.

202

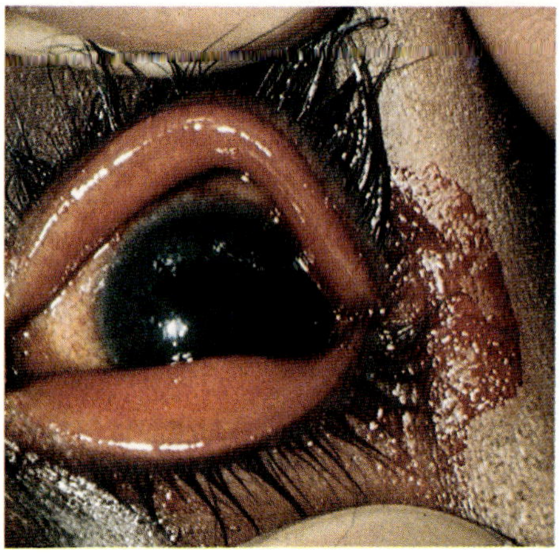

202 Measles keratoconjunctivitis and xerophthalmia. There is xerosis of the conjunctiva stained with 1% rose bengal. Attributable to measles are the slight chemosis, minimal conjunctival infection and corneal erosions stained with 1% fluorescein.

203 Measles keratoconjunctivitis and xerophthalmia. The corneal light reflex is distorted and the pre-ocular tear film is lacking.

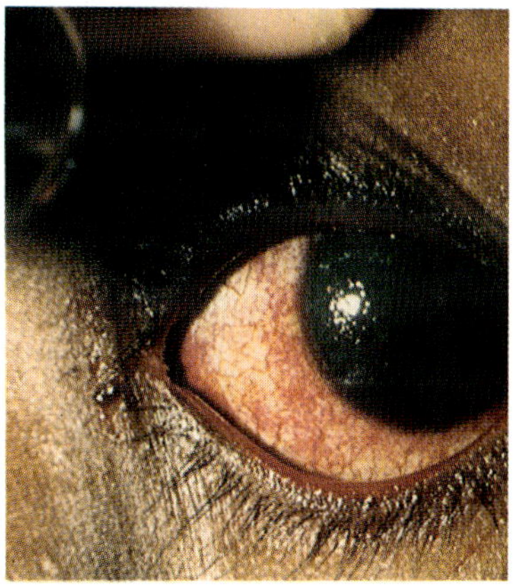

203

204 Conjunctival histology in measles. This should be contrasted with the histological appearance in xerophthalmia (**188, 189**). The epithelium is thickened and hypoplastic and the cells are swollen and have pyknotic nuclei. There is giant cell formation (as in parts of the respiratory tract) and goblet cells are lacking. (*H&E* × 100)

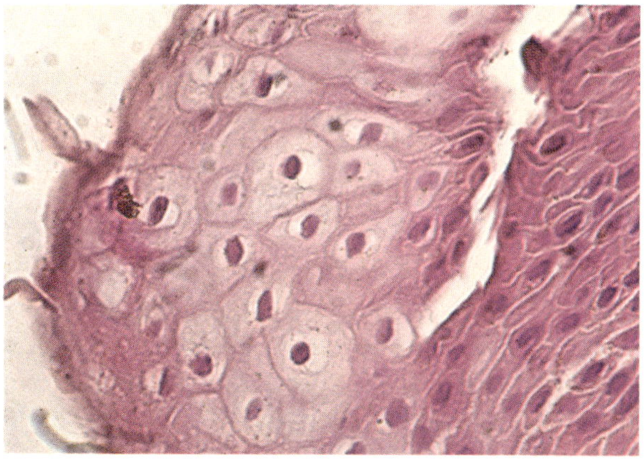

204

205 Marked conjunctival xerosis with corneal xerosis (X1A and X2). The conjunctiva is very dry, thickened and thrown into numerous folds. The cornea is also dry, has lost its normal lustre and its stroma is infiltrated with white cells. From the limbic plexus there is early invasion of the corneal substance by capillaries (neovascularization). There is a superficial erosion situated below the pupillary area, but this has not breached the continuity of the epithelium and has not reached the stage of 'ulceration' (see **206**). Plasma vitamin A was only 3μg/dl (normal 20–50 μg/dl).

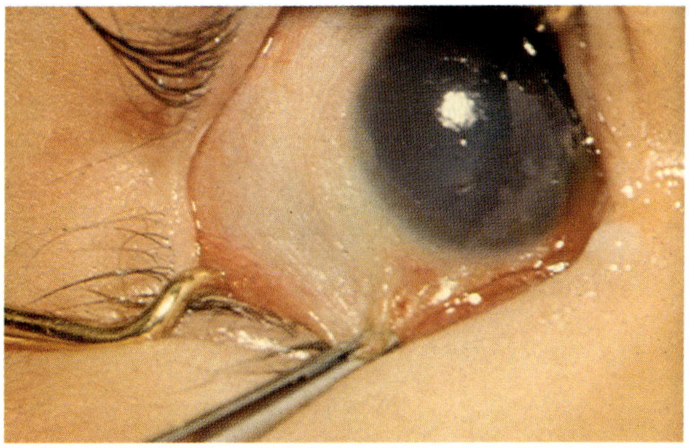

205

206 Corneal 'ulceration' with xerosis (X3A). This is the earliest change in which an irreversible element occurs; some degree of scarring is inevitable. Mucin deficiency in the tears as a result of atrophy of conjunctival goblet cells causes instability of the pre-corneal film, and the 'break-up time' (BUT) is shortened to less than 10 seconds. Ulceration does not imply infection in this context and xerosis of the cornea is a constant feature. It involves loss of substance of a part or of the whole of the corneal thickness. Minimal denudation of the epithelial surface (erosion) without transgression of Bowman's membrane leaves no permanent damage and is not included in this stage. When the ulcer progresses to advanced stromal loss it may result in descemetocele or complete perforation with iris prolapse.

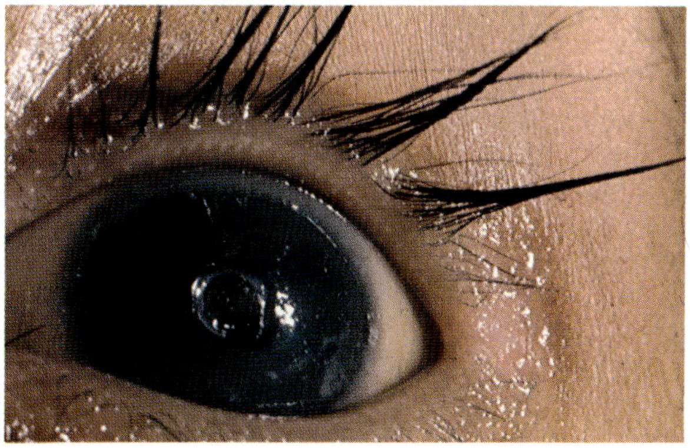

206

207

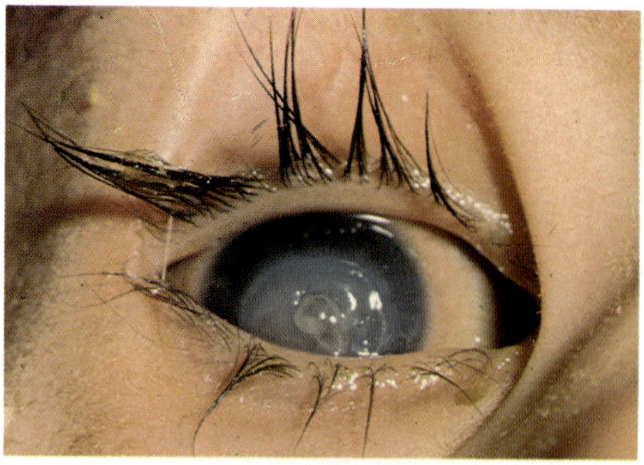

207 Keratomalacia – typical appearance (X3B). Although any part or all of the cornea may be affected, the central area as shown here is most commonly affected when the patient is first seen. Even with prompt vitamin A treatment gross scarring will be inevitable. The precise nature of the pathological process that leads to dissolution of the cornea – termed colliquative necrosis – is not understood. It bears a resemblance to that seen in alkali burns of the cornea. It is probable that instability of the pre-corneal film and keratinization of epithelial cells lead to activation of corneal collagenase and/or other proteases, resulting in liquefaction.

208

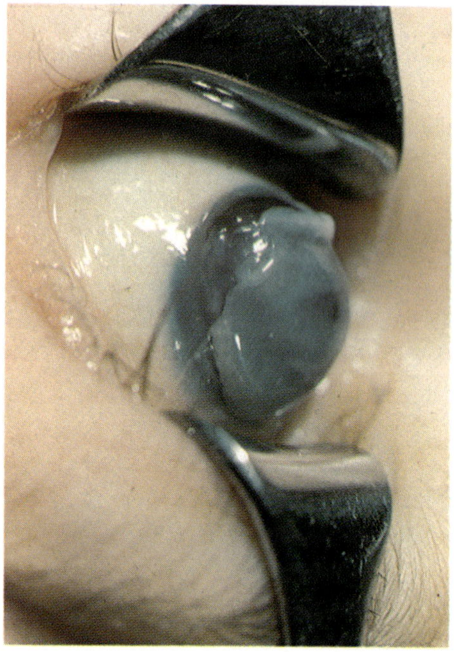

208 Keratomalacia – total (X3B). This is the appearance of one eye of the child in **139**. In the other eye the process was not quite so advanced but sight was also destroyed. The entire thickness of the whole of the cornea is a cloudy, gelatinous mass. Particularly in very young children, keratomalacia may develop very rapidly and, as in this case, there may be complete absence of xerosis and Bitot's spot formation in the conjunctiva. The minimal reaction in the surrounding tissues and lack of discharge are characteristic and assist in the differentiation from other conditions.

209

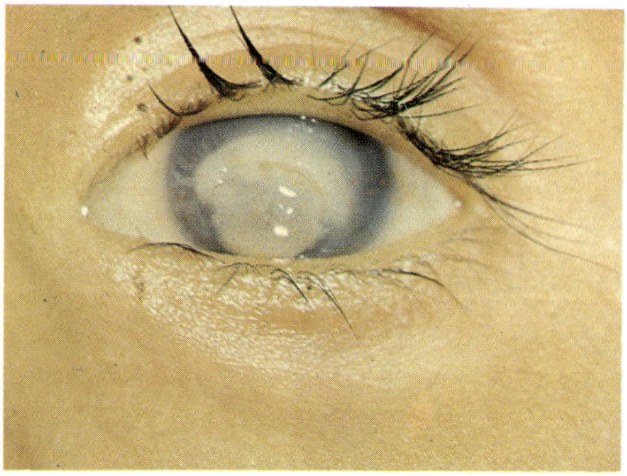

209 Keratomalacia with prolapse of the lens. A serious complication which leads to disorganization of the eye contents and subsequent blindness. The total lack of inflammatory reaction is remarkable but characteristic.

210 Panophthalmitis. Perforation of the cornea in keratomalacia frequently leads to the introduction of secondary infection and destruction of the eye. Fortunately this often occurs in only one eye and useful vision may be preserved in the other with prompt vitamin A therapy.

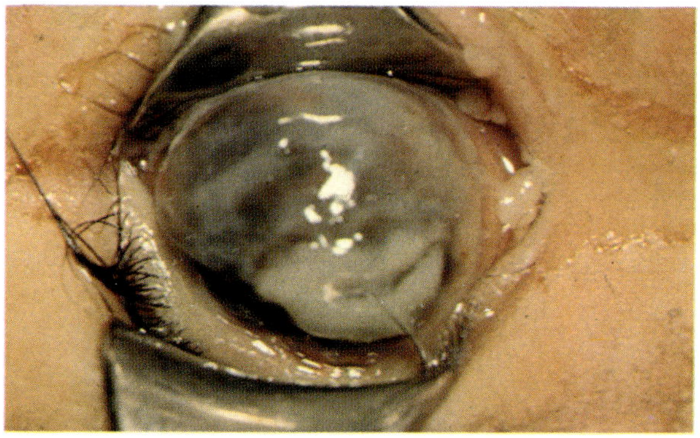

210

211 Ectasia of the cornea (**XS**). During the active stage the softened cornea has bulged forwards due to intraocular pressure. The scar usually consists of a thick epithelial layer lying upon scar tissue that is thinner than the normal stroma. As is the case for all corneal scars, a diagnosis of previous xerophthalmia can only be presumptive, and based on a careful history (see **213**).

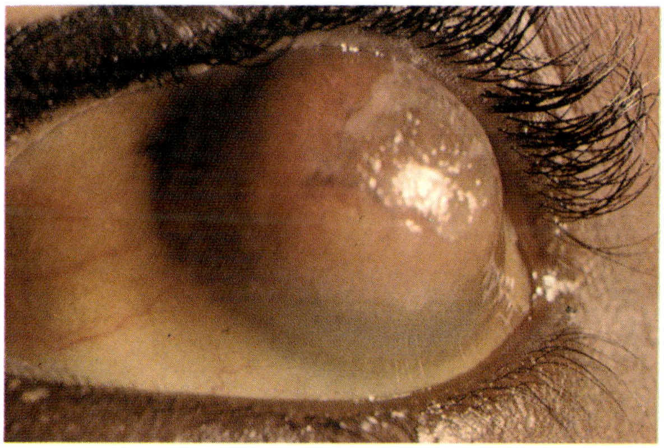

211

212 Anterior staphyloma (**XS**). The extensive corneal defect has been stretched before the scar tissue has consolidated and the wound has been complicated by the incorporation of corneal tissue.

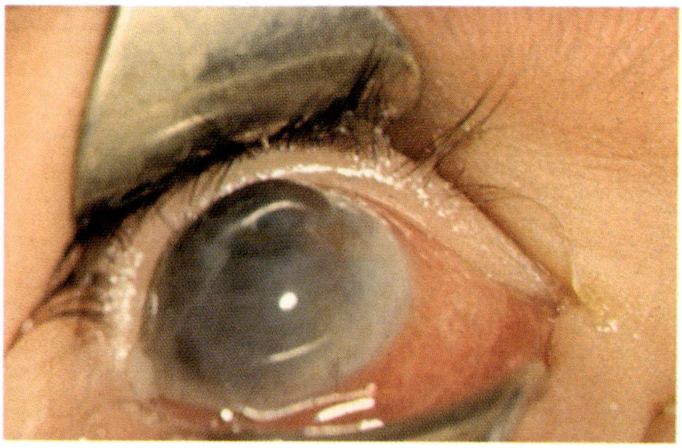

212

213 Corneal scars (**XS**). These are of varying density: very fine (nebula), moderately dense (macula) and very dense (leucoma). They also vary in size, from pin-head to involvement of the entire cornea. The cornea may be scarred from many causes besides previous vitamin A deficiency, including injury and many kinds of eye infection. As they tend to be of higher prevalence than active lesions in communities subject to vitamin A deficiency it is important to distinguish those of nutritional aetiology if possible. A history of the onset of the eye lesions between about 2 months and 5 years of age accompanying general malnutrition is suggestive. Absence of injury, prolonged purulent discharge or severe trachoma in the history supports the likelihood of vitamin A deficiency as the cause. Both corneas are likely to be affected to some degree, and if only part of the cornea is scarred it is frequently the inferior central area that is affected as in this Syrian infant.

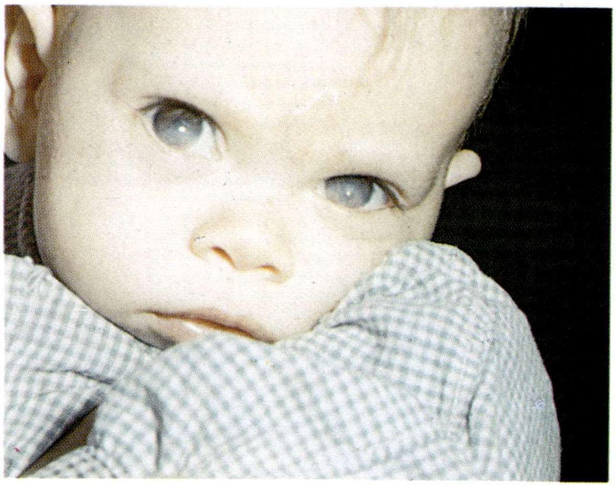

213

214

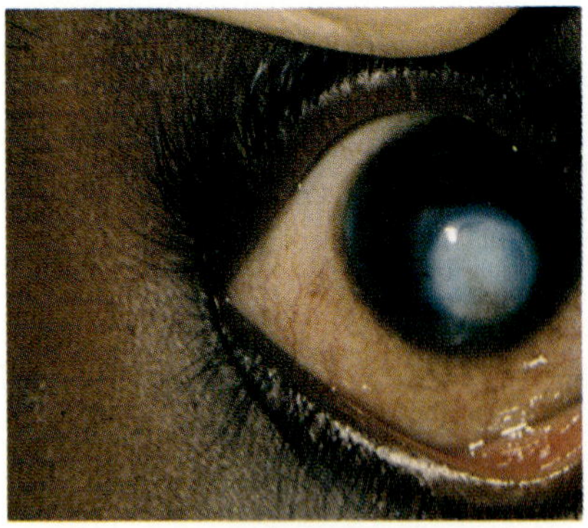

214 Adherent leucoma (XS). The corneal changes have been arrested before perforation but the iris has become adherent to the cornea and the pupil is distorted behind a dense disc-shaped leucoma.

215

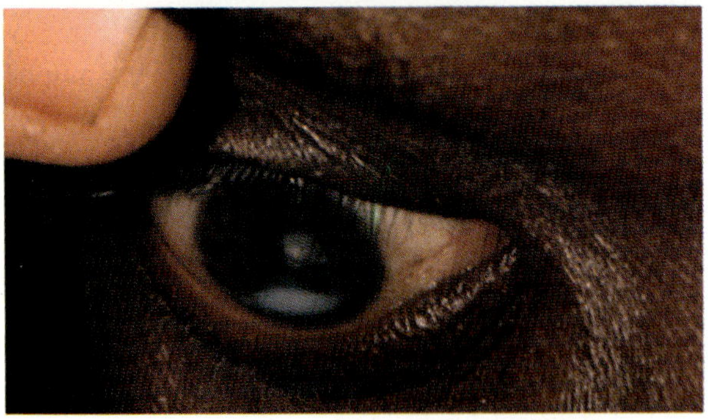

215 Adherent leucoma with anterior polar cataract (XS). The lens is otherwise clear and the pupil is not distorted. The small, dense leucoma is inferiorly situated and some useful vision will be retained.

216

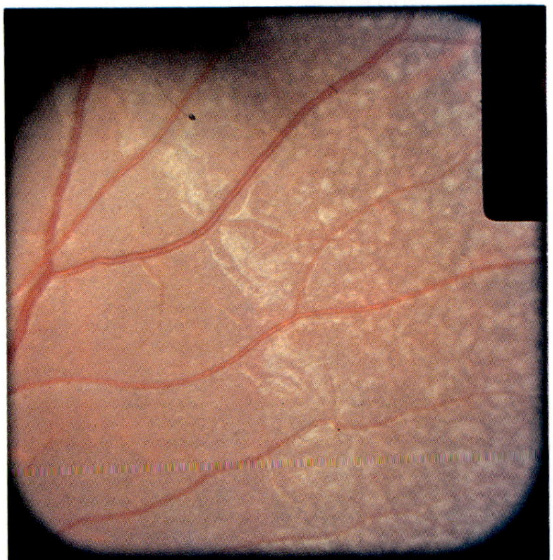

216 Xerophthalmia fundus (XF). Fundus photograph shows the characteristic whitish speckled appearance of the affected retina. Fluorescein angiography revealed 'window' defects which appeared to be in the pigment epithelium. The appearance cleared with vitamin A therapy but some of the window defects remained. Retinitis punctata albescens and fundus albi punctatus are very similar in appearance but do not respond to treatment. Fundus changes are a rare manifestation of vitamin A deficiency and have only been reported from areas of high endemicity, as in Indonesia.

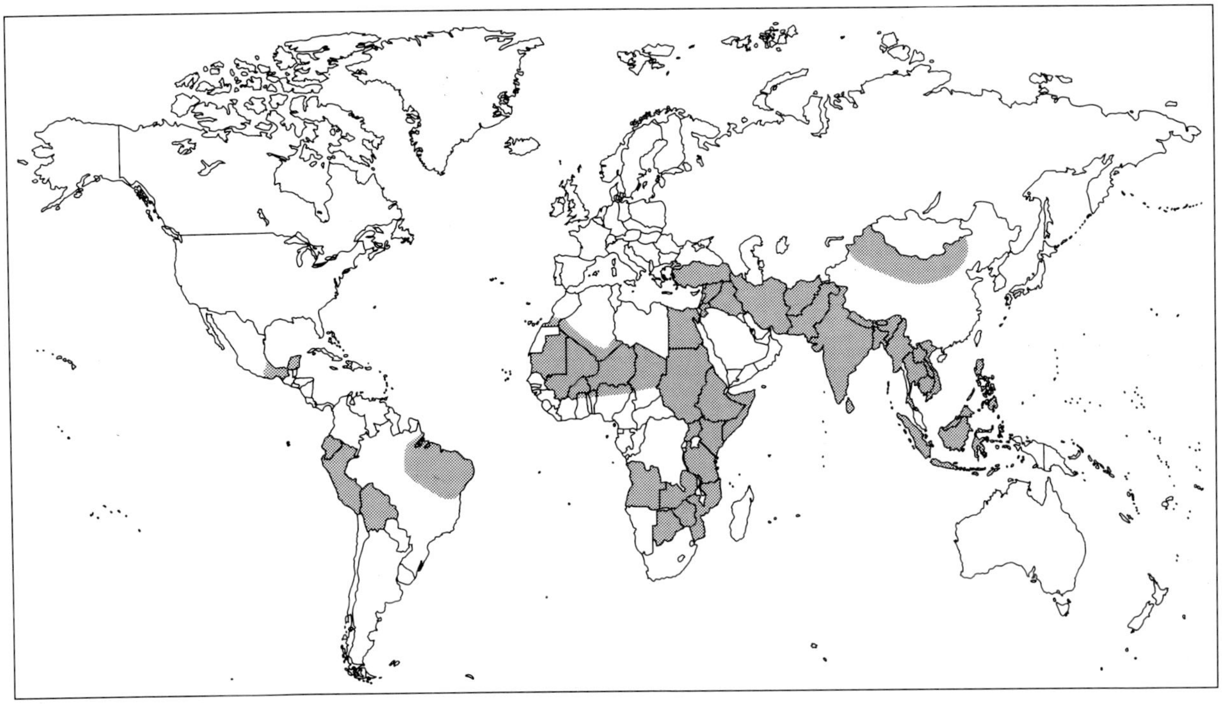

217 The geographical distribution of xerophthalmia and vitamin A deficiency.

Table 43. Prevalence criteria (in percentage of the pre-school-age population, 6 months to 6 years old, at risk) for determining the public health significance of xerophthalmia and vitamin A deficiency.

Criteria
Night blindness (XN) in > 1%
Bitot's spot (X1B) in > 0.5%
Corneal xerosis/corneal ulceration/keratomalacia (X2/X3A/X3B) in > 0.01%
Corneal scar (XS) in > 0.05%
Plasma vitamin A of < 0.35 μmol/l (10 μg/dl) in > 5%

Xerotic changes in the skin, especially affecting the areas surrounding hair follicles on certain parts of the body (**218–221**) have long been associated with deficiency of vitamin A but are non-specific and rarely occur in pre-school age children, the group most at risk.

Table 44 indicates some of the ways in which vitamin A deficiency may be brought about secondary to various diseases.[68-70]

218

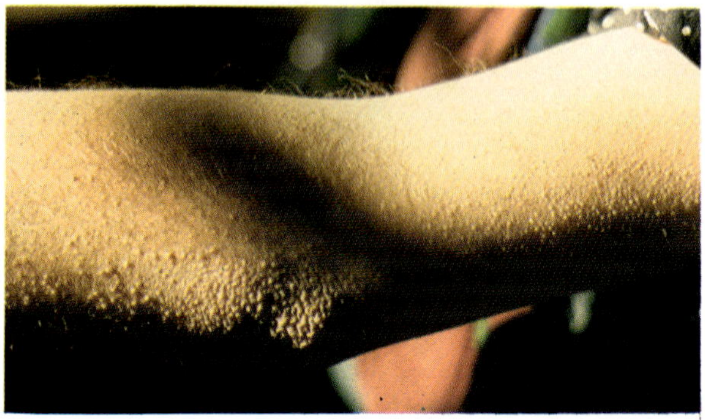

218 Perifollicular hyperkeratosis (phrynoderma, toad skin). Spinous papules appear at the tips of the hair follicles against the background of a generally dry and rough skin. Areas first affected are the posterolateral parts of the arm (as in this case) and the anterolateral aspects of the thighs. There is steady spread to the extensor surfaces of the limbs, shoulders and lower part of abdomen. The chest, back and buttocks are usually only involved in very extensive cases. It is only seen in undernourished subjects and has most frequently been associated with vitamin A deficiency and general undernourishment. It is easily differentiated from the perifollicular haemorrhages of scurvy (**354**). Icthyosis is familial and affects the entire skin. Keratosis pilaris is similar but occurs in well nourished adolescents. Acne vulgaris has a different distribution and features pustulation. Perifollicular hyperkeratosis is not seen before school age.

219

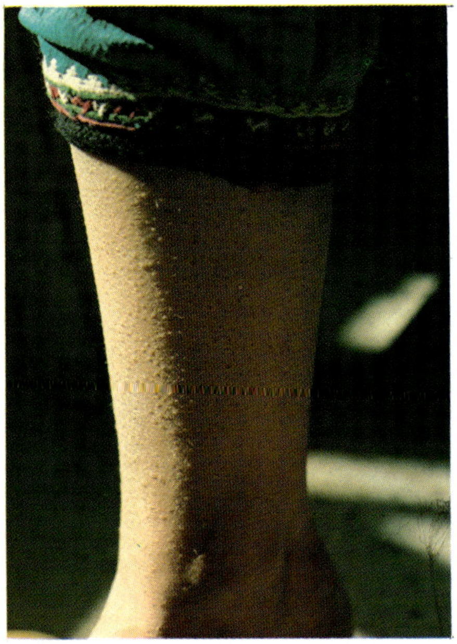

219 Perifollicular hyperkeratosis. The shin is a common site as in this Turkoman child.

220

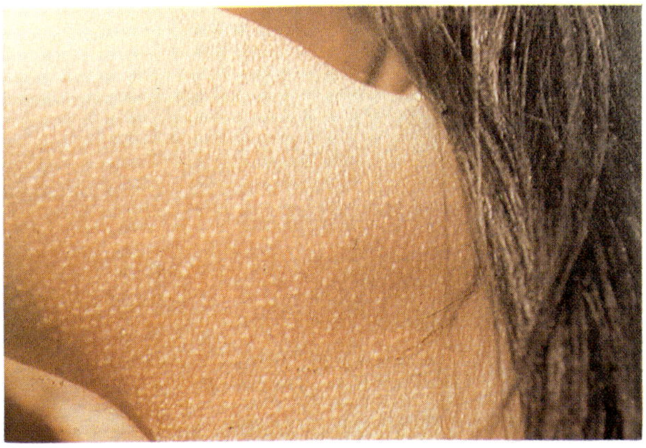

220 Perifollicular hyperkeratosis, prominent over the shoulder region.

221

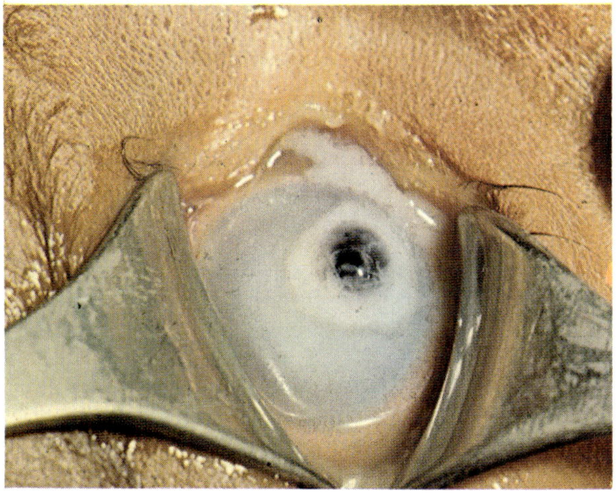

221 Dermomalacia. This was the name given by Pillat to the liquefactive skin changes he observed in severely vitamin A-deficient Chinese soldiers in the 1930s. The gross hyperkeratinization of the skin surrounding the eyes in this infant with severe keratomalacia is an early stage of the condition and is a rare occurrence. (This is the same patient as in **122**).

Table 44. Secondary or endogenous causes of vitamin A deficiency.

Diseases	*Mechanisms*
Coeliac disease, sprue, obstructive jaundice, ascariasis, giardiasis, partial or total gastrectomy	Impaired absorption of lipids including vitamin A
Chronic pancreatitis	In some cases secondary to zinc deficiency
Cystic fibrosis	Excessive faecal loss, unrelated to degree of fat in stools[69]
Enzyme defect	Failure to cleave β-carotene, in small intestine[68]
Chronic liver disease, especially cirrhosis	Zinc deficiency may predispose, most storage in stellate cells, involved in collagen formation and cirrhosis[64]
Heterozygotic reduction of plasma RBP	One case reported of keratomalacia due to reduced transport[70]

Vitamin A Toxicity

This may be either acute or chronic and the clinical manifestations differ considerably (*Table 45*).

Some of the recognized changes are illustrated below (**222–224**).

X-rays of the bones may be helpful in diagnosis of the chronic form, but most help will be obtained from blood sampling and discovery of a markedly elevated plasma retinol (> 3μmol/l).

Table 45. Clinical manifestations of acute and chronic hypervitaminosis A.

Acute	*Chronic*
Nausea	Anorexia
Vomiting	Weight loss
Headache	Dry and scaling skin
Vertigo	Pruritus
Stupor	Alopecia
Blurred vision	Coarsening of hair
Papilloedema	Hepatomegaly
Pseudotumour cerebri	Splenomegaly
Fontanelle bulging (infants)	Anaemia
Fever	Papilloedema
Peeling of skin	Diplopia
	Subperiosteal new bone growth, cortical thickening–especially bones of hands and feet, long bones of legs
	Gingival discolouration

222

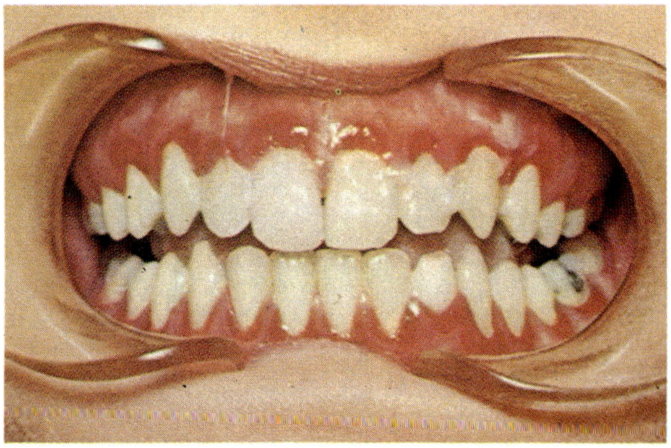

222 **Hypervitaminosis A.** Bright red marginal discolouration of the gingiva as shown here is characteristic.

223 Skull in hypervitaminosis A. Frontal view of a 2-year-old female showing wide sagittal and coronal sutures.

223

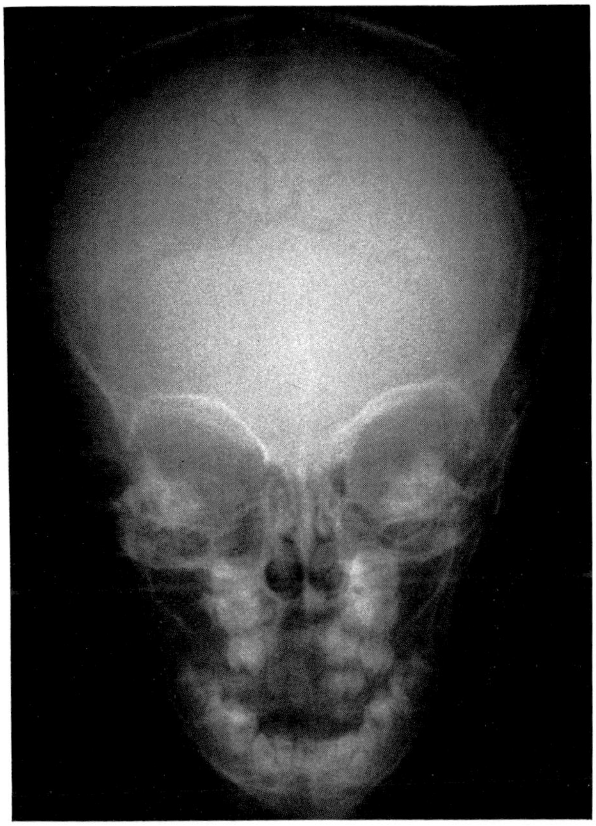

224 Skull in hypervitaminosis A. Lateral view of the same case.

224

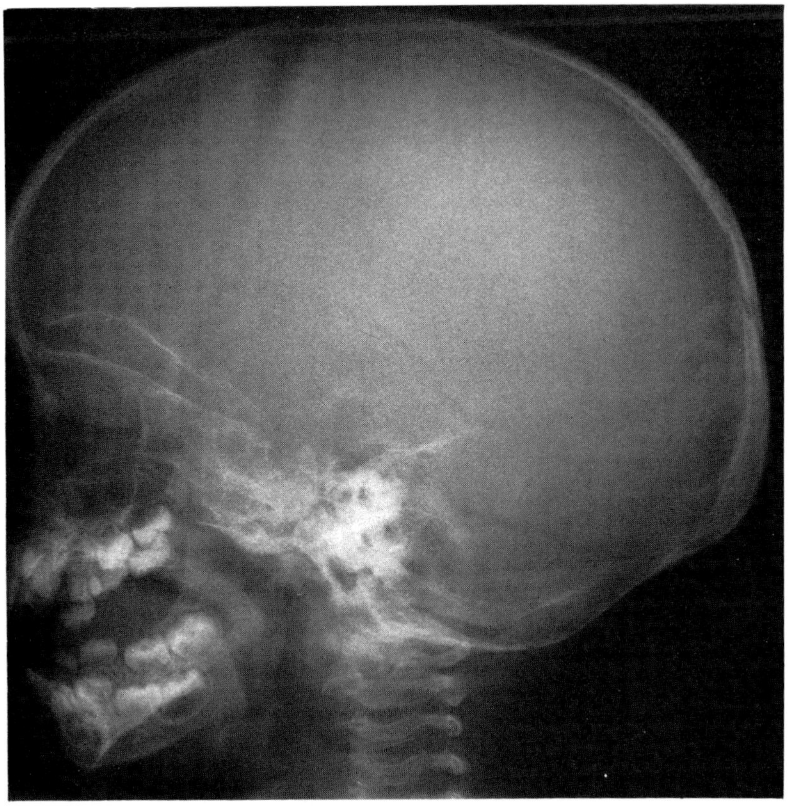

Hypercarotenosis

This is usually a benign condition in which pigmentation of the skin, which gradually fades when excessive intake of carotene is stopped, is the only manifestation (225–227).

225

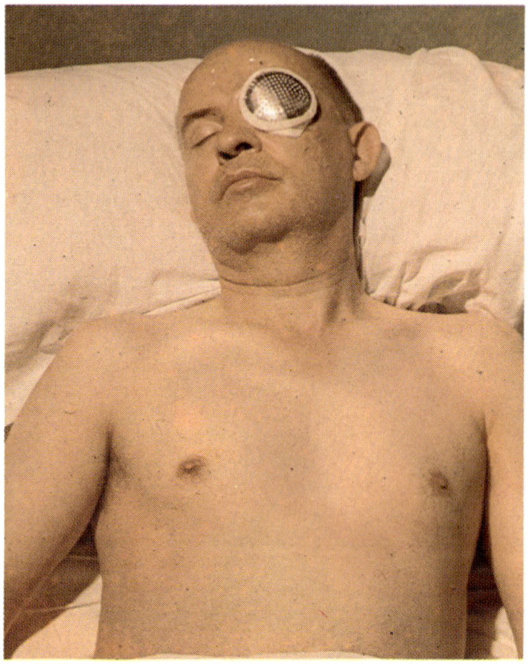

225 Hypercarotenosis. Prolonged excessive ingestion of carotenoids in carrot juice, carrots or dark green leafy vegetables leads to high blood levels and staining of the whole body. The condition is benign and subsides after withdrawal of the source. It may occur secondarily in diabetes mellitus, hypothyroidism or anorexia nervosa.

226

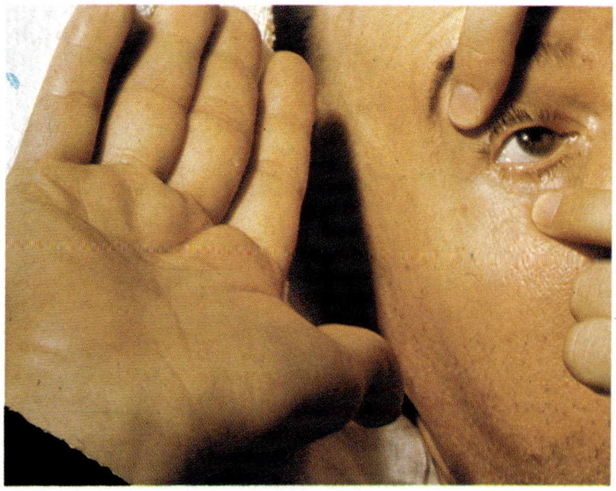

226 Hypercarotenosis. The face, eye and palm of the hand. The sclerae remain clear, distinguishing the condition from jaundice.

227

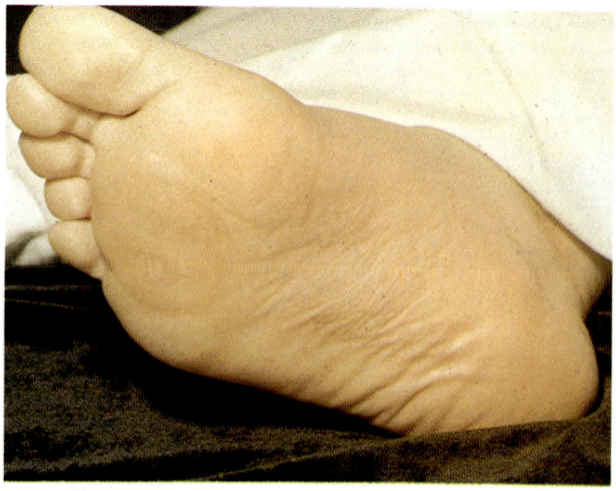

227 Hypercarotenosis. The sole of the foot. The staining is usually heaviest on the palms and soles due to the secretion of carotenoids by sebaceous glands heavily concentrated in these areas.

The carotenes responsible will vary with the source; with red palm oil (see page 102) it will be mainly B-carotene. In the case of a young woman who was a tomato soup faddist it was mostly lycopene, a nonprovitamin carotenoid. More serious have been reports of toxicity from canthaxanthin, another nonprovitamin carotenoid. Several cases of reversible retinopathy have been reported (**228, 229**) from Canada[71] and in the United States one young woman died. from aplastic anaemia. This substance is being sold for giving the skin a tanned appearance and is readily available through commercial tanning salons and mailing advertisements, although it has not been approved by the Food and Drug Administration.

228 **Retinal damage following a course of canthaxanthin.**

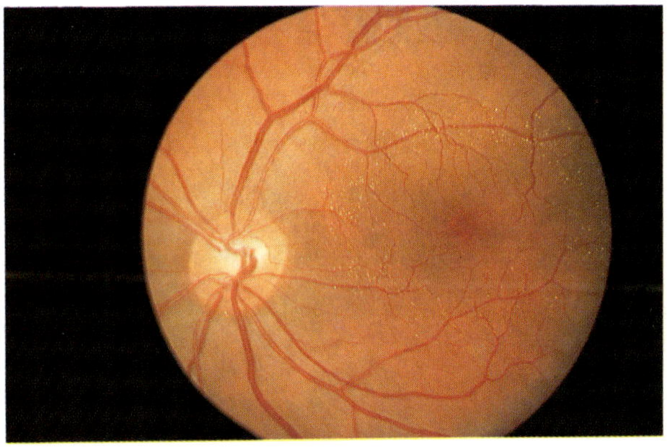

228

229 **The same retina after cessation of treatment** showing considerable regression of pigmentation and white exudates.

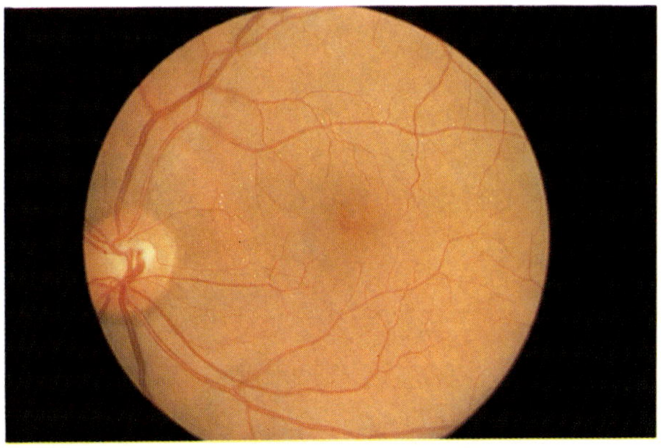

229

Retinoids

The increasing understanding of the role of retinol in epithelial cell differentiation has led to the development by the pharmaceutical industry of a large number of synthetic compounds with retinol-like structure; these are known as retinoids. They have been applied very successfully in the treatment of skin conditions in which epithelial differentiation is disordered. Severe acne often responds well and photo-ageing of the skin which may be precancerous improves markedly with topical tretinoin (**230, 231**).

Many of the patients have been young women and some of them have continued on the treatment after they have conceived. This has resulted in a number of reports of congenital malformations (**232**).[72]

Vitamin A itself has long been known to be teratogenic in experimental animals.

At the present time numerous field and clinical trials are being undertaken using retinoids, together with some of the carotenoids, in efforts either to prevent malignant change in epithelial tissues or as treatment of cancers in the early stages. Preliminary results are encouraging.

230

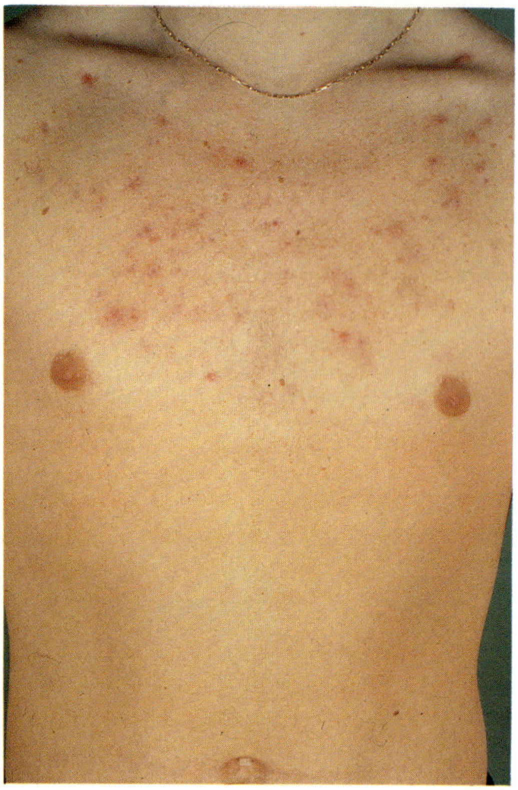

231

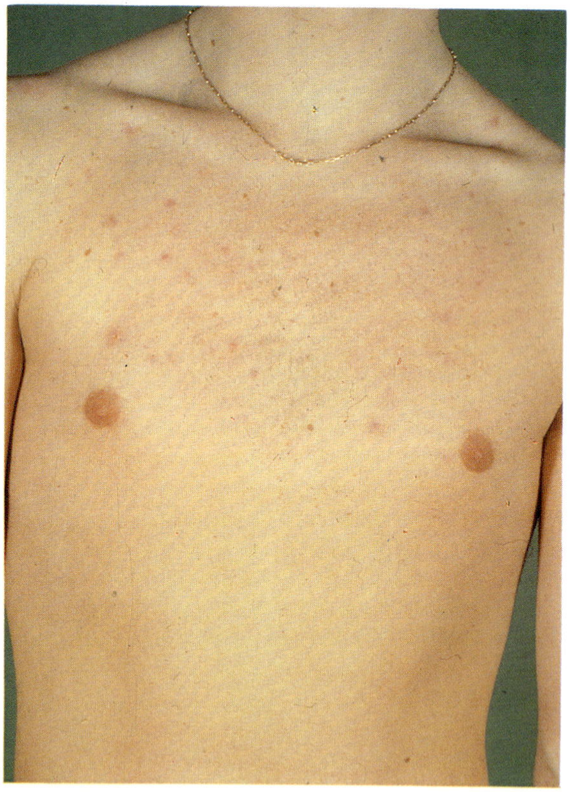

232

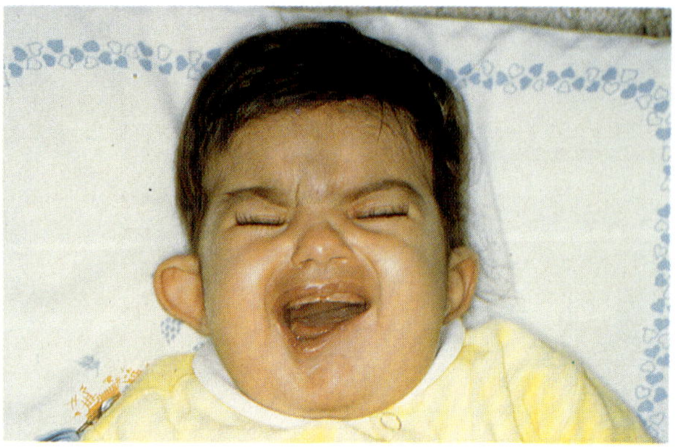

230 Severe acne of the chest before treatment with the retinoid isotretinoin systemically.

231 Same patient as in 230 after 2.5 months of treatment.

232 Retinoid embryopathy. Child born to a 22-year-old Brazilian woman who had been taking etretinate for psoriasis. Visible changes are bilateral lop ears with malformed antihelices, left lower facial nerve paralysis and upsweeping hair line. The cardiovascular abnormality tetralogy of Fallot had to be operated on. The abnormalities in this case have also occurred in offspring of women receiving tretinoin.

Vitamin D (calciferol)

Several compounds have vitamin D activity but only two are of practical nutritional importance. Vitamin D_2, ergocalciferol, is made from ergosterol by fungi and yeasts under the influence of ultraviolet light. It contributes little to the diet and is mainly used by the pharmaceutical industry. Vitamin D_3, cholecalciferol, is produced in skin by ultraviolet irradiation of 7-dehydrocholesterol. This is the main source of the vitamin, but it is present in dairy products naturally and is added to milk and some other products. Fish liver oils are very rich sources. Its sterol chemical structure, mode of formation in the body, and function in calcium homeostasis all indicate that calciferol and its derivatives act like hormones rather than vitamins (*Table 46* and **233**).

Even in less sunny parts of the world the average person obtains most of their vitamin D requirement from synthesis in the skin. It is therefore difficult to set a realistic RDA figure but this is usually given as 10μg for most age groups (Appendix I, Table 4). Blood levels of circulating metabolites are sensitive methods of assessing vitamin D nutritional status (Appendix III, Table 1). Plasma alkaline phosphatase is raised early in deficiency, indicating demineralization of bone. Hypocalcaemia and X-ray changes in bone appear late on in the disease, but are nevertheless useful for monitoring recovery.

Table 46. Actions of vitamin D and its metabolites.

Intestine	
	Enhances transport (absorption) of calcium – the main function of $1{,}25(OH)_2D_3$; phosphate and magnesium
Bone	
	Stimulates mineralization
	Mobilizes calcium to bone fluid compartment (PTH-like effect)
Muscle	
	Maintains integrity (? through Ca and P transfer)
Parathyroid glands	
	Inhibits PTH secretion
Lymphomedullary system	
	Antitumour activity
Other tissues	
	Control of cellular proliferation and differentiation
	? Regulation of intracellular calcium

233

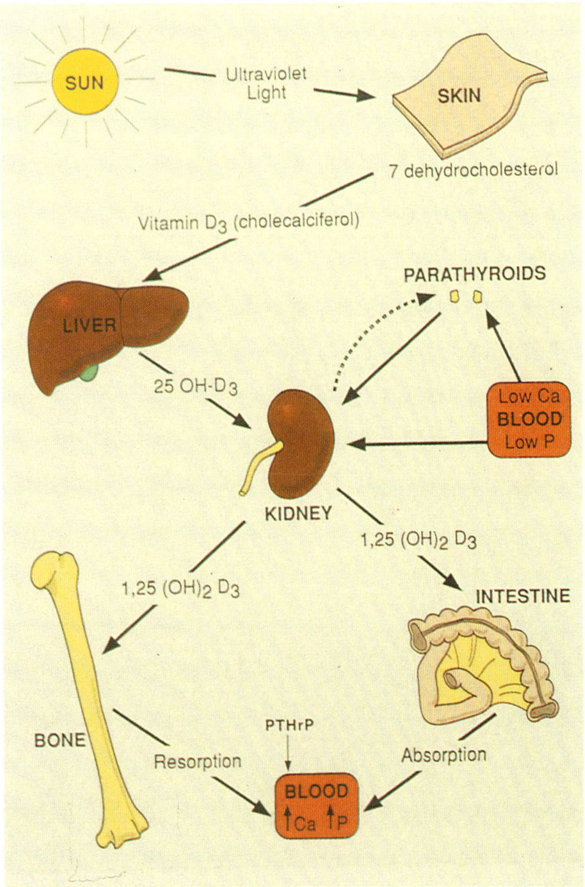

233 Metabolism of vitamin D_3. Vitamin D_3 is produced in the skin and is hydroxylated in the liver to produce 25-hydroxyvitamin D_3 (25-OHD_3). A second hydroxylation in the kidney produces 1,25-dihydroxyvitamin D_3 (1,25 $(OH)_2D_3$) which stimulates calcium absorption in the intestine and calcium resorption in bone. This increases calcium (Ca) in the blood. Low blood calcium stimulates parathyroid hormone secretion which increases production of $1{,}25(OH)_2D_3$ while low blood phosphorus (P) has a direct action on the kidney to stimulate synthesis of 1,25 $(OH)_2D_3$. Parathyroid-hormone-related protein (PTHrP) increases blood calcium.

Deficiency

The disease is called rickets while growth is occurring and osteomalacia in the adult and, as a result, the clinical features differ to some extent. In addition to primary or so-called nutritional rickets which relates to inadequate availability of the vitamin, there are numerous forms of endogenous deficiency (*Table 47*). While primary rickets and osteomalacia respond well to the vitamin (about 40μg daily) the metabolic disorders are sometimes refractory or in other instances respond well to about 1μg/day of the active metabolite $1,25(OH)_2D_3$ or the synthetic analogue 1-α $(OH)D_3$.

It is a mistake to think that rickets is absent from the tropics. In many third-world countries women spend long hours working in the fields or markets in the blazing sun and keep their infants covered (**234**). Swaddling is still practised (**235**).

Table 47. Classification of rickets and osteomalacia.

Deficiency of vitamin D
Dietary lack, lack of exposure to ultraviolet light

Impaired absorption
Malabsorption syndromes, high phytate or phosphate intake

Defects related to production of 25-$(OH)D_3$
Liver disease (advanced parenchymal and cholestatic)
Anticonvulsants (prolonged use of phenobarbital, phenytoin), enzyme induction, impaired absorption (?)

Defects related to action of $1,25(OH)_2D_3$
Vitamin D-dependent (pseudo-vitamin D deficiency) rickets, type I (defect in synthesis of 1,25 α hydroxylase)
Vitamin D-dependent rickets, type II (at least 2 types, receptors for $1,25(OH)_2D_3$ absent or defective)

Other forms
Familial hypophosphataemic (vitamin D-resistant) rickets, an X-linked dominant defect in phosphate transport across renal tubules
Hypophosphataemic bone disease – very rare autosomal dominant defect of phosphate absorption in renal tubules
Fanconi syndrome – autosomal recessive, general defects of absorption in renal tubules
Chronic renal failure (renal osteodystrophy); diabetes mellitus (increased incidence of osteopenia, osteoporosis); pseudohypoparathyroidism

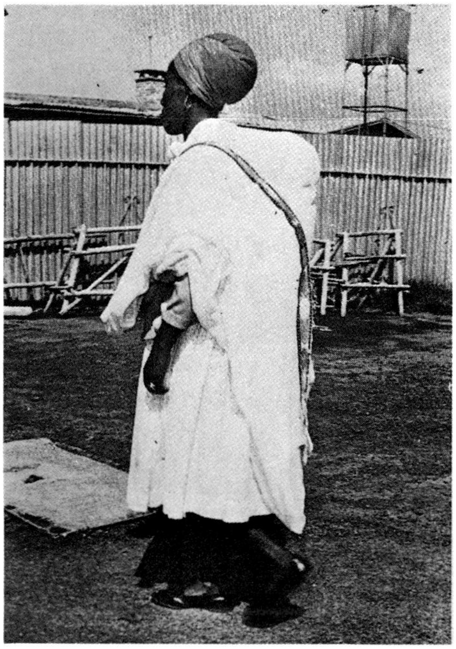

234

234 **Excessive protective clothing.** This Ethiopian mother is preventing the ultraviolet light acting on 7-dehydrocholesterol in the skin of the infant on her back to form its main source of vitamin D. Rickets is by no means uncommon in the tropics for this reason. The practice of purdah in which women in some cultures are largely confined to the house, together with their young children, has a similar result.

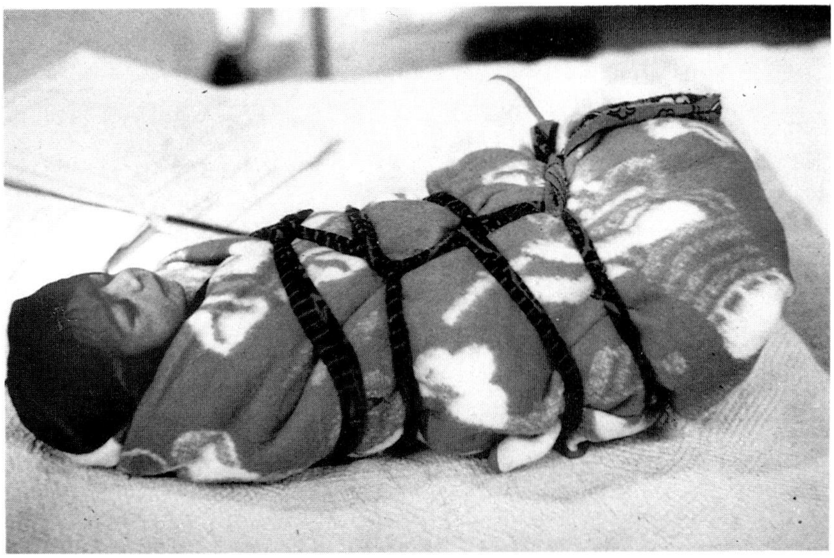

235

235 A Saudi infant characteristically swaddled.

Even in cities and towns young children may spend most of their time in dark basements or tenement buildings. Under these circumstances infantile rickets (**236–246**) often heals once the child is old enough to toddle out into the sunshine and the mother may be preoccupied with a newer arrival (**247**).

236

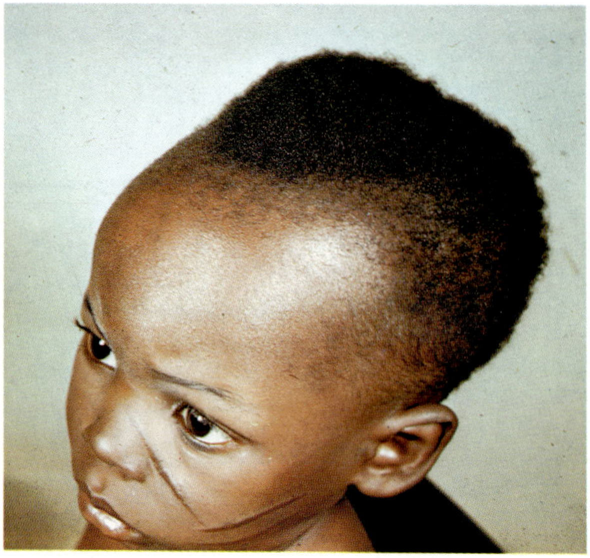

236 The skull in rickets. In infancy the frontal bones are prominent and bossed. The fontanelles are delayed in closing. The skull is soft to the touch and closely resembles pressure on a table tennis ball; the bone depresses then comes out again with eactly the same sensation. This is known as craniotabes. It is physiological at the suture lines and only indicative of rickets when it occurs also away from the suture lines.

237

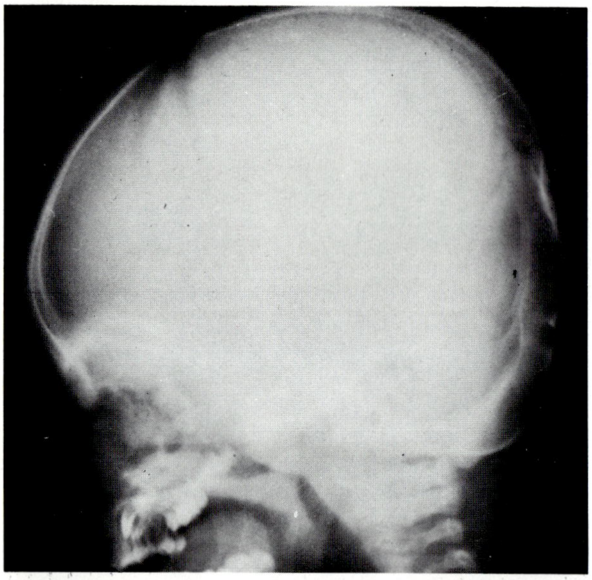

237 Skull X-ray in rickets. Frontal bossing and fontanelle separation are clearly shown.

238

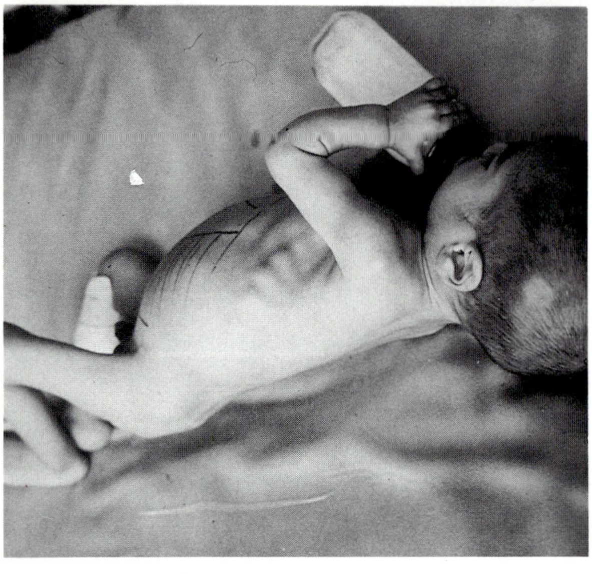

238 A typical rickety rosary of the ribs in a wasted, bottle-fed infant.

239 Harrison's sulcus or groove. This is a bilateral indentation of the lower ribs at the site of attachment of the diaphragm. Other deformities of the thorax, such as funnel chest, which is usually familial, and pigeon chest should not be attributed to rickets.

239

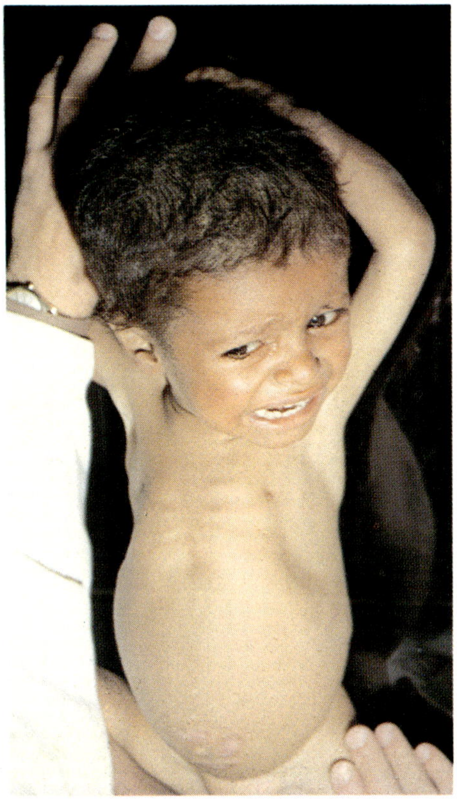

40

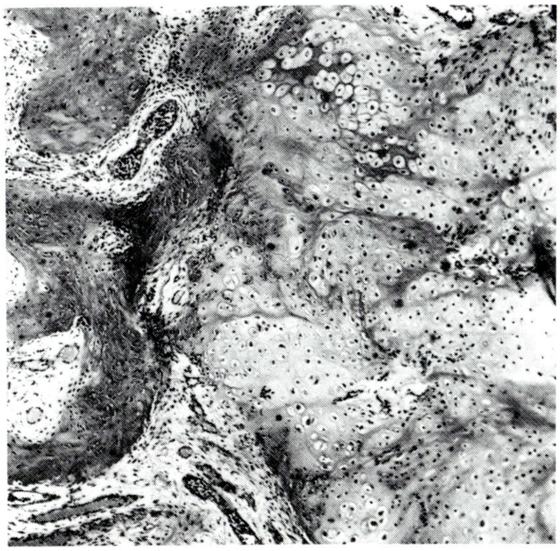

241

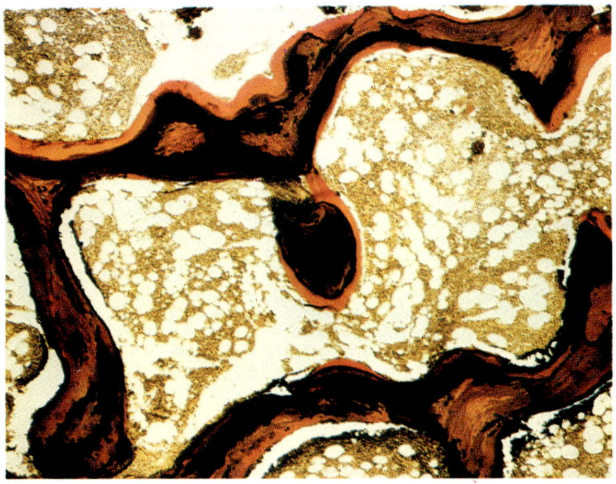

240 Bone in rickets. There is a failure in deposition of inorganic salts in the matrix of epiphyseal cartilage between rows of hypertrophied cartilage cells which are not destroyed and pile up irregularly to many times their normal thickness. This gives rise to the bulky mass of intermediate zone so evident on X-ray (see **243–246**). This zone is easily compressed, deformed or displaced. There may be excessive bone destruction as the result of increased parathyroid activity and the shafts readily bend under pressure.

241 Bone in rickets. In the shafts there are borders of osteoid around the bone trabeculae shown here with the uncalcified osteoid stained red. (*Tripp and McKay stain*)

242

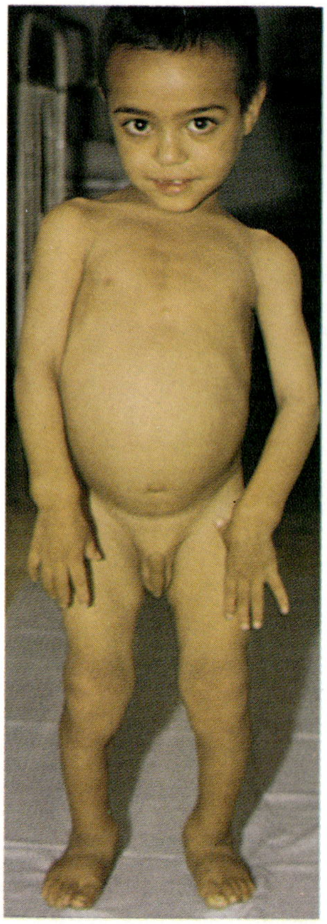

242 Bowlegs in rickets. The typical lateral curvature indicates that the weakened bones have bent after the second year as a result of standing. If severe rickets occurs before the child walks it produces a combination of bowed thighs and knock-knees. Bowing of the arms is less common, although X-ray changes at the wrist (see **243**) are almost invariably present in the infant. It precedes bowing of the legs and indicates active rickets during the last few months of the first year, when the child is crawling and pushing itself towards the erect position.

243 X-ray of the wrists. Some of the most characteristic and early changes take place here. The metaphyses are concave and irregular and the intervening zone of uncalcified osteoid is increased.

243

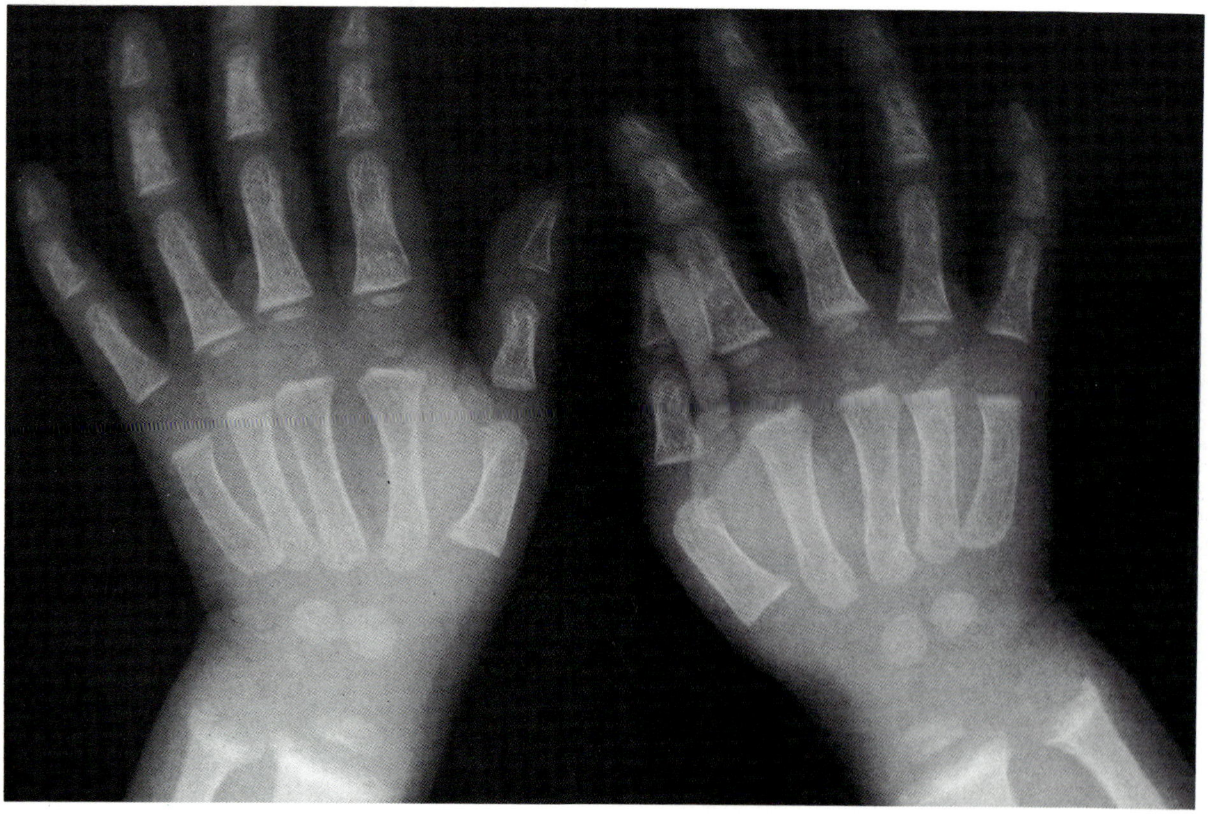

244

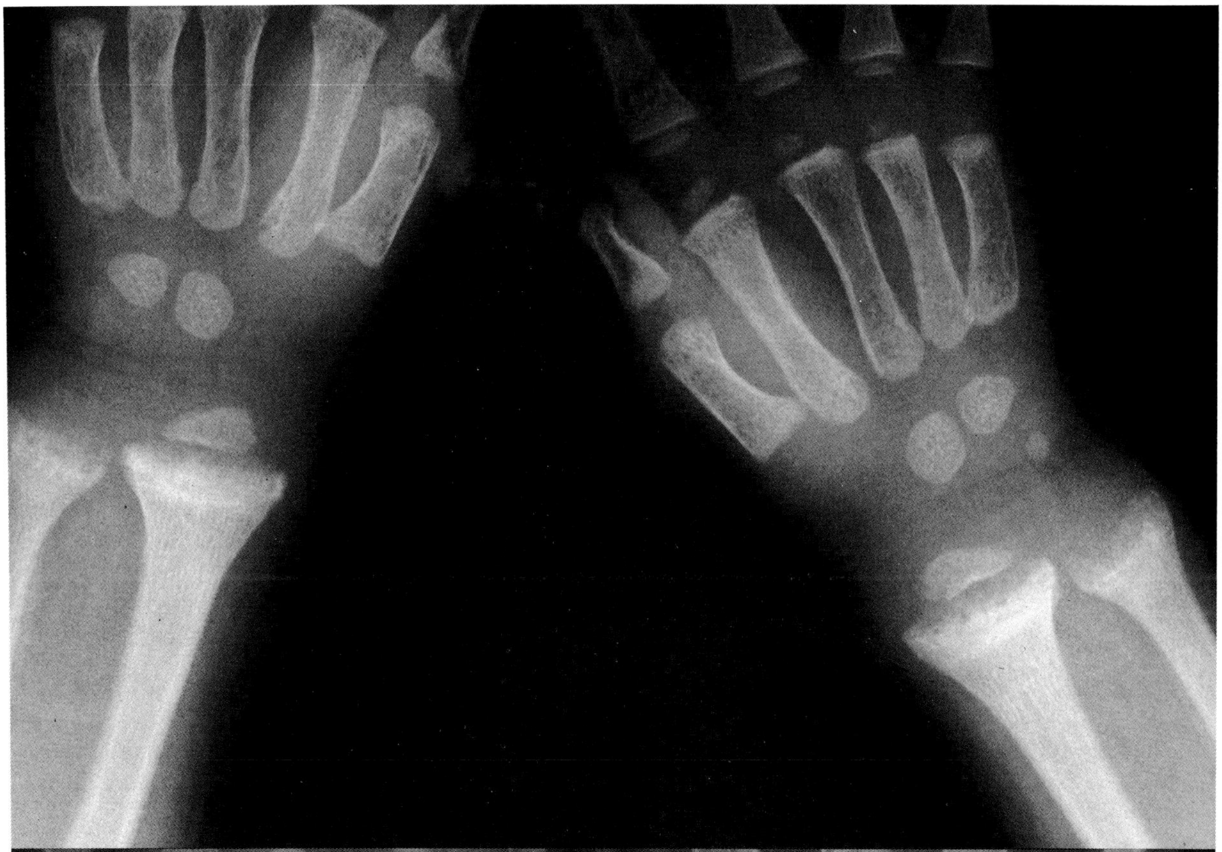

245

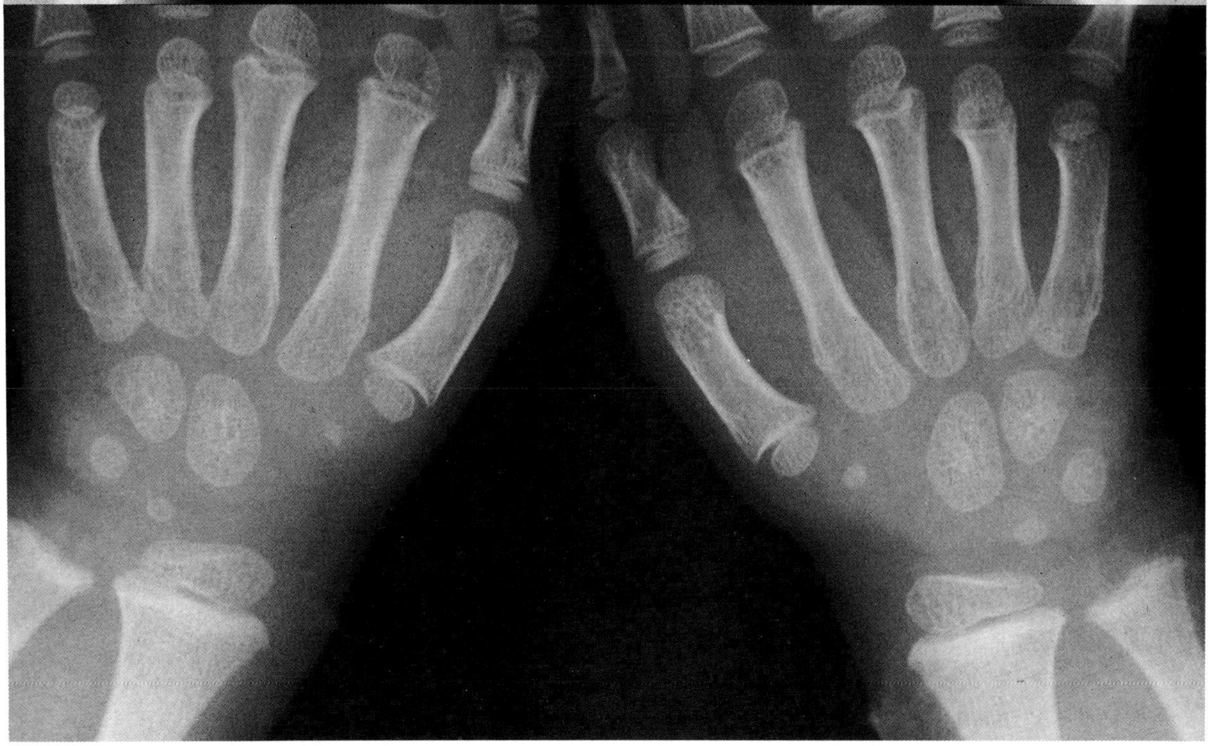

244 X-ray of the wrists. Partial healing after 4 months of treatment.

245 X-ray of the wrists. Complete healing 19 months after previous X-ray was taken.

246

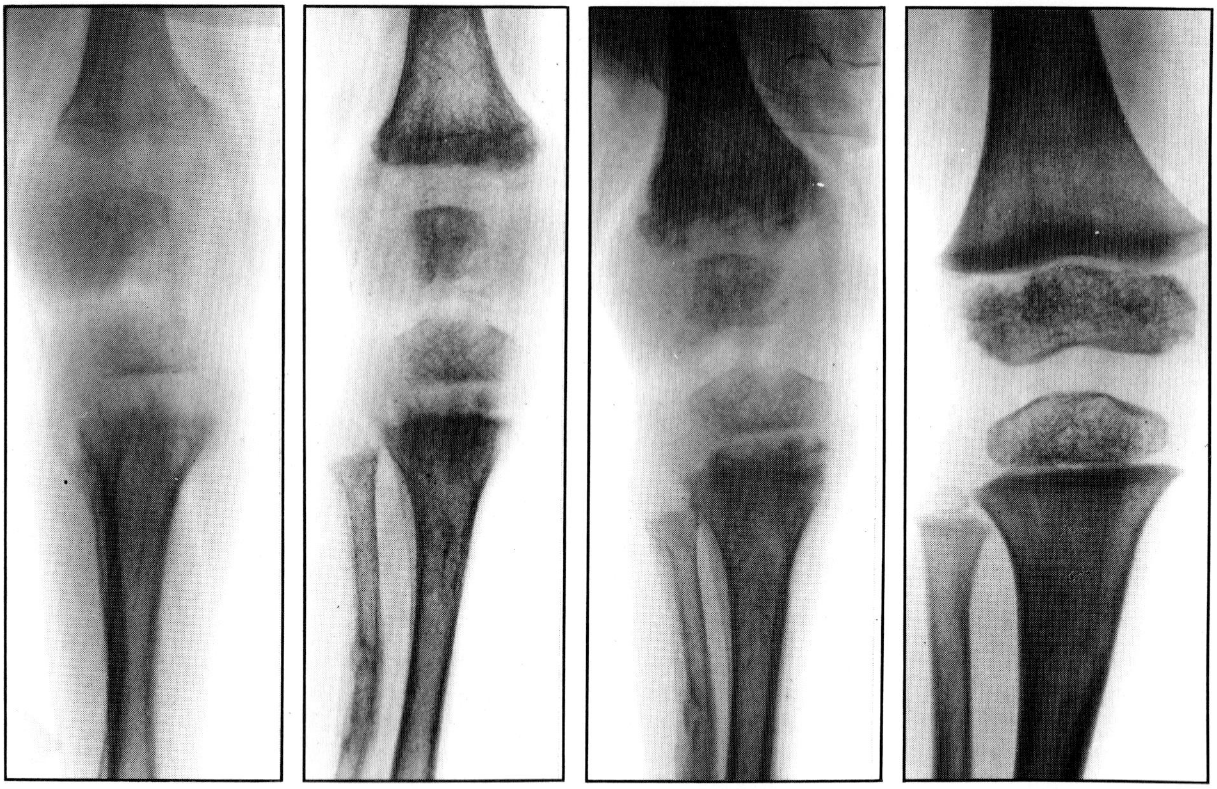

246 Active rickets of the knees. The metaphyses of the bones are concave and irregular and the zone of uncalcified osteoid is enlarged. These X-rays show the progressive changes over a 10-month period during which healing took place in this case.

247

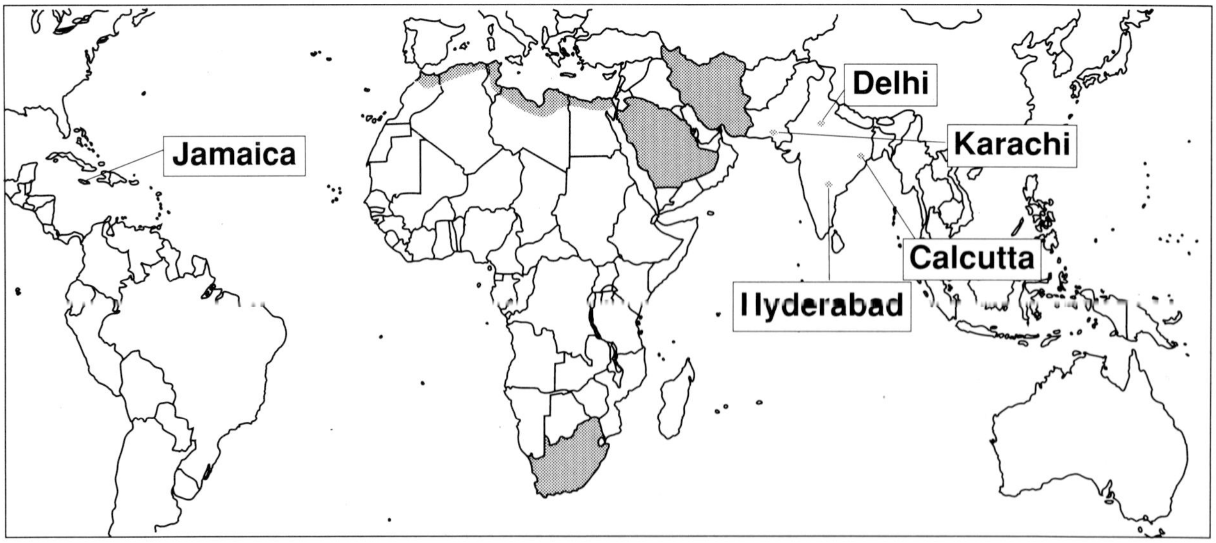

247 Areas of endemic rickets and osteomalacia in the tropics.

Some of the features of metabolic forms of rickets are shown in *Table 48* and **248–251**.

Table 48. Features of pseudohypoparathyroidism.

Hypocalcaemia produces –	Tetany (65%)
	Fits (65%)
	Cramps (40%)
	Laryngeal spasm
	Paraesthesiae
Other features –	Subcutaneous and basal calcification (due to hyperphosphataemia) (60%)
	Cataract (35%)
	Mental defects (10%)
	Skeletal–short metacarpals (70%)
	short metatarsals (40%)
	stocky, overweight (50–70%)
	bone density increased (15%)
	or decreased (15%)
	thickened calvaria (20%)

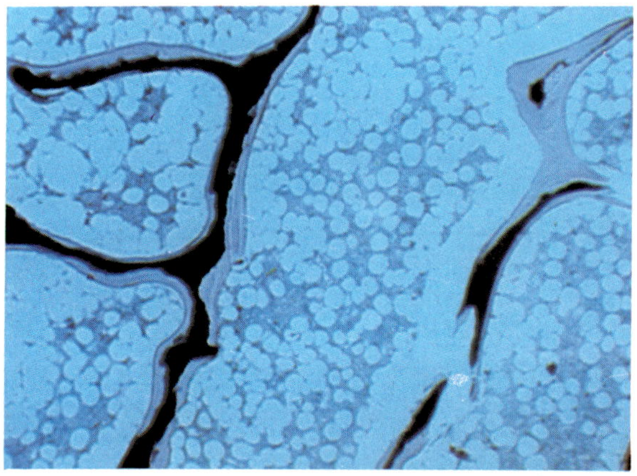

248

248 Vitamin D-resistant rickets. In a number of relatively rare metabolic disorders, rickets identical to that caused by a lack of vitamin D arises from defective hydroxylation of cholecalciferol in the liver or the kidney to the active hormone form 1,25$(OH)_2$ cholecalciferol. Very small daily doses of this compound or a synthetic analogue are often effective in treatment (see *Table 81*).

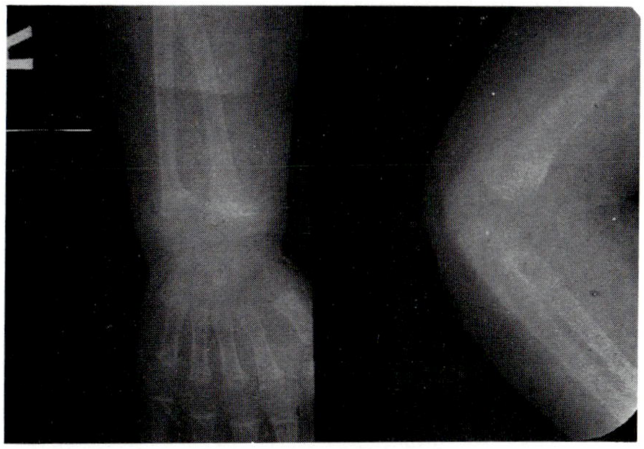

249

Courtesy of Professor Dame S. Sherlock and J.A. Summerfield.

249 Biliary rickets may complicate intrahepatic cholestasis of childhood. The general density of the bones is reduced. The metaphyses are widened and 'cupped' and the depth of the epiphyseal cartilage is increased.

250

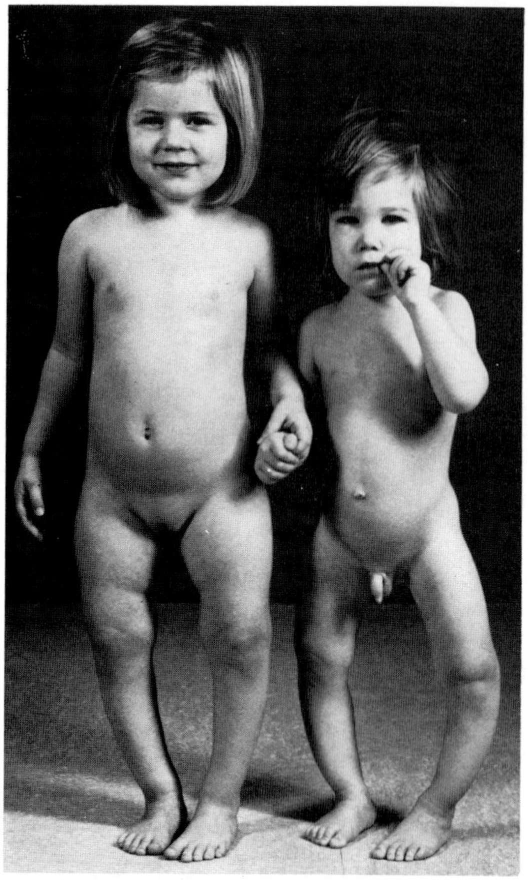

250 Hereditary vitamin D resistant rickets. Two children (of different parents) at ages 5 years and 3 years. Both are 9 cm too short.

251

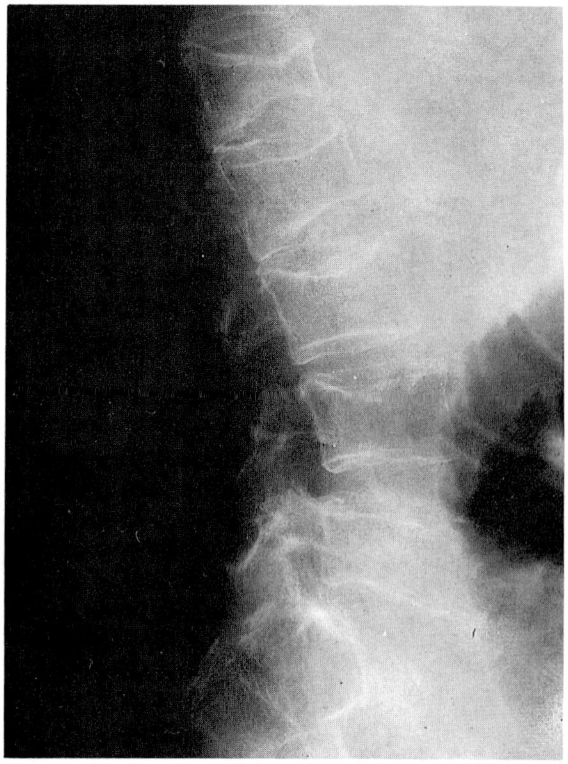

Courtesy of Professor Dame S. Sherlock and J.A. Summerfield.

251 Osteomalacia develops in chronic cholestasis due to abnormal calcium and vitamin D metabolism. Demineralization of the bones has led to crushed and wedge-shaped vertebral bodies in this patient. She had been jaundiced for five years following a benign bile duct stricture. Secondary biliary cirrhosis had developed. Back pain is a prominent complaint. Osteoporosis may also contribute to the bone thinning. Severe osteoporosis develops in cholestatic patients given prednisolone.

Osteomalacia has some distinctive pathological (252) and radiological features (253).

252

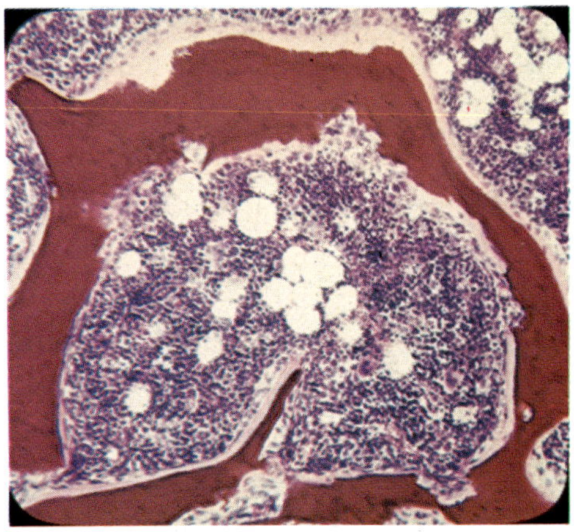

252 Osteomalacia. This is the adult form of vitamin D deficiency rickets. The section shows wide osteoid seams that cover all trabecular surfaces without increased numbers of osteoclasts.

253

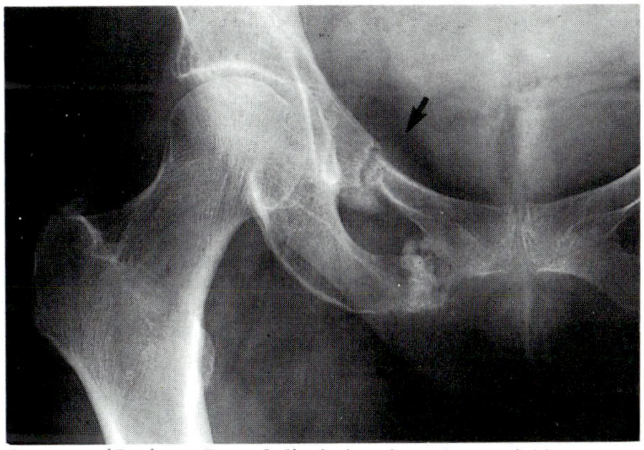

Courtesy of Professor Dame S. Sherlock and J.A. Summerfield.

253 Looser zones (Milkman lines). These radiotranslucent zones shown here in the pelvis, and also often occurring on the axillary border of the scapula, are 'pseudofractures' (there is no bone discontinuity as in true fractures) characteristic of osteomalacia from any cause. Besides nutritional vitamin D deficiency it occurs in patients with liver or kidney disease and secondary to some drugs from interference with vitamin D hydroxylation.

Contracted pelvis due to decalcification may result in obstructed labour after a rapid succession of normal pregnancies and prolonged lactation.

Vitamin D toxicity

Hypercalcaemia is a feature of hypervitaminosis D but has numerous other causes (see *Table 73*). A mild form of vitamin D toxicity is much less common now that the amount of vitamin D with which milk can be fortified is strictly limited. The onset is usually in later infancy. A rare severe form has a poor prognosis and constitutes a syndrome which includes osteosclerosis, hypercalciuria, nephrocalcinosis, mental retardation, 'elfin facies' (254, 255), and anomalies of the great vessels including supraventricular aortic stenosis.

254

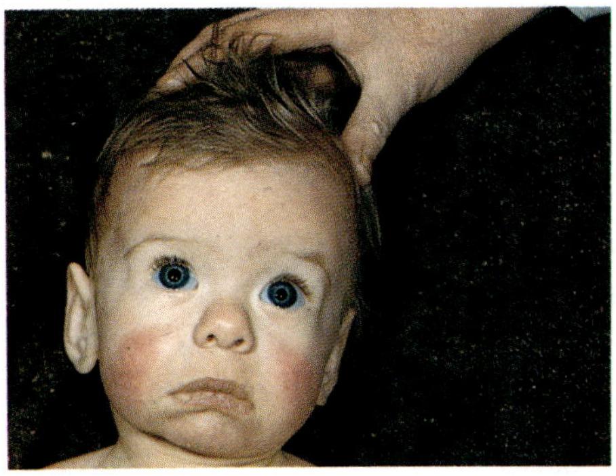

255

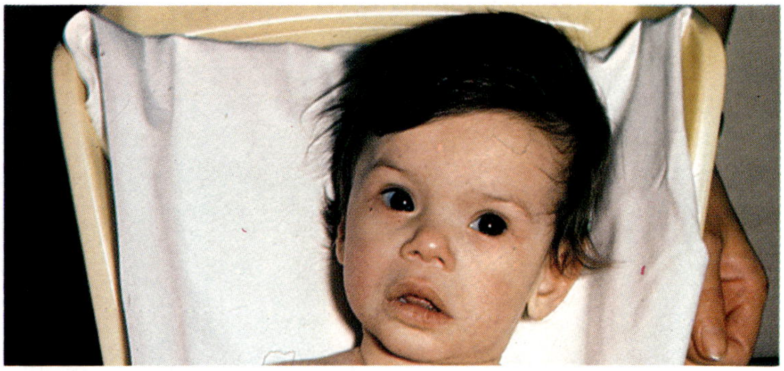

254, 255 Elfin facies of idiopathic hypercalcaemia. The characteristic facial appearance of the severe form of the disease is shown in these two patients. They are unrelated but the similarity of features might suggest a family likeness.

X-ray of the skeleton can be helpful in diagnosis (**256, 257**) and plasma alkaline phosphatase is low.

Treatment consists of commercially available milk low in calcium and without added vitamin D, and acidification of the urine.

256

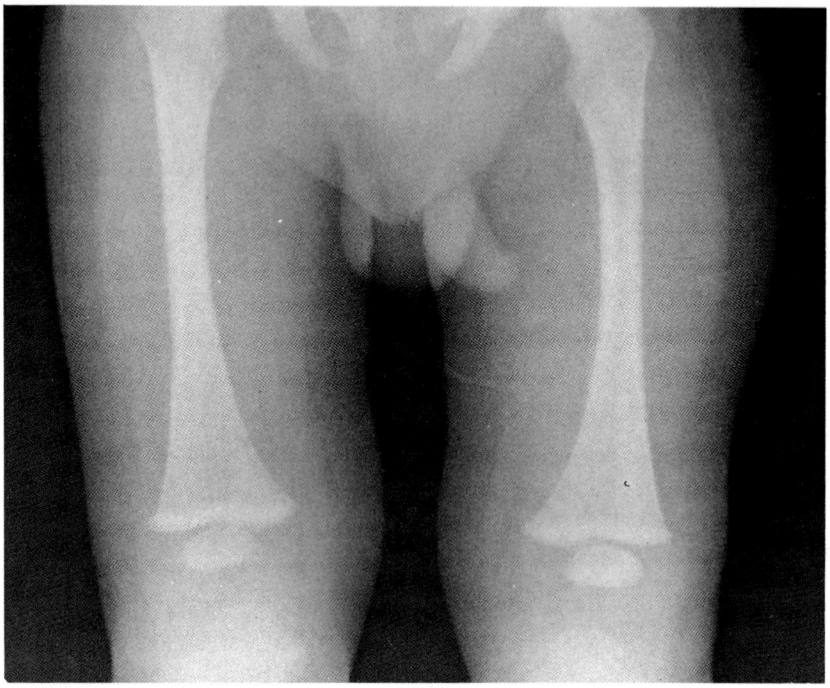

256 Idiopathic hypercalcaemia. X-ray shows increased epiphyseal bone density due to excessive calcium deposition.

257

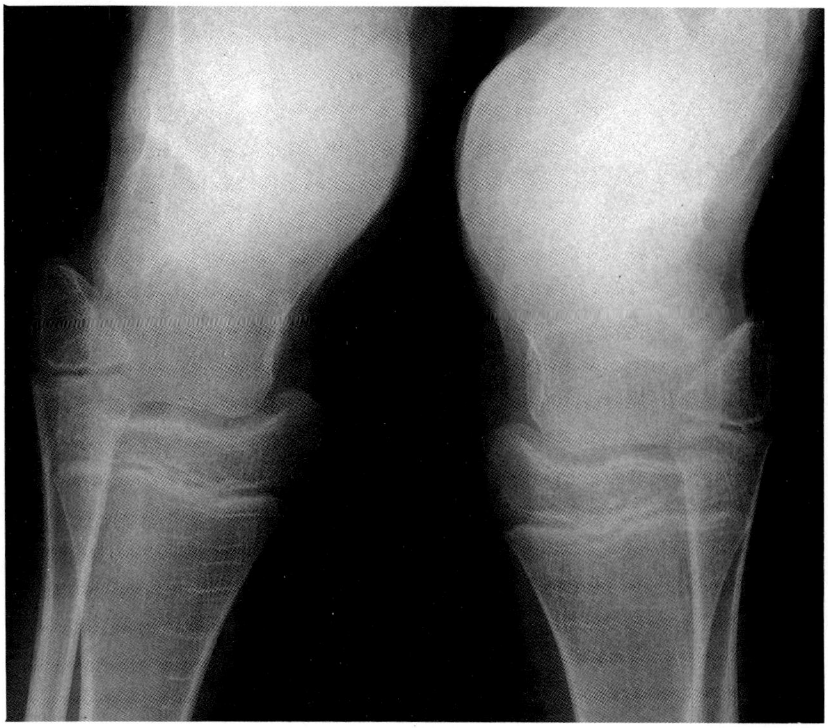

257 Idiopathic hypercalcaemia. There are marked 'growth lines' of excessive calcium deposition in this cured case.

Vitamin E (tocopherol)

Eight tocopherols and tocotrienols have vitamin E activity, the most potent being α tocopherol. It is found mainly in vegetable oils, in amounts roughly proportional to polyunsaturated fatty acids which it helps to protect from oxidation.

Plasma levels (normal 0.8–1.4mg/100ml in adults) reflect nutritional status and are lower in infants and very low in low birthweight infants. Apart from its antioxidant function little is known about the actions of vitamin E, which resemble those of selenium (see page 223) in some respects. The adult RDA is about 10mg α-tocopherol equivalents.

Deficiency

Dietary intake is rarely inadequate, except in early life. Retinopathy of prematurity (ROP) is primarily due to oxygen excess in the treatment of the low birthweight infant but there is some evidence that low vitamin E status may make it worse and that dosing with vitamin E brings some improvement (**258**).

Secondary deficiency due to malabsorption or liver disease has resulted in brown bowel syndrome (**259, 260**) and spinocerebellar degeneration, and is one of the causes of intraventricular or subependymal haemorrhage in the newborn (see vitamin K, page 137).

The retinopathy seen in abetalipoproteinaemia (see **229**) is especially responsive to large doses of vitamin E. In these conditions as much as 100–600mg tocopheryl acetate has been given daily.

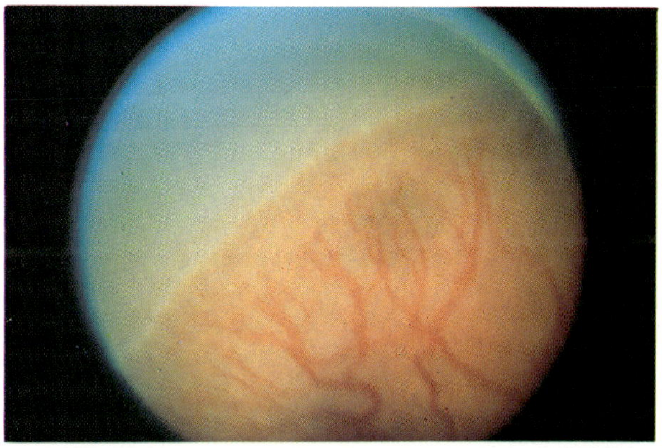

258 **Fundus in an infant with retinopathy of prematurity** (previously called retrolental fibroplasia) showing the abnormal ridge of vascular tissue that forms between the vascularized and non-vascularized temporal retina.

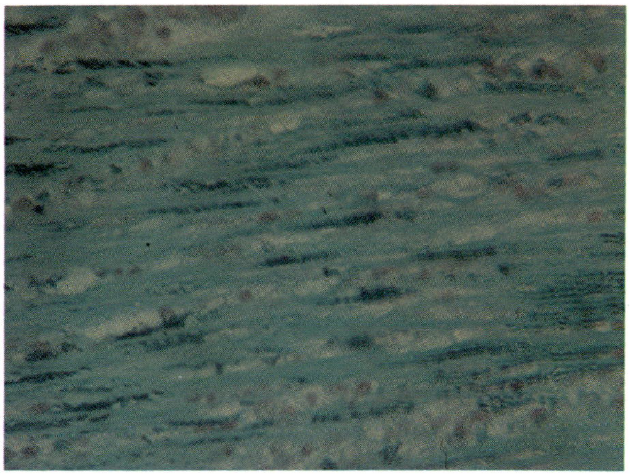

259 **Brown bowel syndrome.** Part of the circular layer of the tunica muscularis of the small intestine showing fusiform accumulation of lipofuscin pigment within muscle cells. Vitamin E deficiency is thought to play a part in this and other disorders in which there is smooth muscle myopathy probably of mitochondrial origin. (*Nile blue*, × 200)

260 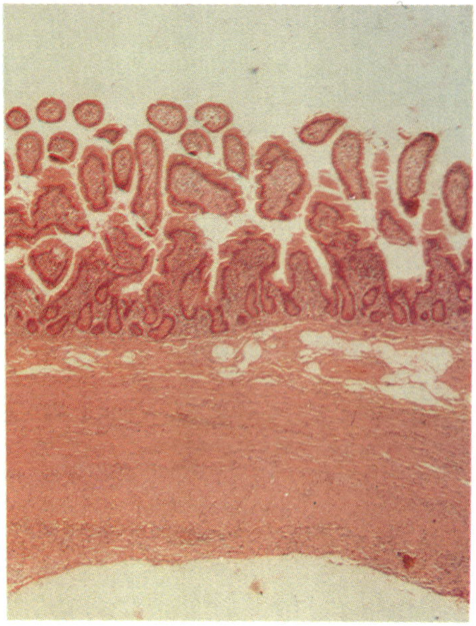

260 Brown bowel syndrome. A transverse section of the jejunum showing normal mucosa, healthy villus pattern and no evidence of mucus gland depletion. The muscularis mucosae is intact and the tunica muscularis shows no oedema or inflammation. (*H&E*, × 180)

Toxicity

In low birthweight infants large doses of a preparation now banned have caused a high rate of sepsis and necrotizing enterocolitis (see *Table 95*) with a high mortality.

Vitamin K (phylloquinone)

This vitamin is unusual in that about half the required amount is synthesized by the normal intestinal flora, the other half coming from the diet, especially dark green leafy vegetables and some fruit, tubers and seeds. It is necessary for the formation of blood coagulation factors II (prothrombin), VII, IX and X by the liver. It acts by inducing the carboxylation of glutamyl residues that give rise to a new amino acid, γ-carboxylglutamic acid, necessary for normal prothrombin formation and calcium binding. About 100μg are required by the adult daily.

For many years vitamin K status was assessed by measurement of the prothrombin time or bleeding and coagulation times of blood, but a more sensitive test is now being generally introduced. It is a monoclonal, monospecific antibody test which measures abnormal proteins that are produced in the absence of vitamin K and is known as PIVKA II (proteins induced in the absence of vitamin K) (see Appendix III, Table 1).

Deficiency

Table 49 indicates the very varied circumstances in which vitamin K deficiency may arise. The newborn is especially susceptible because the gut flora have not been established and enzymes in the liver involved in the synthesis of the coagulation factors may be immature. Vitamin K therapy will overcome the former problem. All newborns should be given prophylactic vitamin K (0.5–1mg phytomenadione) either intramuscularly or orally; alternatively the mother may be dosed before delivery (**261, 262**).

Table 49. Causes of deficiency of prothrombin and other vitamin K-dependent coagulation factors.

Haemorrhagic disease of the newborn
Dietary inadequacy: low-fat diets, PEM
Total parenteral nutrition deficient in vitamin K
Biliary obstruction: gallstones, stricture, fistula
Malabsorption syndromes: e.g. cystic fibrosis, sprue, coeliac disease, ulcerative colitis, Crohn's disease, short bowel syndrome
Liver disease: impaired synthesis – not responsive to vitamin K therapy
Drug therapy: coumarin anticoagulants and related drugs; antibiotics including cephalosporins; megadoses of vitamin E

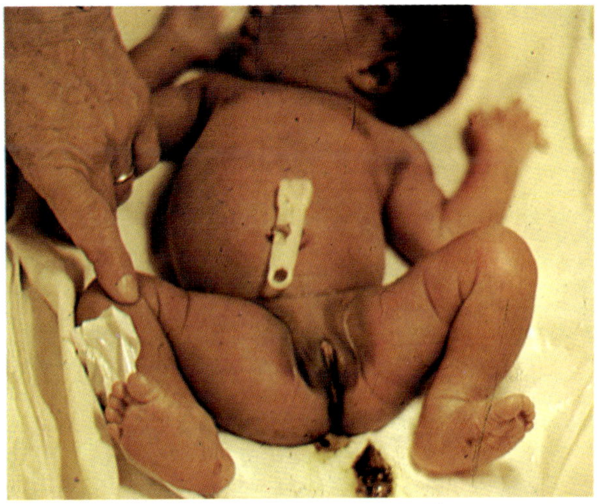

261

261 Haemorrhagic disease of the newborn. The most common sites for bleeding are the gut (producing melaena neonatorum), large cephalohaematomas, the umbilical stump, and from circumcision. Generalized ecchymoses (often without petechiae), and large intramuscular haemorrhages may develop less commonly.

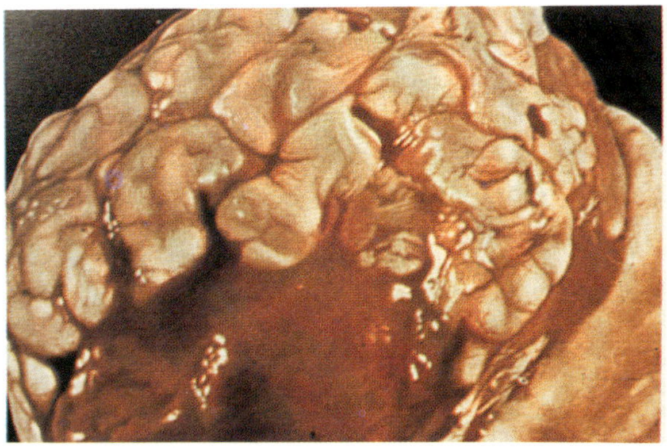

262

262 Haemorrhagic disease of the newborn. Fatal subdural haemorrhage.

Toxicity

Children with glucose-6-phosphate dehydrogenase (G6PD) deficiency and very low birthweight babies are especially susceptible to develop haemolytic anaemia when given the synthetic vitamin K analogue Menadol or its water-soluble derivatives. This drug is still available and warning against its use in children is not always given. Premature infants have occasionally developed the serious condition kernicterus (**263**).

263

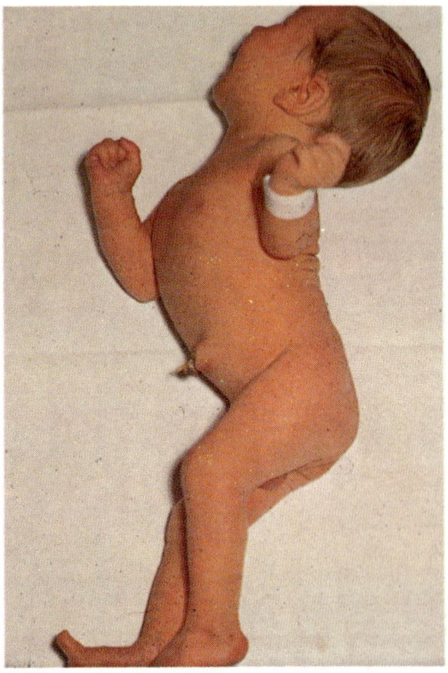

263 Kernicterus (bilirubin encephalopathy). Menadiol and its water-soluble derivatives may cause this in low birthweight infants in relatively high doses (75mg). It is attributed to increased haemolysis and inhibition of glucuronide formation, leading to the deposition of unconjugated bilirubin in the lipid-rich basal ganglia in the midbrain. Vitamin K is free from these effects and should be used in treatment.

The affected infant becomes lethargic, hypotonic and loses the sucking reflex. Later opisthotonos and generalized spasticity develop, followed by irregular respiration, and death results from pulmonary complications. Survivors may suffer from the post-kernicterus syndrome: high-frequency nerve deafness, athetoid cerebral palsy and dental enamel dysplasia. This patient shows neck retraction, hypertonic extensor spasm of the limbs and intense jaundice.

Essential fatty acids (EFA)

Most fatty acids can be interconverted by the body but this is not true for at least three, which must be present in the diet. Fatty acids are usually identified by a shorthand formula that consists successively of the number of carbon atoms, number of unsaturated bonds, and position of the double bond in relation to the terminal methyl group. Arachidonic acid (C20:4 n–6) is present in small amounts in animal tissues but can be synthesized from linoleic acid (C18:2 n–6) which makes up a high proportion of corn oil and other vegetable cooking oils. Prostaglandins, thromboxanes, prostacyclins and leukotrienes are all synthesized in the body from arachidonic acid.

The other essential fatty acid is in another series, the n–3 series, and is α-linolenic acid (C18:3 n–3). Vegetable oils are good sources. In the n–3 series also is eicosapentaenoic acid (C20:5 n–3) which although not essential is present in large amounts in fatty fish and has a thrombolytic effect in the circulation (see Chapter 3).

There is no RDA established for EFAs but intake of linoleic acid should be about 6–8% of total energy intake, as it is in most human diets. A minimum of 1% is advisable for linolenic acid. A sensitive method of assessing EFA status is the triene:tetraene ratio (20:3 n–9/ 20:4) in plasma. Early deficiency is present when this ratio is 0.4 or above, resulting from increased amounts of an abnormal metabolite 20:3 n–9 and diminished 20:4 acids.

Deficiency

It is becoming evident that linoleic acid deficiency affects mainly the skin, while deficiency of linolenic acid is associated mainly with neurological changes.

Prolonged parenteral nutrition which was lipid-free has been associated with a dry, flaky skin which precedes scaling, eczematoid dermatosis, usually starting on the nasolabial folds and eyebrows and spreading across the face and neck (**264, 265**). Anaemia and enlarged fatty liver have also been reported. Intralipid providing 100–300 g linoleate was curative in such cases and has been routine in parenteral nutrition for some years.

Linolenic acid deficiency in man is not fully substantiated. Following extensive gut resection a few patients with neurologic changes including paraesthesiae, weakness, inability to walk, pain in the legs and blurred vision have been reported to respond to incorporation of linolenic acid into the parenteral therapy.

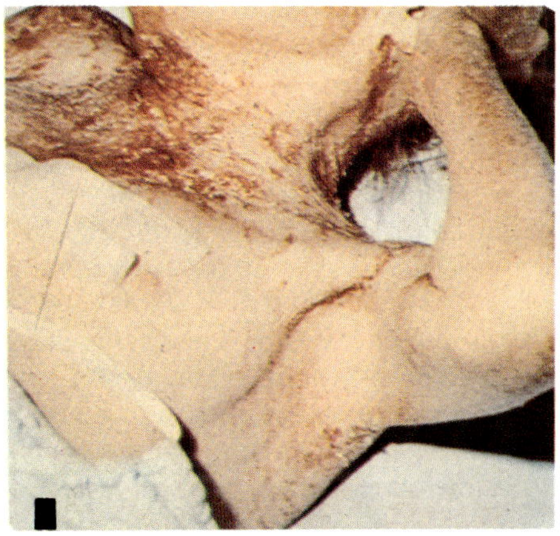

264

264 Essential fatty acid deficiency. Linoleic, linolenic and arachidonic acids are essential dietary constituents and in this respect resemble vitamins. They are necessary for growth, membrane formation and integrity of the skin. They are precursors of the prostaglandins.

Clinical deficiency is rare as most normal dietaries supply the body's requirements. Patients receiving fat-free parenteral nutrition have developed biochemical abnormalities and skin lesions as shown here.

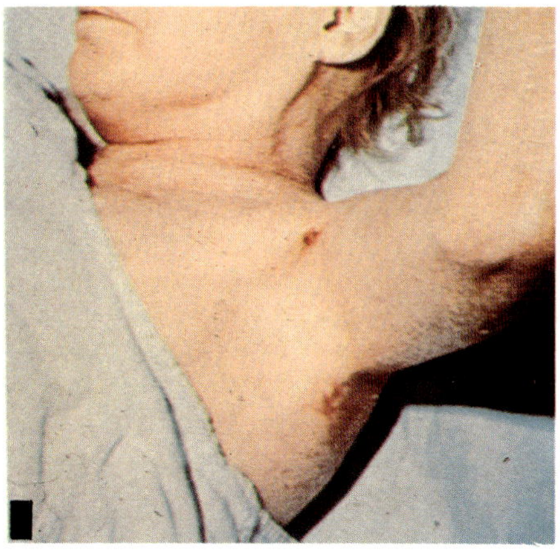

265

265 Essential fatty acid deficiency. Complete resolution in the same patient after 2 weeks of treatment with Intralipid.

Thiamin (vitamin B_1)

Thiamin is mainly found in cereals but it is also present in meat, fish and dairy products. Thiamin content in food is considerably reduced in cooking by heating, oxidation and leaching.

Thiamin pyrophosphate (TPP, cocarboxylase) is the coenzyme of carboxylase which plays an important role in carbohydrate metabolism in the decarboxylation of pyruvic and α-ketoglutaric acids. Thiamin also activates transketolase, an enzyme in the direct oxidative pathway for glucose. Transketolase activity in red blood cells may be used for assessment of thiamin status; direct measurement of TPP in plasma is more sensitive but is not in general use at present (Appendix III, Table 1). The adult RDA is about 1.0 mg.

Deficiency (beriberi)

This tends to arise under two strikingly different circumstances – rice-dependent third world cultures and chronic alcoholism in industrialized societies.

Oriental beriberi is nearly always associated with the consumption of non-parboiled commercially milled rice as staple food. In rice, as in other cereals, thiamin and other B group vitamins are present mainly in the germ, pericarp and endosperm; they are largely removed by commercial milling but remain intact after home pounding. Parboiling before pounding, has the effect of dispersing the vitamins and so preserving them. As diets have become more diversified beriberi has tended to diminish.

Beriberi is the most common and serious nutritional deficiency affecting chronic alcoholics. A combination of factors is responsible – poor and monotonous diet; impaired absorption, tissue storage, and phosphorylation in the liver; and increased requirements for thiamin due to a high energy consumption (ethanol = 7kcal/g).

Beriberi takes three main clinical forms. The highly fatal infantile beriberi results from exclusive breastfeeding by mildly deficient mothers. The symptomatology may take different forms as shown in **266**. Dry (neurological) beriberi in its least serious form consists of chronic peripheral neuropathy, with wrist drop and/or foot drop as prominent features (**267**).

Response to thiamin is not uniformly good; there is some improvement with multivitamin therapy that suggests that deficiency of other vitamins may also be involved. Complete recovery is often not achieved.

266

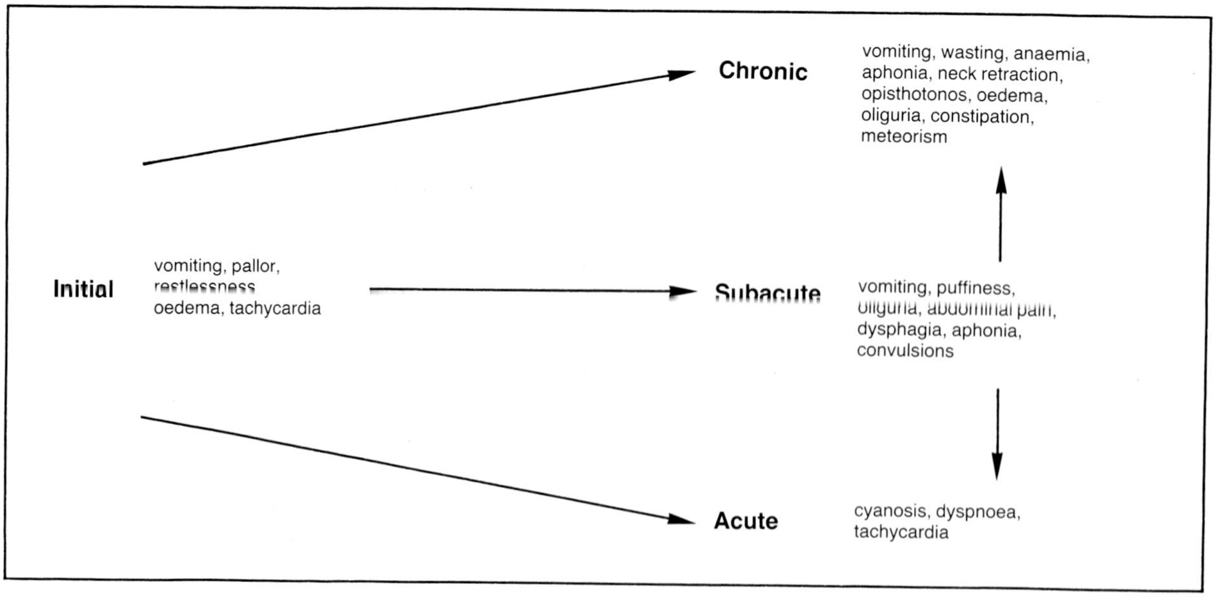

266 Infantile beriberi. Forms and progression of the disease.

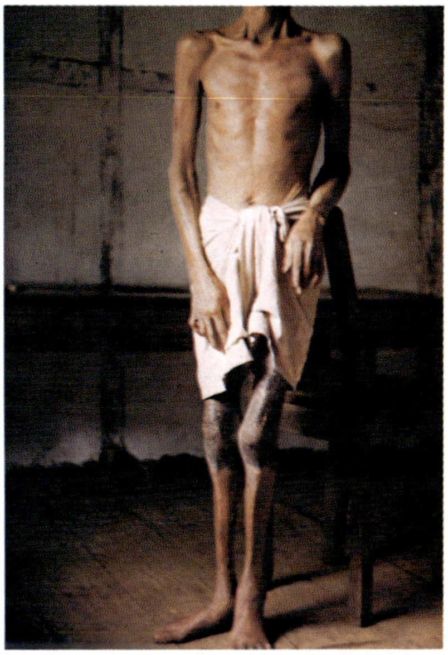

267

267 Wrist drop and foot drop. This patient has chronic polyneuritic 'dry' beriberi. In these patients there is also loss of tendon reflexes, joint position sense, and vibration sense, tenderness in the calf muscles on pressure, anaesthesia of the skin especially over the tibia, paraesthesiae in the legs and arms, and motor weakness.

More serious are the central nervous system changes known as Korsakoff's psychosis and Wernicke's encephalopathy, or sometimes as the Wernicke–Korsakoff syndrome[73] (**268, 269**).

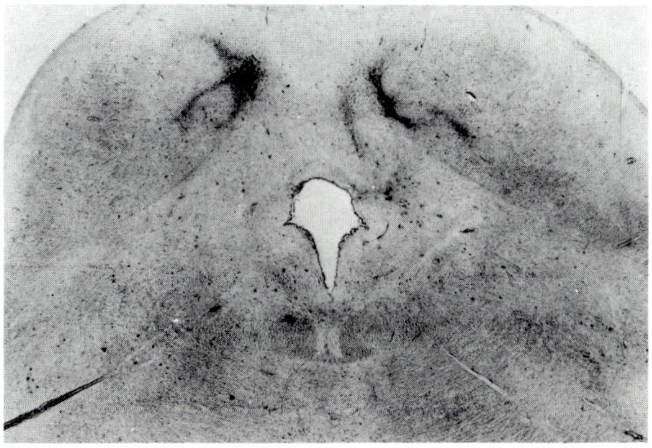

268

268 Wernicke–Korsakoff syndrome. Mental confusion, aphonia and nystagmus progress to bilateral 6th nerve paralysis and coma. Polyneuropathy is frequent. This section shows symmetrical haemorrhages in the corpora quadrigemina. Small petechiae are also present in the peri-aqueductal grey matter. (*H&E*, × 4)

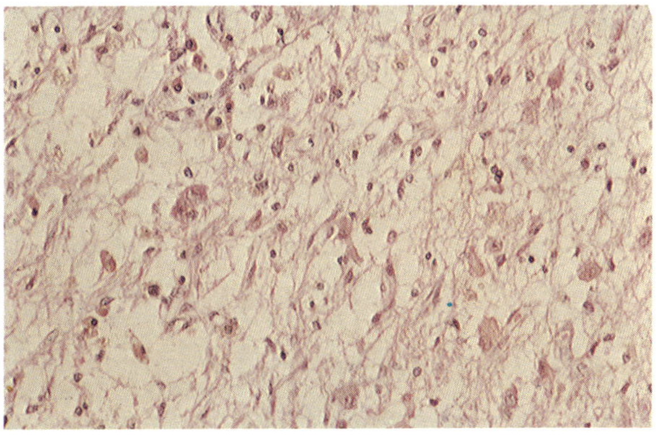

269

269 Wernicke's encephalopathy. Spongy degeneration in the mammillary body, with loss of nerve cells and astrocytic reaction. Some macrophages contain haemosiderin as the acute haemorrhagic stage is past (*H&E*, × 160).

The general progression of symptoms and signs appears to be from the Wernicke state to Korsakoff amnesic-confabulation and, in those who survive, a permanent amnesic defect.[74] Treatment consists of large doses, about 100mg daily, at first intravenously, and initial response is usually dramatic. In Korsakoff's psychosis the response is only partial and alcoholism itself may play a part in neurotoxicity (see Chapter 9). Wet (cardiovascular) beriberi is also an acute medical emergency requiring intravenous thiamin (**270–274**).

There is evidence[75] that severe lactic acidosis, due directly to the block in carbohydrate metabolism, is responsible for the high fatality rate, rather than cardiac failure as has been generally supposed.

Thiamin deficiency may underly many cases of what has been called 'sudden cardiac death' (see Chapter 2).

270

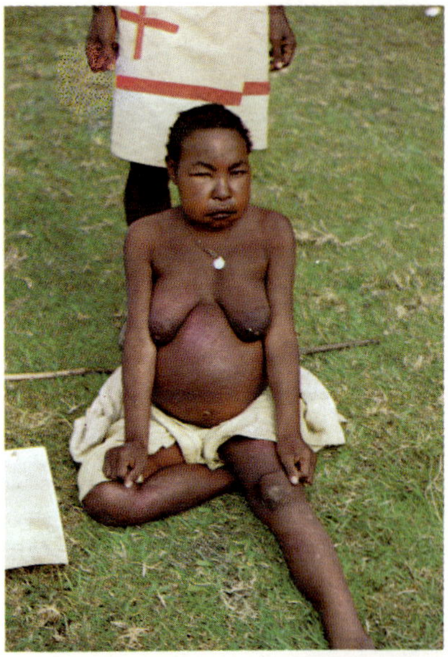

270 **'Wet' or cardiac beriberi.** Generalized oedema results from biventricular heart failure with pulmonary congestion. Peripheral vasodilatation, mainly in skeletal muscle, leads to high output failure with increased right ventricular pressure and left ventricular filling pressure. Pyruvate and lactate are important substrates for oxidation in cardiac muscle, and the decarboxylation of pyruvate and its subsequent oxidation in the citric acid cycle are blocked in thiamin deficiency.

271

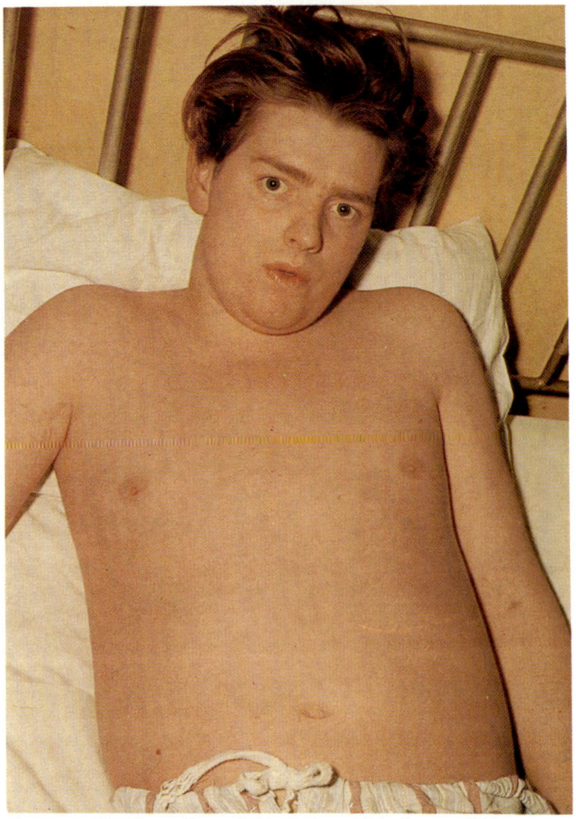

Courtesy of Professor Dame S. Sherlock and J.A. Summerfield.

271 Cardiac beriberi in a patient with chronic alcoholism. There is pitting oedema up to his chest.

272 Cardiac beriberi. Enlarged right atrium and ventricle.

272

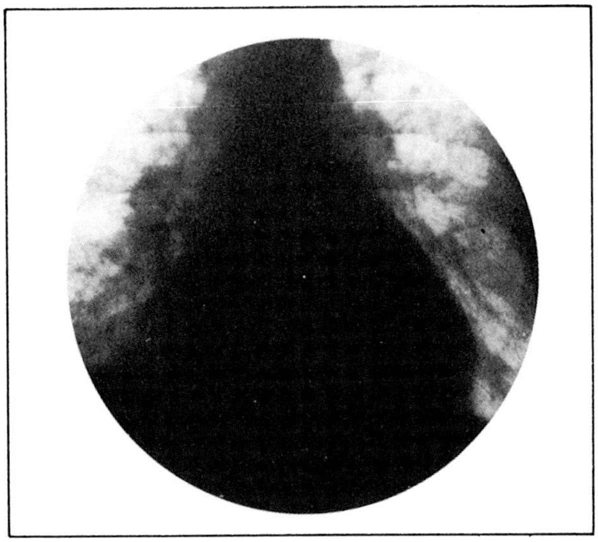

273 Cardiac beriberi. Some improvement after 1 week of thiamin therapy.

273

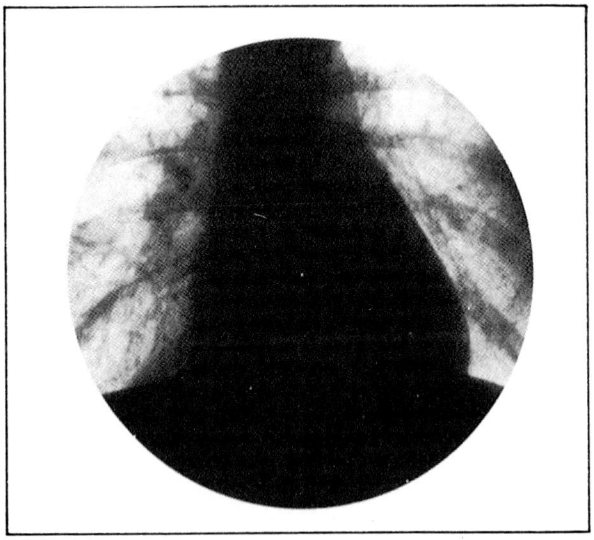

274 Cardiac beriberi. Considerable reduction in heart size after 3 weeks' treatment.

274

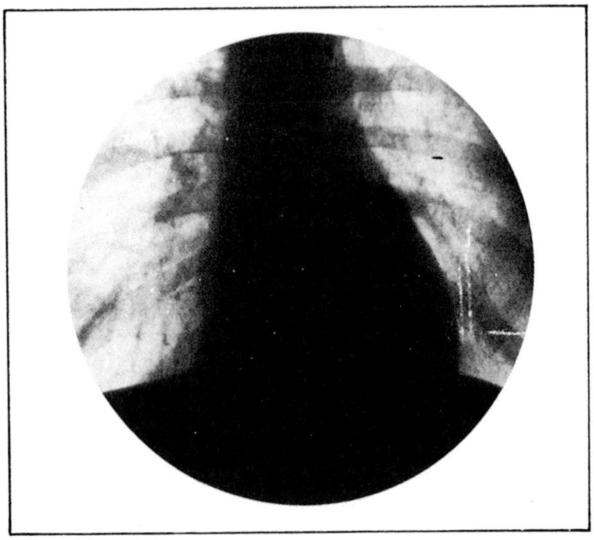

Niacin (nicotinic acid)

Niacin is very stable in solution and is found mainly in yeast, liver, meat, poultry and legumes. Although milk and eggs are low in niacin they are rich in the amino acid tryptophan, from which the body is able to obtain about half its daily requirements by conversion. An unavailable form of niacin, niacytin, occurs in cereals such as maize, and deficiency may result unless alkali is used in food preparation, as it is in the making of tortillas.

Niacin is involved in a series of oxidation–reduction reactions essential to life (similar to nicotinamide in NAD (nicotinamide adenine dinucleotide, coenzyme I) and NADP, the phosphate, coenzyme II). Excretory products in the urine are usually measured to assess nutritional status (Appendix III, Table 1) and the RDA for the adult is about 18mg niacin equivalents (Appendix I, Table 4).

Deficiency (pellagra)

The dermatosis is the most characteristic clinical feature and the appearances should be studied carefully and used in differential diagnosis (**275–286**). The tongue changes may be helpful. Dementia in a patient with a dermatosis should suggest pellagra until ruled out. In some countries inmates of prisons or of mental asylums may be there because of pellagra or have developed it there.

275

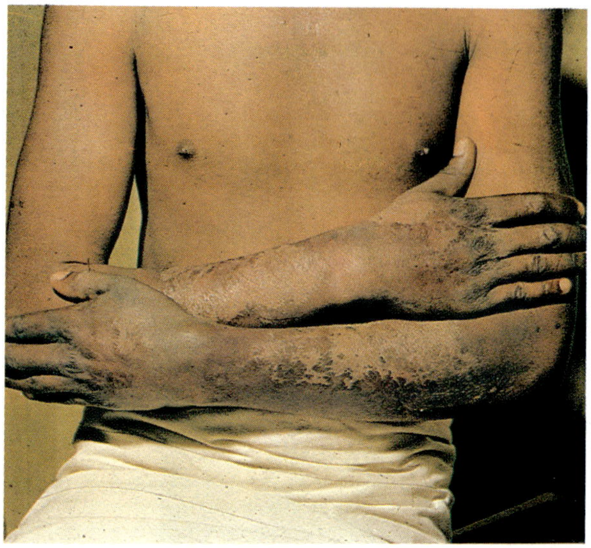

275 **Early pellagra affecting the arms.** The dermatosis begins as an erythema with pruritus and burning. Blebs may run together to form bullae and burst. At the slightly later stage shown the skin becomes hard, rough, cracked, blackish and brittle. In the dark skinned, as in this young Tanzanian male, the dermatosis may be easily overlooked. The symmetrical distribution on parts of the body exposed to the sun is characteristic but lesions are not necessarily confined to these areas. In this case the only other hyperpigmented areas were over those parts of the toes rubbed by ill-fitting shoes.

276 Casal's necklace. This fairly broad band or collar of dermatosis running right round the neck, and sometimes extending downwards like a bib, is a classic sign of pellagra. Other parts of the body exposed to the sun are usually also affected.

276

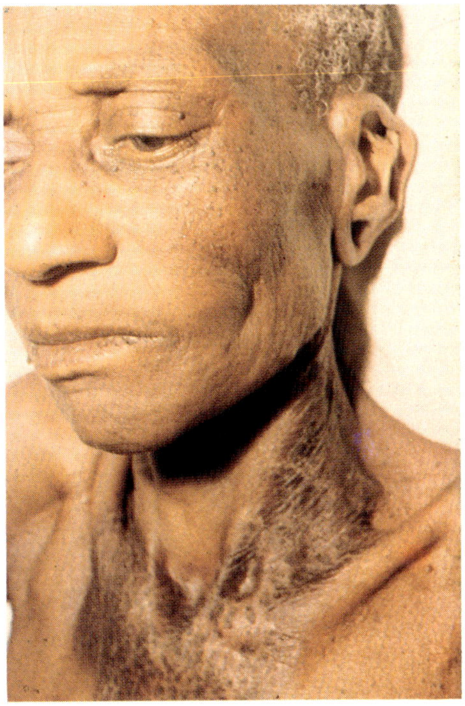

277 Extensive pellagrous dermatosis. The symmetrical involvement of the exposed parts of the body and the clear demarcation of the lesions from the normal skin on unexposed parts are striking in this elderly African female patient. It is not clear why the face is frequently unaffected.

277

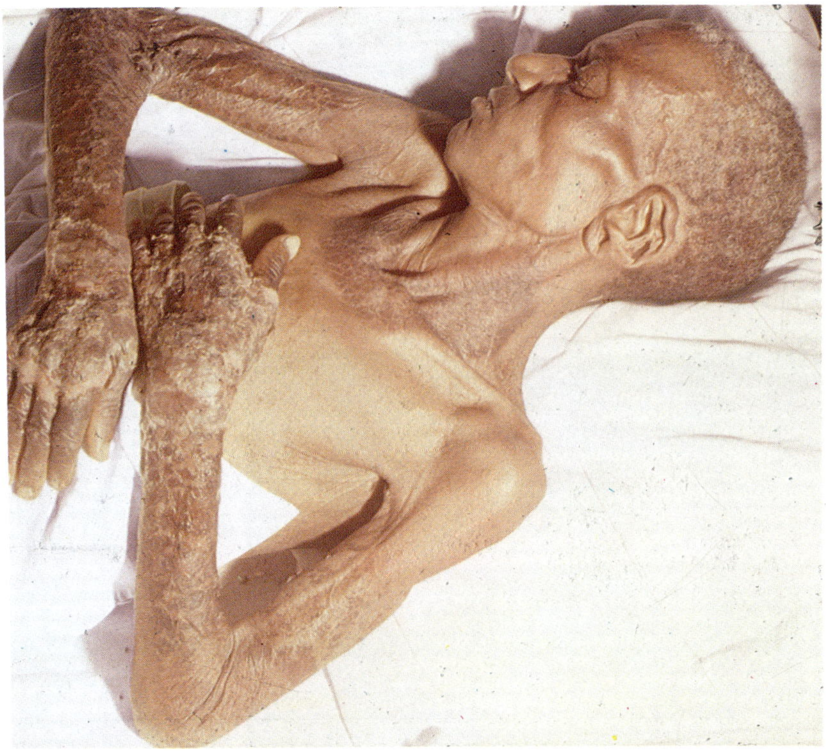

278

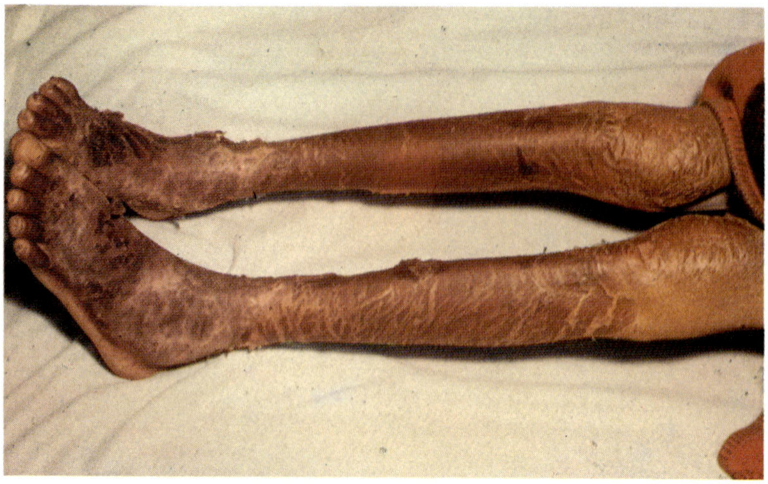

278 **Dermatosis of pellagra.** The symmetrically equal involvement of the skin of the legs is quite characteristic.

279

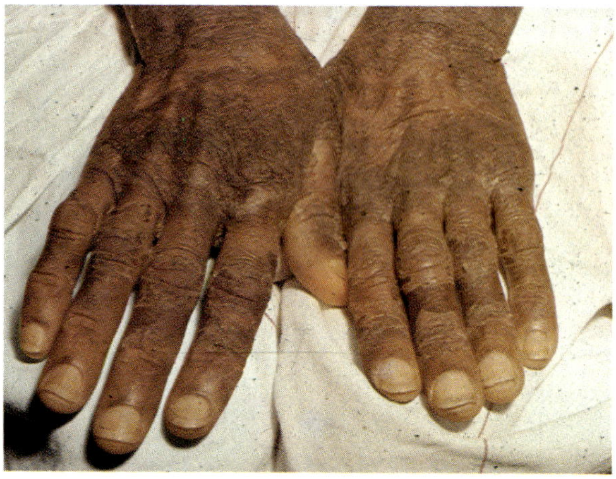

279 **Dermatosis of pellagra.** The backs of the hands and fingers are often the most severely involved parts of the body. The lesions are healing here and the dead skin is being exfoliated.

280

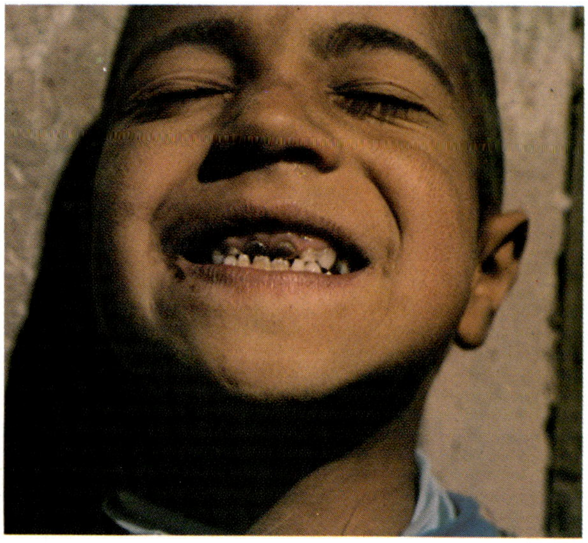

280 **Chapped cheeks.** This roughening and hyperpigmentation is sometimes mistaken for pellagra. Account should be taken of the influence of exposure, and examination of the classical sites for pellagra will serve to differentiate.

281 Symmetrical chapping of dorsum of hands. This is a common site for the skin changes of pellagra to occur. A careful history and full examination will permit the distinction to be made.

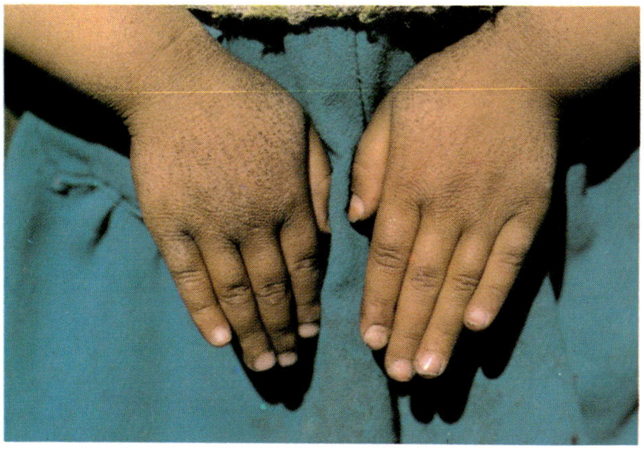

281

282 Scarlet tongue. The tongue in pellagra is frequently scarlet in appearance and extremely painful. However, this may occur in many non-nutritional conditions and other signs, especially those in the skin, have to be present to make the clinical diagnosis. Fissuring of the tongue alone is not of significance.

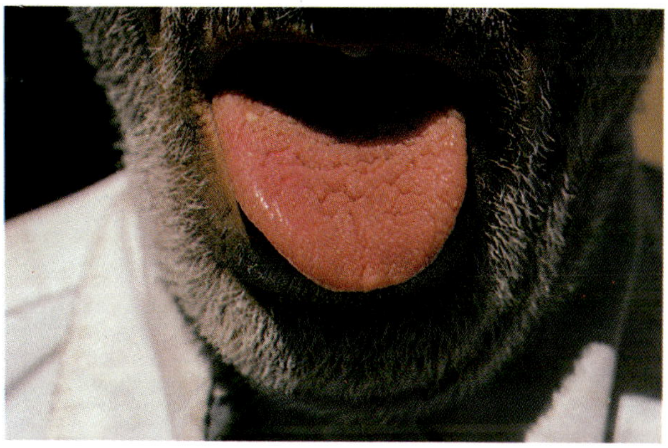

282

283

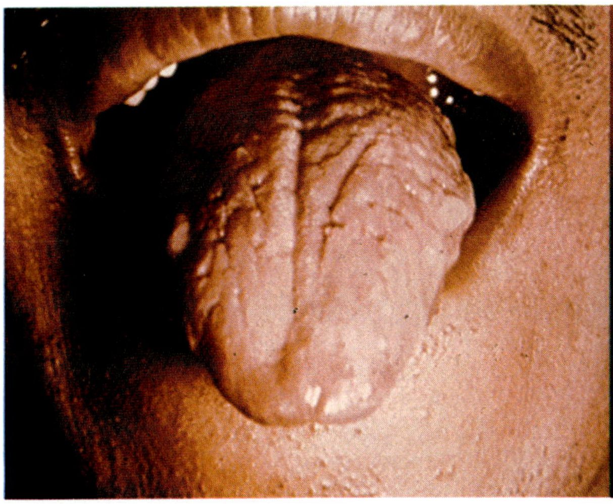

284

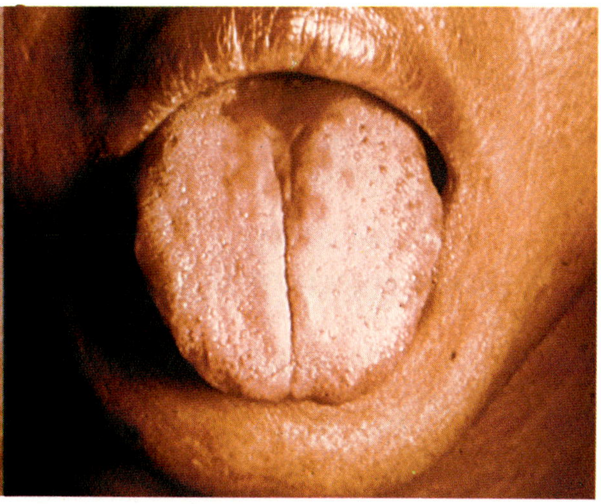

283 Filiform papillary atrophy. This is often seen in deficiency of niacin, folic acid, vitamin B_{12} or iron. It sometimes occurs in well nourished people wearing dentures. The filiform papillae are low or absent, giving a smooth or slick appearance, which remains after scraping lightly with an applicator stick.

284 Fungiform papillary hypertrophy. The condition can be seen and felt as a tongue blade is drawn lightly over the anterior two-thirds of the tongue. Hyperaemia may give the tongue a berry-like appearance. The condition is non-specific and may be due to general undernutrition.

285 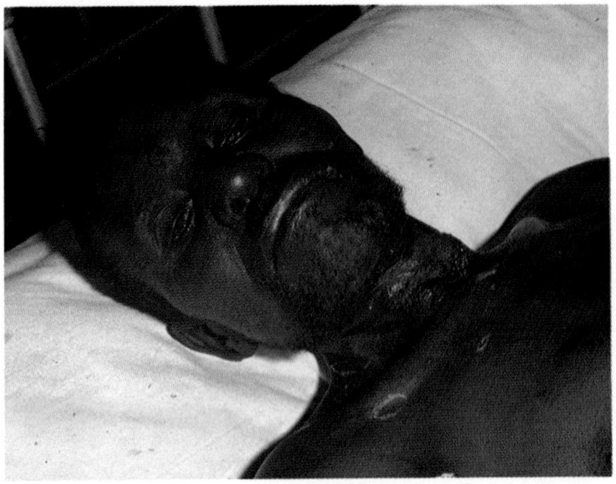

285 Encephalopathy of pellagra. In the late stages this is identical with that of Wernicke (**268, 269**), but responds to niacin. Early features are depression, apprehension, insomnia, headache and dizziness. Later, tremulous movements or rigidity of the limbs increase and finally, loss of tendon reflexes and numbness and paresis of the limbs progressively incapacitate the patient. The skin changes of pellagra, around the neck in this patient, assist in the differential diagnosis.

286 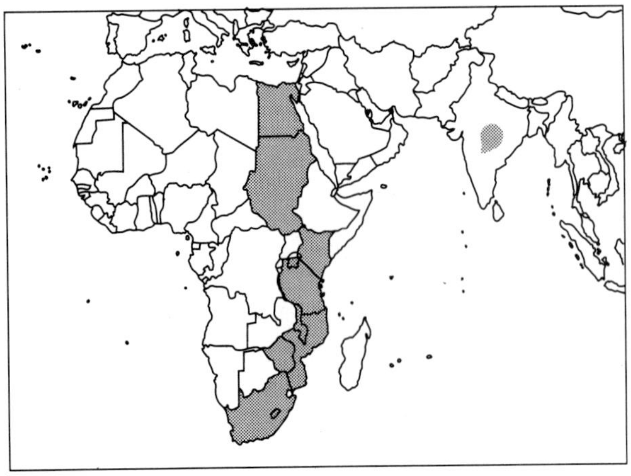

286 Present-day endemic areas of pellagra.

Toxicity

Reports from the United States have suggested that sustained release niacin causes liver damage.

Riboflavin (vitamin B_2)

Riboflavin is widely distributed in animal and vegetable foods. In staple cereals the quantities are low except after germination, when they are eaten in snacks in the Far East providing a rich source of the vitamin. Glutathione reductase is activated by riboflavin and this activity in red cells is used as a sensitive method for assessing riboflavin status (Appendix III, Table 1). Like niacin it acts as a coenzyme in oxidation–reduction reactions, this time as part of various flavoproteins with enzyme activity. The adult RDA is about 1.5mg.

Deficiency

Surprisingly, in view of its role in key enzyme reactions, death or even serious disease has never been attributed to riboflavin deficiency in man, although complete deprivation of riboflavin in experiments on animals is uniformly fatal. It is one of the most common vitamin deficiencies in developing countries but is invariably mild.

The tongue and lips are usually affected, but the signs are by no means pathognomonic (287–296). The genitals, the vulva in the female and the scrotum in the male (297–299), may become scaly and inflamed and the skin in areas rich in sebaceous glands shows a quite distinctive appearance called dyssebacia (300–302). Rapid recovery follows riboflavin 10mg daily by mouth.

287

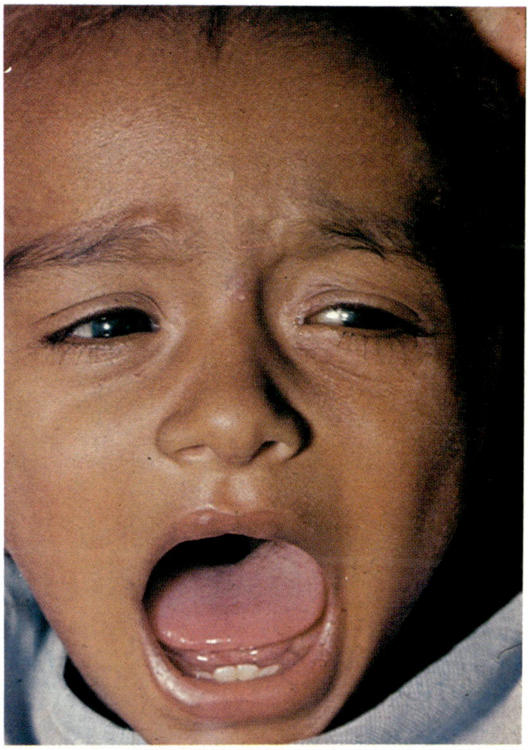

287 **Magenta tongue.** The purplish-red colouration of the tongue, as in this child, is generally regarded as being characteristic of riboflavin deficiency. The tongue is usually sore but other morphologic changes are usually absent.

288 **Tongue in riboflavin deficiency.** The patient was an inn-keeper who presented with a number of the features of chronic alcoholism. His main complaint, however, was his very sore tongue, which is seen to be markedly swollen and oedematous and to have a light magenta colour.

289 The same patient as in the previous figure with the tongue returned to its normal size and colour and painless several weeks after large doses of vitamin B complex were administered.

8

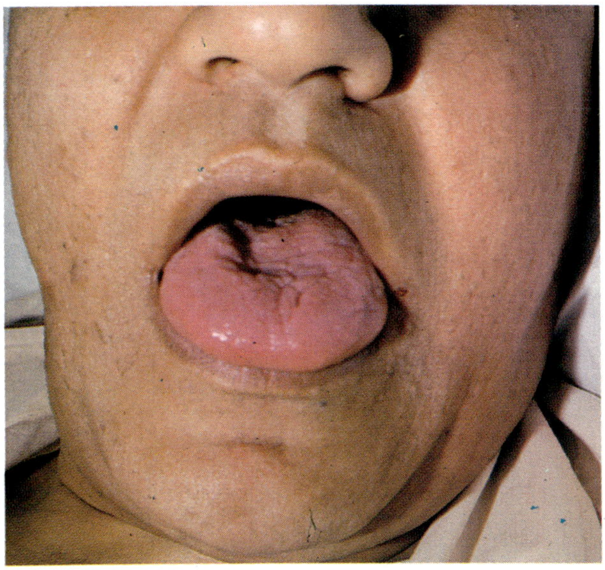

289

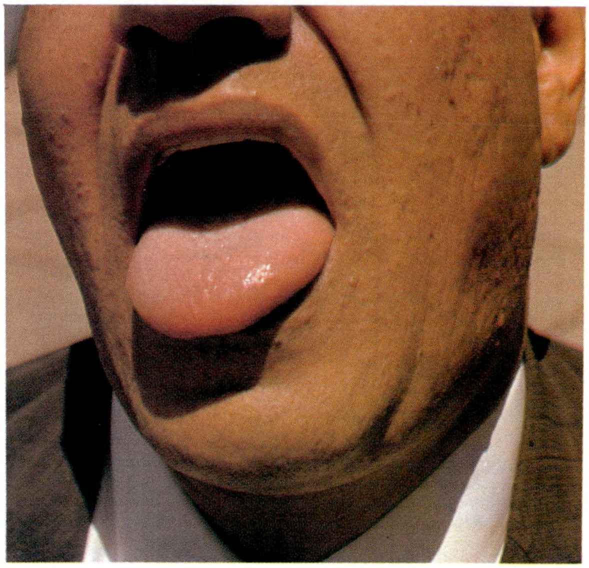

290

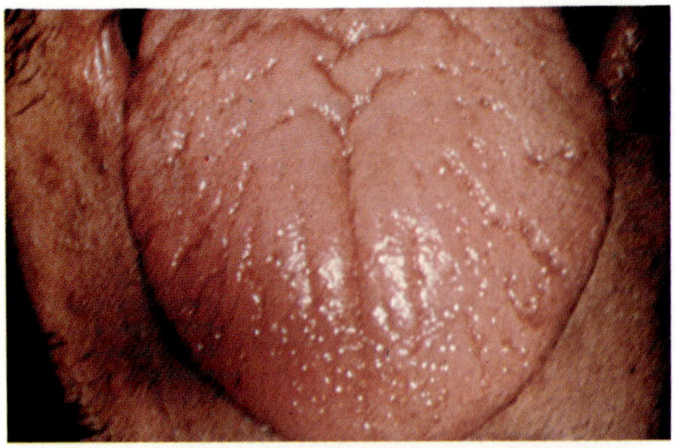

290 Glossitis. A painful and inflamed tongue may occur in other nutritional deficiency states besides pellagra; most notably of riboflavin, folic acid, vitamin B_{12}, pyridoxine or iron. The filiform papillae are atrophic and the fungiform papillae hypertrophic. The differential diagnosis includes uraemia, diabetes mellitus, antibiotic administration, monilial infection, aphthous stomatitis and malignancy. Moeller's glossitis appears as circular, sharply demarcated, denuded areas and is transitory.

291

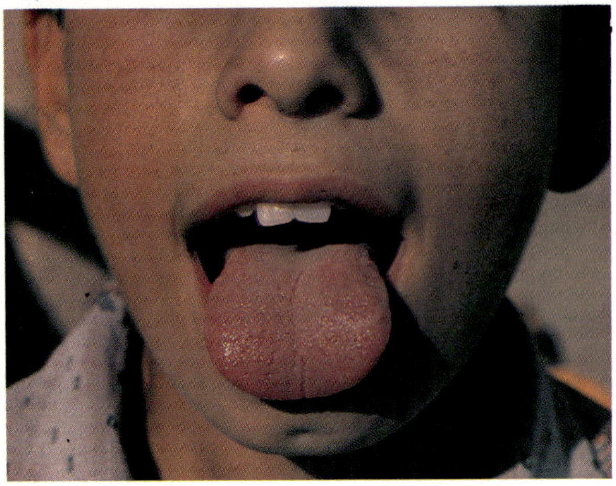

291 Geographic tongue. There are irregularly distributed patchy areas of denudation and atrophy of the epithelium. It is painless and symptomless. The aetiology is obscure, there is no evidence that nutritional factors are involved and it should not be attributed to deficiency of riboflavin or other members of the B vitamin complex.

292

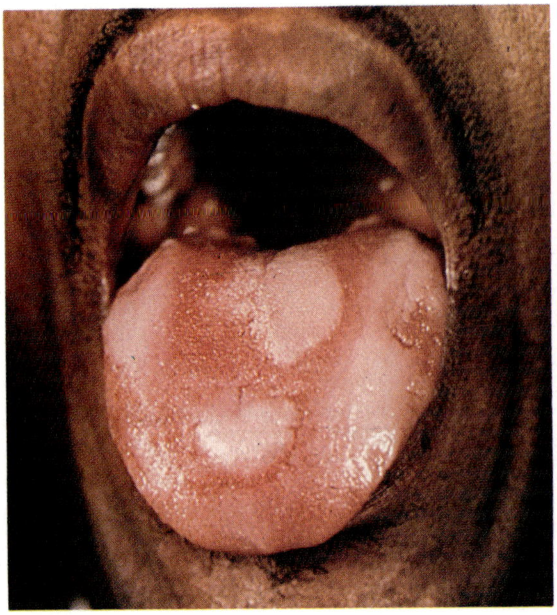

292 Geographic tongue. This patchy denudation of the tongue is often wrongly attributed to riboflavin deficiency. It is of no nutritional significance.

293 Angular stomatitis. The mucocutaneous junctions at the angles of the mouth are sodden, macerated and excavated with fissuring. Both angles are affected but often unequally. On healing, angular scars or rhagades occur (**295**) and must be differentiated from those that follow congenital syphilis. Besides riboflavin deficiency it may also occur in other B vitamin deficiencies and in iron deficiency. Ill-fitting dentures may be responsible. The angles of the eyelids may also be affected – angular palpebritis.

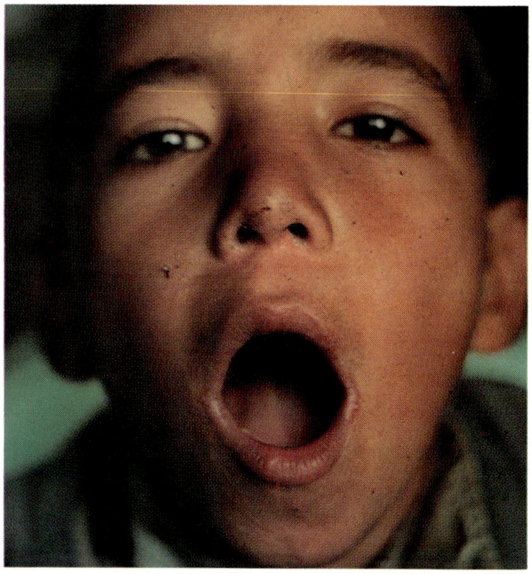

293

294 Perlèche. In cases of neglect the lesions of angular stomatitis may be colonized by *Candida albicans* giving rise to an exuberant yellowish growth of fungal material. The mucocutaneous junction of the nose is similarly affected in this young child.

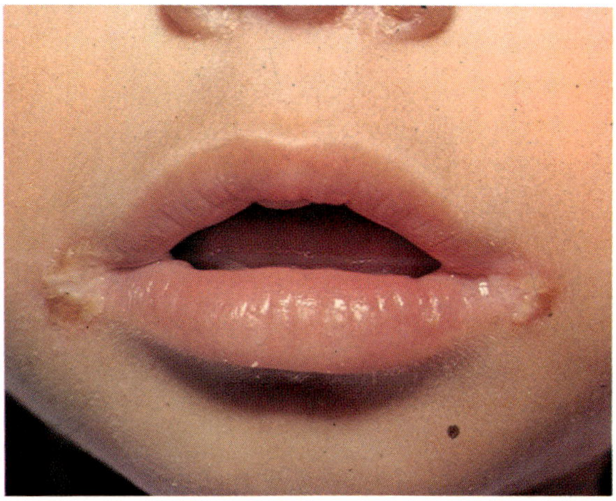

294

295 Rhagades. Chronic erosions and scarring at the angles of the mouth in a schoolboy in the north-east of Iran where widespread riboflavin deficiency has recently been demonstrated biochemically.

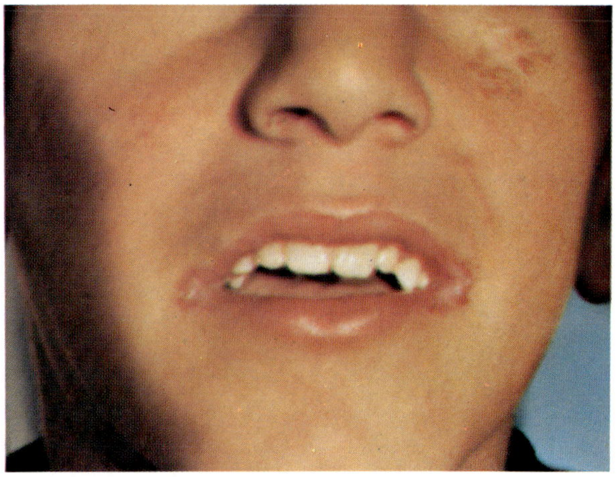

295

296

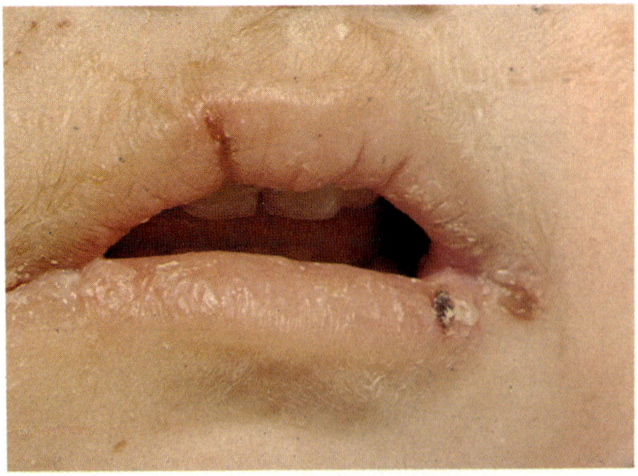

296 Cheilosis. This term should be reserved for vertical fissuring, later complicated by redness, swelling and ulceration of the lips, other than the angles. The centre of the lower lip is usually most affected. Climatic factors, such as cold and wind, may sometimes be responsible.

297

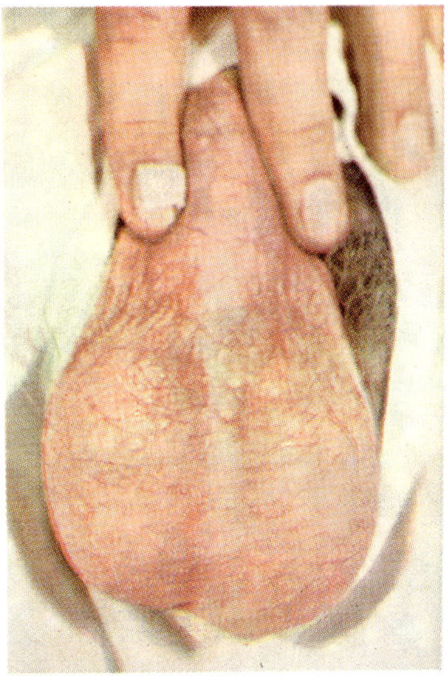

298

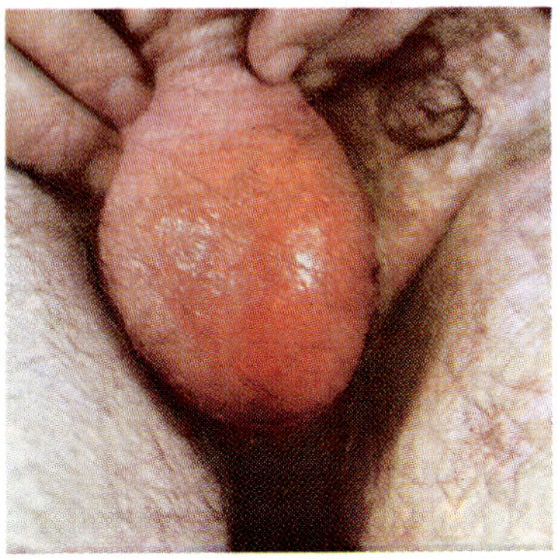

299

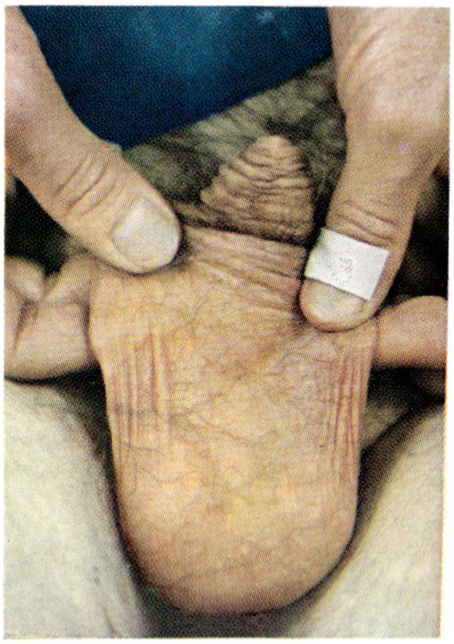

297 Experimental riboflavin deficiency. Early phase of scrotal dermatitis after 175 days on diet that provided 0.51mg riboflavin per day.

298 Experimental riboflavin deficiency. More severe lesion of scrotum observed in another patient after 288 days on diet that provided 0.55mg riboflavin per day. There was no appreciable healing of this lesion until riboflavin supplementation was provided 21 days later.

299 Experimental riboflavin deficiency. Demonstrates recovery of the same scrotum as that in **298**, 1 week after the subject was supplemented with 6mg of riboflavin per day.

300 Dyssebacia (shark skin). The lesion consists of greasy, filiform excrescences, greyish or yellowish-white in colour, most commonly situated on the nasolabial folds, but also occurring on the bridge of the nose, eyebrows and backs of the ears. It is produced by plugging of the enlarged sebaceous glands by retained inspissated sebum.

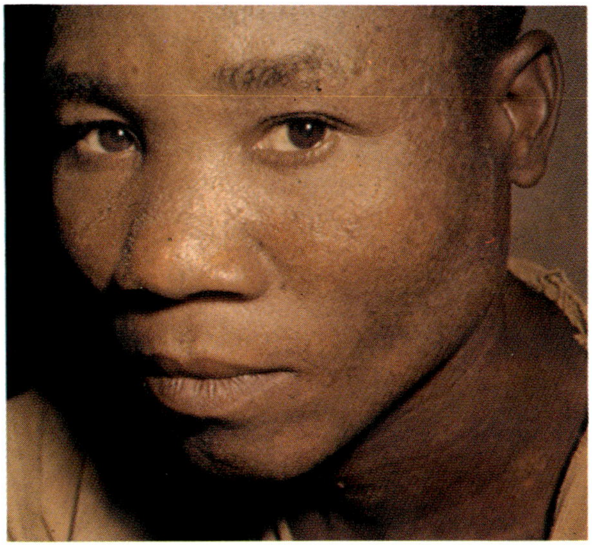

300

301 Extreme dyssebacia of the face. There is also corneal infiltration and early corneal vascularization. This alcoholic African patient also had multiple peripheral neuropathy. A combined vitamin B complex deficiency was suspected in this patient but the lesions shown were most likely to have been due to riboflavin deficiency.

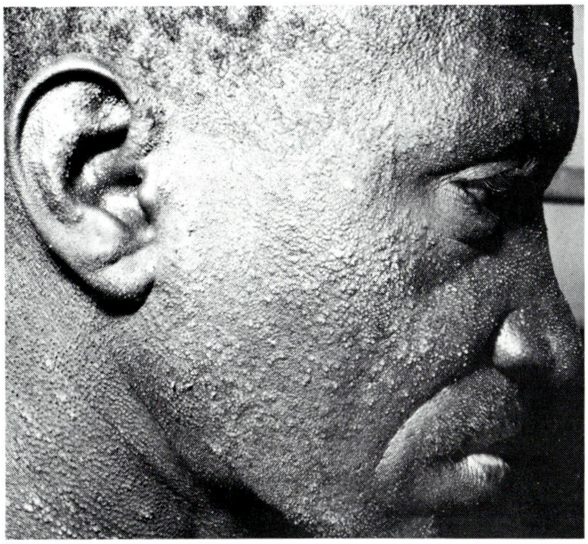

301

302 Extreme dyssebacia on the face. The same patient as in the previous figure after 10 days on a good diet and B complex therapy. There is considerable improvement.

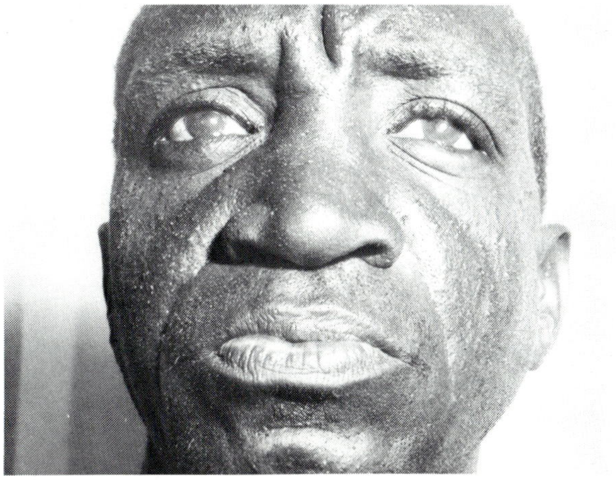

302

Pyridoxine (vitamin B_6)

Pyridoxine, pyridoxal, and pyridoxamine are equally effective in the body in transamination, decarboxylation and other functions in amino acid and protein metabolism. Most classes of foodstuffs provide pyridoxine, and pure dietary deficiency is rare. Vitamin B_6 status has been related to urinary excretion of metabolites but may now be assessed by plasma levels (Appendix III, Table 1). The adult RDA is about 2.0mg.

Vitamin B_6 dependency is the most common form of vitamin dependency and is considered in Chapter 7.

Deficiency

Hyperirritability, convulsions and anaemia occurred in young infants fed exclusively on a milk formula in which pyridoxine had been inadvertently destroyed during processing (**303, 304**).

Experimental deficiency in man has been studied (**305, 306**).

Some drugs interfere with one or other of the coenzyme forms of the vitamin. Among these are isoniazid (used in the treatment of tuberculosis), hydralazine (the antihypertensive), and penicillamine (used to chelate copper in Wilson's disease) (see page 218), causing neuropathy.

Pyridoxine deficiency is one among many causes of sideroblastic anaemia, usually severe microcytic hypochromic in form and resulting from abnormal utilization of iron, leading to iron overload and a characteristic picture in the marrow (**307**). Both congenital and acquired cases respond only partially to vitamin B_6, 50mg t.i.d. orally.

303

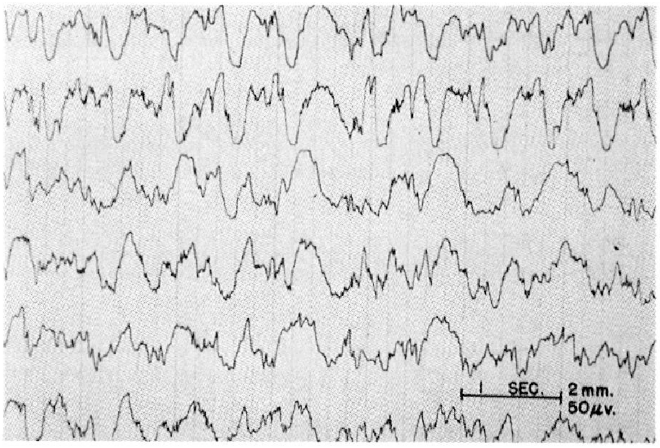

303 Pyridoxine deficiency. Electroencephalogram of infant during convulsions caused by pyridoxine deficiency.

304

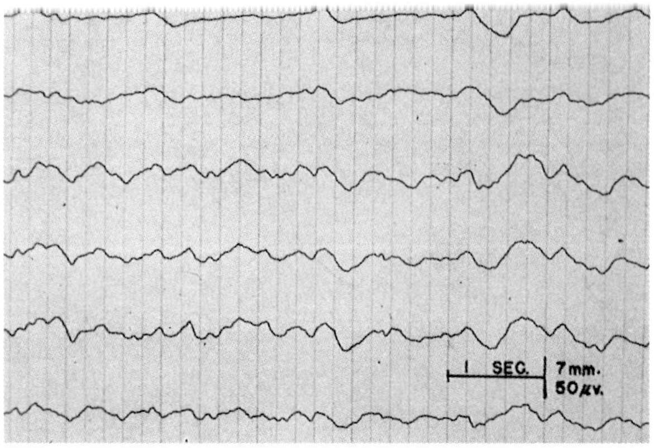

304 Normal EEG five minutes after pyridoxine administration; the colour improved and the infant slept.

305 Pyridoxine deficiency. The scaling seborrhoea-like dermatosis in this patient and the glossitis in **306** were induced in volunteers by giving the pyridoxine antagonist desoxypyridoxine. Such lesions have not been proved to occur spontaneously although it is suspected that some instances are due to pyridoxine deficiency.

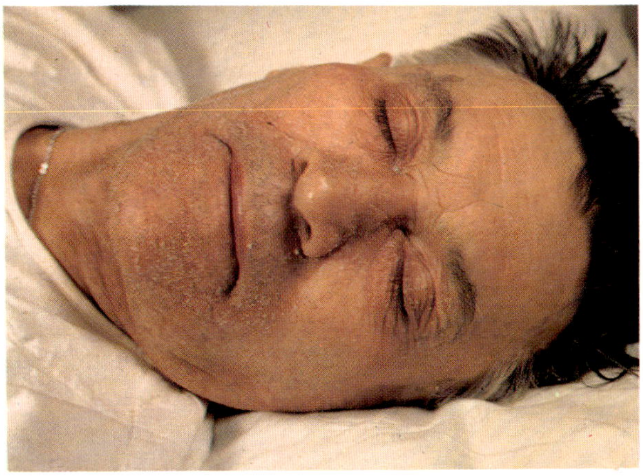
305

306 Glossitis in pyridoxine deficiency. This is indistinguishable from that due to deficiency of other B group vitamins (**282**, **287**, **290**, **310**, **324**).

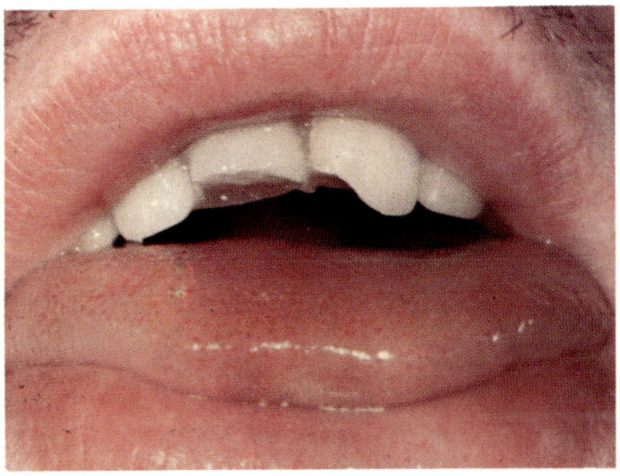
306

307 **Ringed sideroblasts in bone marrow.** These are seen in many conditions in which there is a failure in iron reutilization and hyperferraemia. Pyridoxine deficiency is one of these. (Prussian blue, × 100)

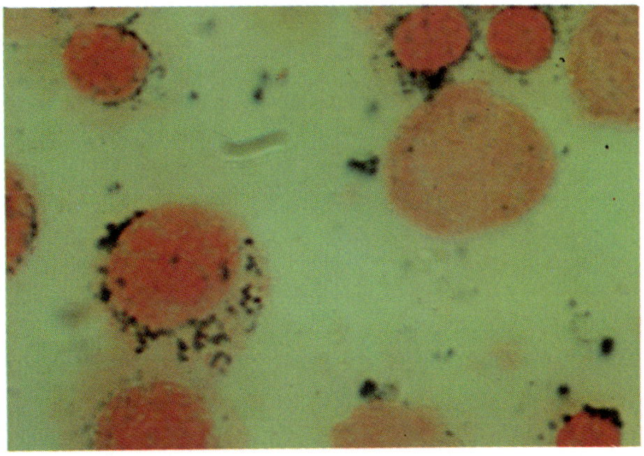
307

Toxicity

Patients receiving large doses of pyridoxine gradually developed sensory ataxia and profound lower limb impairment of position and vibration sense. It is not fully clear whether or not an impurity in the pharmacological product might have been responsible.[76]

Folic acid (pteroylglutamic acid)

In both plant and animal tissue folic acid is quite widely distributed in unstable forms, reduced methyl or formyl polyglutamates, that are subject to losses in cooking, canning and on exposure to light.

Polyglutamates in food are readily broken down and absorbed rapidly by an active process in the jejunum in small amounts, but by passive diffusion in therapeutic doses. Serum, liver and other tissues contain the coenzyme form 5N-methyl tetrahydro folate. Vitamin C helps prevent coenzyme oxidation. The coenzyme assists in transfer of one-carbon units, such as in early purine and pyrimidine synthesis, generation and use of formate, and amino acid conversions.

Plasma folate is much influenced by recent dietary intake and red cell folate should be measured to assess status (Appendix III, Table 1). The adult RDA is 400μg.

Deficiency

The system most commonly affected is the haemopoietic (**308, 309**).

308

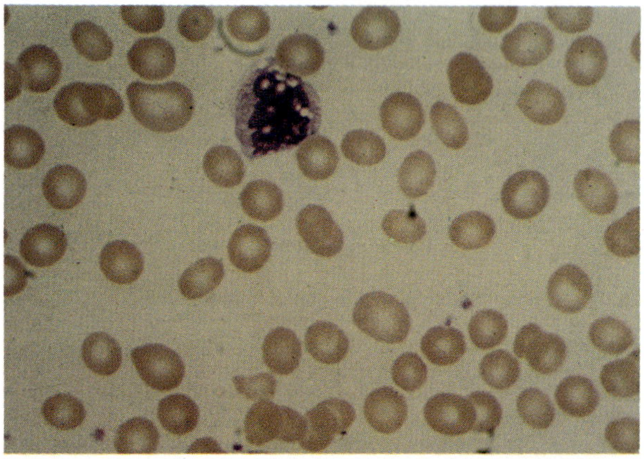

308 Peripheral blood in folic acid deficiency. The erythrocytes are larger than normal (macrocytosis) and consequently the mean corpuscular volume (MCV) is greater than normal, usually > 96 μm^3. Many red cells are irregularly shaped (poikilocytosis). Dimorphic anaemias, in which iron deficiency is also present, may result in normalization of the red cell indices but the peripheral blood film reveals the characteristic morphology.

Polymorphonuclear leucocytes are usually reduced in number and frequently have more lobes than the normal number of five or six maximum. There is thrombocytopenia and many platelets appear in giant form. (× 100)

309

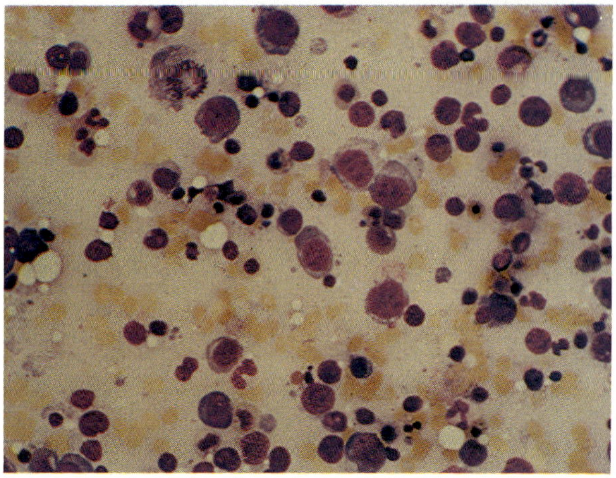

309 Bone marrow in folic acid deficiency. Haemopoiesis is characteristically megaloblastic. Megaloblasts are large cells with very lacy chromatin strands that have distinct parachromatin spaces between them. Mitotic figures are seen as in the upper left area here. The granulocyte nuclei have a similar appearance. The full expression of the megaloblastic appearance may be retarded by concomitant iron deficiency. The morphologic changes in peripheral blood and bone marrow are identical in deficiency of folic acid and vitamin B_{12}, and biochemical tests have to be relied upon for differential diagnosis (× 40).

The tongue may be red and painful (**310**) or pale if the anaemia is marked and other problems coexist (**311**).

The skin may be hyperpigmented as it is in vitamin B_{12} deficiency (see page 165) but in both instances this is a rare sign (**312**). Folic acid deficiency in animals readily causes congenital malformations of the spinal cord and several studies have suggested that it may be responsible for human neural tube defects (**313**). A large Medical Research Council trial recently completed confirmed the relationship with an impressive two-thirds reduction for pre-pregnancy dosing with folic acid.[77]

0

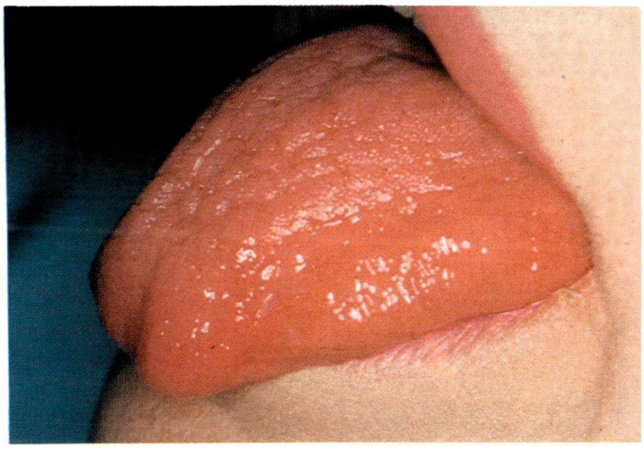

311

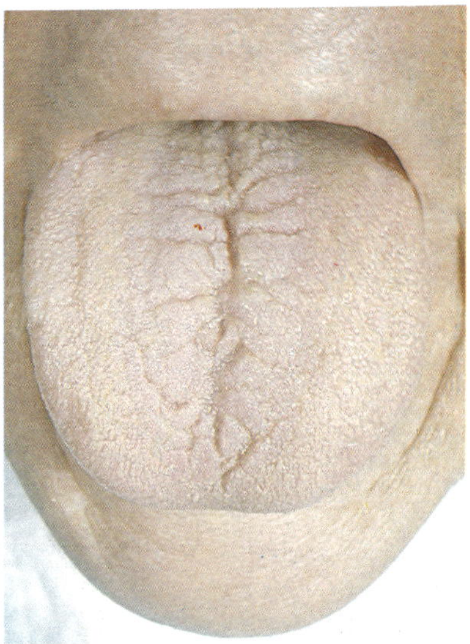

310 The tongue in folic acid deficiency. The most marked oral manifestation is often a glossitis. The tongue becomes very red and painful and the papillae atrophy, leaving a shiny, smooth surface.

311 Folic acid deficiency. An 82-year-old woman with marked anaemia and largish white tongue suggesting hypothyroidism with coexistent anaemia. Thyroid indices were reduced.

312

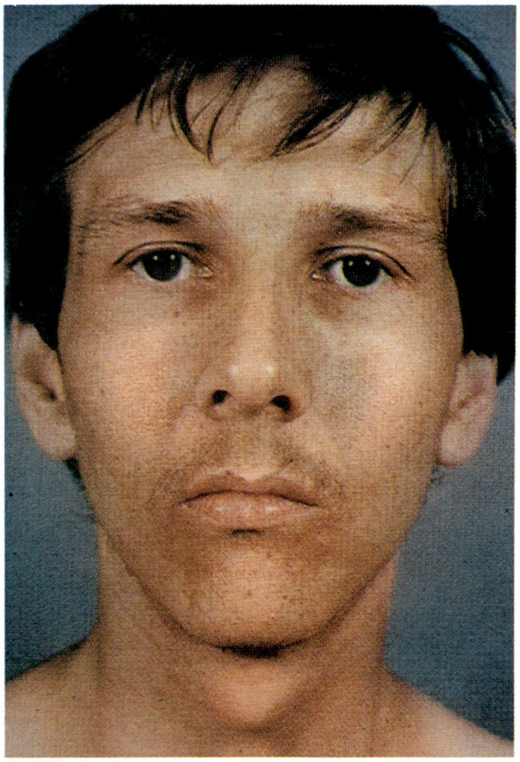

312 Hyperpigmentation of the skin. This patient also had a megaloblastic anaemia and recovery, including the skin, resulted from treatment with folic acid. Similar pigmentation occurs in vitamin B_{12} deficiency (**327**).

313

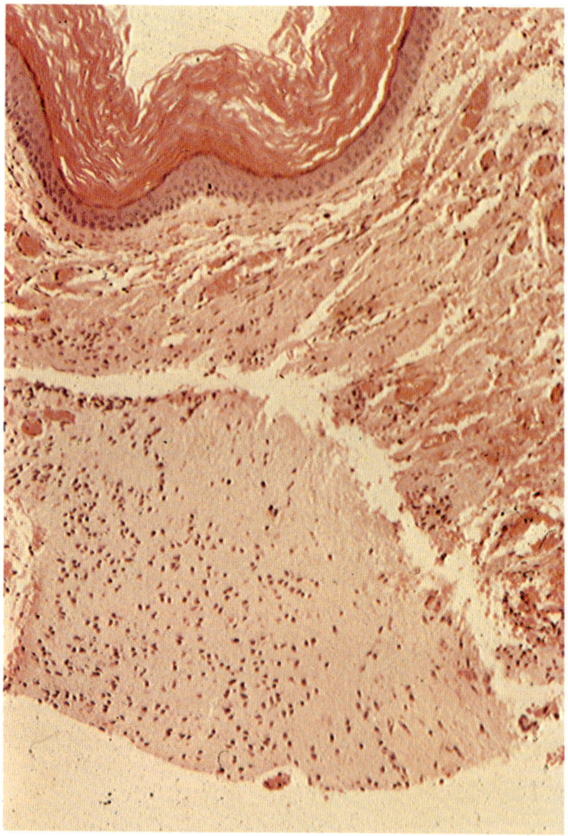

313 Meningomyelocele. Biopsy showing neural tissue, mainly glial, with some distorted neurons deep to the subcutis. The epidermis may be intact, as here, or ulcerated. (*H&E*, × 35)

Causes of folic acid deficiency are related to problems with ingestion, absorption, utilization, or increased requirement or excretion (*Table 50*).

Liver disease predisposes to folate deficiency in a variety of ways (*Table 51*).

Table 50. Some causes of folic acid deficiency.

Inadequate ingestion
Poor diets–lacking unprocessed, fresh, lightly cooked food; nutritional megaloblastic anaemia; chronic alcoholism

Inadequate absorption
Malabsorption syndromes
- coeliac disease
- other chronic disorders involving upper small intestine
- drugs–especially alcohol, anticonvulsants and others

Specific malabsorption for folate
- congenital or acquired enzyme defects, blind loop syndrome

Inadequate utilization
Folic acid antagonists
Enzyme deficiencies
Vitamin B_{12} deficiency (reduces folate uptake and retention by red cells)
Alcohol
Ascorbic acid deficiency

Increased requirement
Parasitization (including fetus, breastfed infant, malignant tissue)
Infancy (for growth)
Increased haemopoiesis
Increased metabolism

Increased excretion
Renal dialysis
Chronic exfoliative dermatitis

Table 51. Mechanisms of folate deficiency in liver disease.

Decreased intake:	of rich sources such as fresh green leafy vegetables, pulses, oranges, bananas, nuts, bread, and offal
Decreased absorption:	of pteroyl polyglutamates following deconjugation, reduction, and methylation
Decreased liver uptake and storage:	as 5-methyl tetrahydrofolate or increased liver 'trapping'
Decreased utilization:	of folate in haemopoiesis, leading to increased excretion of formiminoglutamic acid
Decreased affinity:	for folate-binding protein, leading to increased urinary folate excretion

Herbert has mapped out in detail the evolution of folic acid deficiency[78] (**314**) and this should be compared with his similar scheme for vitamin B_{12} deficiency (**315**).

In treatment the usual dose is 1mg/day but if there is coincident vitamin B_{12} deficiency this latter vitamin must also be given if neurological deterioration is to be avoided.

314

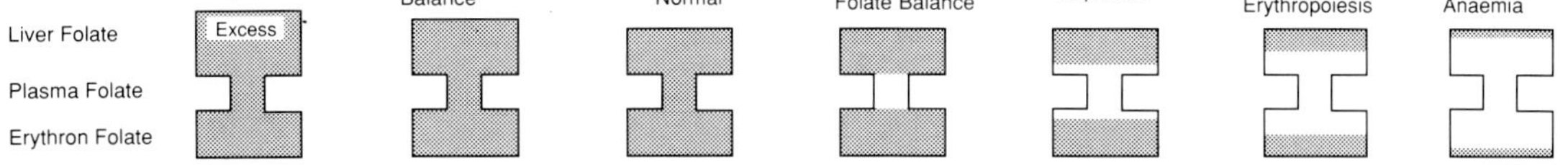

	Excess*	Positive Folate Balance	Normal	Negative Folate Balance	Folate Depletion	Folate Deficiency Erythropoiesis	Folate Deficiency Anaemia
Serum Folate (ng/ml)	>10	>10	>5	<3	<3	<31	<3
RBC Folate (ng/ml)	>400	>300	>200	>200	<160	<120	<100
Diagnostic dU Suppression	Normal	Normal	Normal	Normal	Normal	Abnormal	Abnormal
Lobe Average	<3.5	<3.5	<3.5	<3.5	<3.5	>3.5	>3.5
Liver Folate (µg/g)	>5	>400	>3	>3	<1.6	<1.2	<1
Erythrocytes	Normal	Normal	Normal	Normal	Normal	Normal	Macro-ovalocytic
MCV	Normal	Normal	Normal	Normal	Normal	Normal	Elevated
Haemoglobin (g/dL)	>12	>12	>12	>12	>12	>12	<12
Plasma Clearance of Intravenous Folate	Normal	Normal	Normal	Normal	Normal	Increased	Increased

* Dietary excess of folate reduces zinc absorption

314 Sequential stages in the development of folate deficiency.

Vitamin B_{12} (cobalamin)

This is the latest and probably last vitamin to be discovered (1948–9) and has the largest molecule (about 1500 daltons). It is also unique in two ways: it is the only known biologically active form of cobalt; and it is synthesized in nature only by micro-organisms. Animal foods are by far the main source, the gut flora of animals being the ultimate source. Vegans (see Chapter 2) may obtain a little from root nodules or contaminated vegetables.

Absorption can only occur after combination with the intrinsic factor, a glycoprotein secreted by the parietal cells of the gastric mucosa. Absorption is restricted to the terminal part of the ileum, which is often removed in surgery. Specific proteins, transcorrin I and II, carry the active coenzyme forms, methylcobalamin and 5'deoxyadenosylcobalamin, and also the inactive hydroxocobalamin to the tissues. Sufficient amounts to meet daily requirements for many years (about 3μg) are stored in liver and other tissues. Normal plasma level is 140–750 picograms/ml (Appendix III, Table 1). A low plasma level is not sufficient to make a diagnosis – it occurs in some patients as a result of folate deficiency.

In the bone marrow vitamin B_{12} is necessary for synthesis of thymine, the characteristic base of DNA, from deoxyuridine, and its function is bound up with that of folic acid. In the nervous system, however, it acts alone in the maintenance of myelin.

Deficiency

Vitamin B_{12} deficiency, like folic acid deficiency, has many possible causes (*Table 52*). Because of the small requirements and large stores this deficiency evolves over a longer period of time than in any other nutritional deficiency (**315**).

Table 52. Some causes of vitamin B_{12} deficiency.

Inadequate ingestion
- Veganism, food faddism, religious tenets (certain Hindus, Catholic orders, Seventh Day Adventists), chronic alcoholism

Inadequate absorption
- Gastric disorder causing inadequate or absent production of intrinsic factor:
  - Addisonian pernicious anaemia – various types
  - Gastrectomy and diseases of the stomach
    - Diseases affecting the small intestine, especially the terminal ileum
    - Pancreatic disease
    - Competition for vitamin B_{12} by parasites or bacteria

Inadequate utilization
- Congenital or acquired enzyme deficiency
- Abnormal B_{12}-binding protein in serum
- Inadequate B_{12}-binding protein
- Vitamin B_{12} antagonists

Increased requirement
- Hyperthyroidism, infancy, parasitization

Increased excretion
- Liver disease, ? renal disease

Increased destruction by antioxidants
- Pharmacological doses of vitamin C

315

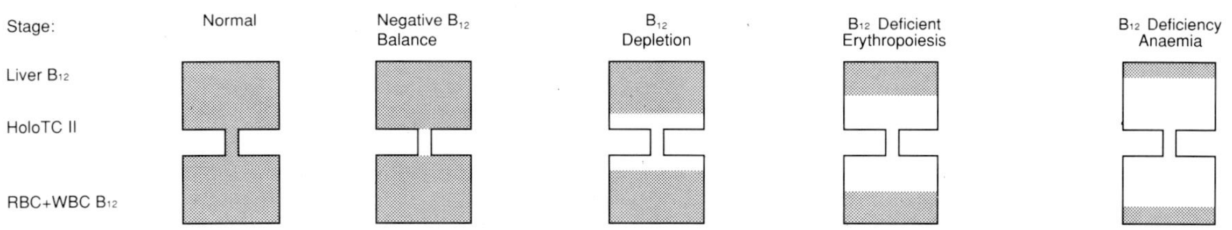

Stage:	Normal	Negative B_{12} Balance	B_{12} Depletion	B_{12} Deficient Erythropoiesis	B_{12} Deficiency Anaemia
HoloTC II	>30 pg/ml	<20 pg/ml	<20 pg/ml	<12 pg/ml	<12 pg/ml
TC II % sat.	>5%	<5%	<2%	<1%	<1%
Holohap	>150 pg/ml	>150 pg/ml	<150 pg/ml	<100 pg/ml	<100 pg/ml
dU suppression	Normal	Normal	Normal	Abnormal	Abnormal
Hypersegmentation	No	No	No	Yes	Yes
TBBC* % sat.	>15%	>15%	>15%	<15%	<10%
Hap % sat.	>20%	>20%	>20%	<20%	<10%
RBC Folate	>160 ng/ml	>160	>160	<140	<140
Erythrocytes	Normal	Normal	Normal	Normal	Macro-ovalocytic
MCV	Normal	Normal	Normal	Normal	Elevated
Haemoglobin	Normal	Normal	Normal	Normal	Low
TC II	Normal	Normal	Normal	Elevated	Elevated
Methylmalonate	No	No	No	?	Yes
Myelin damage	No	No	No	?	?

315 Sequential stages in the development of vitamin B_{12} deficiency. The biochemical and haematologic sequence of events as negative vitamin B_{12} balance progresses. Holo TC II is holotranscobalamin II (i.e., transcobalamin II with cobalamin on it). Without cobalamin, it is apotranscobalamin II. TC II % sat is % of total TC II that has cobalamin on it. Holohap is holohaptocorrin (i.e., haptocorrin with cobalamin on it). Synonyms for haptocorrin are cobalaphilin and transcobalamin (I and II).

Key: dU suppression: diagnostic test of ability of cells (bone marrow cells, peripheral blood lymphocytes) to make DNA.
Hypersegmentation: increase in number of lobes in granulocytic white cell nuclei.
TBBC % sat: % of total B_{12} binding capacity of plasma that has B_{12} on it.
RBC: red blood cell.
MCV: mean corpuscular volume of red cells.

Pernicious anaemia, due to lack or abnormality of the intrinsic factor, is probably the commonest cause (**316–320**). The fish tapeworm infests certain communities and may interfere with absorption (**321, 322**). Neurologic disease is made worse if folic acid is given without vitamin B_{12}, as previously mentioned (page 159), (**323**).

316

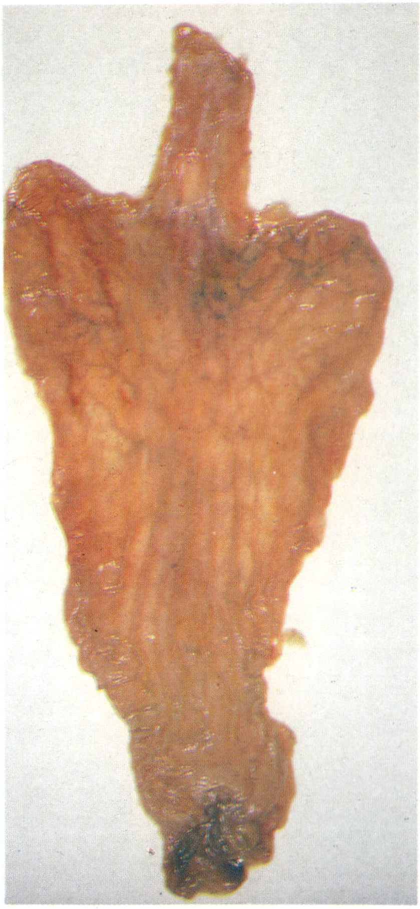

31

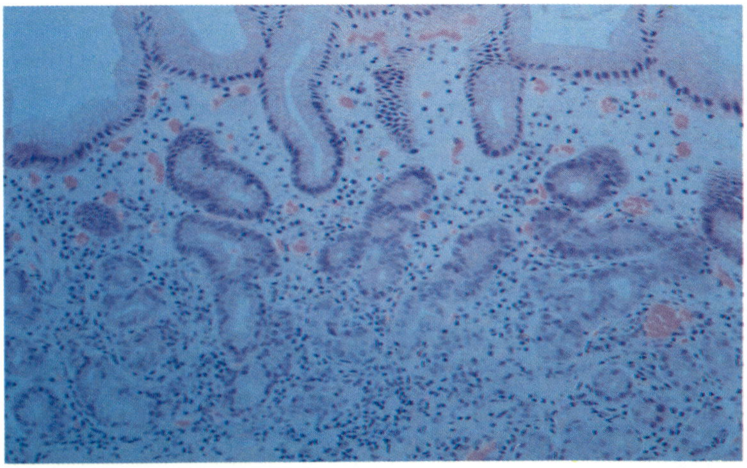

317 Pernicious anaemia. The mucosa of the gastric body in a patient with pernicious anaemia. The specialized glands have been replaced by antral-type glands which can be shown by immunohistochemistry to contain gastrin cells (normally only found in the antrum). This is part of the generalized, probably reactive, increase in gastrin cells in this condition. The lamina propria shows an increase in chronic inflammatory cells.

316 Pernicious anaemia. The loss of gastric folds and pale atrophic mucosa are particularly prominent in the body of this stomach.

318

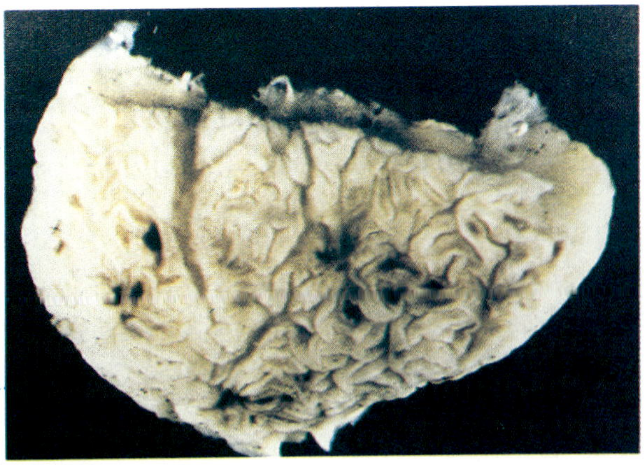

3

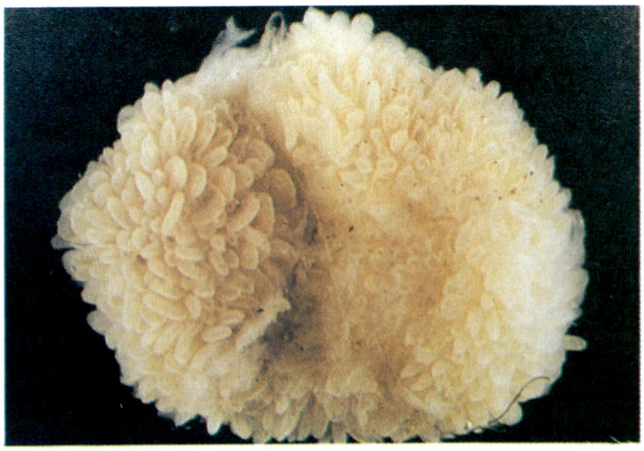

318 Vitamin B_{12} deficiency. Complete atrophy of the gastric mucosa in a vegan who had no food of animal origin for about 16 years.

319 Gastric biopsy from a normal individual.

320 Pallor of pernicious anaemia. There is a pronounced lemon-yellowish tint to the skin together with faint icterus of the sclerae due to hyperbilirubinaemia. The skin is often velvety smooth, yet inelastic. It is remarkable how frequently patients have blonde or prematurely grey hair and light-coloured irides.

320

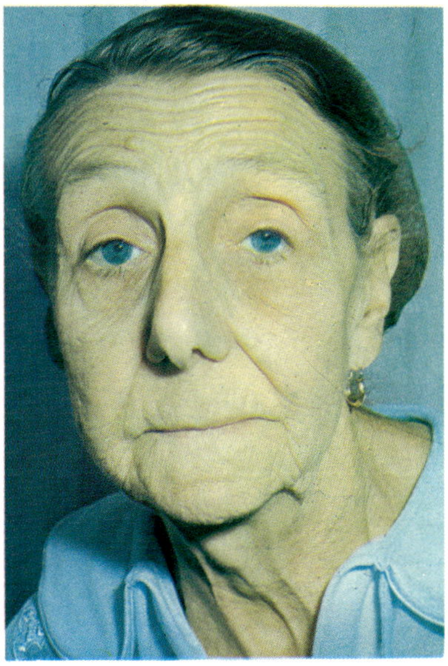

321, 322 Cross-section of head, and segments of adult tapeworm. The fish tapeworm, *Diphyllobothrium latum*, is common around large lakes in Europe, North America and elsewhere. A mature adult may reach 10m in length. The head and mature proglottids are readily distinguished from those of *Taenia* in man. Mature worms may produce one million eggs daily. (× 8)

321

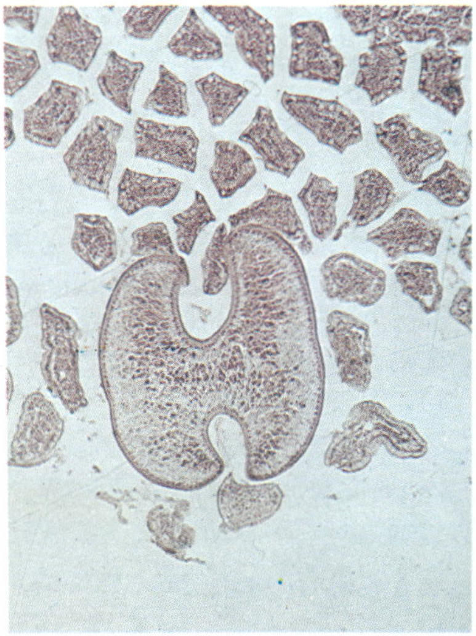

322

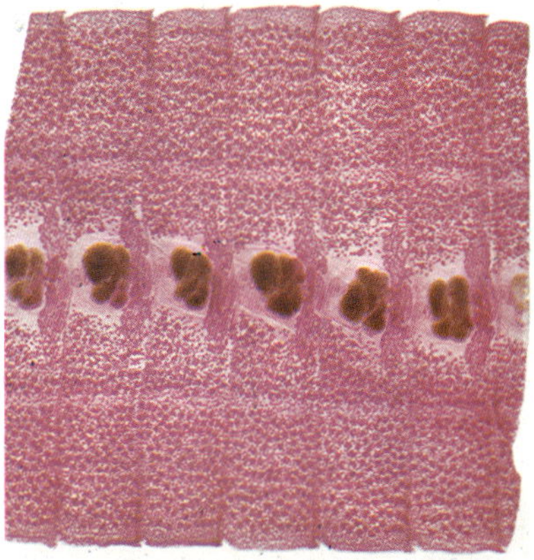

323

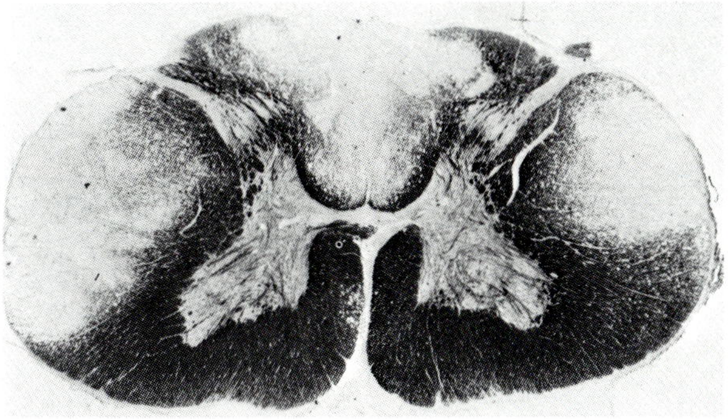

323 Subacute combined degeneration of the cord. Severe myelin degeneration affecting the posterior columns (sparing part of the cuneate tract) and lateral corticospinal tracts. Early involvement of the left anterior corticospinal tract is present. (*Weigert-Pal*, × 12)

Other changes are sore tongue (**324–326**) and hyperpigmentation of the skin (**327, 328**). Neither is pathognomonic of vitamin B_{12} deficiency.

324

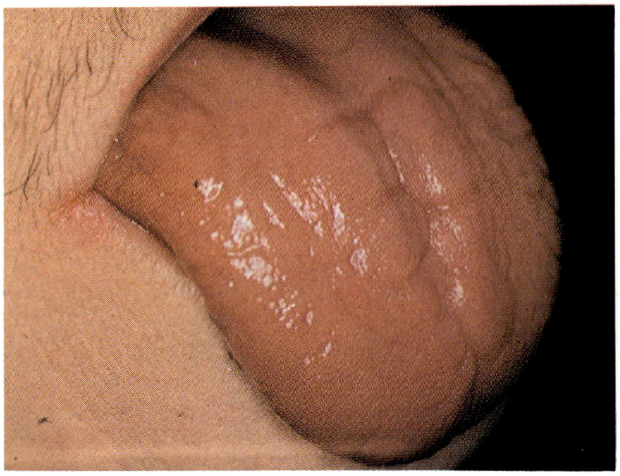

324 A common initial sign in vitamin B_{12} deficiency. The red sore tongue with atrophy of the papillae is often present in pernicious anaemia and, in the case illustrated, angular stomatitis is also present.

32

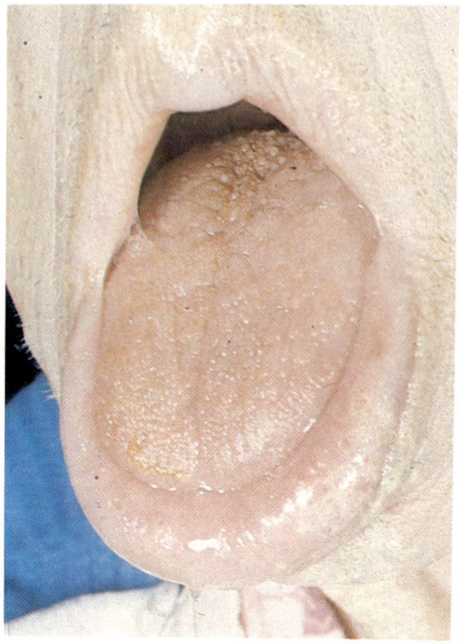

325 Gross vitamin B_{12} deficiency. Pale pink tongue of an 83-year-old woman. Blood and bone marrow examinations confirmed the diagnosis. Note atrophy of the edge of the tongue consistent with gastric atrophy. Her three sisters have pernicious anaemia.

326

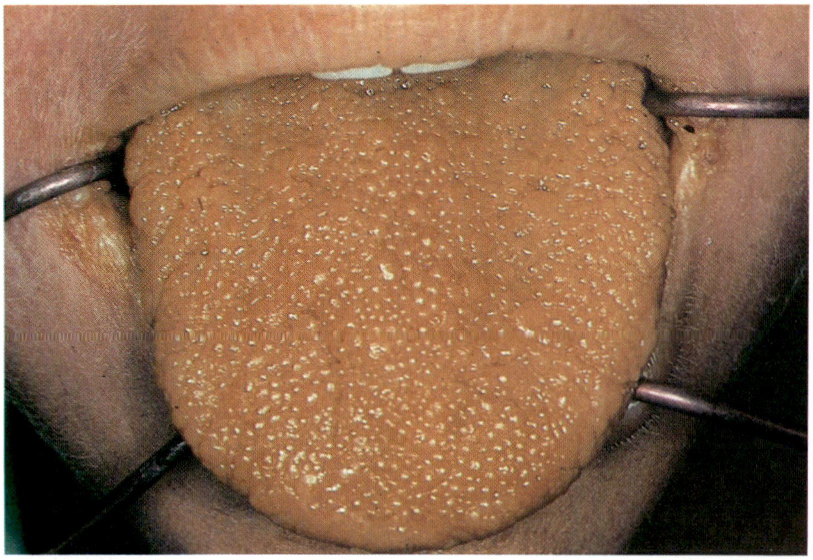

326 Berry-like red tongue. Very acute painful glossitis related to nutritional deficiencies (i.e. vitamin B complex).

327

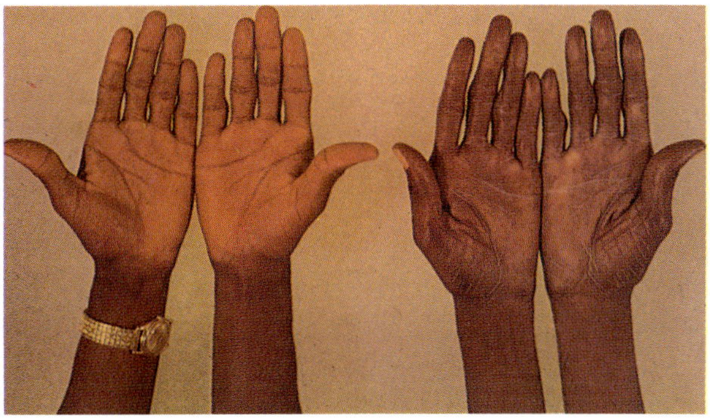

328

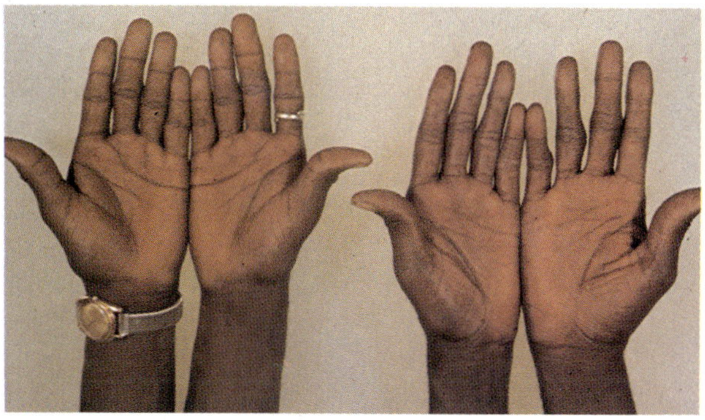

327 **Hyperpigmentation of the skin.** The hands of the patient on the right should be compared with those of his normal brother. A similar change has been described in folic acid deficiency (**312**).

328 **Normal pigmentation.** This picture shows that after treatment with vitamin B_{12} the hands of the patient have become the same colour as those of his brother.

Biotin (vitamin H)

Biotin in food is usually found attached to protein, both animal and vegetable; it is also produced by intestinal bacteria. Diets are rarely deficient; the few human cases have arisen either experimentally or following consumption of large quantities of raw egg containing avidin, which firmly binds biotin in the intestine and inactivates it.

Biotin acts as a coenzyme in a diverse series of metabolic processes. There is insufficient evidence to set an RDA for biotin, but the 'estimated safe and adequate daily dietary intake' for adults lies between 30 and 100μg.

Deficiency

The changes described are seen in other deficiency states also (**329–332**) and symptoms complained of, such as depression, lassitude, and muscle pain, are quite non-specific. Biotin dependency is discussed in Chapter 7.

329

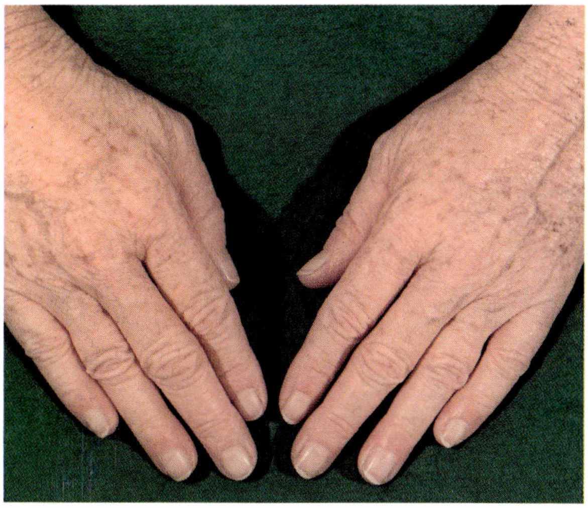

329 Biotin deficiency. This rarely occurs on a natural diet but has been reported, occasionally, as in this case, in patients consuming large quantities of raw egg. This contains avidin which antagonizes the action of biotin. This patient also had cirrhosis of the liver. The skin of the hands is shiny, dry and scaly before treatment.

330

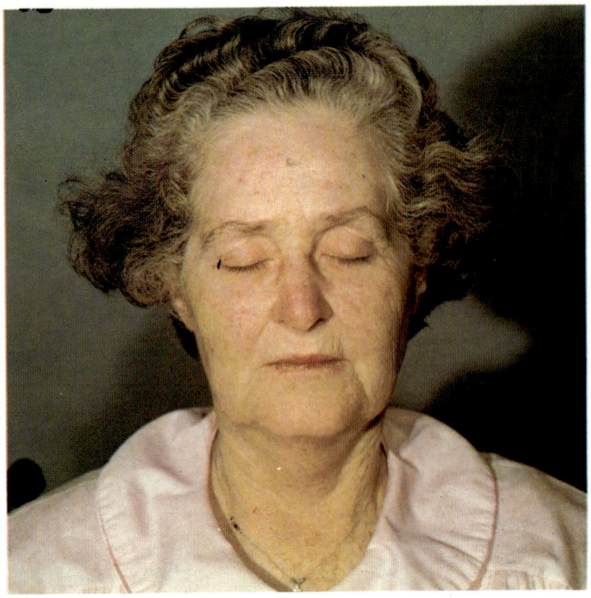

330 **Biotin deficiency.** The face of the same patient before treatment.

3

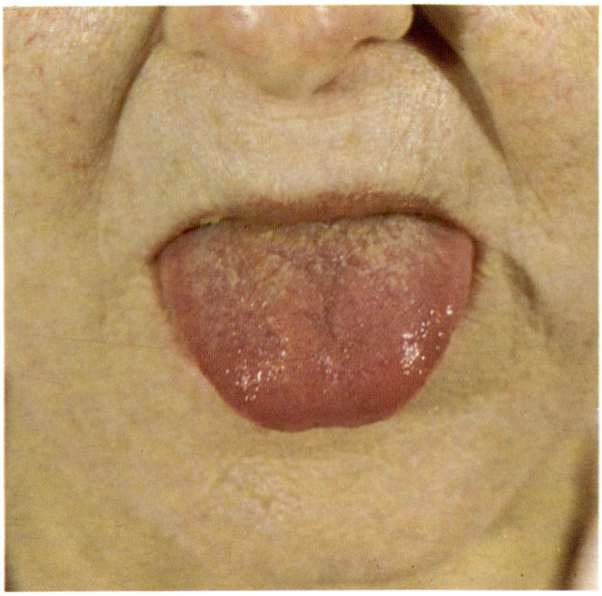

331 **Biotin deficiency.** The tongue of the same patient returned to normal after treatment with biotin as did the skin.

332

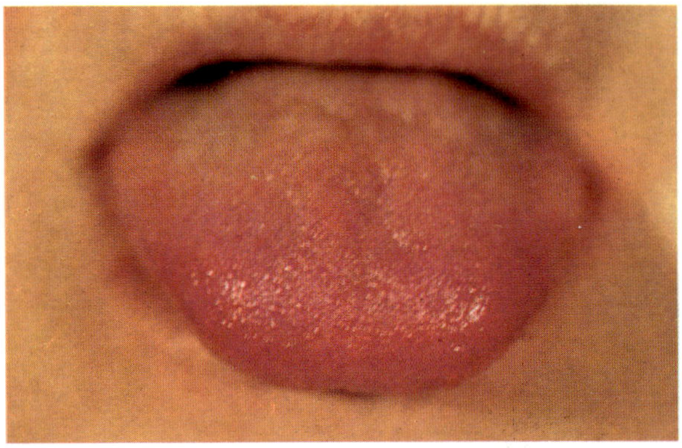

332 **Biotin deficiency.** The oral mucosa is reddened and sore and the tongue is a magenta colour, swollen and painful before treatment.

Vitamin B complex

Vitamins of the B complex are frequently found together in foodstuffs and it is therefore to be expected that deficiency will often be multiple. Moreover, their functions are often interrelated[79] (333).

333

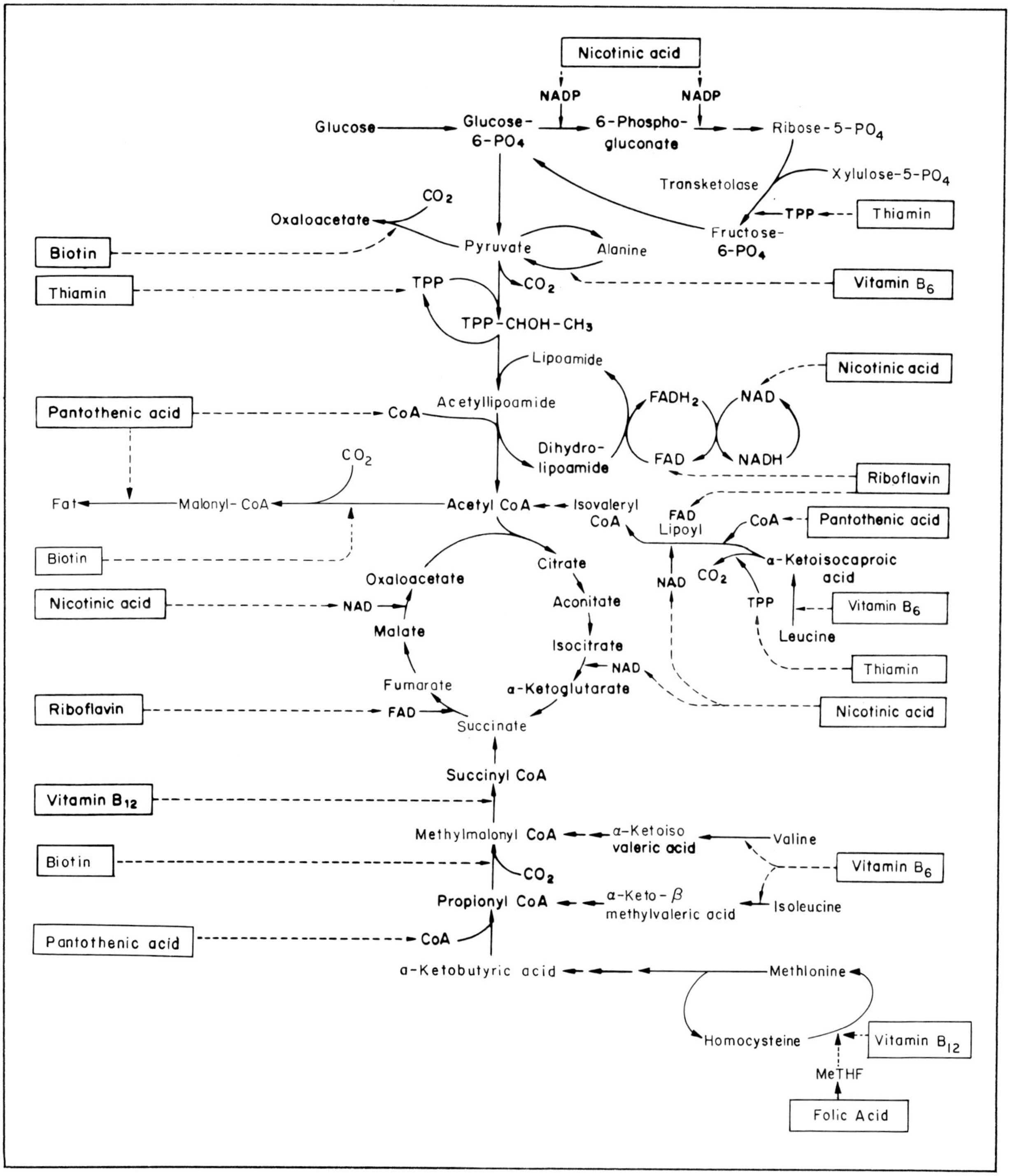

333 **Coenzyme function of B group vitamin derivatives** in some major pathways in the liver.

Among the signs that have been attributed to vitamin B complex deficiency are the oral appearances shown (**334–336**) and nutritional amblyopia (**337**). The latter may have, in addition to the deficiency element, a toxic component involving cyanide, either from pipe tobacco smoke or improperly treated cassava (see also Chapter 9).

334

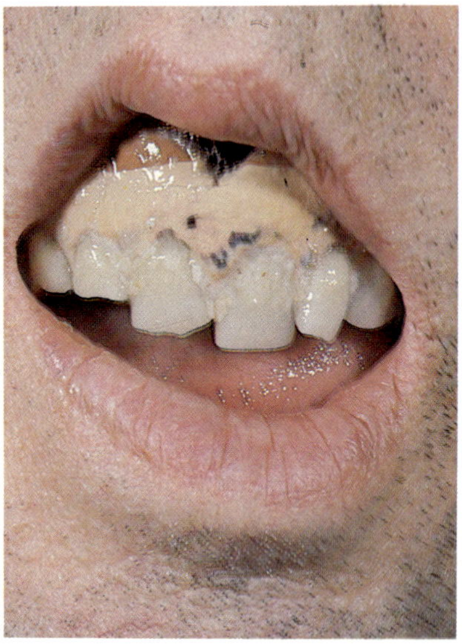

335

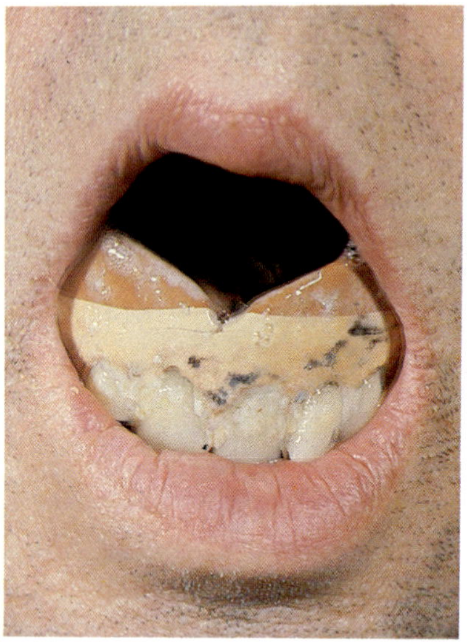

334, 335 **'Portcullis syndrome'.** A good example of this in an elderly European male with recent weight loss and poorly-fitting, out-dated 30-year-old dentures which have not been relined. These are dropping to guard the entrance to his mouth as he goes to sleep, and the lower jaw opens. Such loose dentures and 'portcullis syndrome' are invariably associated with nutritional deficiencies just visible in glossitis at the tongue tip.

336

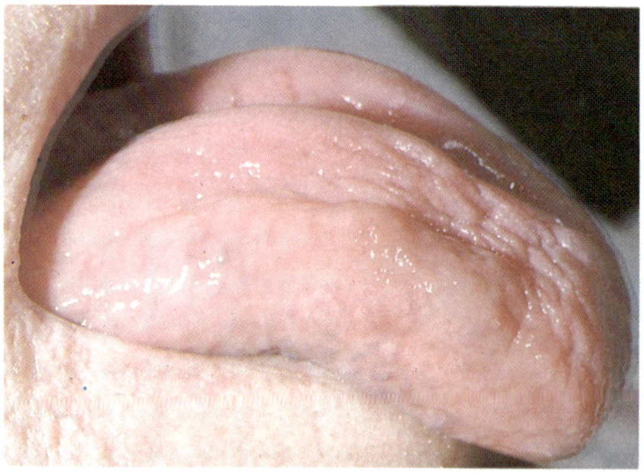

336 **'Portcullis syndrome'.** The tongue of an elderly female where atrophy of filiform papillae dominates the clinical picture, giving rise to a smooth pale tongue and iron deficiency anaemia.

337 **Nutritional retrobulbar neuropathy.** Increased pallor of the temporal aspect of the optic disc is accompanied by pain behind the eyeball, photophobia and visual field defects consisting of central or centrocaecal scotomata. The papillomacular bundle of the optic nerve shows degenerative changes.

Patients are frequently deficient in vitamin B_{12} but thiamin deficiency may sometimes be responsible.

337

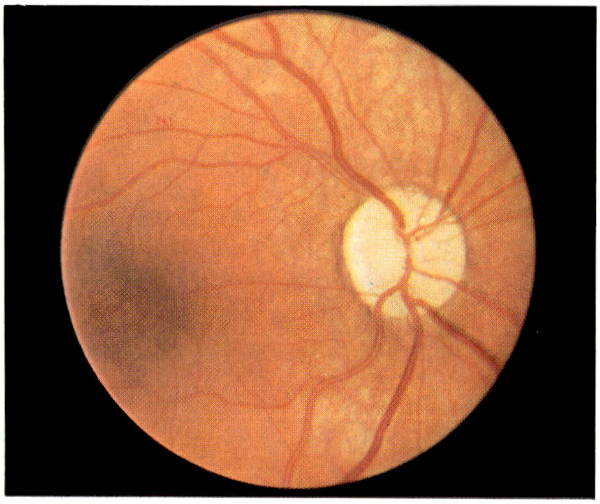

Vitamin C (ascorbic acid)

Man is among the relatively few animals that cannot synthesize ascorbic acid (see Chapter 1). In his diet most ascorbic acid comes from fresh citrus fruits and vegetables like broccoli, brussel sprouts and potatoes, none of which are rich in the acid, but they are all eaten in large amounts. It is the vitamin most readily destroyed in large scale cooking or food processing.

Ascorbic acid is involved in intracellular electron transfer, being readily oxidized and reversibly reduced. It is also necessary for normal fibrous collagen to be formed and in connective tissue it takes part in the hydroxylation of protocollagen proline and lysine to collagen hydroxyproline and hydroxylysine. It is one of the most potent enhancers of non-haem iron absorption in the small intestine.

Contrary to some suggestions, it is not generally accepted that vitamin C in megadoses (i.e. many grams/day) decreases the incidence or severity of the common cold or prevents cancer. Vitamin C status is better reflected in the level in the leucocytes of the blood (the 'buffy coat') than in the plasma concentration (Appendix III, Table 1). The RDA has been set at different levels in different countries at different times but at present is about 60mg for the adult (Appendix I, Table 4).

Deficiency (scurvy)

Deficiency of vitamin C is common in arid areas during the 'hungry' season and in famines when all age groups may be affected. Elsewhere a high-risk group is infancy (Barlow's disease) especially if vitamin supplements and fruit juice are not given and if artificial milk is boiled and the vitamin C destroyed (338–345). Many of these changes are not seen in the adult.

338

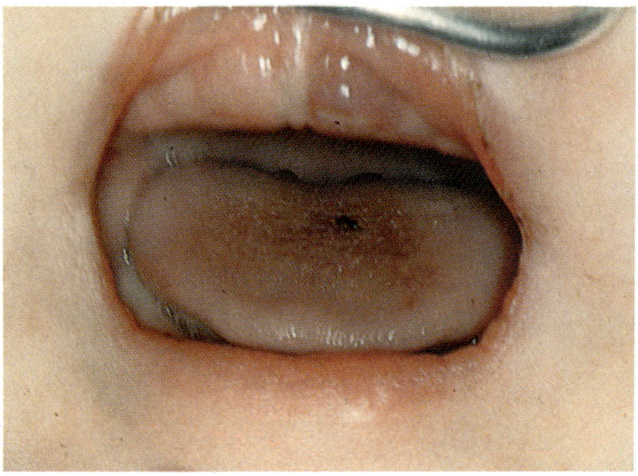

338 **Gum changes in infant scurvy.** The swelling and haemorrhages are confined to the areas of gum surrounding the erupting teeth.

339

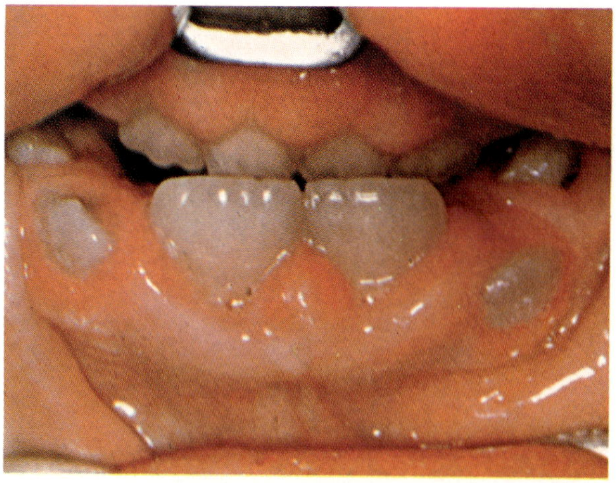

339 Dilantoin toxicity. This should be distinguished from scorbotic gum lesions. Among the side effects of dilantoin (phenytoin sodium, diphenylhydantoin sodium) is gingival hyperplasia, occurring in about 20% on long-term therapy. It is probably the most common toxic effect in children and adolescents. The hyperplasia appears to involve altered collagen metabolism. Toothless portions of the gums are not affected. It can be minimized by good oral hygiene and does not necessitate withdrawal of medication.

340

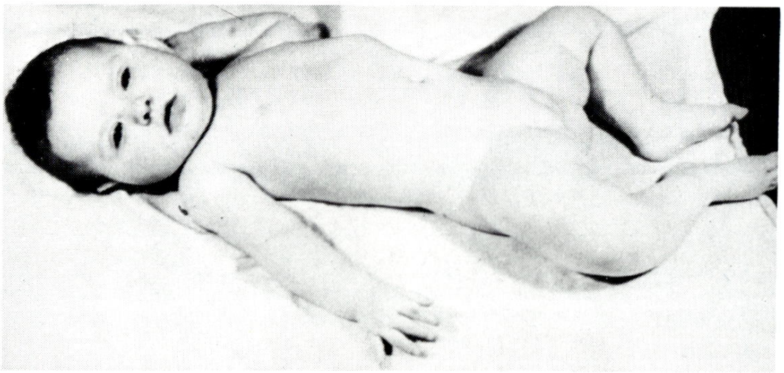

340 The 'pithed frog' position. The characteristic pseudo-paralysis of the limbs, with the legs flexed at the knees and the hips partially flexed and externally rotated, is due to the extreme pain experienced on their movement due to haemorrhages under the periosteum and sometimes infraction of an epiphysis.

341

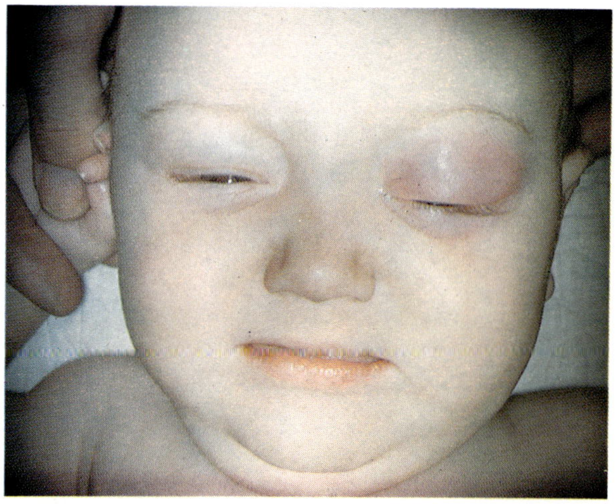

341 Orbital haemorrhage. This is a dramatic but infrequent sign of scurvy. There is complete clearing with treatment.

342 Bone in scurvy. Defective formation of mesenchymal tissue results from failure of deposition of intercellular ground substance by fibroblasts. In the shafts of long bones osteoid is not deposited by osteoblasts, the cortex is thin, trabeculae are diminished in size and haemorrhages occur under the periosteum.

342

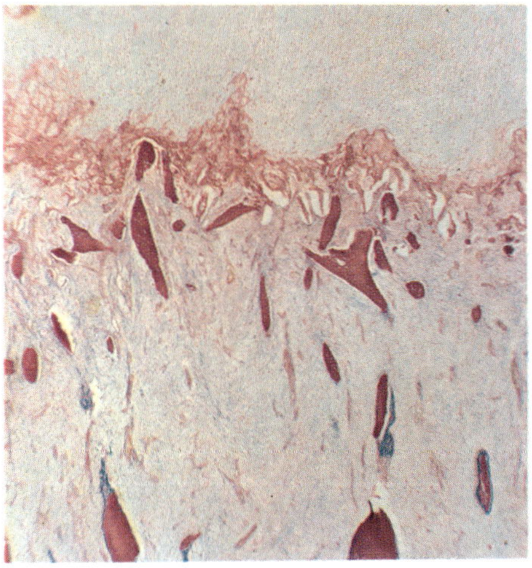

343 Bones in active scurvy. The earliest X-ray changes appear at the sites of most active bone growth: sternal ends of the ribs, distal end of the femur, proximal end of the humerus, both ends of tibia and fibula, and distal ends of radius and ulna. Several characteristic signs are shown here. A zone of rarefaction immediately shaftward of the zone of provisional calcification gives rise to the 'corner fracture' sign. Atrophy of the trabecular structure and blurring of trabecular markings cause the bone to have a 'ground glass' appearance. Widening of the zone of provisional calcification causes a dense shadow at the end of the shaft (the white or Frankel's line). It also occurs at the periphery of the centres of ossification ('halo' epiphysis or 'pencilled effect') (see *Table 53*).

343

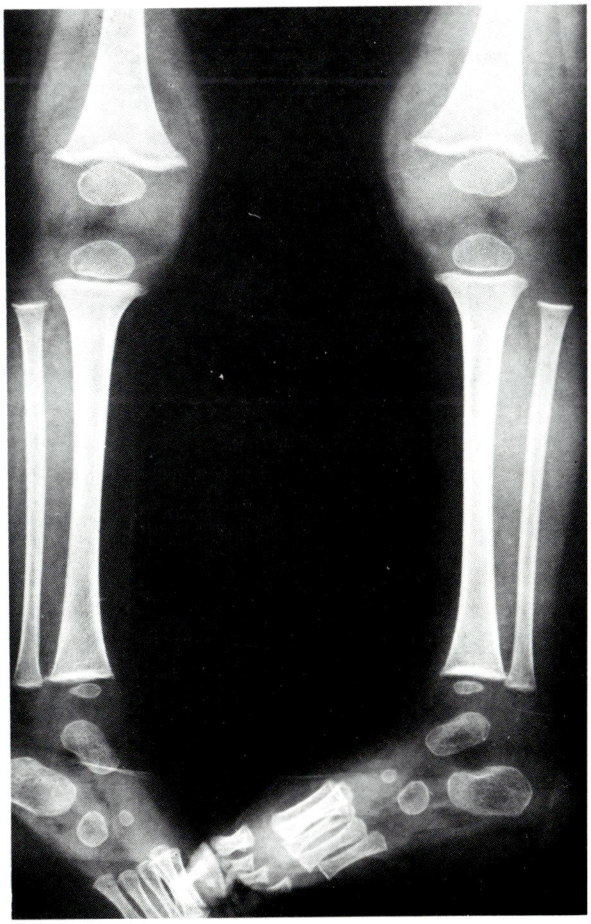

344

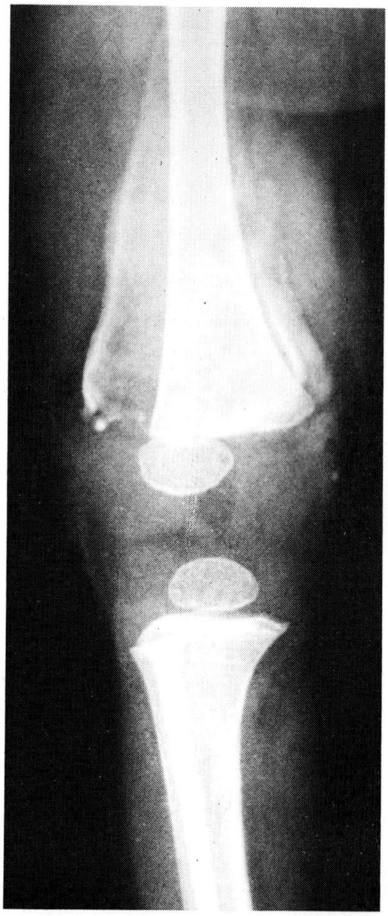

344 Bones in healing scurvy. Calcification is occurring in the region of subperiosteal haemorrhage in an infant two weeks after treatment with vitamin C. The femoral epiphysis is displaced. Even the grossest deformities resolve, but radiological evidence may persist for several years.

345

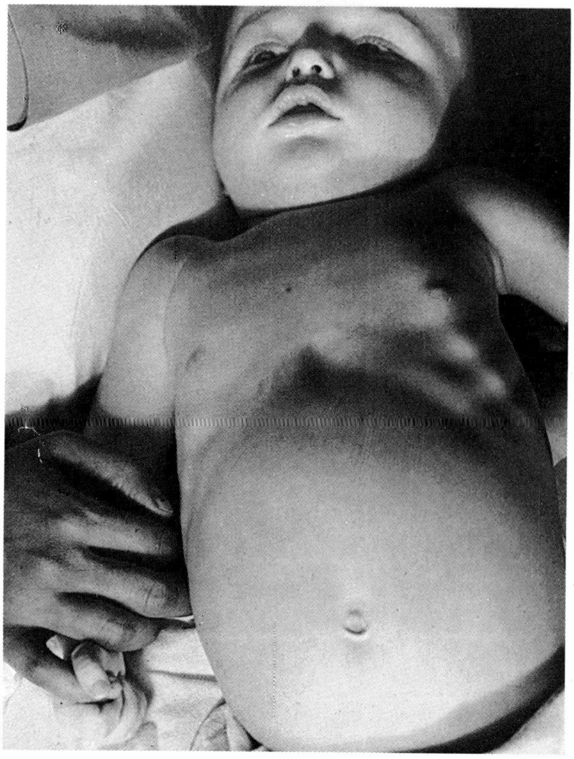

345 Active scorbutic rosary. The cartilaginous thoracic wall is pulled in by the respiratory effort.

There are numerous characteristic X-ray appearances which assist in diagnosis (*Table 53*).

The other group singled out is the elderly, in particular men living on their own or handicapped – it has been termed 'bachelor's' or 'workhouse' scurvy. Among advanced changes are bleeding, spongy gums (**346, 347**), splinter haemorrhages (**348**) and impaired wound healing (**349–351**).

Table 53. X-ray appearances in infantile scurvy.

First affected are sites of rapid bone growth: sternal ends of ribs (scorbutic rosary), distal end of femur, proximal end of humerus, both ends of tibia and fibula, distal ends of radius and ulna
Corner sign – earliest sign; cleft underneath epiphyseal line due to pulling away of abnormal scorbutic lattice, especially at lower ends of tibia and radius
White line – dense zone of provisional calcification at epiphyseal end of diaphysis
Zone of rarefaction (Trummerfeld of Fraenkel), area of broken down bone trabeculae and connective tissue
Ground glass appearance of osteoporotic shaft
Halo or pencilled outlining of epiphyses from dense cortex and atrophic trabeculae
Subperiosteal haemorrhage with laminated calcification on healing

346

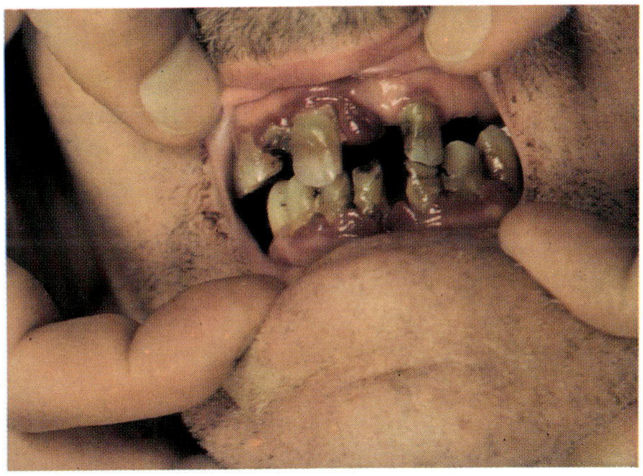

347

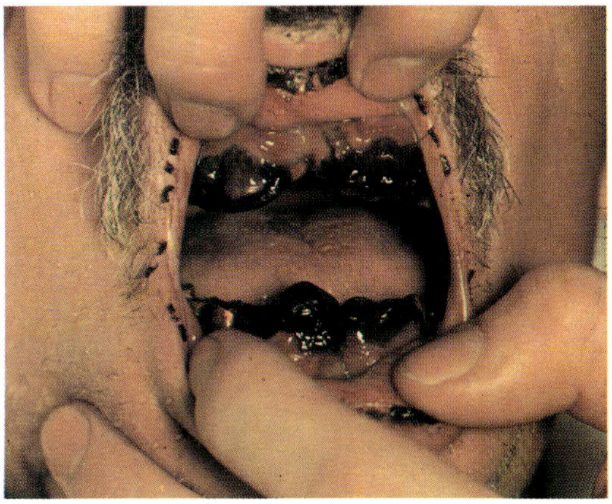

346 Gums in scurvy. The gums are blue-red and grossly swollen in this patient with severe scurvy. The earliest changes are swelling of the interdental papillae and tendency to bleed easily. Lesions occur only in relation to teeth and so in young infants and edentulous adults they are absent. In advanced cases there is usually an element of infection, and antibiotics as well as vitamin C are required for healing.

347 Very advanced gum lesions in scurvy.

348

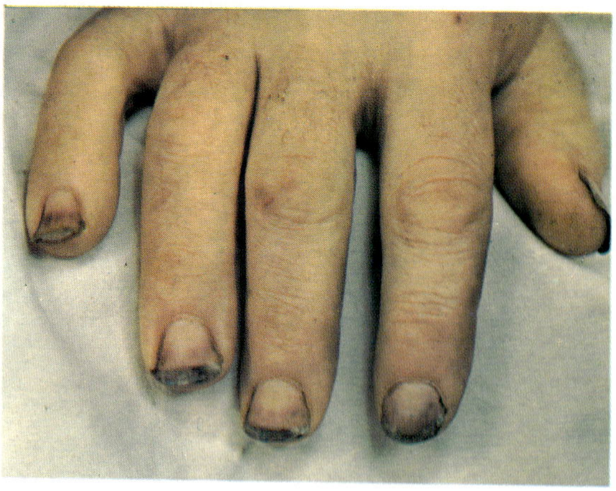

348 Splinter haemorrhages. In this unusual sign in scurvy the haemorrhages are arranged in a semicircular lattice involving the nail beds. They are more extensive than those in subacute bacterial endocarditis.

349

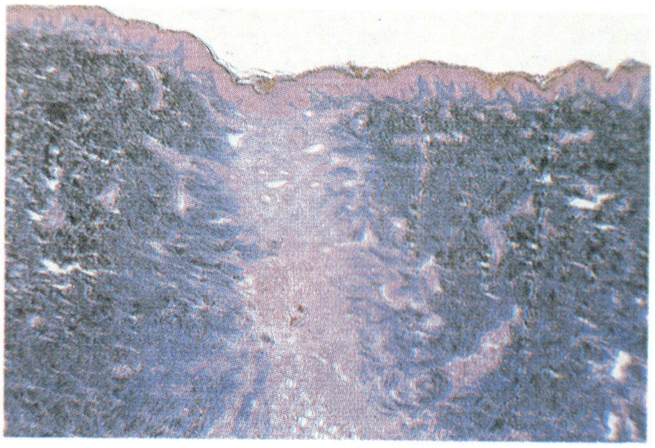

349 Impaired wound healing. In 1940 J.H. Crandon placed himself on a vitamin C-free diet. After 3 months when the ascorbic acid level in the blood had been zero for 44 days, a wound was made in the mid-back region. Biopsy 10 days later shows suboptimal healing (see **351**).

350

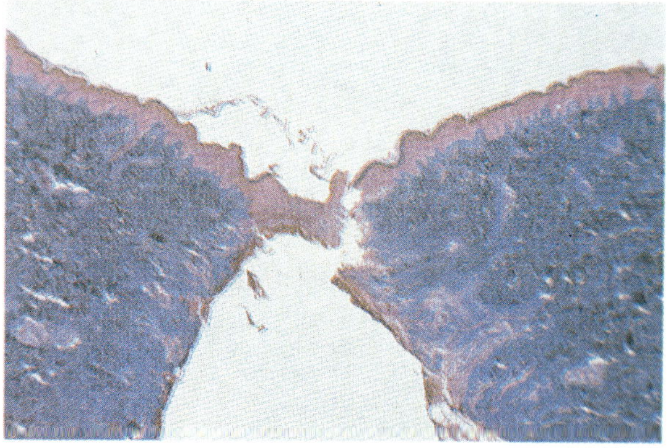

350 Impaired wound healing. After 6 months of the scorbutic diet another wound was made. Biopsy 10 days later shows no healing except of the epithelium (gap in tissue was filled with a blood clot).

3

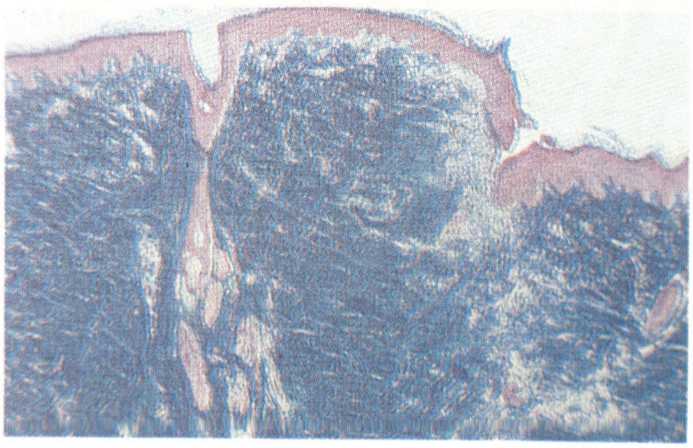

351 Impaired wound healing. After 10 days of vitamin C treatment, another biopsy of the second wound shows healing with abundant collagen formation, considerably more than occurred in the first wound.

Osteoporosis in scurvy is occasionally seen (**352**). Bone changes are much less common in the adult than in childhood (**353**).

352 Bone changes of scurvy in Bantu of South Africa. These have been described in association with iron overload (see page 187).

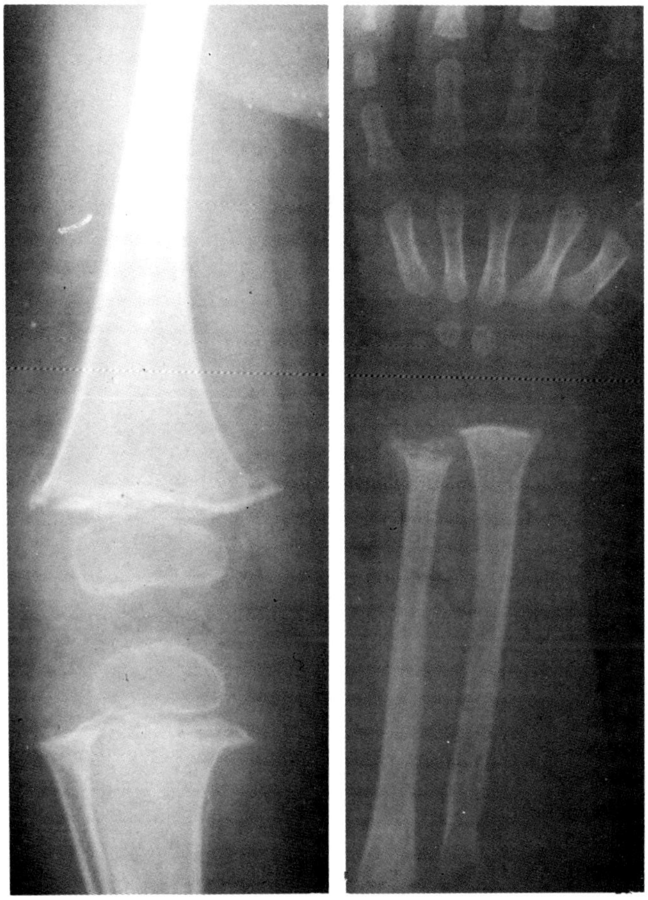

352

353 **Scorbutic rosary** in the healed stage in a boy who had had scurvy off and on since infancy. The sharp edges at the costochondral junctions are easily visible and this appearance is said to differentiate the scorbutic from the rachitic rosary, in which the enlarged costochondral junctions are smooth and rounded. Nevertheless, rickets and scurvy coexist not infrequently.

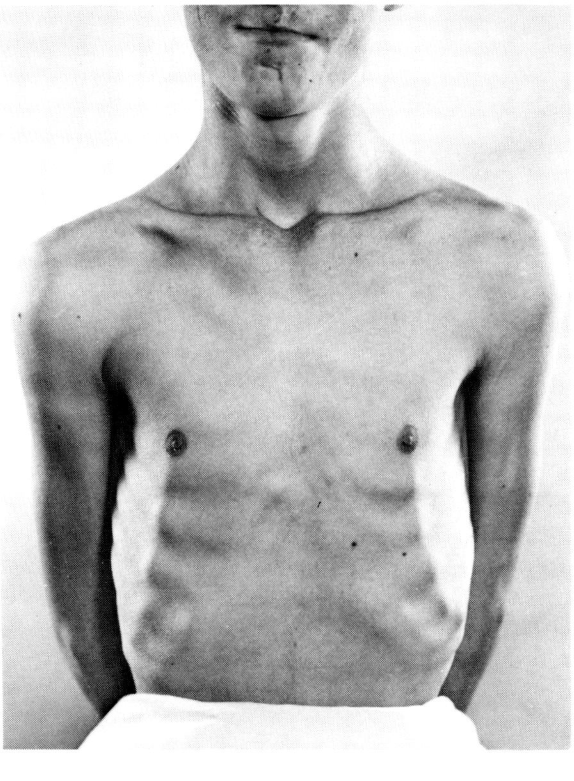

353

Important clinical changes for early recognition of deficiency include perifollicular petechiae (**354**) and 'swan neck' deformity of hairs (**355**); ecchymoses are a later extension of petechiae (**356**).

Rapid response follows 100mg vitamin C t.i.d. until 4g have been given. Weakness and bleeding cease within 24 hours, gum and skin changes disappear in about 2 weeks, but bone healing takes 1–2 months.

354

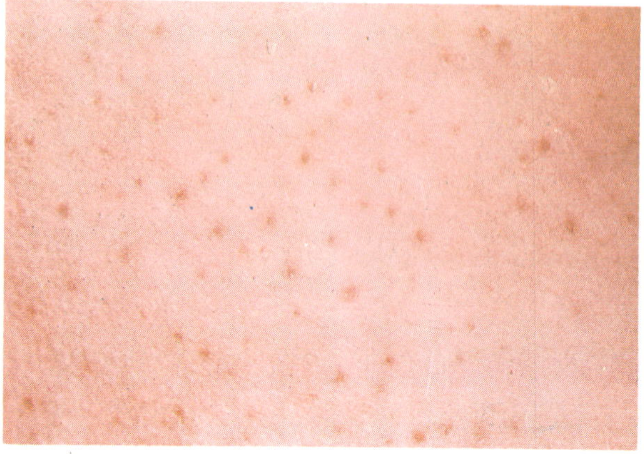

354 Perifollicular petechiae. Minimal bleeding into the hair follicles is pathognomonic of vitamin C deficiency and is often one of the earliest clinical manifestations. In vitamin K deficiency, thrombocytopenia and other conditions petechiae are situated in areas of skin unrelated to the hair follicles. In perifollicular hyperkeratosis (**218**, **219** and **221**) there is no bleeding and hyperkeratosis is present. Ecchymoses develop in more advanced deficiency and are the most frequent sign in 'workhouse' scurvy in old men.

355

355 'Swan neck' deformity of the hairs characteristic of the early stages of adult scurvy.

356

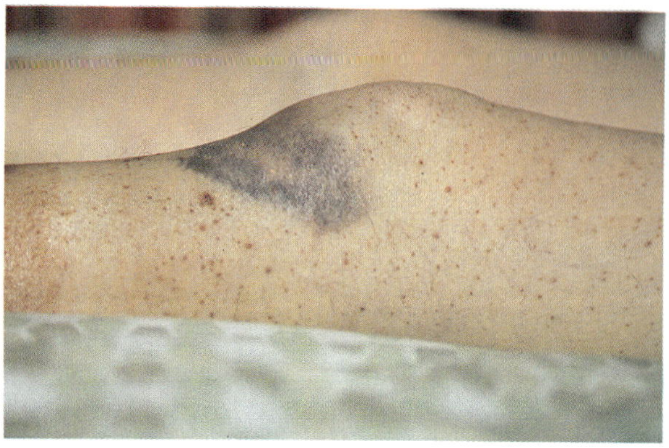

356 Ecchymoses like this may occur anywhere in the skin in advanced scurvy.

6. Element, Water and Electrolyte Deficiency and Toxicity

Of the 92 natural chemical elements more than 50 are found in body tissues and fluids of man. About 96.5% of body weight is made up of just four of these – oxygen, hydrogen, carbon, and nitrogen. Hydrogen and oxygen in the form of water account for about 60% of body weight. The remaining 4% is made of essential elements, most of which are minerals, and also traces of mineral contaminants from the environment. Over recent years many elements that were in the last category have been 'promoted' to the former because they have been found to be essential in trace amounts for animals and/or man. The relative positions in the Periodic Table (357) of the elements that appear below suggest that the process is not yet completed.

It is convenient to classify elements that are found in the body into five categories:

1. **Essential macroelements** – required in amounts of 100mg/day or more: calcium, phosphorus, sodium, potassium, chlorine, magnesium, and sulphur.
2. **Essential micro- or trace elements** – required in amounts of no more than a few mg and sometimes only a few µg/day: iron, copper, cobalt, zinc, manganese, iodine, molybdenum, selenium, and chromium.
3. **Essential microelements necessary for animals but not proved for man:** tin, silicon, vanadium, and most recently arsenic and possibly cadmium and lead.
4. **Trace contaminants with no known function:** mercury, barium, strontium, aluminium, lithium, beryllium, rubidium, gold, silver, and others.
5. **Indeterminate status:** fluorine – requirement not proved, but protective against dental caries and possibly osteoporosis; boron – requirement not proved, but enhances action of other elements against osteoporosis.

Some elements in the fourth category with no known function can be notoriously toxic and their occurrence and effects in food are considered with other food toxins in Chapter 9.

357

																H	He
(2.2) Li	(36) Be											(48) B	**C**	**N**	**O**	(3300) F	Ne
Na	**Mg**											(100) Al	(1100) Si* 1972	**P**	**S**	**Cl**	Ar
K	**Ca**	Sc	(9) Ti	(10) V* 1971	(3) Cr* 1959	(14) Mn* 1931	(4000) Fe* 17thC	(1.3) Co* 1935	(8) Ni* 1973	(60) Cu* 1928	(2000) Zn* 1934	Ga	(20) Ge	(14) As* 1975	(21) Se* 1957	(200) Br	Kr
(320) Rb	(340) Sr	Y	(340) Zr	(120) Nb	(13) Mo* 1953	Tc	Ru	Rh	Pd	(0.8) Ag	(34) Cd* 1976	In	(42) Sn* 1970	(6) Sb	(7) Te	(15) I* 1850	Xe
(1.4) Cs	(22) Ba	La	Hf	Ta	W	Re	Os	Ir	Pt	Au	(13) Hg	(7) Tl	(122) Pb* 1979	(0.2) Bi	Po	At	Rn
Fr	Ra	Ac															

357 **Periodic table of elements,** showing the relative positions of essential and non-essential elements. (The lanthanoid and actinoid series have been omitted.) The symbols for essential elements present in greater than trace quantities are in large letters; those for trace elements currently recognized as essential are in smaller letters followed by asterisks and with the years in which they were first reported to be essential †. Symbols for trace elements not currently known to be essential are shown in smaller letters. Quantities (mg) of the trace elements found in the average 70-kg human are given in parentheses.

Iron

Iron is probably the most studied microelement. It is found in most usual foodstuffs; only 10% or less of the non-haem iron from vegetable sources is absorbed and absorption is impaired by phytate but improved by animal protein and ascorbic acid. Haem iron is much more readily absorbed and uninfluenced by other dietary components.

The metabolism of iron is outlined in 358.

358

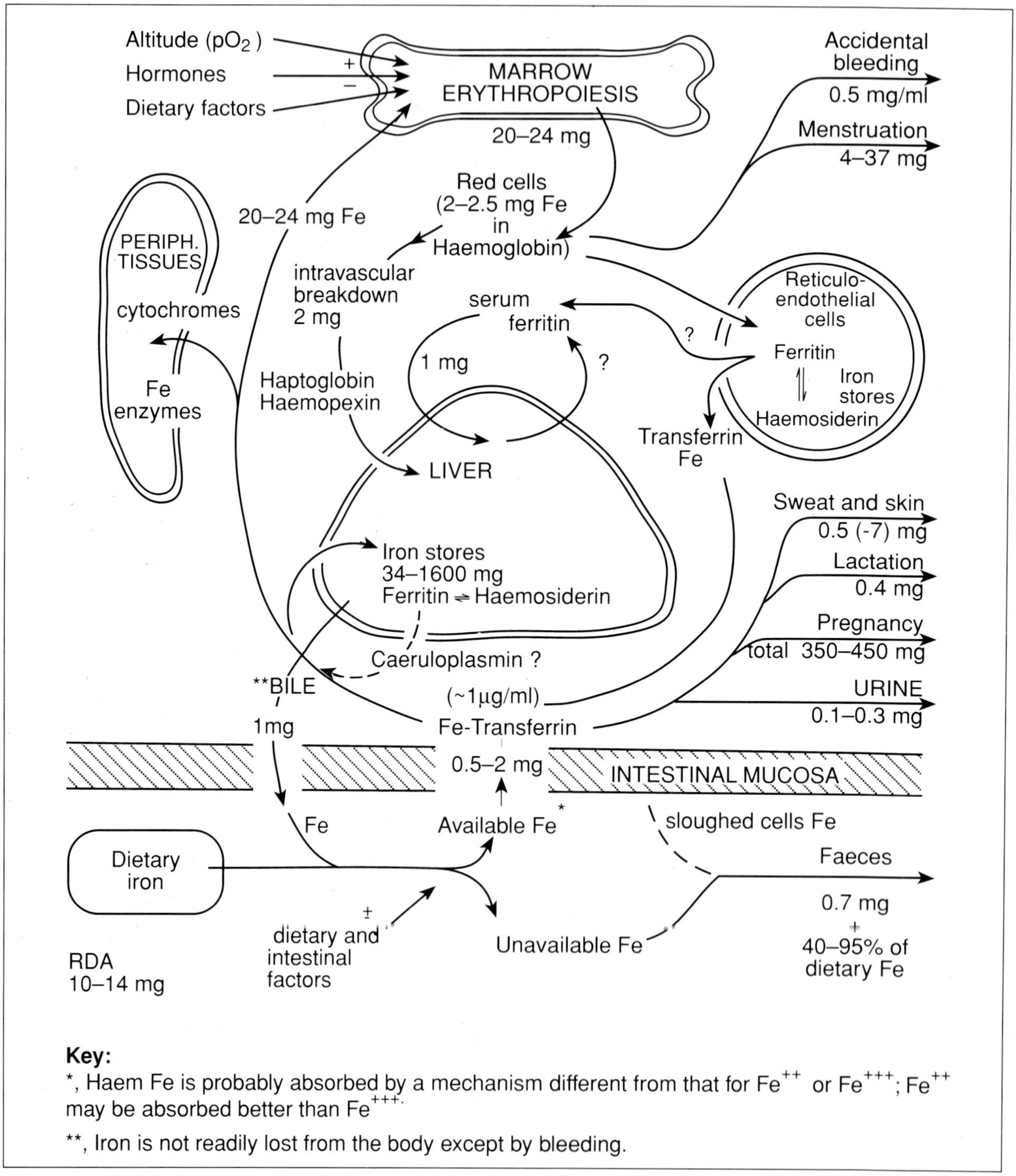

358 Nutrition and metabolism of iron. Quantities are average values per day. Total body iron is 2.5–3.5g.

The minute amount of ferritin in serum (normal male 14–31 µmol/l; female 11–30 µmol/l) is a sensitive measure of iron status (Appendix III, Table 2).

The relative sensitivity of various tests in assessing iron status is shown diagrammatically in 359. The adult RDA is 10mg in the male and 18mg in the female.

359

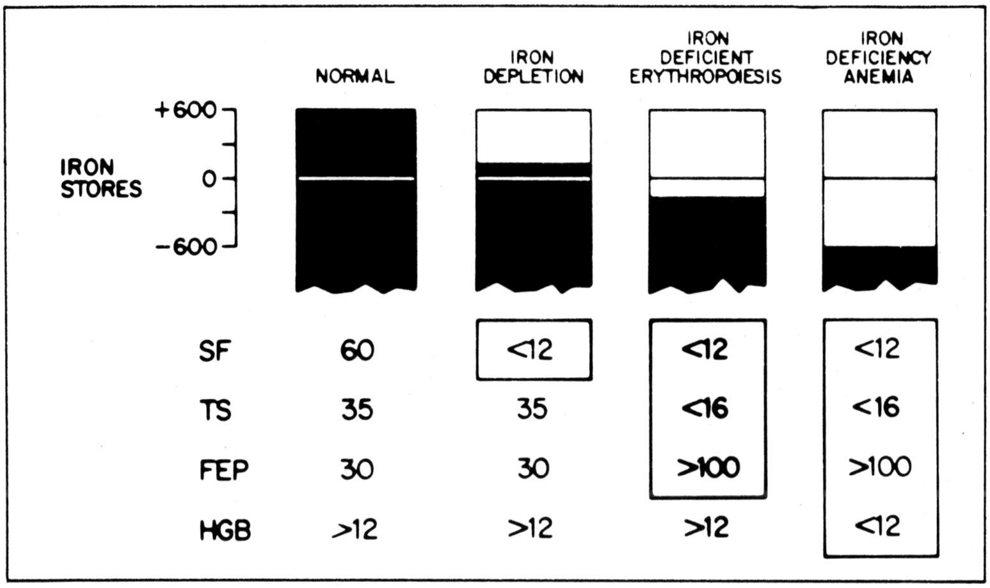

359 Iron status in relation to body iron stores. Various measures of body iron status are shown in relation to body iron stores in milligrams (shaded areas). Negative iron stores represent depletion from circulating red cells. **Key:** SF, serum ferritin (µg/l); TS, transferrin saturation (as a percentage); FEP, free erythrocyte protoporphyrin (µg/100ml red cells); and HGB, haemoglobin (g/dl).

Deficiency

Although iron deficiency is usually thought of together with anaemia, it is being increasingly recognized that certain clinical features may precede the development of anaemia (*Table 54*).

Table 54. Signs of iron deficiency unrelated to anaemia.

Glossitis – red, painful in 40%
Angular stomatitis
Koilonychia
Dysphagia – in 10%, mostly women, with postcricoid webs leading occasionally to cancer
Splenomegaly, in 10%
Atrophy of gastric mucosa, achlorhydria
Intestinal mucosal atrophy
Fatigue in absence of anaemia (possibly related to impairment of cytochrome oxidase and other enzyme systems)
Immune system – treatment of iron deficiency tends to increase infections (bacterial and some other)
Impaired intellectual function, especially in young children

Table 55. Causes of iron deficiency.

Increased requirements	
	Infancy (especially low birthweight)
	Adolescence
	Menstruation
	Pregnancy and lactation
Reduced dietary intake	
	Diet high in cereal content, low in animal protein
	Veganism
	Elderly
Defective absorption	
	Geophagia (pica), especially young children and pregnant women
	Malabsorption syndromes (e.g. coeliac disease)
	Chronic diarrhoea
	Partial or total gastrectomy
	Gastric bypass surgery for refractory obesity
	Atrophic gastritis and achlorhydria
	Elderly
Blood loss	
	Gastrointestinal: often occult, most commonly peptic ulcer, hiatus hernia, oesophageal varices, salicylate ingestion, intestinal diverticula, tumours, helminthiasis, regional enteritis, ulcerative colitis
	Other sites: e.g. urinary tract, menorrhagia
Reduction in availability of Fe for Hb synthesis	
	Idiopathic pulmonary haemosiderosis
	Paroxysmal nocturnal haemoglobinuria
	Chronic inflammation, malignancy (failure of reutilization)
	Congenital atransferrinaemia
Idiopathic	
	March haemoglobinuria
	Elite long distance running

The main causes of iron deficiency are given in *Table 55*.

The well-known haemopoietic system features are shown in **360–362**.

360 Hypochromia and microcytosis of iron deficiency anaemia. These changes are evident only when iron deficiency is severe and they are also very nonspecific. Mean corpuscular volume (MCV) < 80μm^3 is a sensitive index of microcytosis but is nonspecific as to cause. Early indications of iron deficiency are generally considered to be serum iron concentration < 50μg/dl or transferrin saturation < 15% in adults. (× 100).

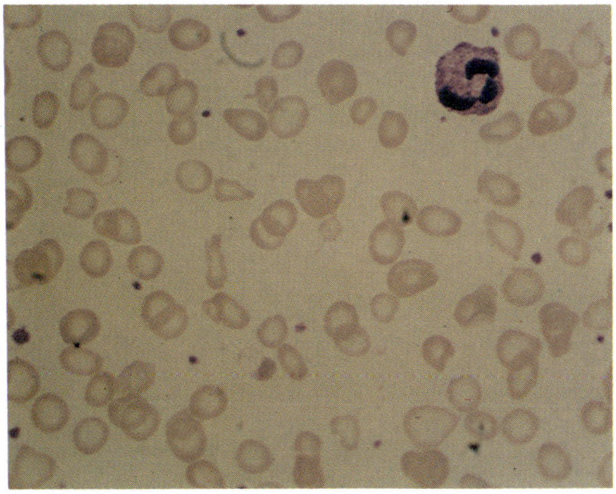

360

361 Bone marrow in iron deficiency. Erythroid hypoplasia and nuclear dysplasia are present. In sections stained with Prussian blue little stainable iron will be evident. Serum ferritin is in equilibrium with storage iron in marrow, liver and other tissues and is a good early indication of iron state (normal male 14–31μmol/l, normal female 11–30μmol/l). (× 100)

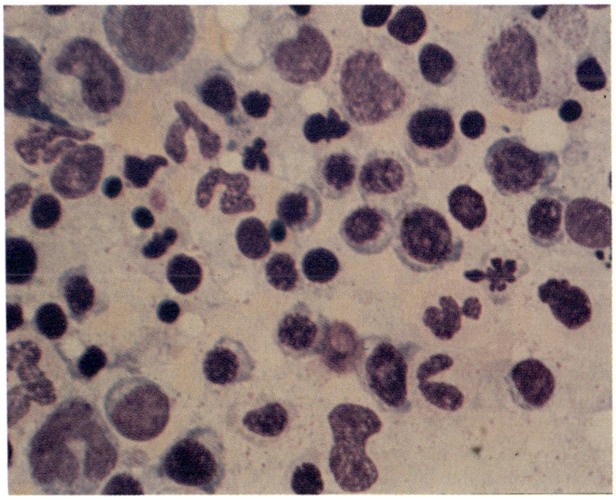

361

362 Iron deficiency anaemia. The electron microscopic appearance of the small and poorly filled erythrocytes. (× 8900)

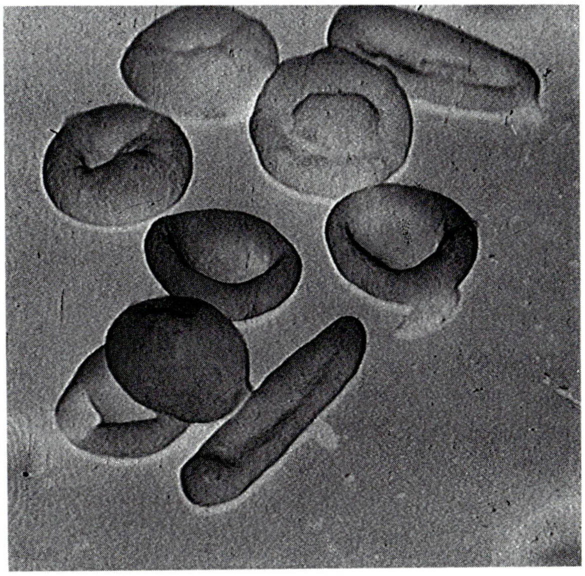

362

363

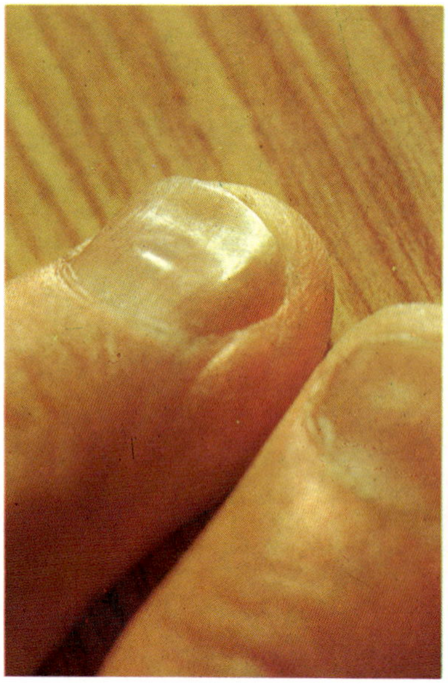

Characteristically the nails show koilonychia (**363, 364**), but other causes have also been reported (*Table 56*).

363 **Koilonychia.** Thinning, flattening and finally a concave or spoon-shaped appearance of the nails, as here, is typical of advanced iron deficiency. Brittle or longitudinally ridged nails are nonspecific, Koilonychia is thought to be rare in young children with iron deficiency, but it was present in at least one study in a considerable proportion. The mechanism is not clear, nor is it understood why it does not occur in other forms of anaemia. It may result from prolonged exposure to soap suds and other caustic agents. When associated with fungal diseases of the skin the nails are irregularly pitted. Spoon-shaped toenails are common in bare foot communities and are of no significance.

364

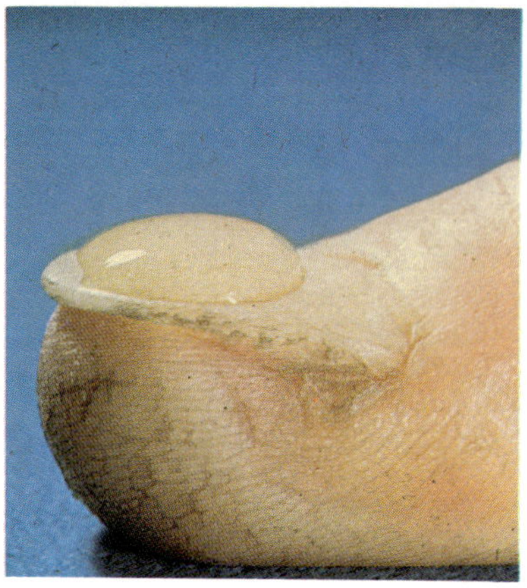

364 **Drop of water test for koilonychia.**

Table 56. Factors in koilonychia.

Iron deficiency, severe (most common)
Deficiency of sulphur-containing amino acids as in severe PEM
Diabetes mellitus of long standing, especially in men
Raynaud's disease (uncommon)
Developmental abnormality

365 Skull in iron deficiency. Frontal X-ray of the skull in a young child with iron deficiency anaemia demonstrating non-uniform widening of the diploic space with a 'hair-on-end' appearance.

365

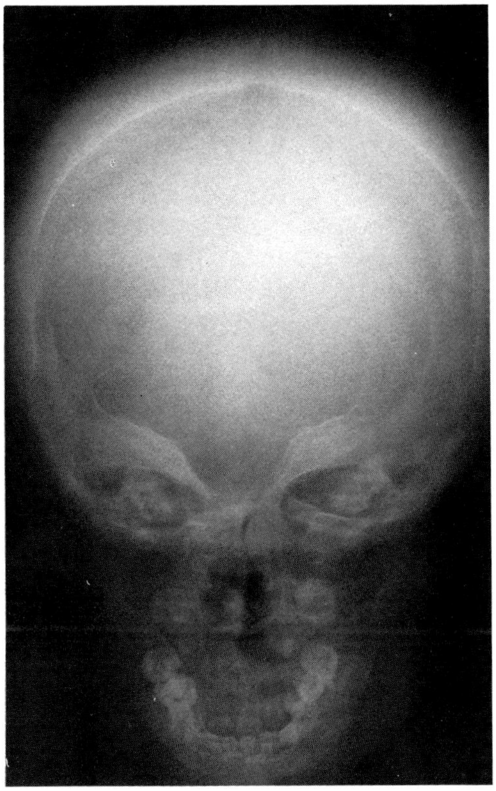

366 Skull in iron deficiency. Lateral view of the same patient.

366

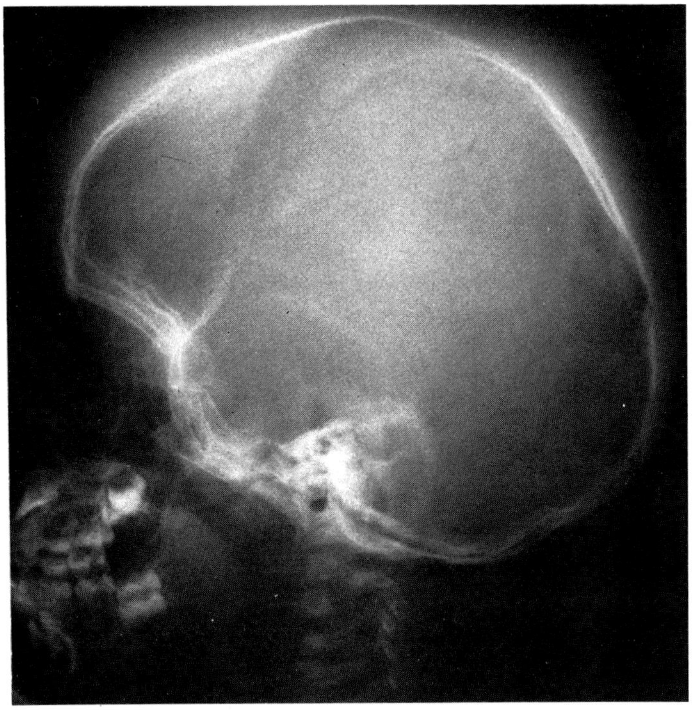

The gastrointestinal tract shows mucosal atrophy (**367**) and changes in the tongue which are not diagnostic (**368**).

Glossitis, angular stomatitis and postcricoid changes causing dysphagia and which may go on to carcinoma are features of the Plummer–Vinson (Paterson–Kelly) syndrome, much less common in women than it used to be in the earlier part of this century (**369–374**).

367

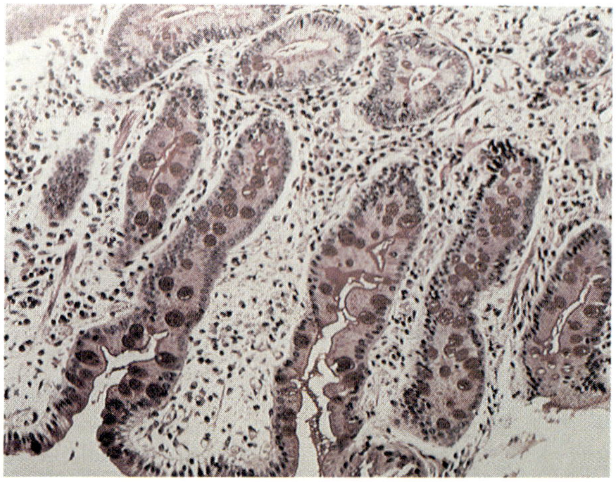

367 **Iron deficiency and the stomach.** This patient had iron deficiency for several years. The section shows intestinalization of the stomach which is considered to be premalignant.

368

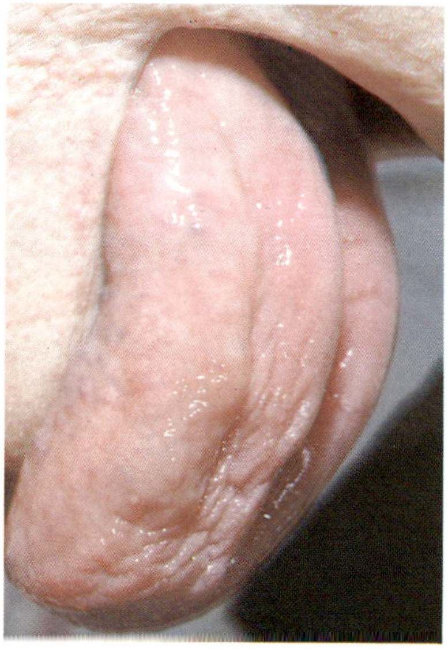

368 **Atrophy of filiform papillae** leading to a smooth pale tongue may have been caused by iron deficiency or 'portcullis syndrome' (see **336**).

369 Plummer–Vinson (Paterson–Kelly) syndrome. There is usually a longstanding history of sideropenic anaemia, angular stomatitis, brittle nails (often koilonychia) and dysphagia. Six months before admission of this 71-year-old woman (cases are almost always female) X-ray showed typical postcricoid webs.

369

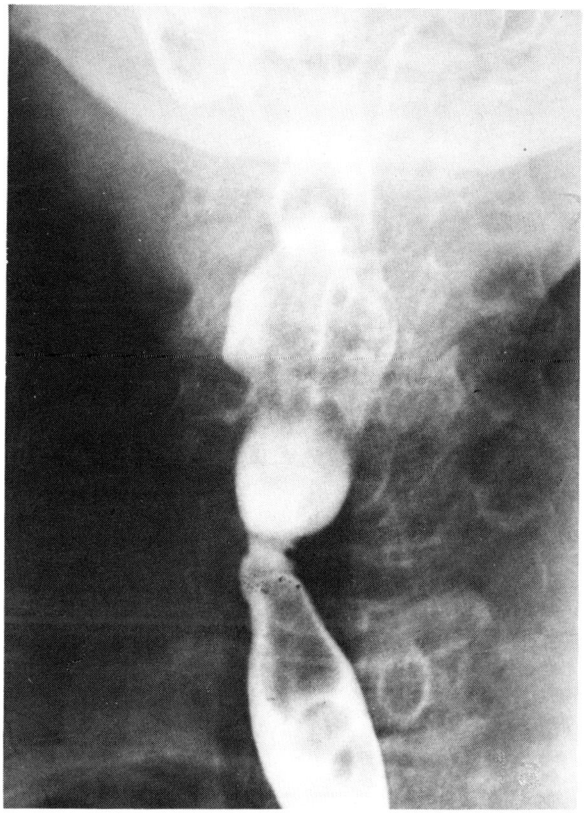

370 **Plummer–Vinson syndrome.** Another X-ray view of the same patient taken at the same time.

371 **Plummer–Vinson syndrome.** The same patient as before in whom an X-ray taken 6 months later reveals an extensive hypopharyngeal carcinoma involving both upper and lower part. The haemoglobin and serum iron were normal.

70

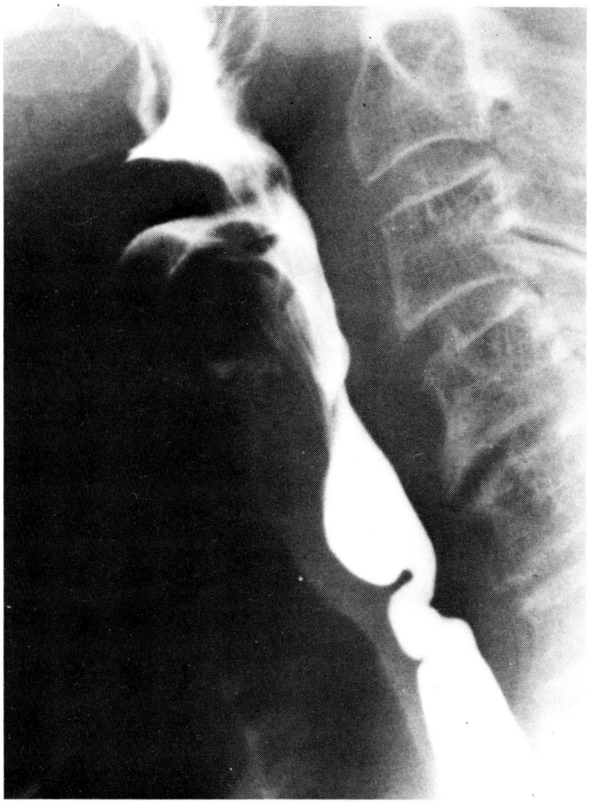

371

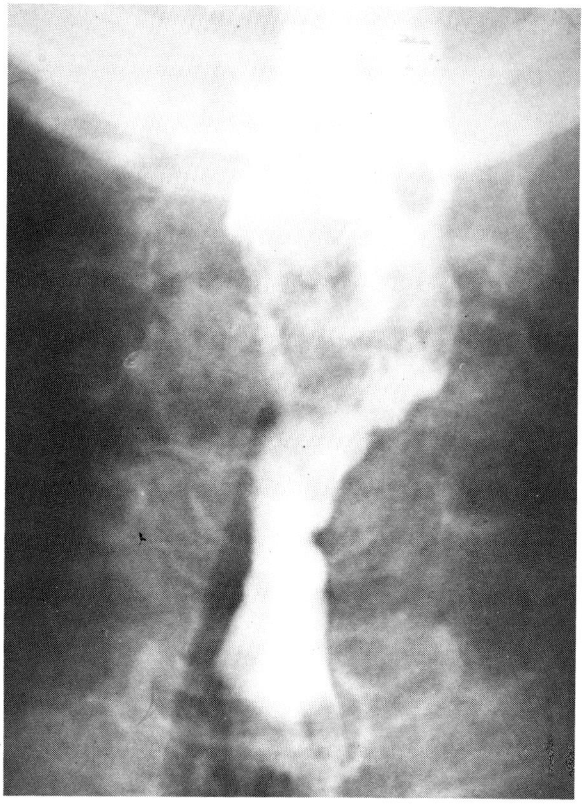

372

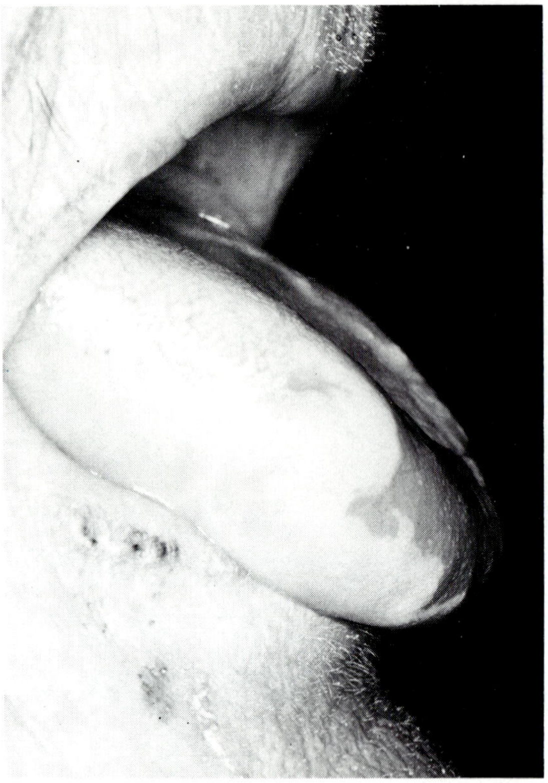

373

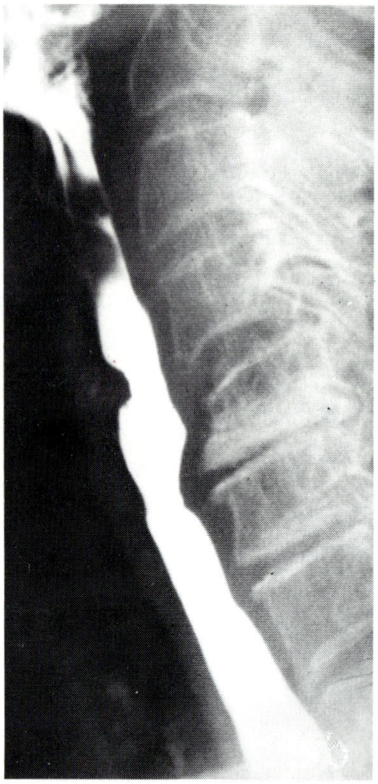

372 Plummer–Vinson syndrome. A 74-year-old woman with thick leukoplakia covering a large part of the tongue and pronounced mucosal atrophy of other parts.

373 Plummer–Vinson syndrome. The same case as pictured previously. There is a slight precricoid stricture in the hypopharynx.

374

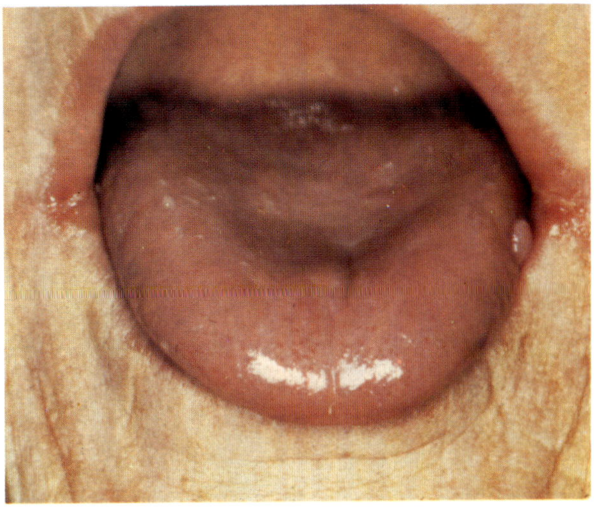

374 Plummer–Vinson syndrome. Angular stomatitis, glossitis, papillary atrophy of the tongue and a small benign squamous cell papilloma on the left border of the tongue are present.

Toxicity

Acute poisoning, often fatal, usually results from young children swallowing iron tablets in the mistaken belief that they are sweets. Vomiting, upper abdominal pain, diarrhoea, cyanosis, shock and coma may occur, and death may follow.

Chronic iron overload (haemochromatosis) may arise in various ways (*Table 57*). Only about 1–2% of all cases are primary or familial. Certain tissues are predominantly the sites of excess iron deposition (375–380).

Treatment consists of greatly reduced intake, venesection if severe and use of the chelating agent desferrioxamine to mobilize iron from the tissues for excretion.

Table 57. Classification of iron overload (haemochromatosis or haemosiderosis).

Primary haemochromatosis	
Usually autosomal recessive trait in neonate, child or adult	
Secondary haemochromatosis or haemosiderosis	
Increased parenteral intake – repeated transfusions, iron dextran i.m.	
Increased iron absorption	
Increased ingestion –	Bantu siderosis (alcoholic beverages), also genetic factor
	Ethiopian (tef cereal)
	Alcoholic cirrhosis
	Oral iron therapy
	Kaschin–Beck disease
Increased absorption from a normal intake – anaemia with erythroid hyperplasia; possibly megadoses of vitamin C	
Focal haemosiderosis	
Idiopathic pulmonary haemosiderosis	
Renal haemosiderosis	
Porphyria cutanea tarda with hepatic haemosiderosis	

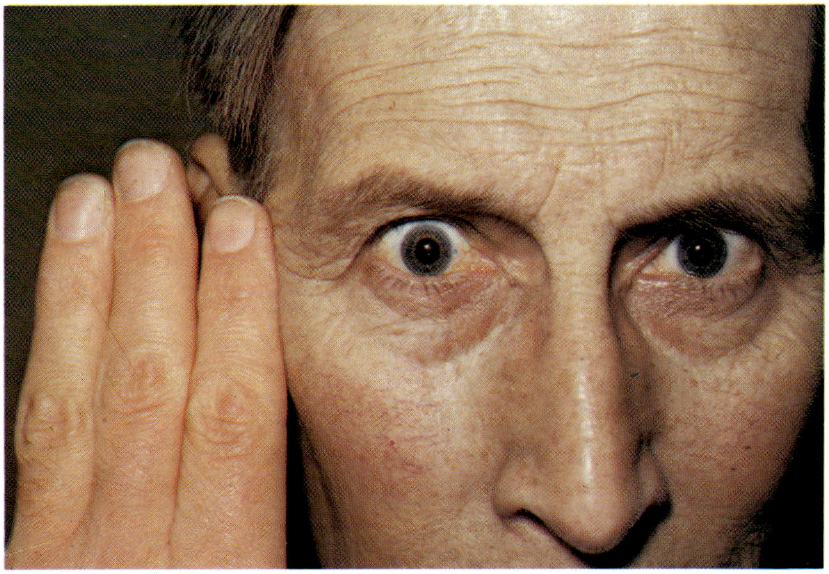

375

375 Haemochromatosis. The slate grey skin of haemochromatosis (face) compared with normal skin (hand).

376

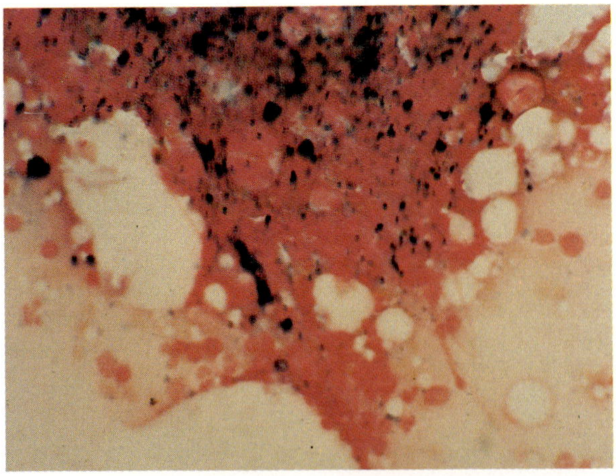

376 **Bone marrow in iron overload.** Prussian blue staining reveals an excess of stainable iron, mostly in the form of haemosiderin. (× 40)

377

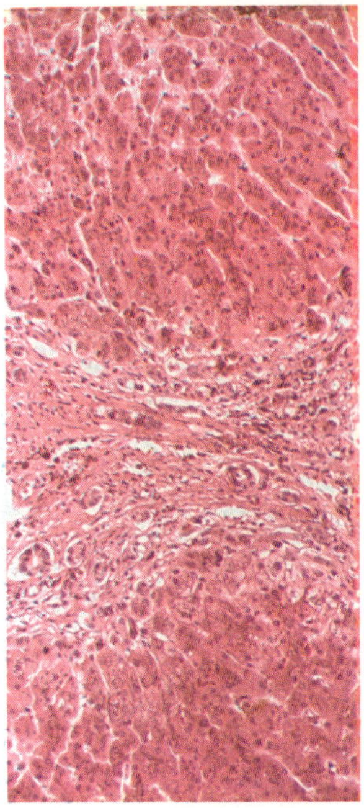

378

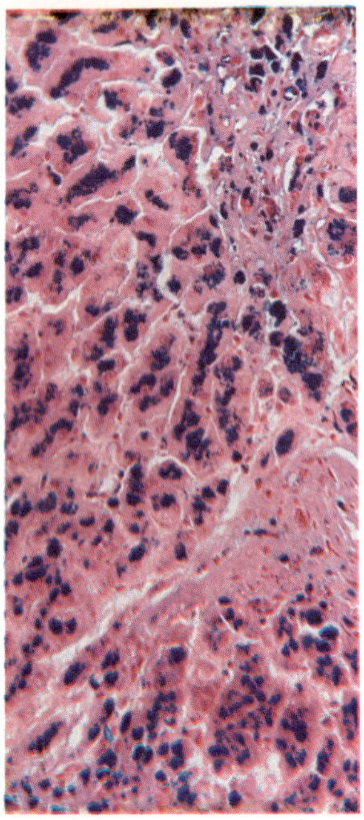

377 **The liver in haemochromatosis.** The liver is finely nodular, the nodules being created by finely interlacing strands of connective tissue which tend to interconnect portal triads but which also penetrate the individual lobules to separate small islands of liver substance. (*H&E*).

378 **The liver in haemochromatosis.** Large accumulations of haemosiderin occur within lymphocytes, Kupffer cells, bile duct epithelium and in the interlacing fibrous scars. The pigment is often extracellular within the scars as well as within the fibroblasts. (*Prussian blue*)

379

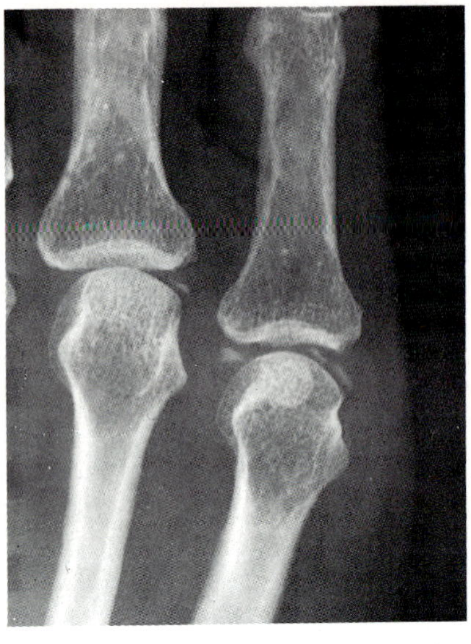

379 **Haemochromatosis.** Chondrocalcinosis in haemochromatosis, in the cartilage overlying the metacarpophalangeal joints of the fingers. There was no evidence of hyperparathyroidism, gout or pseudogout, osteoarthritis, or Wilson's disease, all of which may be associated with calcification in cartilage.

380 **Haemosiderosis of the liver.** Most of the iron staining is confined to the reticuloendothelial (Kupffer) cells in the parasinusoidal spaces. It may also be localized to lungs or kidneys. The term haemosiderosis implies absence of tissue damage; when the latter occurs the term haemochromatosis is used (375–379).

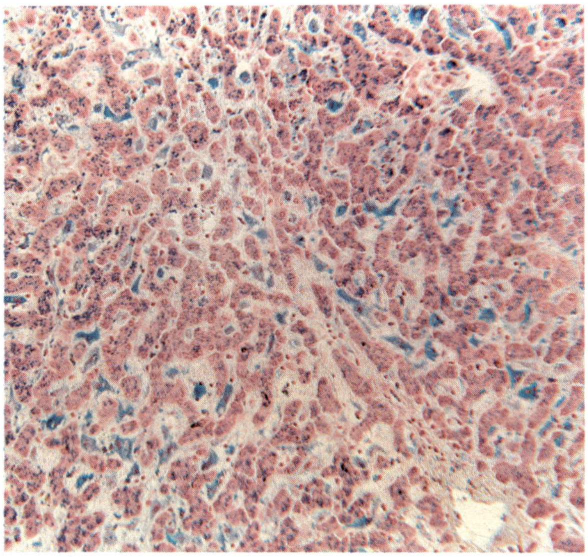

380

Iodine

It has long been known that iodine is required for normal thyroid function and that colloid or endemic goitre occurs in deficiency. Only in recent years have other health aspects come to the fore.

Most soils are poor in iodine and consequently most foodstuffs are not rich sources, but there is a high concentration in seafoods of all kinds. Iodine is readily absorbed, stored as thyroglobulin and released into the circulation as thyroid hormones T_3 and T_4. In the circulation most is present in plasma as protein-bound iodine (Appendix III, Table 2). Through the function of thyroid hormones iodine plays a part in cellular oxidation and hence overall metabolism. The RDA in the adult is about 150μg. **381** summarizes iodine physiology.

381

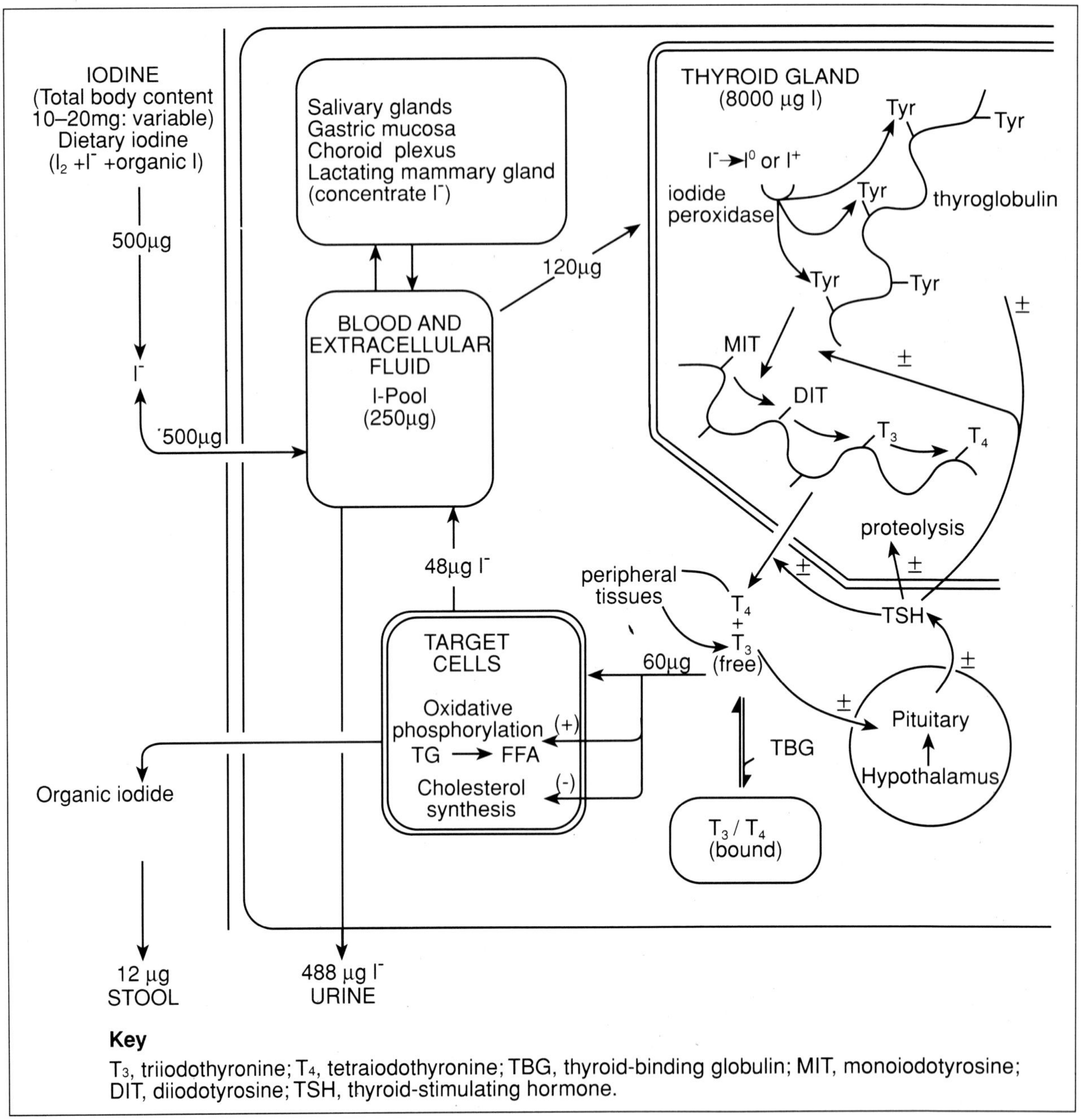

381 Nutrition and metabolism of iodine (total body content 10–20 mg, variable).

Deficiency

The term iodine deficiency disorders (IDD) has been introduced in recent years[80] to indicate the widespread scope and significance of lack of the element (*Table 58*).

The generally accepted grading of goitre follows the scheme shown in *Table 59*.

In field studies goitre incidence correlates with urinary iodine concentration (*Table 60*, **382–387**).

Table 58. The scope of iodine deficiency disorders.

Hypothyroidism – in fetus, neonate, child or adult
Goitre – in neonate, child, adolescent or adult (including complications)
Cretinism, neurological or myxoedematous – in fetus or child
Impaired mental function* – in fetus, child, adolescent, or adult
Abortion*, stillbirth*, congenital abnormalities*, increased perinatal and infant mortality*

* These features may be attributable to many other disease states

Table 59. Grading of goitre.

Grade 0	0a:	Thyroid not palpable, or if palpable, not larger than normal
	0b:	Thyroid palpable, but usually not visible with the head in a normal or raised position
Grade I		Thyroid easily palpable and visible with the head in either a normal or raised position
Grade II		Thyroid easily visible with the head in a normal position
Grade III		Goitre visible at a distance
Grade IV		Monstrous goitres

Table 60. Public health criteria of an iodine deficiency problem.

Classification	*Percentage of population with goitre*	*Urinary iodine* (μg/g creatinine)
Mild	5–20	50–100
Moderate	30–50	25–50
Severe	> 50	< 25

382 Colloid goitre, Grade 1. The thyroid gland is enlarged four or five times at this stage. Thrusting the head back makes the gland appear more prominent. A normal gland is usually described as feeling no larger than a walnut. The neck, in a relaxed position should be palpated with the fingers of both hands from behind the subject.

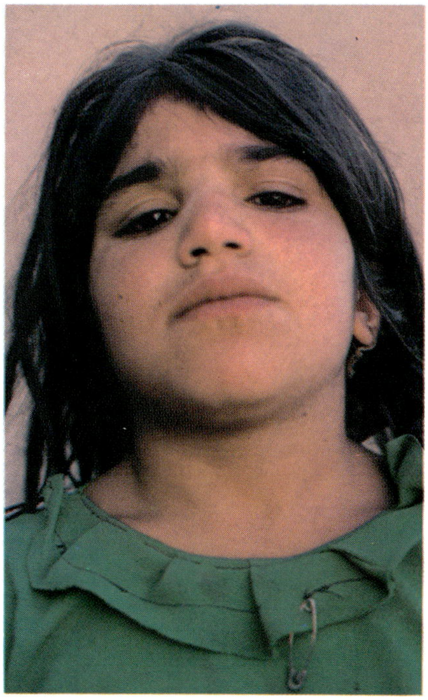

382

383

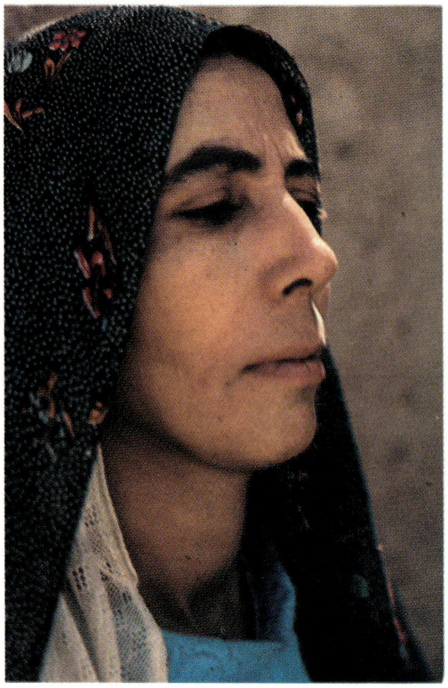

383 **Colloid goitre, Grade 2.** The goitre is easily visible with the head in the normal position.

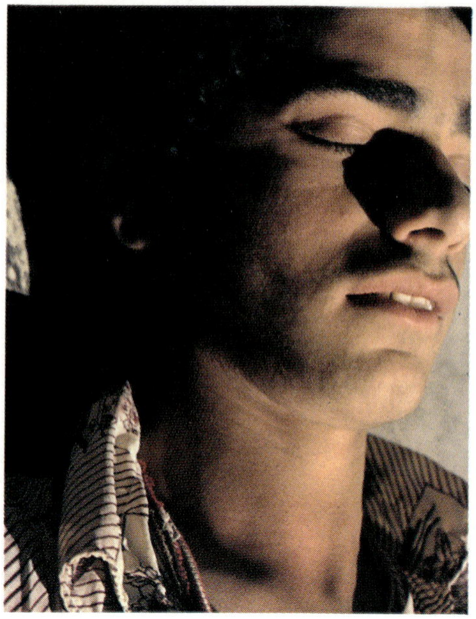

384 **Colloid goitre, Grade 3.** The goitre is large, visible even at a distance, disfiguring, and may cause mechanical difficulties with respiration.

385

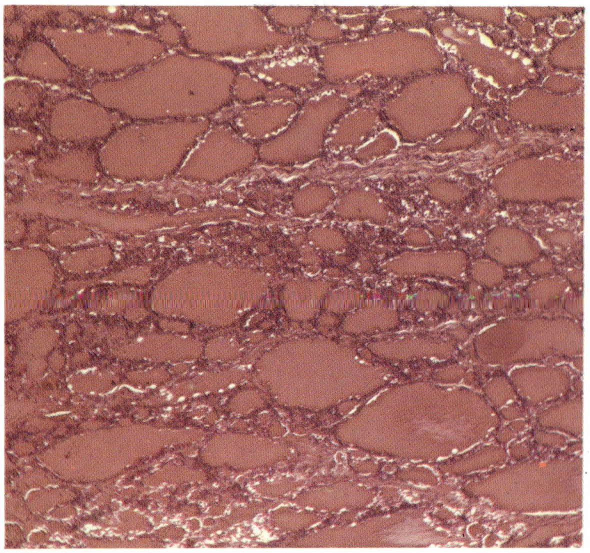

385 **Colloid goitre.** The follicles are distended with colloid and the epithelial lining is flattened. There is a scant amount of interacinar connective tissue devoid of significant lymphoid infiltrate. Vascularization is diminished.

386 **Colloid goitre.** The thyroid gland is considerably enlarged and follicles of varying size can be seen distended with colloid.

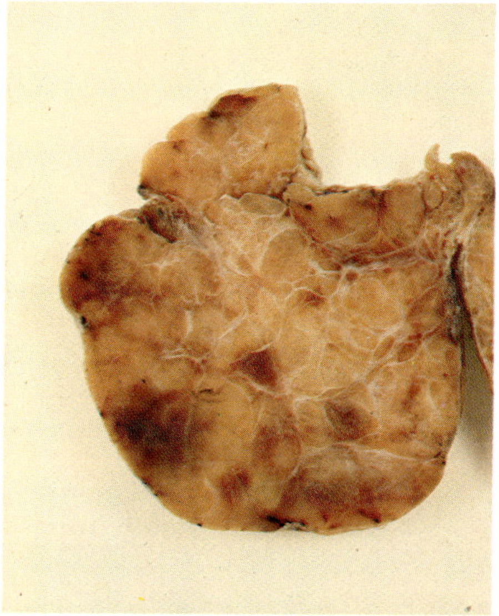

386

387 **Toxic goitre.** This is not due to iodine deficiency. There are signs of increased metabolism. This is hyperthyroidism (Graves' disease, exophthalmic goitre, thyrotoxicosis).

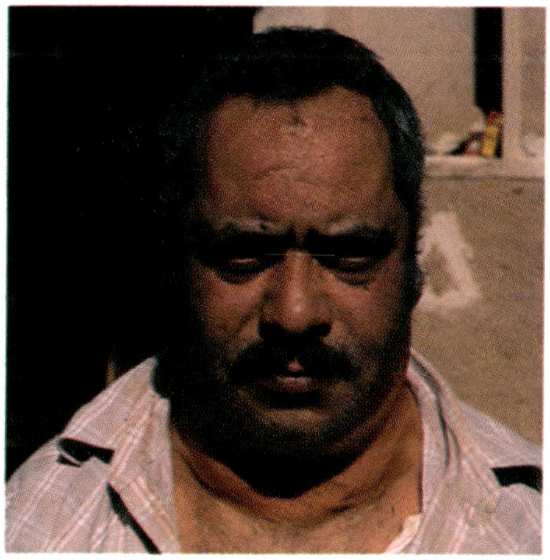

387

Endemic cretinism is indicative of severe iodine deficiency in pregnancy and takes two distinct forms in the offspring (*Table 61*, **388–391**).

Table 61. Features of the two types of cretinism.

Feature	*Myxoedematous cretinism*	*Neurological cretinism*
General features	Coarse, dry skin, protuberant abdomen, umbilical hernia, and large tongue	No signs of hypothyroidism
Stature	Severe growth retardation	Usually normal
Mental retardation	Present, often severe	Present, often severe
Deaf-mutism	Absent	Usually present
Strabismus	Absent	Often present
Cerebral diplegia	Absent	Often present
Reflexes	Delayed relaxation	Excessively brisk
X-ray of limbs	Epiphyseal dysgenesis	Normal
ECG	Small voltage QRS complexes and other abnormalities of hypothyroidism	Normal
Effect of thyroid hormones	Improvement	No effect

388

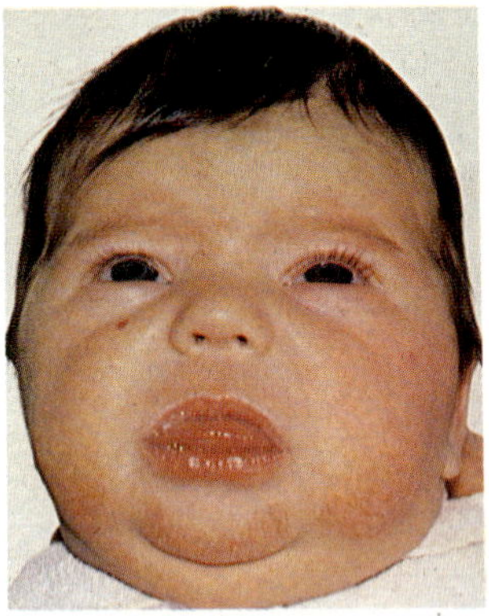

389

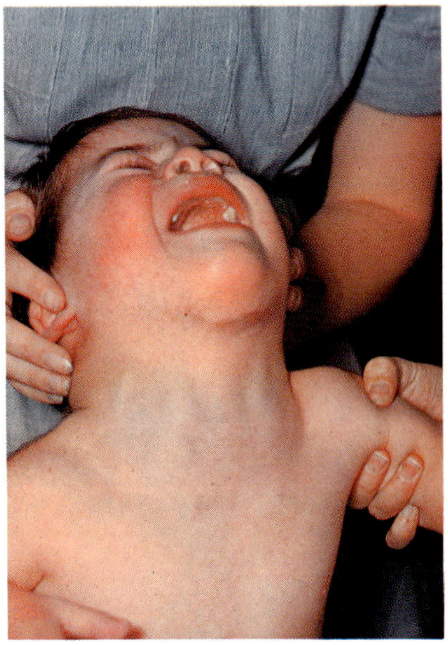

390

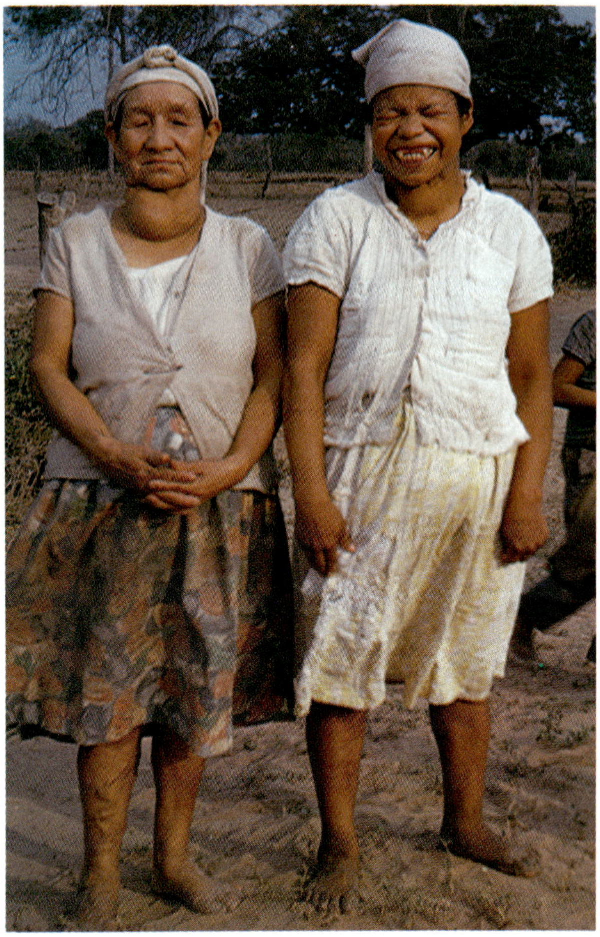

388 Cretinism in infancy. The characteristic facial appearance with protruding tongue and coarse features may not be obvious until several months after birth. Other causes of mental retardation and umbilical hernia, another feature of cretinism, must be differentiated.

389 Cretinism. Five-year-old with large goitre. Mentally deficient. Several members of the family were similarly affected. They lived in an area where cretinism was endemic.

390 Endemic goitre and cretinism in Bolivia. The mother, on the left, is goitrous but otherwise normal. The daughter is goitrous, mentally retarded, and a deaf mute, but of normal stature and clinically euthyroid.

391 Hypothyroidism – cretinism. Skeletal growth and maturation depend on thyroid hormone among other factors. If thyroid hormone is lacking from birth, cretinism is the result. It is rarely seen now in developed countries. The examples shown are of an untreated patient who presented in adult life.

(a) Skull.

The bones of the vault (A) and base (B) are thickened. The sutures are prominent and a few sutural (wormian) bones can be seen (C).

(b) Lateral thoracic and lumbar spine showing gross platyspondyly.

All of the vertebrae are flattened and some of the apophyses (A) have not fused. The sacral segments (B) are still separate.

These changes and the changes in the epiphyses resemble certain of the mucopolysaccharidoses. This patient was originally thought to have gargoylism (MPS I) and thyroid treatment was not given. Hence the full-blown appearance in adult life.

391

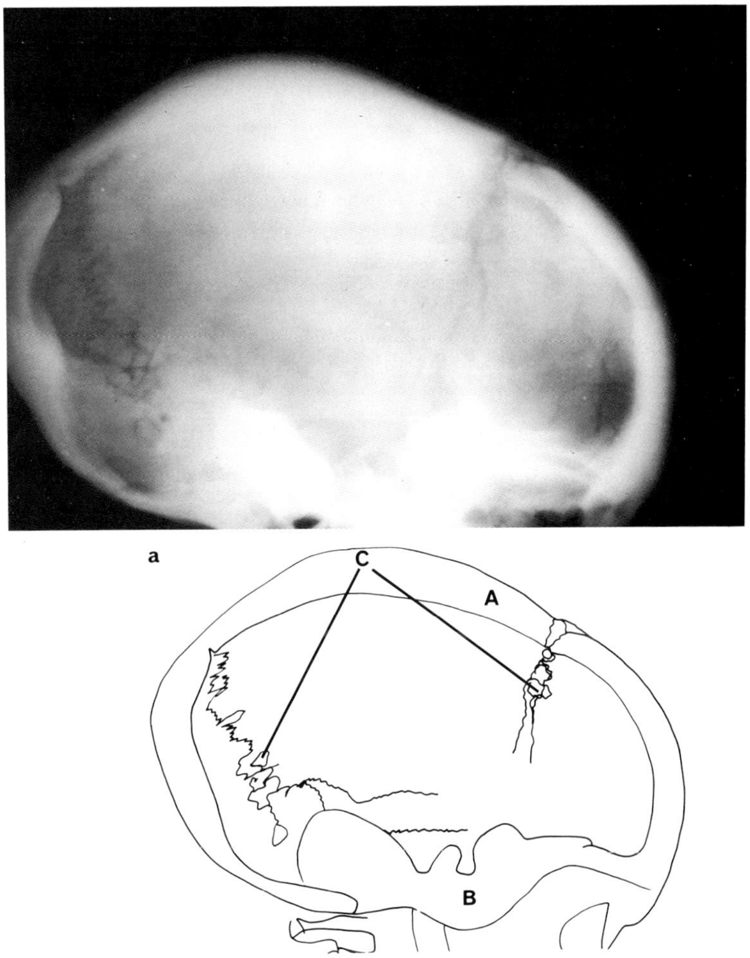

a

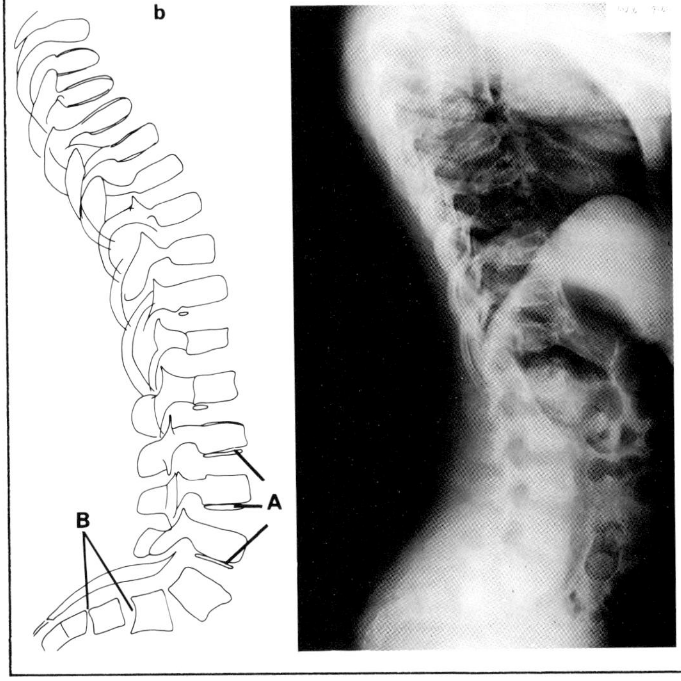

b

In most areas the neurological form is much more common. Highly endemic areas include the Andean regions of South America, parts of Central America and of central and eastern Africa, the Himalayan region of Asia, and Papua New Guinea (**392**).

In recent years evidence has been accumulating that lesser degrees of iodine shortage during pregnancy may be very widespread and an important cause of retardation of fetal physical growth and brain development[80].

392

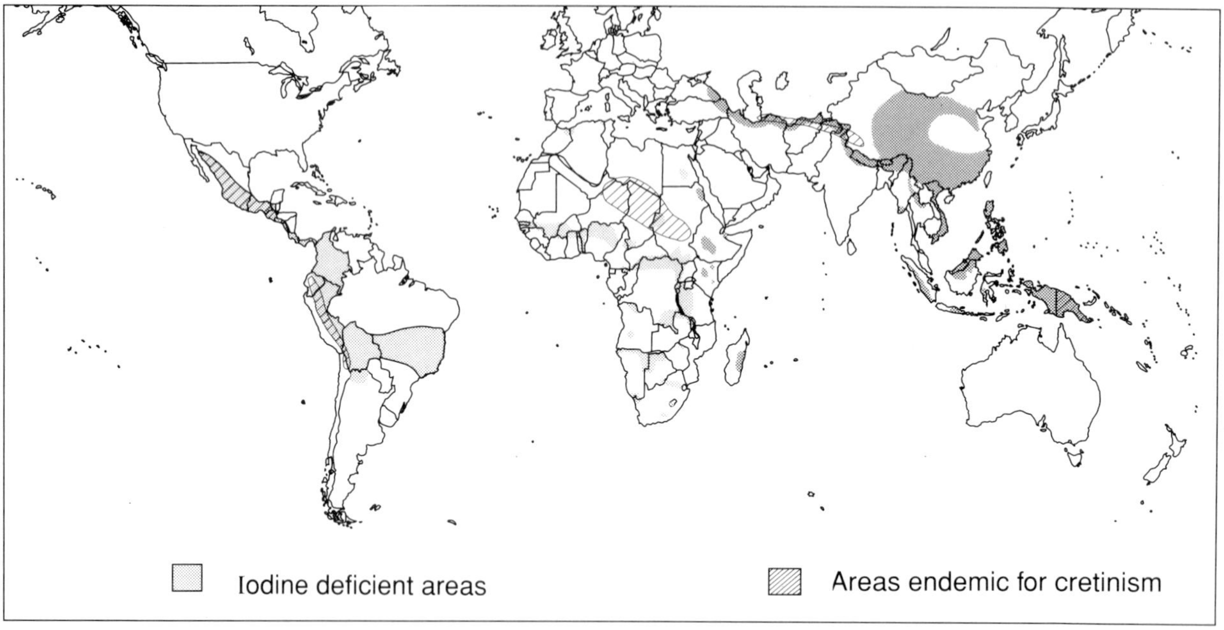

392 Distribution of iodine deficient areas in developing countries.

Toxicity

Prolonged intake of iodine about 20-fold in excess of requirements results in iodide-goitre or myxoedema (Wolff-Chaikoff effect) especially if Hashimoto's thyroiditis pre-exists. In China the cause is very high iodine levels in drinking water in some regions,[81] in the United States many fast foods are responsible, and in the UK the use of iodine-containing compounds in the dairy industry for antisepsis is increasing mean iodine intake alarmingly[82].

Fluorine

Like boron, fluorine does not yet fit neatly into the scheme of elements (see page **177**). Evidence is so far lacking for its essentiality in animals, including man, but low intake is associated with disease, as is toxicity.

Fluorine is widely distributed in nature and the level in drinking water is of key importance. The body treats fluoride like chloride and it is dispersed throughout the extracellular space. Teeth and bone contain the highest concentrations.

Deficiency

Epidemiological studies have shown an inverse relationship between the levels of fluoride in drinking water and the incidence of dental caries (**393**).

Levels of 1.0–1.5 ppm are associated with minimal caries and no mottling. Fluoridation of water supplies to this concentration is the aim of public health measures (**394, 395**).

In addition fluoride rinses, tablets and, especially

in the United Kingdom, fortified toothpastes have played important roles.[83]

Fluoride increases trabecular bone density and may be of benefit in osteoporosis[84] (see Chapter 11).

393

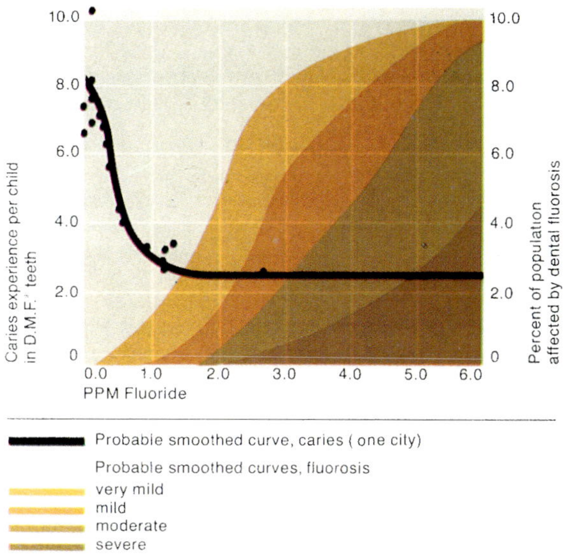

393 Dental caries and dental fluorosis in relation to fluoride in public water supplies. (* DMF = decayed, missing and filled.)

4

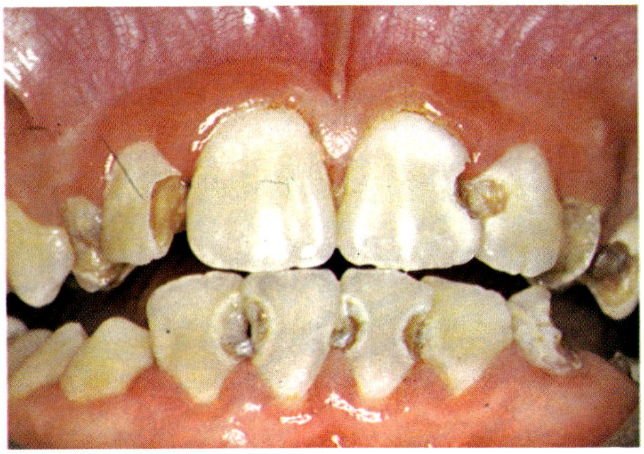

394 Dental caries. This is a localized progressive loss of tooth substance initiated by demineralization of the tooth surface by organic acids. These are produced by enzymes of cariogenic bacteria (especially *Streptococcus mutans*) that ferment sugars trapped in the tooth-adherent bacterial film called dental plaque. Oral hygiene is clearly of paramount importance in prevention but fluoride ions have been shown to inhibit caries by replacing some of the hydroxyl ions in tooth hydroxyapatite to form a relatively acid-insoluble fluorhydroxyapatite.

395

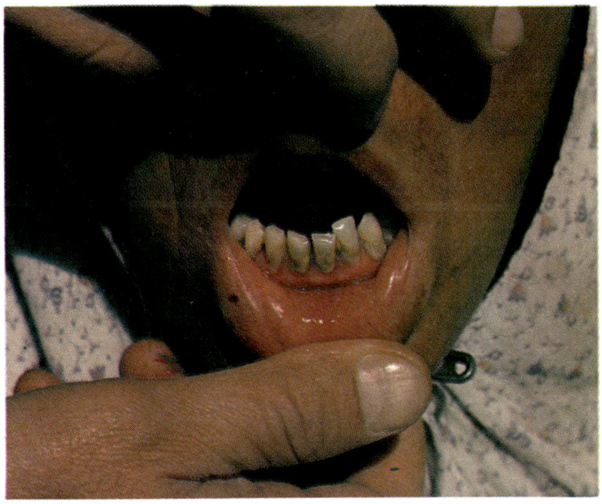

395 Pyorrhoea or periodontitis. There is an inflammatory breakdown of the supporting structures of the roots (gingiva and periodontal ligament) with a resultant loss of alveolar bone. The gums are hyperaemic and bleed easily but there is no hypertrophy. Although common in undernourished subjects there is no evidence that nutritional deficiency plays a part, and it must be distinguished from scurvy (**346, 347**).

Toxicity (fluorosis)

Both teeth (**396–398**) and bone (**399, 400**) can be damaged by prolonged excessive fluorine intake.

396

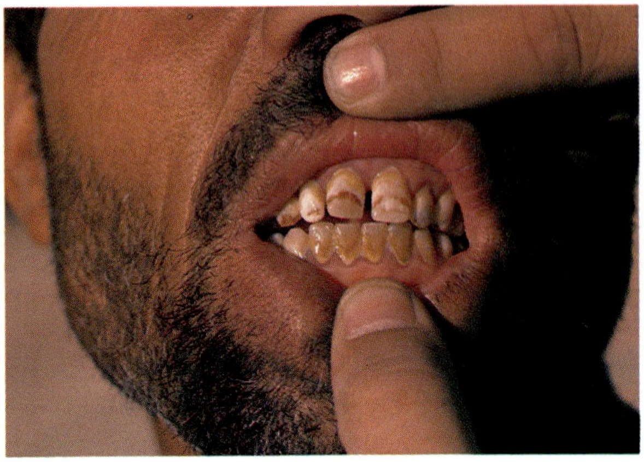

396 **Mottled enamel in fluorosis.** The affected areas are 'paper-white', yellowish or brownish and are usually situated on or near the tips of cusps or incisal edges. They shade off imperceptibly into the surrounding normal enamel. Fluorosis is most frequent on teeth that calcify slowly (cuspids, bicuspids, second and third molars) and is less marked on lower than upper incisors. Usually seen on six or eight homologous teeth, it is extremely rare on deciduous teeth. This degree of discolouration usually follows several years of constant exposure to concentrations up to about 10 times the normal (about 1 ppm) of fluorine in the drinking water. The teeth of most inhabitants of such an area are affected by school age. There is no damage to teeth at this stage.

397

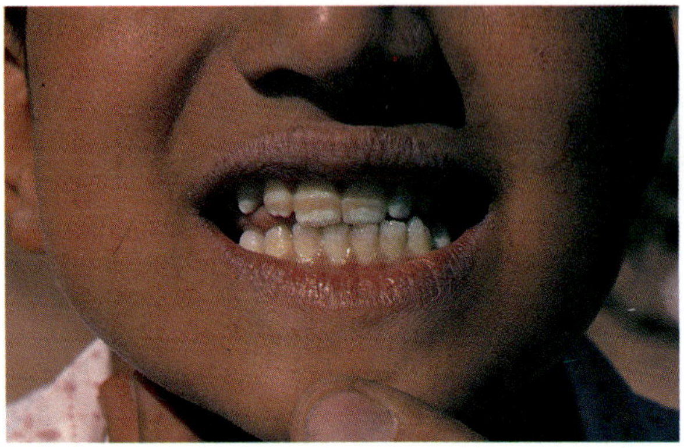

397 **Enamel hypoplasia.** The central part of the upper incisors is usually affected as in this case. It is not known to be related to nutritional deficiency. It can be distinguished from the mottling of fluorosis by the pigmentation being present at the time of eruption and by the etched and roughened surface of the enamel.

398

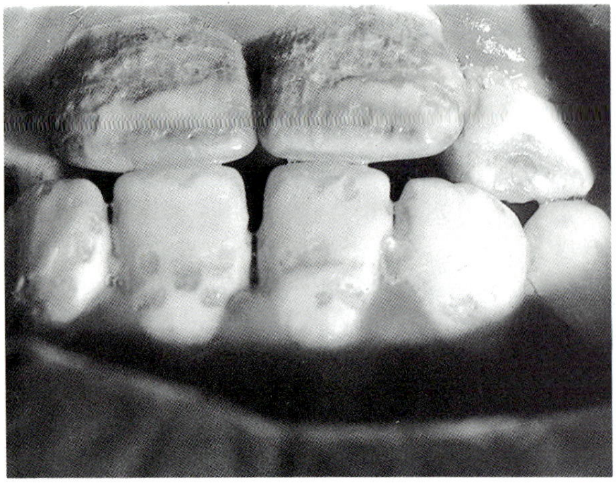

398 **Pitting and mottling of the teeth.** In prolonged and extreme fluorosis the weakened enamel is lost, resulting in pits. As in the earlier stage of mottling alone the upper incisors are more severely affected with the confluence of isolated pits into bands of erosion.

399

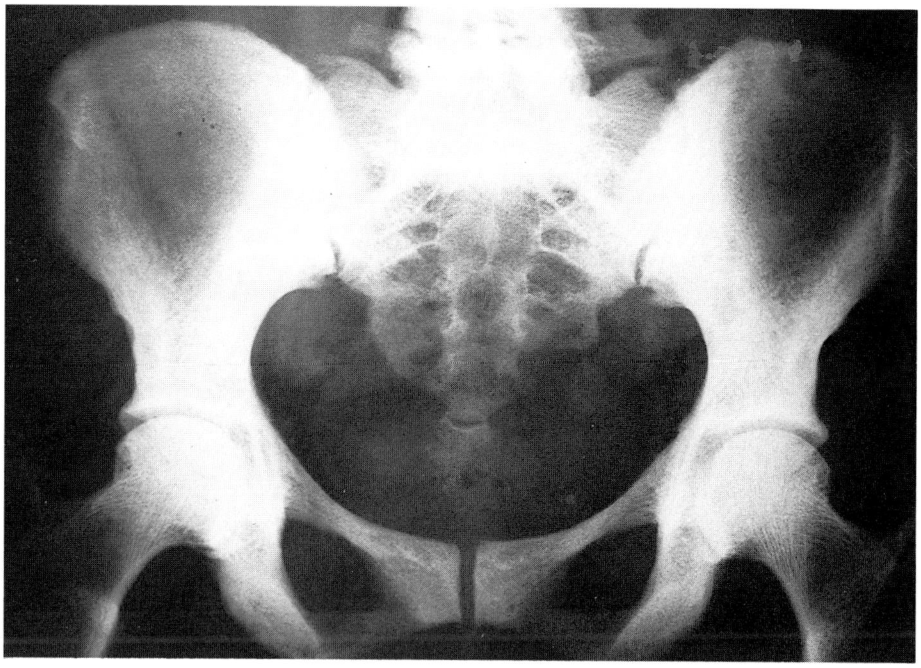

400

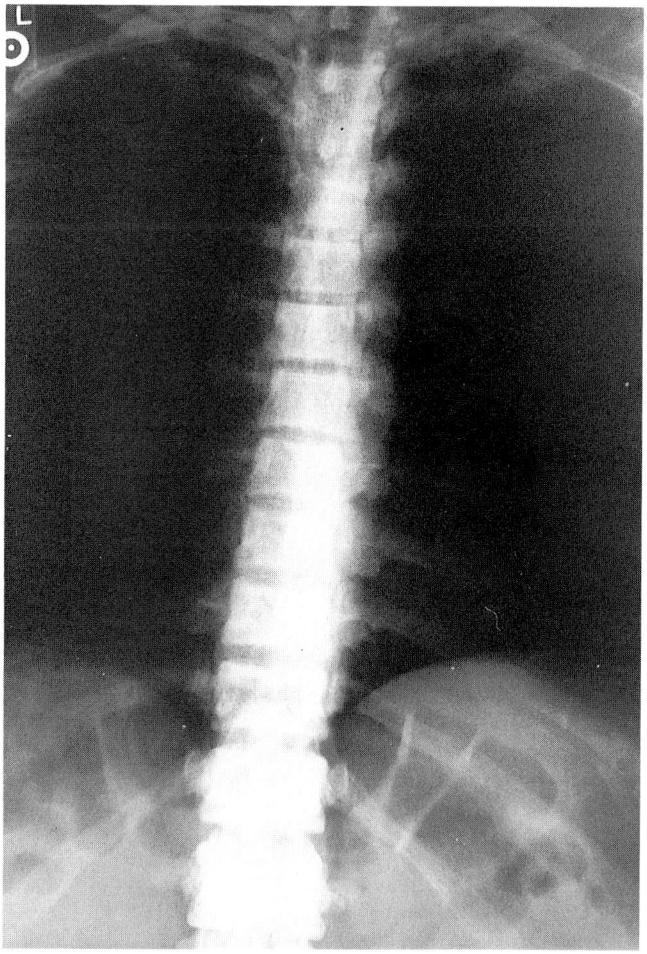

399 Skeletal fluorosis. In parts of India, the Arabian Gulf and Africa lifelong consumption of drinking water with many times the normal concentration of fluorine results in skeletal fluorosis. Marked osteosclerosis of the spine causes severe pain and limitation of movement; marked genu valgum also occurs. This pelvic X-ray shows dense bones and coarse, trabecular pattern.

400 Skeletal fluorosis. X-ray of the spine shows some exostoses and calcification of tendons and ligaments and some loss of distinctness between individual vertebrae.

Electrolytes and water

Although water is not a nutrient in the strictest sense it merits some consideration here on several grounds. Besides comprising about 60% of the body it constitutes the medium, both intra- and extracellularly, in which all the metabolic processes of the body take place and as a result of which some water of metabolism is formed. Water forms part of the diet in two ways: it is consumed in solid food because vegetable and animal tissues are watery, and it is drunk in a variety of liquid forms. Finally, there is a minimal daily requirement for water sufficient to excrete waste products in urine, the minimal daily output of which has to be about 830ml. For health a balance needs to be maintained within a wide range of intake and output[85] (*Table 62*).

Disorders of water balance cannot be considered in isolation from those affecting the main electrolytes. These are present in ionic form in both extracellular fluid including plasma, and within cells. Cations are Na^+, K^+, Ca^{2+}, Mg^{2+} and anions are Cl^-, HCO_3^-, $H_2PO_4^-$, HPO_4^{2-}. Although they all have to be provided by the diet just like any other nutrients they have attracted little attention in this role until recently. This is probably because in the short term their maintenance at quite precise levels is vital for survival, and homeostatic mechanisms exist for this purpose. Deficiency or excess rarely arises from purely dietary causes and corrective measures are rapidly brought into play by the body. Nevertheless, the long-term consequences of lifelong high or low levels of consumption of electrolytes like sodium, calcium, potassium or magnesium on blood pressure (Chapter 3) and bone density (Chapter 11) are attracting intense interest at the present time.

Table 62. Daily water balance of a young man leading a sedentary life and consuming a diet providing 2110 kcal (8.8MJ)/day.[85]

Mean of five daily measurements	*Water (ml/day)*
Intake	
Water content of solid food	1115
Liquid drunk	1180
Metabolic water	279
Total	2574
Output	
Urine	1295
Faeces	56
Evaporative loss	1214
Total	2565
Balance	+9

Water deficiency (dehydration)

This has many causes (*Table 63*) and is especially serious in young children as they have a relatively high water content and are unable to respond readily to the urge of thirst in order to increase water intake. In the third world dehydration in this age group is frequently accompanied by malnutrition (**401**).

Table 63. Common causes of water depletion.

Reduced intake	
Water unavailable	Various kinds of disasters
Inability to obtain water	Infants, elderly, debilitated or unconscious
Inability to swallow	Diseases of mouth, neck, oesophagus
Increased losses	
From the gastrointestinal tract	Prolonged diarrhoea, vomiting, fistulae
In the urine	Diabetes insipidus, renal insufficiency, osmotic diuresis – in diabetes mellitus, hyperosmotic feedings
From the skin	High ambient temperature, strenuous exercise, pyrexia, thyrotoxicosis
From the lungs	Hyperventilation, as in fever, high altitude, etc.

401

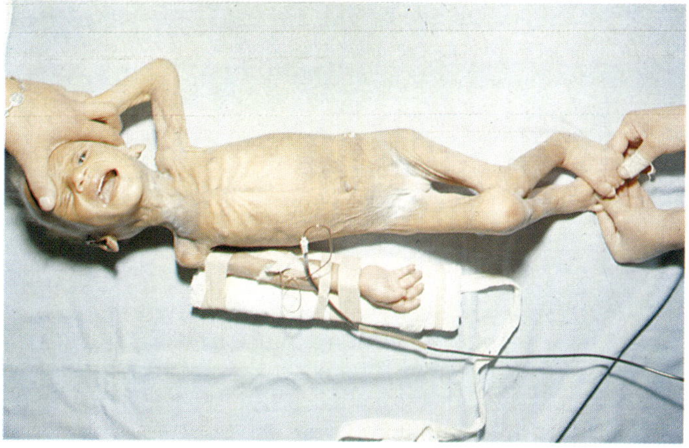

401 Severe dehydration and malnutrition.

Water excess (Hypo-osmolar syndromes)

This is usually linked with a build-up of sodium in the body (hypernatraemia) and is accounted for mainly by impaired water diuresis. Oedema may not be present and the syndrome may be asymptomatic. Symptoms include confusion, lethargy, headache, anorexia, vomiting, weakness and, rarely, convulsions (**402**).

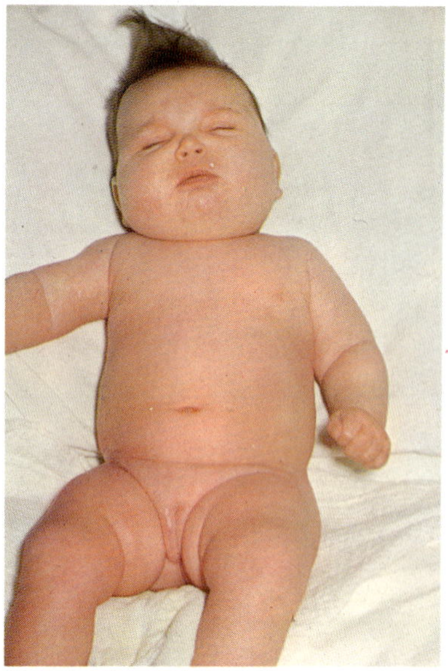

402

402 Overhydration. Girl of 2 months, weight 5500g (75th centile for 4 months). Birthweight was 3200g. The feeding formula contained excess of carbohydrates and lack of protein, leading to increased fluid retention and apparent plumpness easily lost during recurrent illness.

Sodium

Sodium is widely distributed in small amounts in foods and is often added during the processing and cooking of food. Dietary intake is very variable and the implications of this in relation to blood pressure are discussed in Chapter 3. Most excess sodium is excreted in the urine. The level in plasma is an accurate assessment of status (Appendix III, Table 2).

Sweating in relation to physical work and ambient temperature is an important regulatory component of sodium balance. Acclimatization to heat results in a more dilute sweat and conserves electrolytes. There is no mechanism comparable to thirst to warn the body of impending salt depletion.

Sodium serves many functions including a part in acid–base and water balance and in transmission of nerve impulses.

There is no RDA but the estimated safe and adequate intake is considered to be 1–3 g for adults.

Sodium deficiency (hyponatraemia)

Table 64 shows the main causes of hyponatraemia.

Sudden correction of hyponatraemia may precipitate Wernicke's encephalopathy (Chapter 5) or central pontine myelinolysis (Chapter 9). Symptomatic hyponatraemia with plasma Na$\leq$ 128 mmol/l in both adults and children may cause permanent brain damage or may even be fatal.

Table 64. Causes of hyponatraemia (normal range in plasma 135–143 mmol/l).

Extracellular water	*Urinary concentration of Na*		
	Decreased	*Increased*	*Variable*
Increased	Conditions associated with oedema (heart failure, cirrhosis, nephrosis) Increased water intake	Acute renal failure Chronic renal failure Inappropriate ADH secretion Infections, burns Chlorpropamide, vincristin	
Decreased	Inadequate sodium intake Excessive extrarenal losses (gastroenteritis, sweating)	Pituitary insufficiency Hypo- and pseudohypo-aldosteronism Obstructive uropathy Diuretics Prematurity	
Normal			'Essential' Hyponatraemia Malnutrition Tuberculous meningitis

Sodium excess (hypernatraemia)

This dangerous condition (**403–405**) has a variety of causes (*Table 65*).

Table 65. Principal causes of hypernatraemia.

Loss of hypotonic fluid (desiccation) without adequate water replacement:
- Excessive sweating and insensible losses (often comatose patients, or infants without access to water)
- Respiratory losses with fever, dry oxygen, tracheotomy, hyperventilation of dyspnoea, or metabolic acidosis
- Skin losses with burns, or prolonged exposure to dry heat
- Diarrhoeal disorders (especially in children)

Abnormally large volume of dilute urine without water replacement:
- Diabetes insipidus: pituitary ADH deficiency, nephrogenic (ADH unresponsive)
- Osmotic diuretics: marked glycosuria, urea diuresis due to high-protein tube feedings, chronic renal failure
- Recovery phase of acute renal failure
- Hypercalcaemia, hypokalaemia, sickle cell anaemia

403

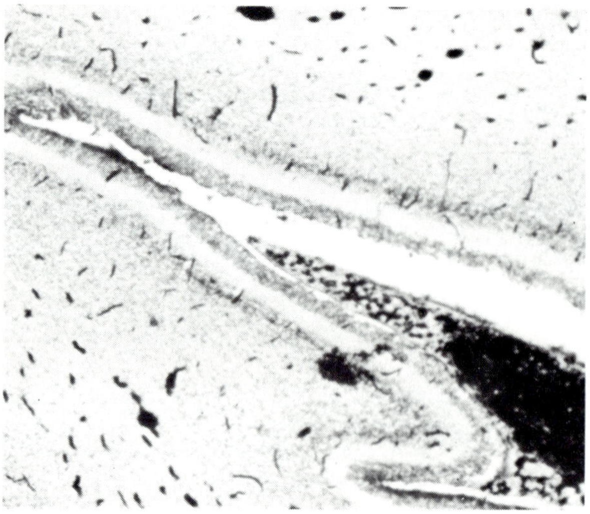

403 Hypernatraemia. Section through the cerebellum in a fatal case of salt poisoning showing a subarachnoid haemorrhage, vascular dilatation and congestion and a small cortical haemorrhage. (*Pickworth-Lepehne stain*, × 50).

404

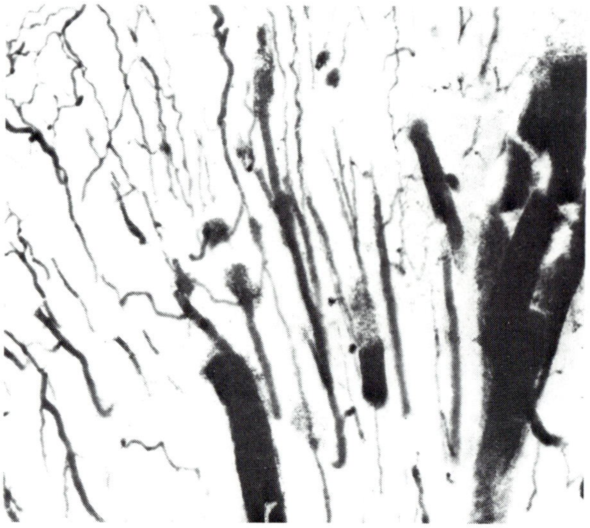

404 Hypernatraemia. Section through the cerebral cortex and subcortical white matter showing widespread capillary and venous congestion with red blood cell diapedesis and small haemorrhages. (*Pickworth-Lepehne stain*, × 50).

405

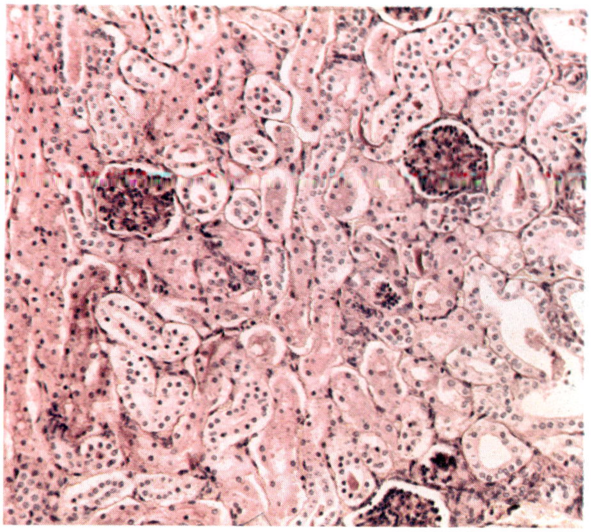

405 Hypernatraemia. Section of the kidney of an infant who died 3 days after salt poisoning, showing extensive sub-basilar vacuolation in renal tubules at all levels of the nephron. Note that the cytoplasm may be lifted off the basement membrane and the lumen obliterated.

Chloride

Chloride is usually found in association with sodium in nature and in the diet but occasionally there is a differential loss (*Table* 66) or accumulation (*Table* 67) of chloride.

There is some evidence, mostly experimental, that chloride as well as sodium may play a part in chronic rise in blood pressure.

Table 66. Main causes of hypochloraemia (plasma Cl < 95mmol/l).

Expanded extracellular fluid in trauma, wasting diseases or water retention with accompanying hyponatraemia
In vomiting, gastric suction or salt loss from any level of gastrointestinal tract
From diuretics causing greater loss in urine of chloride than sodium
In adrenal steroid administration causing sodium retention and chloride and potassium loss
Compensating mechanism in chronic respiratory acidosis
Elevated plasma carbon dioxide and pH and low potassium in hypokalaemic hypochloraemic alkalosis
Acute and chronic renal failure

Table 67. Causes of hyperchloraemia (plasma Cl > 110mmol/l).

Excessive use of ammonium chloride, hydrochloric acid or sodium chloride
Carbonic anhydrase inhibitors absorbed from burns
Hypernatraemia in excess solute loading, diabetes insipidus, brain stem injury or desiccation dehydration
Ureterointestinal anastomoses with reabsorption of chloride from bowel, made worse by renal insufficiency

Potassium

Potassium is the major intracellular cation and therefore plasma sampling (normal 3.3–4.7 nmol/l) may not accurately reflect status (Appendix III, Table 2). Potassium is widespread in nature but different samples of the same foodstuff vary considerably in content. Its distribution tends to be reciprocal to that of sodium in food. This may be important in relation to the opposite effects these ions have on blood pressure (Chapter 3). A safe limit has been set for the adult at about 1.8–5.6g/day.

Potassium deficiency (hypokalaemia)

Table 68 shows the common causes of hypokalaemia.

Table 68. Common causes of hypokalaemia (plasma K < 3.5mmol/l).

Decreased intake	—	Dietary as in PEM Infusion
Intracellular potassium shifts	—	metabolic or respiratory alkalosis Administration of insulin or B_2-agonists Familial hypokalaemic paralysis
Gastrointestinal losses	—	Diarrhoea (20–30 mmol K/l) Prolonged vomiting or gastric suction Small bowel fistulae
Renal losses	—	Tubular disorders (Fanconi syndrome, Bartter's syndrome, etc.) Polyuria following obstruction or acute renal failure, diuretics following trauma, anaesthesia or surgery Diuretics, antibiotics and other drugs affecting tubular function
Metabolic changes with secondary K loss in urine	—	Acute surgical trauma, injury and sepsis Antidiuresis following acute ECF volume depletion Hypochloraemic metabolic alkalosis High circulating levels of cortisol, aldosterone and adrenaline

Potassium excess (hyperkalaemia)

Causes of hyperkalaemia are shown in *Table 69.*

In practice it may be necessary to consider both of these states in coming to a diagnosis and the respective symptoms and signs are compared and contrasted in *Table 70.*

Table 69. Common causes of hyperkalaemia (plasma K > 6.0 mmol/l).

Excessive intake or administration –	Oral or intravenous Potassium-containing drugs (penicillin and derivatives) Transfusions
Massive release of K from cells –	Crush injury, major surgical operations, severe metabolic or respiratory acidosis, cardiogenic or hypovolaemic shock, gastrointestinal haemorrhage and release of K from red blood cells, gram negative bacterial septicaemia
Decreased renal excretion –	Renal diseases, extrinsic renal causes such as hypoaldosteronism, diuretics and other drugs
'False' causes –	Prolonged ischaemia during venipuncture, haemolysis, pseudohyperkalaemia

Table 70. Clinical manifestations of potassium deficiency and toxicity.

Deficiency	
	Muscle weakness
	Respiratory failure
	Paralytic ileus
	Hypotension
	Impaired renal concentration
	Cardiac arrhythmias: ECG shows ST segment depression and increased P and T wave amplitude
Toxicity	
	Flaccid paralysis occasionally but usually asymptomatic until cardiac toxicity occurs
	Shortening of Q-T interval on ECG with tall, peaked T waves. With serum K > 6.5mmol/l: nodal and ventricular arrhythmias, widening of QRS complex, P-R interval prolongation, disappearance of P wave and ventricular asystole or fibrillation.

Magnesium

Here too the electrolyte is of widespread occurrence in food and deficiency is of endogenous origin. About 70% of body magnesium occurs in bone and its absorption from the gut and deposition in bone appear to be closely associated with the metabolism of calcium but the details are not understood. Magnesium is mainly an intracellular ion and plasma level (normal =, 0.75–1.05mmol/l) is not a precise guide to status. The RDA for the adult is about 300mg. **406** illustrates the mechanisms for homeostatic control of magnesium.

406 Magnesium balance in adult man. The major features of homeostasis are: (a), the relatively poor absorption from the intestinal tract; (b), its distribution into several tissue pools of which a major one is bone; and (c) dependence on the kidney for excretion.

406

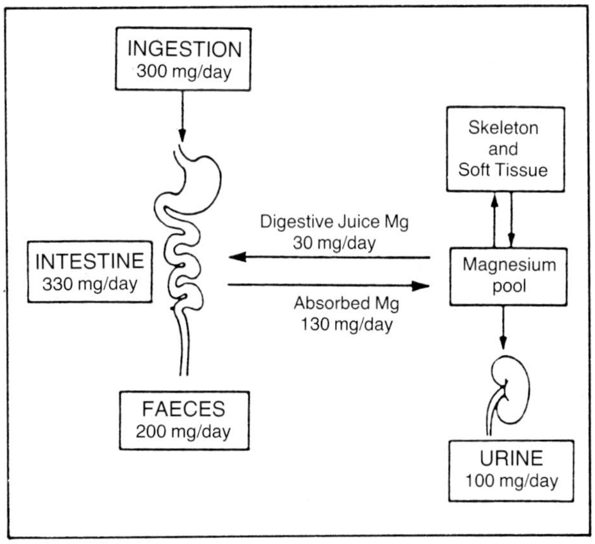

Deficiency (hypomagnesaemia)

The major causes of hypomagnesaemia are listed in *Table 71*.

In clinical practice it is constantly accompanied by hypocalcaemia and frequently hypokalaemia. The symptoms and signs are primarily neuromuscular; increased excitability as evidenced by the signs of Trousseau and Chvostek, muscle fasciculations, muscle spasm, and anorexia, nausea and vomiting. Convulsions, with or without coma, occur in young children.

Table 71. Causes of hypomagnesaemia (serum Mg < 0.7mmol/l).

Inadequate intake
Hypercatabolic states (trauma, burns)
PEM
Prolonged lactation
Alcoholism
Genetic disorders or familial factors
Primary idiopathic hypomagnesaemia
Bartter's syndrome
Renal wasting syndromes
Maternal diabetes or hyperparathyroidism
Endocrine disorders
Hyperthyroidism
Hyperaldosteronism
Hyperparathyroidism with hypercalcaemia
Renal tubular disorders
Metabolic, hormonal and drug related
Gastrointestinal disorders
Malabsorption in inflammatory bowel disease, coeliac disease, short bowel syndrome, etc.

Toxicity (hypermagnesaemia)

This is usually iatrogenic, as in patients with renal failure receiving magnesium-containing drugs or children with chronic constipation treated with magnesium sulphate enemas.

Signs include loss of deep tendon reflexes and ECG changes consisting of prolonged PR interval, QRS complex and widened increased T wave amplitude. With very high blood levels hypertension, respiratory depression, narcosis and death in cardiac arrest occur. Food supplements as well as antacids high in magnesium may cause chronic diarrhoea[86].

Calcium

In the typical western diet about 75% of the intake of calcium comes from milk and milk products and the rest about equally from meat, fish, eggs, cereal products, beans, fruits and vegetables. Vegetarians can meet their requirements if they consume adequate amounts of the non-dairy items. Only about 20–30% of calcium is absorbed but calcium homeostasis is under the control of vitamin D, parathyroid hormone and to a less extent calcitonin (**407**).

Although most of the calcium in the body is involved in the structure of bone and teeth the very small amounts within cells are concerned with many regulatory processes including nerve impulse transmission and muscle contraction. Plasma calcium *per se* is not a reliable indication of calcium status but the corrected ionized fraction is (Appendix III, Table 2). The RDA for the adult has been set at different levels, mainly due to lack of consensus concerning the influence of calcium intake on bone density and prevention of osteoporosis (Chapter 11). However, 800mg for the male and 1200mg for the female are often used.

407

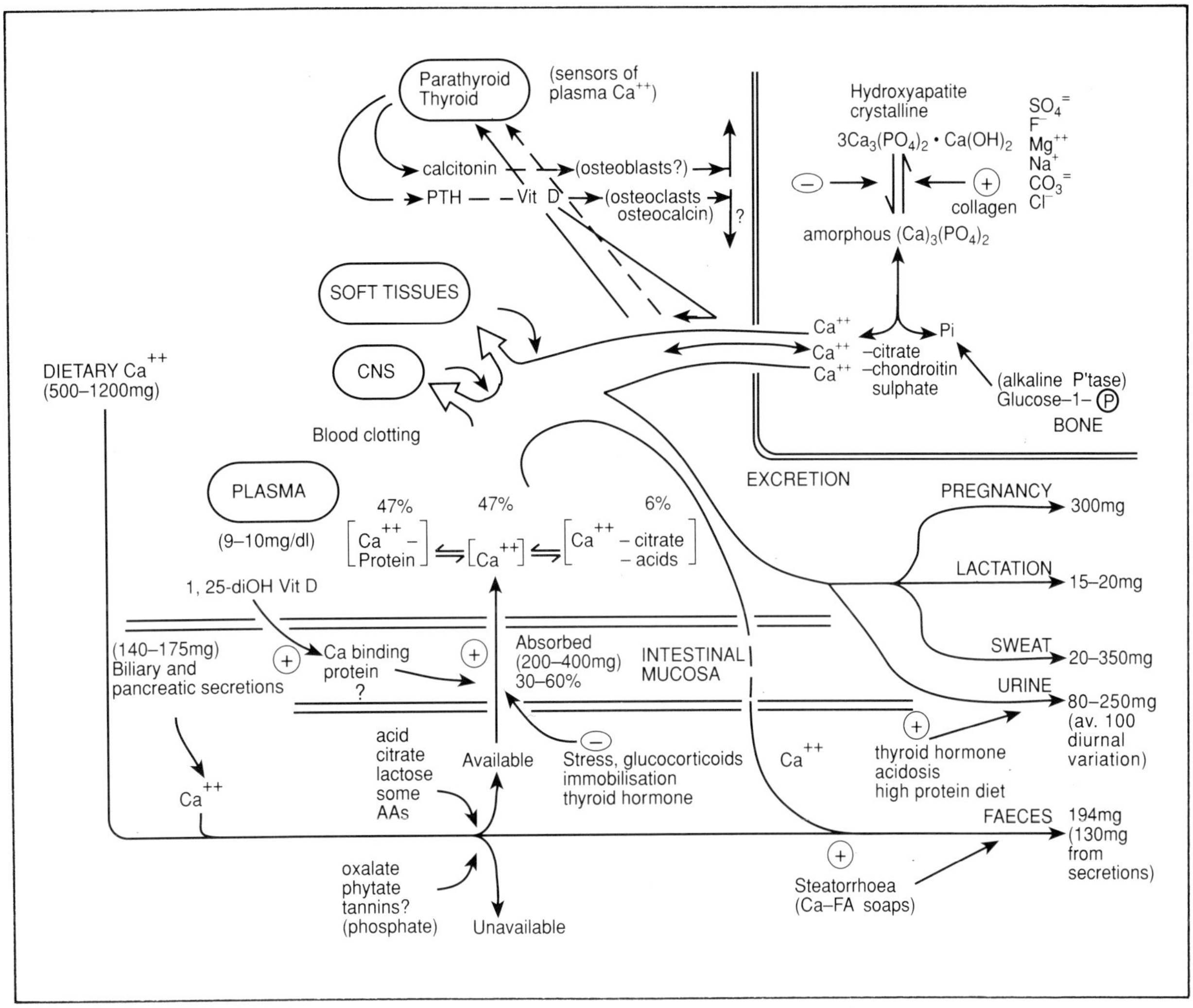

407 Nutrition and metabolism of calcium of which the total amount in the body is about 1200g. Hypocalcaemia (< 7mg/dl plasma), tetany. Hypercalcaemia (> 12–15mg/dl plasma), nonspecific symptoms. '+' indicates stimulation; '–' indicates depression.

Calcium deficiency (hypocalcaemia)

It is almost unheard of for a diet to be so deficient in calcium as to cause clinical disease. Hypocalcaemia has been attributed to a variety of causes as shown in *Table 72*.

The most characteristic syndrome is tetany, consisting of:

- paraesthesiae of the lips, tongue, fingers, and feet;
- carpopedal spasm, resulting in 'obstetrician's hand', a deformity that may be painful and prolonged (**408**);
- muscle aching;
- spasms of the muscles of the face.

Chronic deficiency may lead to depression and psychosis. In the infant convulsions or heart failure may occur.

Table 72. Causes of hypocalcaemia (serum Ca < 2.25mmol/l (7.0mg/dl)).

Parathyroid hormone deficiency or absence	
	Hypoparathyroidism
	Idiopathic hypoparathyroidism
	Pseudohypoparathyroidism
Vitamin D deficiency	
	Nutritional
	Metabolic
	Secondary to other diseases
Hypomagnesaemia	
Malabsorption syndromes	
Acute pancreatitis	
Hypoproteinaemia from any cause	
Increased calcium utilization	
Tumours producing vitamin D 'antagonists'	

408

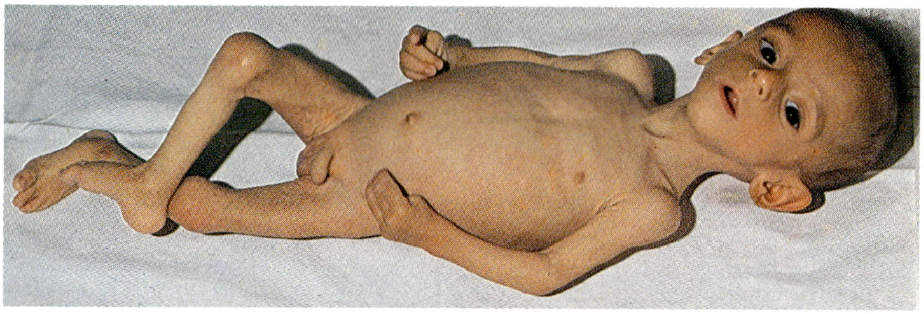

408 Main d'accoucheur. The characteristic contraction of the hands in this marasmic infant is indicative of accompanying tetany. This may be due to calcium deficiency, magnesium deficiency or a combination of both.

Calcium excess (hypercalcaemia)

Hypercalcaemia also has many possible causes (*Table 73*).

Mild hypercalcaemia is often asymptomatic and only discovered during laboratory screening. Manifestations include constipation, anorexia, nausea, vomiting and abdominal pain. Renal function impairment evidenced by polyuria and nocturia progresses if unchecked to nephrocalcinosis and renal failure. In severe disease psychosis may be followed by stupor and coma. Skeletal muscle weakness is common.

Table 73. Principal causes of hypercalcaemia (serum Ca > 2.5mmol/l (10.1mg/dl)).

Increased Ca mobilization	
	Parathyroid hormone excess
	Humoral hypercalcaemia of malignancy
	Malignancy with bone metastases
	Hyperthyroidism
	Vitamin D intoxication (infantile hypercalcaemia)
	Immobilization
Excessive calcium intake and/or absorption	
	Milk-alkali syndrome
	Vitamin D intoxication
	Sarcoidosis and other chronic granulomatous diseases
Uncertain mechanism	
	Myxoedema, Addison's disease, Cushing's disease, acromegaly
	Drugs: thiazides, chlorthalidone, lithium, tamoxifen
	Infections, e.g. tuberculosis, histoplasmosis
Artifactual	
	Elevated concentration of plasma proteins
	Prolonged venous stasis while obtaining blood sample
	Exposure of blood to contaminated glassware

The osteopetroses (Albers-Schönberg disease; marble bones)

This is a group of rare genetic disorders characterized by increased bone density and abnormalities of skeletal modelling (**409, 410**).

They are not related to calcium intake and their aetiology is unknown. Restriction of calcium intake appears to be of benefit in some cases.

409

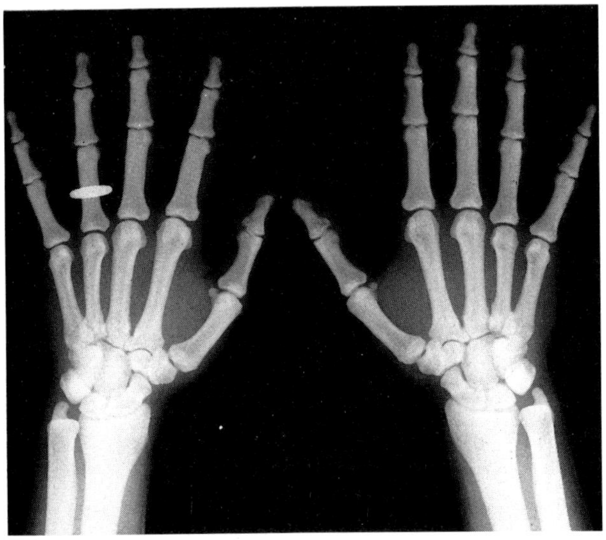

410

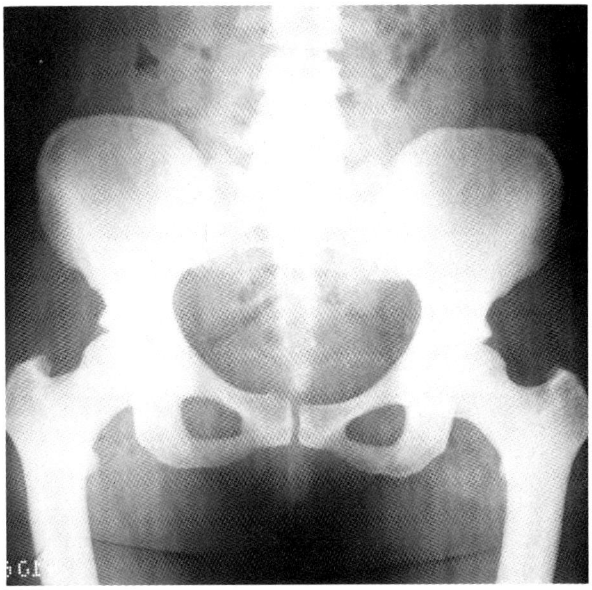

409, 410 Osteopetrosis or marble bone disease. A severe recessive form of this uncommon condition often leads to death in infancy. A milder dominant form is diagnosed in later childhood or adolescence. X-ray of the wrists, hands and pelvic region reveals marked density of bone and lack of moulding. Treatment consists of a low calcium diet combined with corticosteroids and splenectomy.

Phosphorus

Nearly all foods are good sources of phosphorus and dietary deficiency does not occur. It is a component of phytic acid in whole grain cereals which binds with calcium and impairs absorption. About 80% is present in bone and teeth. In combined form it takes part in acid–base balance in plasma and urine and is a component of nucleic acids and several B group vitamins. Phosphate ester is an essential step in carbohydrate breakdown. ATP (adenosine triphosphate) is a concentrated source of energy for cells and cyclic AMP and GMP (adenosine monophosphate and guanine monophosphate) are intracellular messengers. 2,3-diphosphoglycerate (2,3-DPG) shifts the oxygen dissociation curve of haemoglobin to the right, increasing oxygen availability to the tissues.

Inorganic phosphate in plasma is used to assess status (Appendix III, Table 2) and the adult RDA is the same as that for calcium (Appendix 2).

Phosphate depletion (hypophosphataemia)

It has been estimated that between 2 and 10% of all hospitalized patients have this in a mild form. It has often been overlooked in the past, perhaps because the symptoms and signs are not dramatic. They consist mainly of anorexia, muscle weakness and bone pain. Possible causes are numerous (*Table 74*) but it should be guarded against especially in patients suffering from diabetic ketoacidosis, acute alcoholism and those receiving total parenteral nutrition.

Table 74. Symptoms and signs of phosphate depletion.

System	*Manifestations*
General	Anorexia, nausea, vomiting, malaise, debility, lethargy
Nervous system	Confusion, seizures, coma, decreased motor and sensory conduction, peripheral neuropathy
Blood vascular	Red cell rigidity, impaired oxygen release due to 2,3-DPG deficiency, haemolytic anaemia, impaired phagocytosis, thrombocytopenia, haemorrhage
Metabolic	Insulin resistance and glucose intolerance
Gastrointestinal	Dysphagia, ileus, impaired liver function
Musculoskeletal	Rickets or osteomalacia, arthralgia, muscle weakness, true myopathy, rhabdomyolysis
Renal	Glycosuria, magnesuria, renal tubular acidosis

Hyperphosphataemia

This nearly always results from a chronic decline in renal function and is usually asymptomatic. In the past, besides dietary restriction of phosphorus, oral phosphate-binding compounds of aluminium were prescribed but because of toxic effects these have been discontinued (see Chapter 9).

Trace elements

Zinc

Most diets provide adequate zinc but much of it in cereal products is poorly absorbed. Both phytic acid and dietary fibre make it unavailable. The physiology of zinc is outlined in **411**.

At one time analyses of hair were much used for trace element status but these have been heavily criticized more recently, mainly for being difficult to interpret and open to commercial abuse. They have special value for detecting poisoning.[87] Plasma levels reflect status (Appendix III, Table 2) and the adult RDA is 15mg. Zinc appears to have many functions and these are reflected in the deficiency signs in its absence (see below).

411

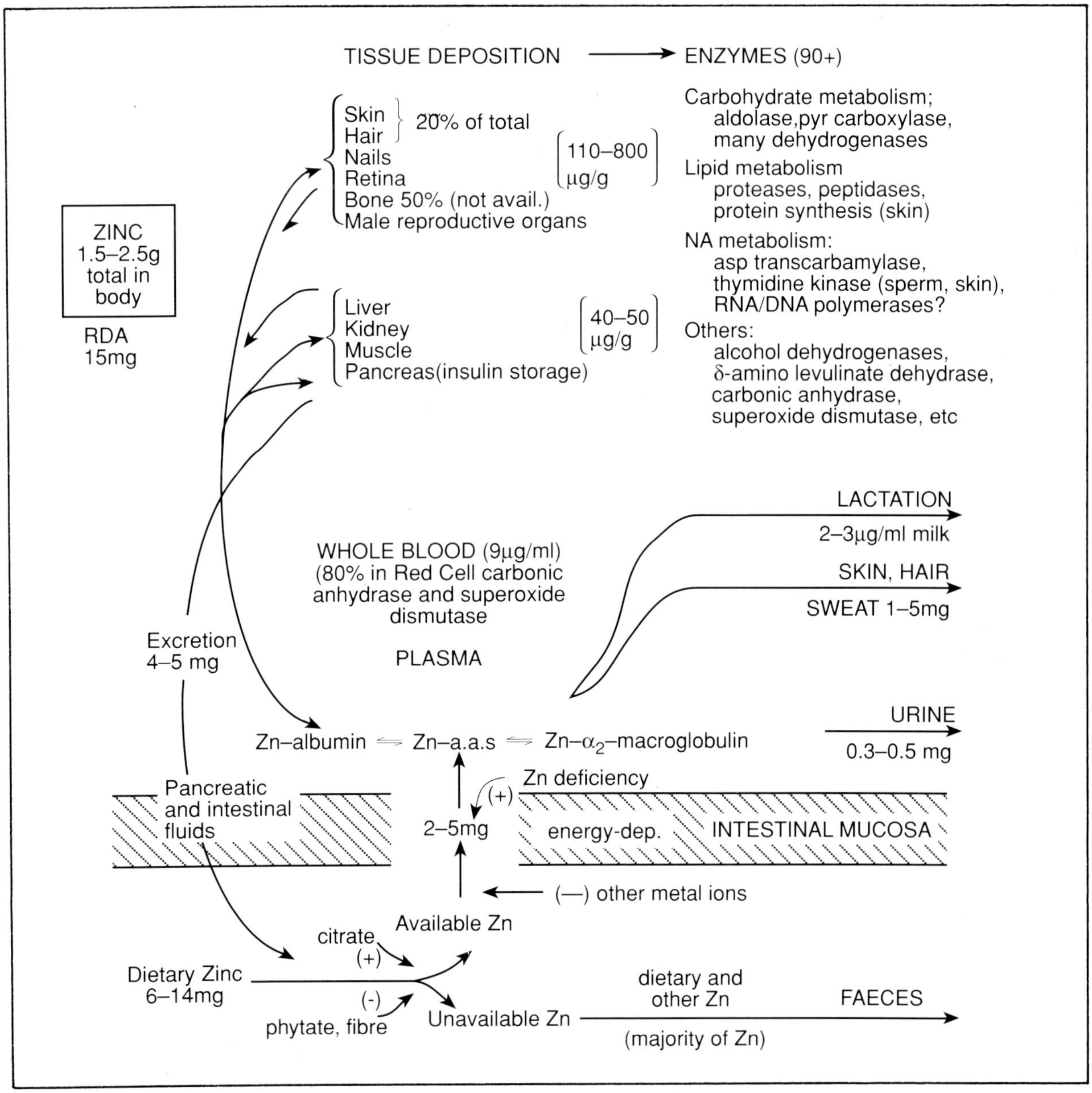

411 Nutrition and metabolism of zinc (1.5–2.5g total in the body).

Deficiency

The symptoms of zinc deficiency are given in *Table 75*.

There are many clinical states that predispose to deficiency as illustrated in *Table 76* and **412**.

Recently the possible significance of zinc in disease has broadened with evidence that deficiency may have a role in an important group of causes of blindness due to macular degeneration for which hitherto no cause has been found (**413**).

Table 75. Symptoms and signs of zinc deficiency.

Anorexia
Impaired taste (hypogeusia) and smell
Diarrhoea
Skin lesions – especially over hands, perineum and cheeks
Hair growth arrest
Nails (growth arrest, loss, Beau's lines)
Paronychia with superinfection with monilia
Growth retardation
Hypogonadism (impotence in renal dialysis patients)
Photophobia, night blindness
Wound healing delay

Table 76. Causes of zinc deficiency.

Inadequate dietary intake
Anorexia nervosa
Anorexia of malignant disease
PEM
Chronic uraemia
Decreased absorption
Diet high in phytate
in fibre
in iron
Geophagia (pica)
Acrodermatitis enteropathica (specific defect)
Malabsorption syndromes
Decreased utilization
PEM
Alcoholic cirrhosis
Increased loss
Intestinal, pancreatic and liver diseases
Alcoholism
Oral D-penicillamine therapy
Burn exudation
Exfoliative dermatitis
Increased requirements
Physiological – infancy, pregnancy, lactation
Neoplastic diseases

412

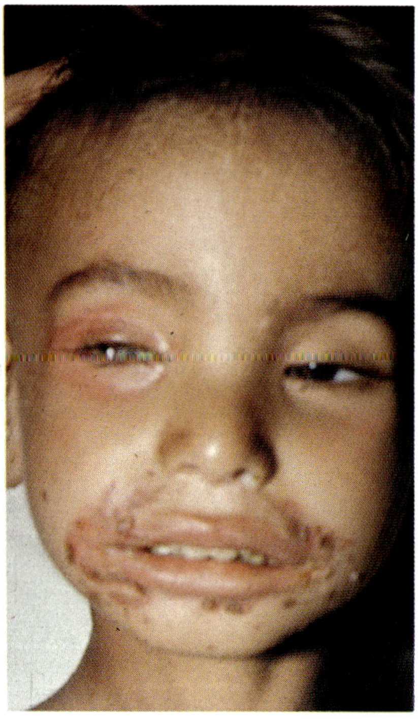

412 Acrodermatitis enteropathica. This is an inherited, previously fatal, disorder characterized by a psoriasiform dermatitis, often affecting the whole body, diarrhoea, hair loss, paronychia and growth retardation. It is due to a defect in the absorption of zinc and responds dramatically to this trace element.

A syndrome of growth retardation and hypogonadism responding to zinc has been described in the Middle East. Low zinc status may occur in many diseases and is probably sometimes responsible for failure to thrive and hypogeusia (impaired taste) in children, and night blindness in adults with liver disease or malabsorption.

413 Age-related macular degeneration (AMD) affects almost 30% of those over the age of 75 and has become the leading cause of vision loss in the elderly. The degenerative changes affect the retinal pigment epithelium in the macular area, which is responsible for central vision.

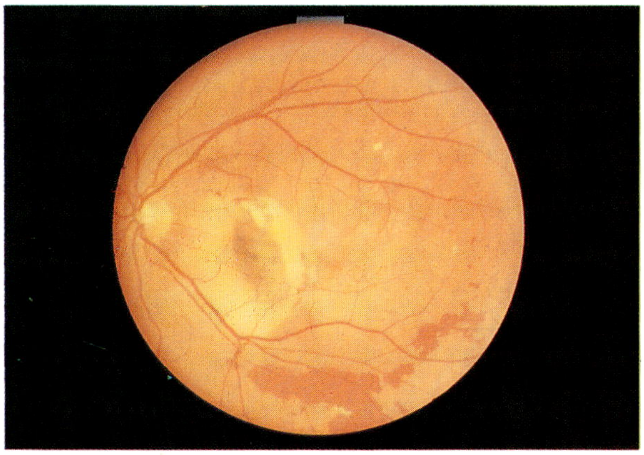

413

Toxicity

Until recently zinc toxicity was largely associated with exposure in industry to fumes of zinc oxide. Several reports have described bone marrow depression and sideroblastic anaemia from zinc-induced copper deficiency as a result of excess zinc ingestion in food supplements or coins (**414**).[88]

414 Zinc toxicity. Abdominal X-ray shows a rounded metallic mass of coins which was removed from the stomach at operation. The coins had been ingested over a period of 12 years by a chronic paranoid schizophrenic patient in the belief that they would protect him from harm. Complete recovery occurred after removal of the source of excess zinc. The anaemia and bone marrow depression were attributable to zinc-induced copper deficiency. This is probably the most notable instance to date of the adverse effect of one nutrient upon another.

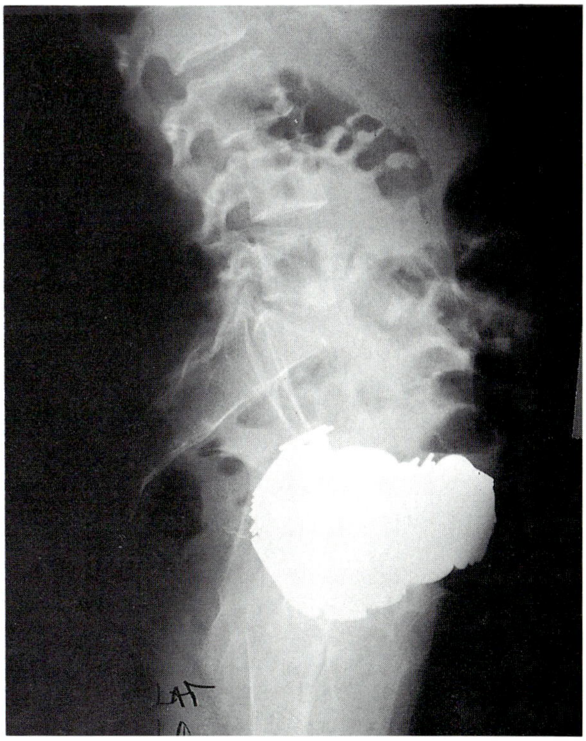

414

Copper

Rich dietary sources are organ meat, oysters, nuts, dried legumes and whole grain cereals. Milk is a poor source and infants are susceptible to deficiency. The metabolism of copper in the body is shown in **415**.

Except as a component of metallo-enzymes the functions of copper are unclear. Plasma copper is used to assess status (Appendix III, Table 2) and a safe and adequate intake for the adult is considered to be 2–3mg.

415

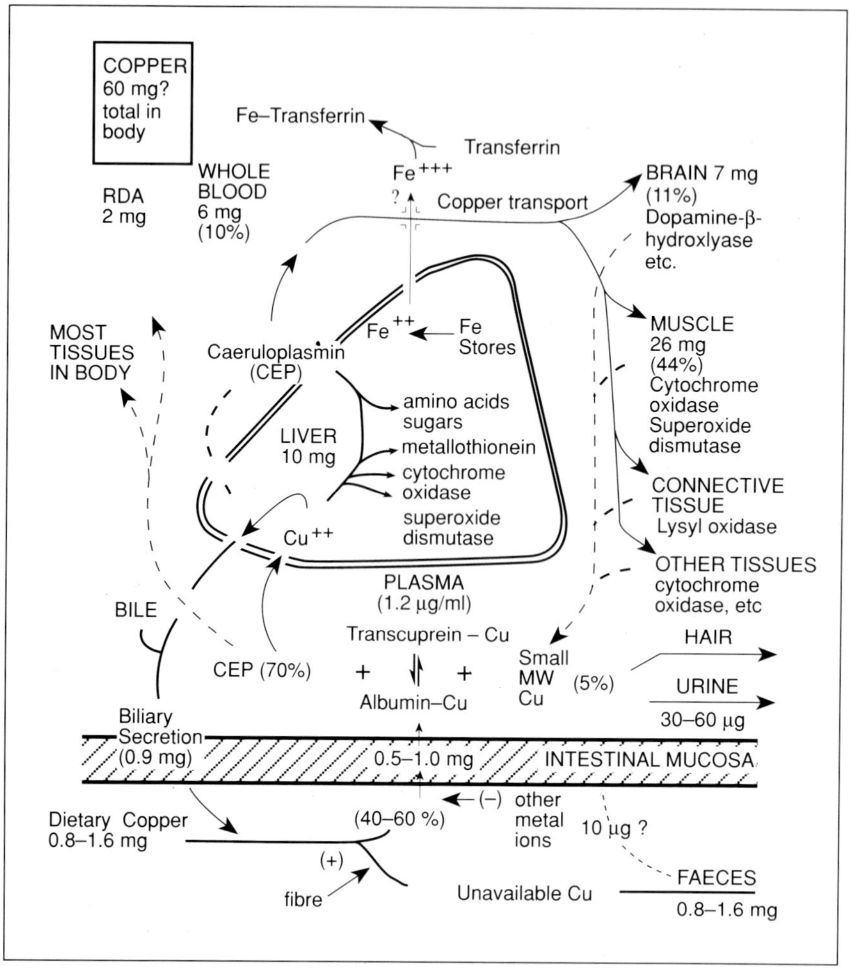

415 Copper metabolism and nutrition.

Deficiency

Table 77 lists the main predisposing conditions leading to copper deficiency.

Several systems are affected by copper deficiency, suggesting that it has widespread functions (*Table 78*, **416**).

Menkes' steely (kinky) hair syndrome results from an inborn error of copper absorption (**417**).

Table 77. Causes of copper deficiency.

Decreased intake	**Increased loss**
Cows' milk-based infant formulae	Intestinal disease: coeliac disease, sprue, Crohn's disease, nephrotic syndrome
Long-term total parenteral nutrition lacking copper	Burns and scalds
Decreased absorption	Primary hyperparathyroidism
Excessive zinc intake	**Increased requirement**
High intake of vitamin C	Low birthweight, pregnancy, lactation
Chronic oral alkali treatment	**Decreased utilization**
Menkes' steely hair syndrome	Menkes' steely hair syndrome
Chronic infantile diarrhoea	
Intestinal disease – short bowel syndrome, jejunoileal bypass	PEM

Table 78. Clinical features of copper deficiency in man.

Microcytic hypochromic anaemia; neutropoenia
Skeletal demineralization; subperiosteal haemorrhages
Depigmentation of hair and skin*, seborrhoeic dermatosis
Defective elastin formation: – arterial aneurysms, decreased tensile strength of skin
Apathy, psychomotor retardation, cerebral and cerebellar degeneration
Hypothermia

* Pili torti or kinky hair is seen only in Menkes' disease, not in acquired copper deficiency

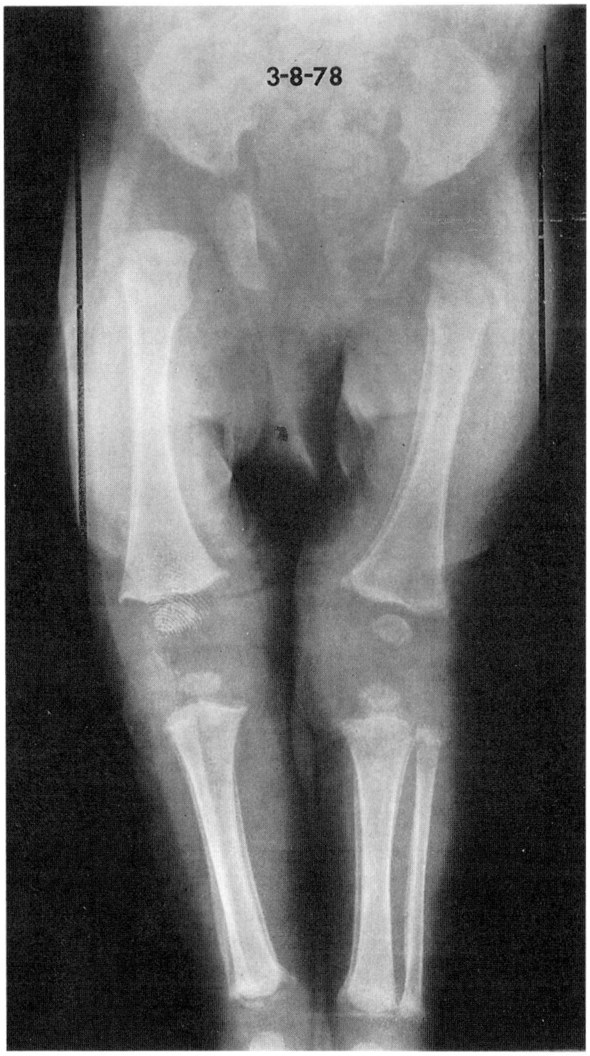

416

416 Infantile nutritional copper deficiency. Antero-posterior view of lower limbs; marked osteoporosis and subperiosteal new bone are present in long bones and ilia. Metaphyses have a wavy and irregular outline. Distal femoral and tibial metaphyseal infractions are present. Note bucket-handle deformities of distal metaphyses of tibiae.

417

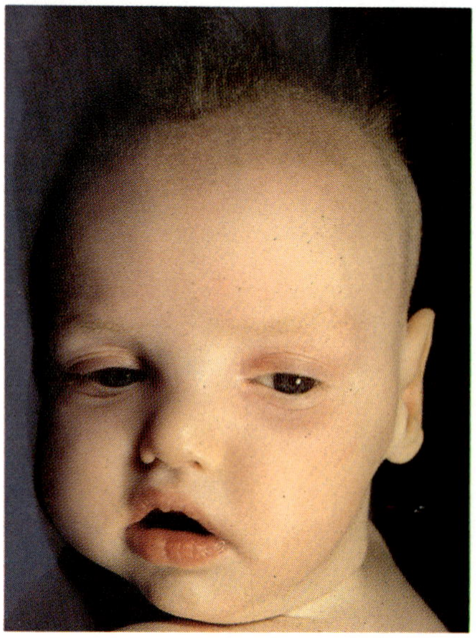

417 **Menkes' steely (kinky) hair syndrome.** The typical appearance of the face and sparse, brittle hair in this sex-linked disorder are caused by a defect in intestinal copper absorption. There is also retarded growth, progressive cerebral degeneration, arterial lesions and scurvy-like bone changes. Early treatment with copper salts intravenously daily may alleviate the condition.

Toxicity

Wilson's disease, hepatolenticular degeneration, is a rare, often familial progressive disorder resulting from accumulation of excess copper in tissues, especially liver, brain, kidneys, and red cells (**418–425**).

418

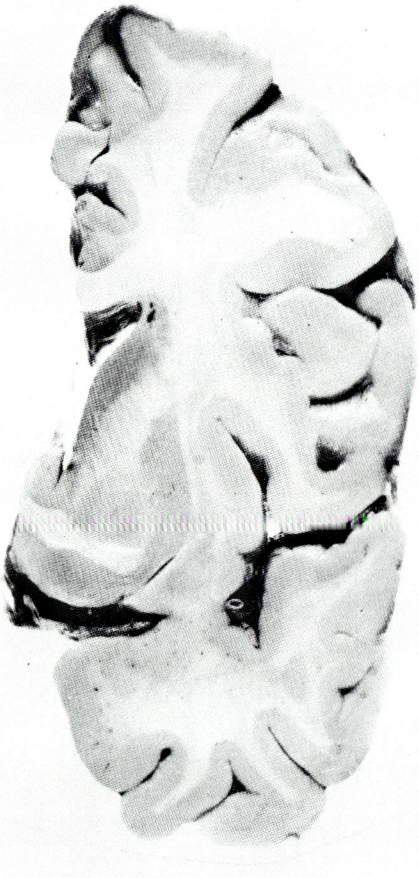

418 **Hepatolenticular degeneration (Wilson's disease).** Right cerebral hemisphere in coronal section to show shrinkage of the putamen and globus pallidus. (× 1.6)

419 Hepatolenticular degeneration (Wilson's disease). The trapezoid body of the pons shows microcystic degeneration, astrocytic hyperplasia and several Opalski cells, which have pink granular cytoplasm and characteristically small round or ovoid nucleus. (*H&E*, × 160)

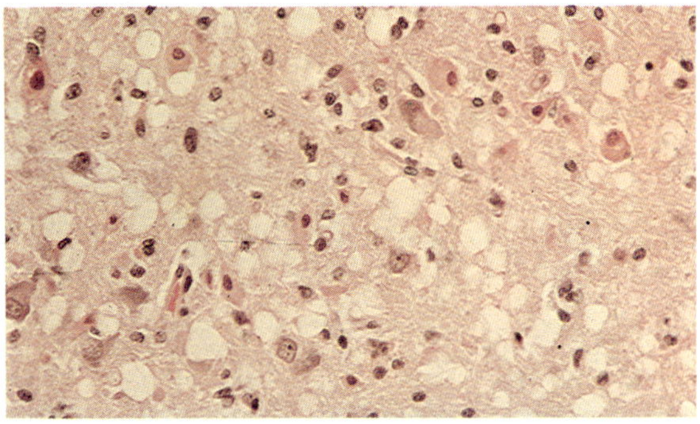

419

420 Cornea in Wilson's disease. Copper deposits in Descemet's membrane in the corneal periphery produce the pathognomonic Kayser-Fleischer ring. This is a complete or incomplete brown to green ring near the limbus, most noticeable superiorly and inferiorly, best seen in the early stages with the gonioprism.

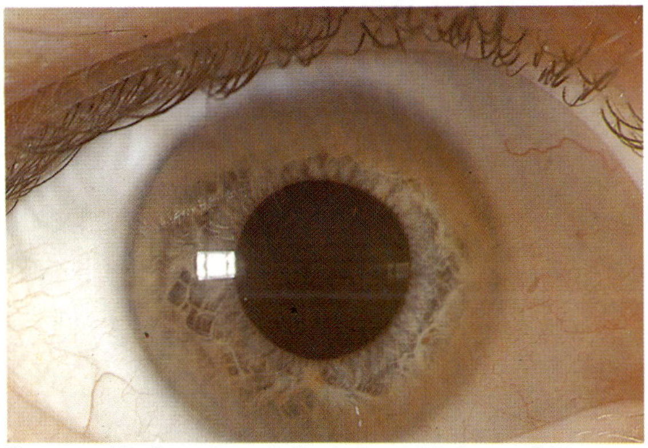

420

Courtesy of Professor Dame S. Sherlock and J.A. Summerfield.

421 The lens in Wilson's disease. Copper deposition is present, resulting in the characteristic 'sunflower' cataract.

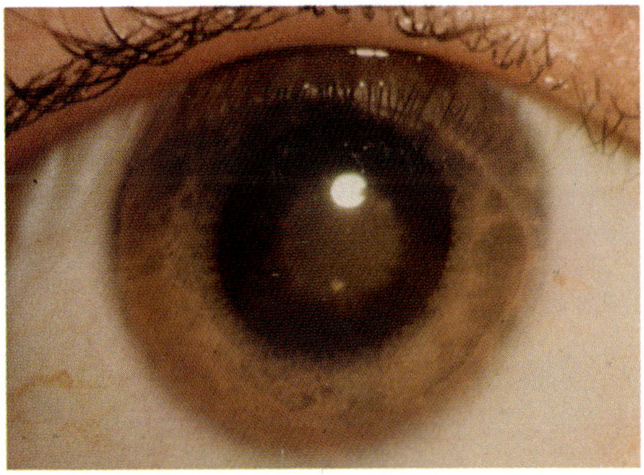

421

422 The lens in Wilson's disease. A painting (by Mr T.R. Tarrant) of the same eye as in the previous figure, of the anterior and posterior surfaces of the lens and the optical section of the lens (*arrowed*).

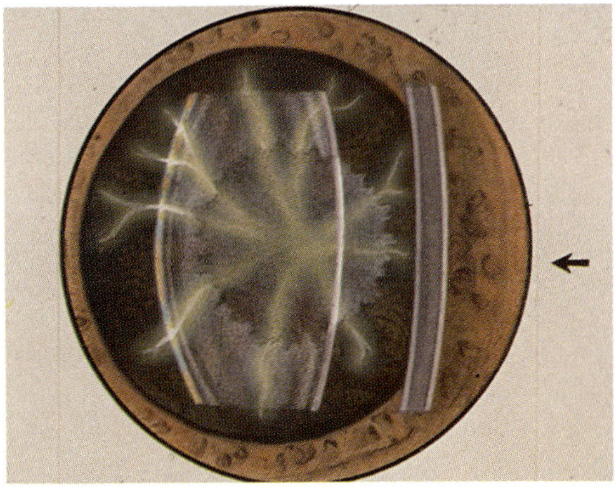

422

423

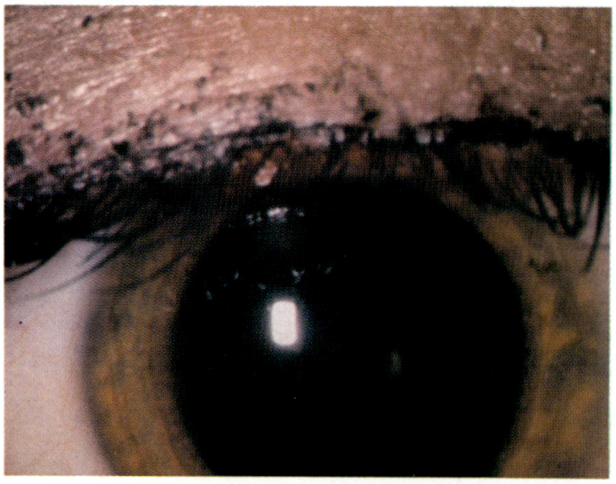

42

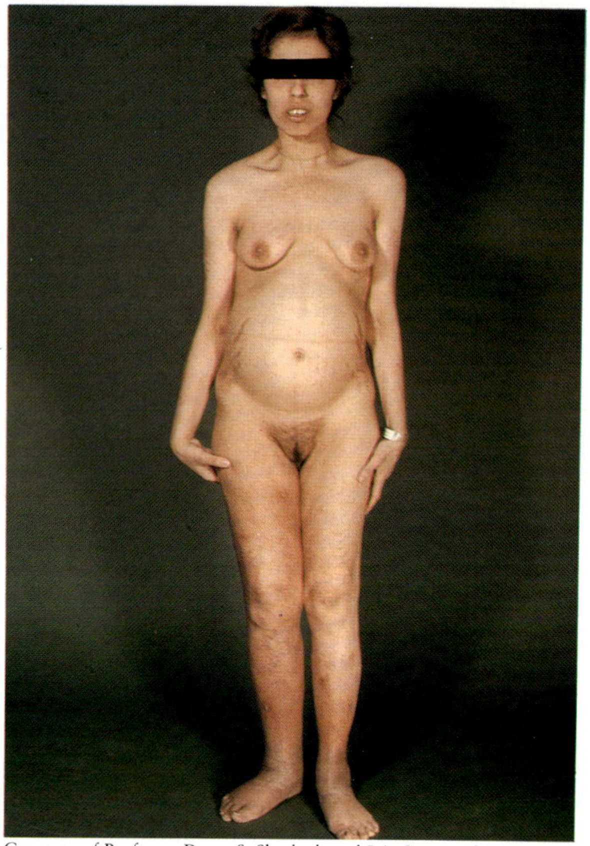

Courtesy of Professor Dame S. Sherlock and J.A. Summerfield.

423 The lens in Wilson's disease. The lens has been photographed as in **421** after 5 years of treatment with penicillamine. There is total clearing of the copper deposits.

424 Wilson's disease may present with an episode of jaundice due to haemolysis or as a well compensated cirrhosis. Alternatively Wilson's disease can mimic chronic active hepatitis, as in this young woman. Note the abdominal striae and leg oedema. The posture and fatuous expression in this patient are due to the basal ganglia changes of Wilson's disease, which usually develop some years after the liver disease.

425

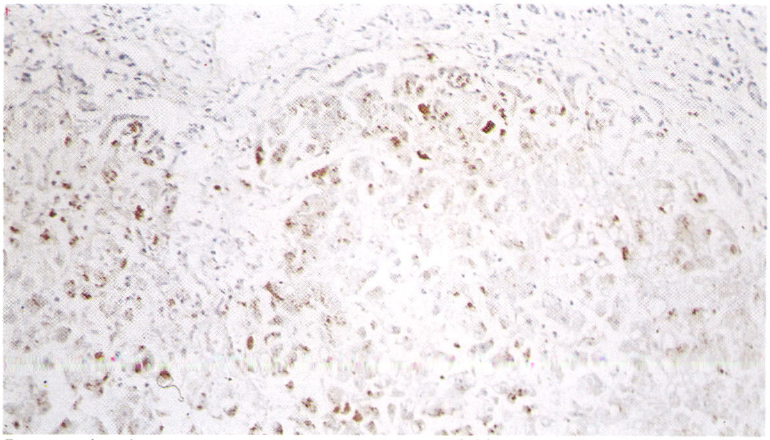

Courtesy of Professor Dame S. Sherlock and J.A. Summerfield.

425 Wilson's disease. The large accumulation of copper in the liver cells has been stained reddish-pink in this biopsy. Histological stains for copper are unreliable for the diagnosis of Wilson's disease. (*Rhodanine*, × 40)

In recent years evidence has been obtained that infantile biliary cirrhosis, most often seen in Indian families, is caused by the practice of feeding animal milk contaminated with copper by boiling and storing in brass or copper pots (**426, 427**).

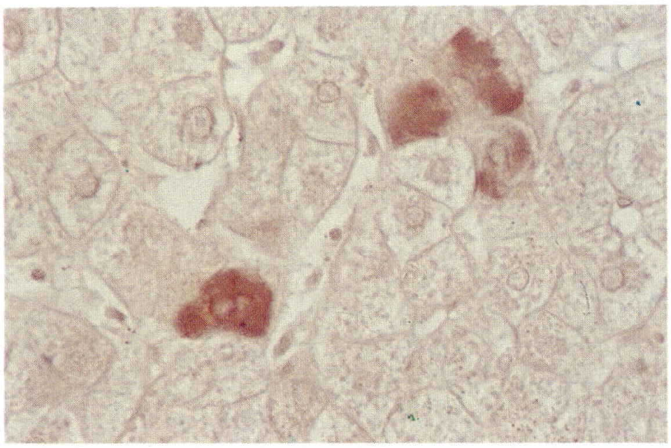

426

426 Indian infantile biliary cirrhosis. Typical HB surface staining in cytoplasm of four liver cells. Biopsy from HB_s seropositive Indian child with chronic active hepatitis (reduced by ⅓ from × 400).

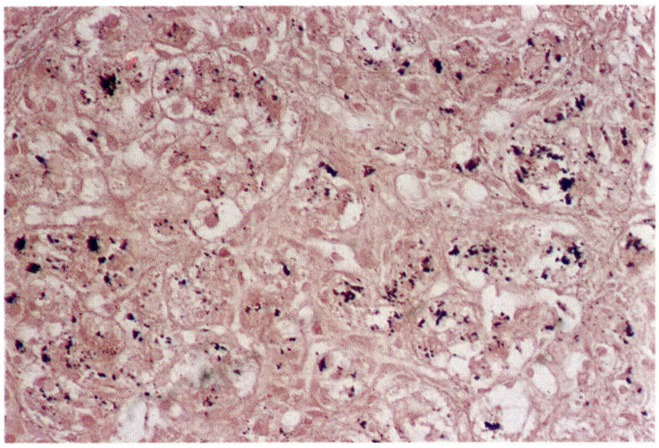

427

427 Extensive granular deposits of copper in Indian childhood cirrhosis (reduced by ⅓ from × 400), stained by orcein method.

Cobalt

As far as is known, cobalt is only utilized in the body to form vitamin B_{12}. Rich sources of the vitamin therefore provide cobalt. Plasma cobalt is used to assess status (Appendix III, Table 2). No safe and adequate limit has been set.

Deficiency other than that of vitamin B_{12} has not been described.

Toxicity

Cobalt has sometimes been recommended for the treatment of the anaemia of chronic nephritis and infection, where it has been reported to cause goitre, myxoedema and congestive heart failure. Cardiomyopathy with a high mortality has occurred after industrial exposure, during renal dialysis, and after consumption of beer that was contaminated with cobalt during processing (**428–433**).

428

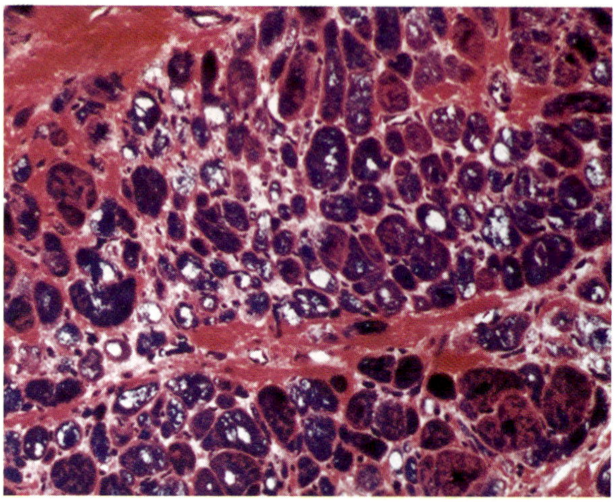

4

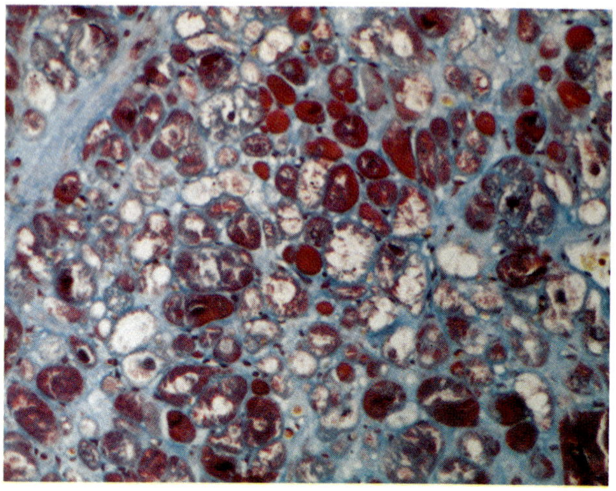

428, 429 Cobalt cardiomyopathy. These sections show the characteristic areas of myocardial necrosis, with vacuolated fibres that have lost their striations, and irregular, very large nuclei. Neutron activation analysis for cobalt showed about 40 times the normal concentration.

430

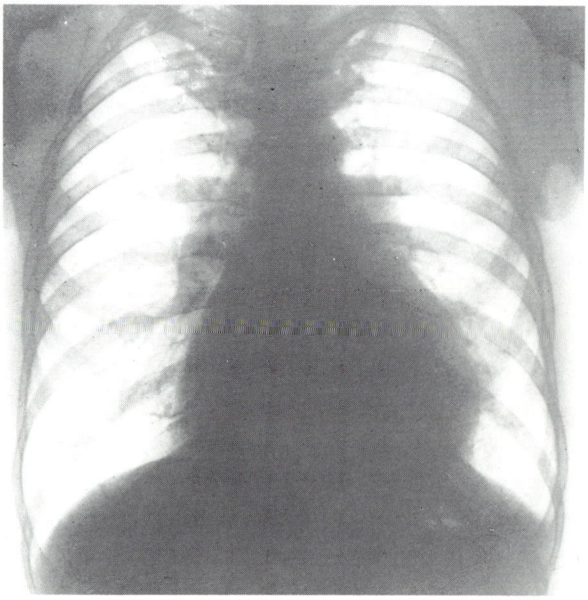

4

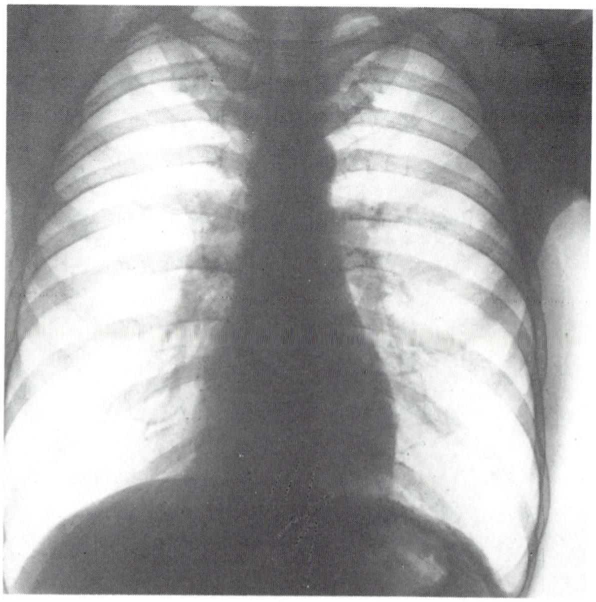

430 Cobalt toxicity. X-ray of the chest on admission showing a grossly dilated heart.

431 Cobalt toxicity. The same patient 4 months after discharge showing the return of the heart to normal size.

432 Cobalt toxicity. Electrocardiogram taken on admission showing prominent P waves and low voltage in the upper tracing.

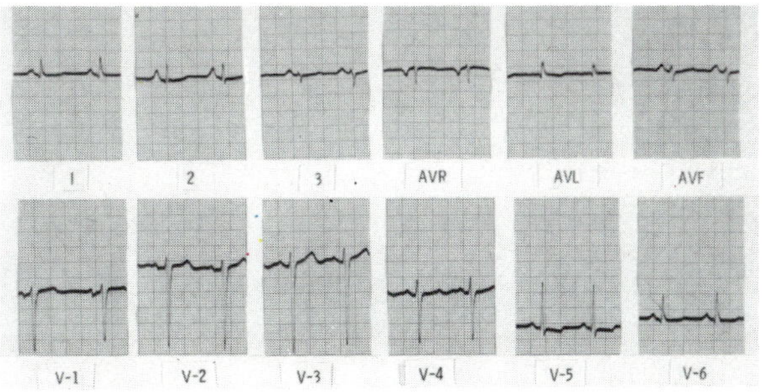

432

433 Cobalt toxicity. The record of the same patient 9 months later showing considerable improvement.

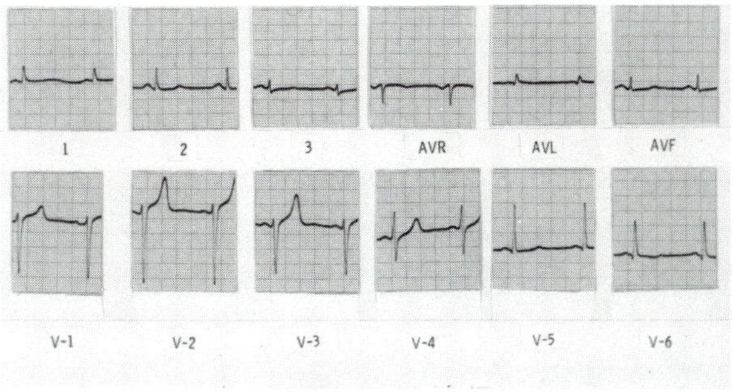

433

Selenium

The food content is influenced by that of the soil in which the food is grown. Most foods provide some. Functions are not clear, but the requirement for selenium by glutathione peroxidase provides a method for assessment of status using plasma as well as measuring selenium there (Appendix III, Table 2). The safe and adequate intake is the same as for chromium, 0.05–0.2mg.

Deficiency

Patients on long-term total parenteral nutrition have developed cardiomyopathy, muscle pain and tenderness, dyschromotrichia, white fingernails and a macrocytic anaemia, which have responded to selenium (**434A**).

From China an endemic cardiomyopathy in young children and women of childbearing age has been given the name Keshan disease after its place of origin. Results of dosing with selenium have been favourable.

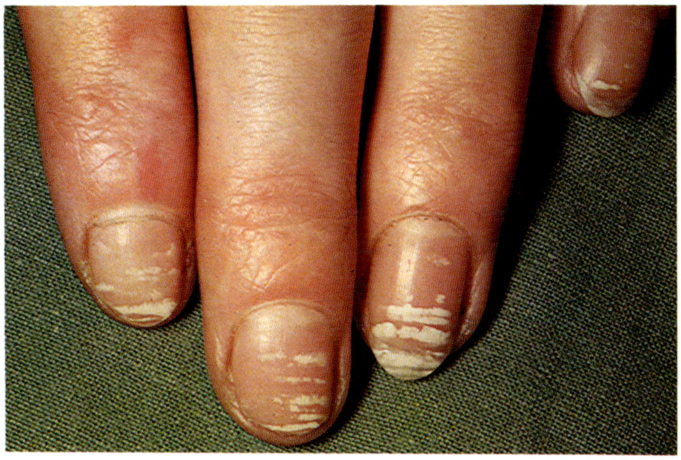

434A

434A Striate leuconychia. Similar to the changes reported in selenium deficiency.

Toxicity (selenosis)

Other areas of China have high levels of selenium and in the United States food supplements have produced symptoms and caused several fatalities. The symptomatology is quite distinctive: metallic taste, odour of garlic due to methylation of selenium, mucosal irritation, gastroenteritis, paronychia, and red pigmentation of nails, hair and teeth (**434B, C**).

434B

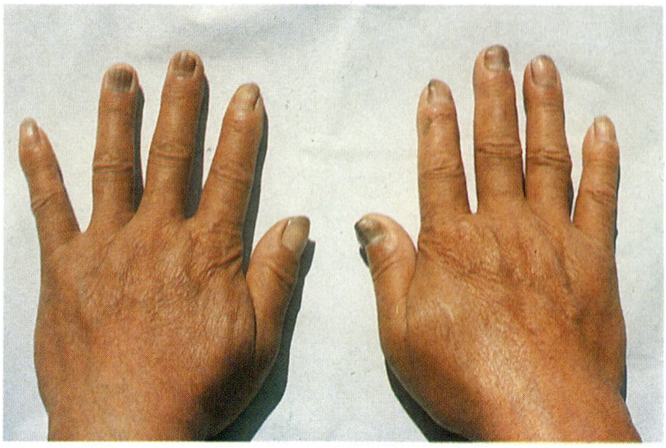

434B Selenium toxicity. Patient in Enshi, China, where average dietary Se intake is 1300μg/day (normal is about 200μg/day) and mean plasma Se is 1.51 ± 0.05μg/ml) (normal is 0.1–0.2μg/ml). The nails are discoloured, thickened and deformed.

434C

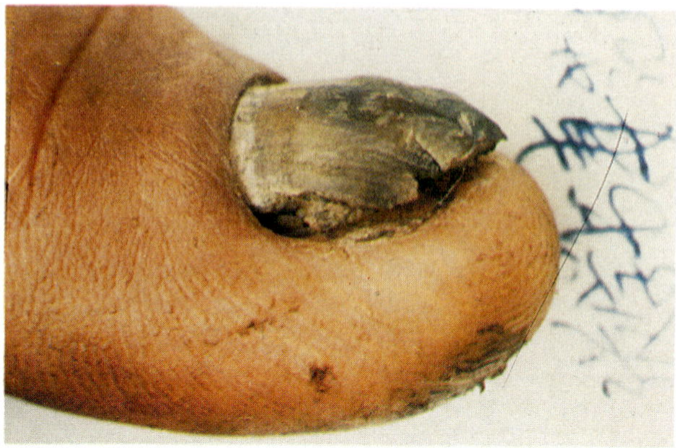

434C Selenium toxicity. Another Chinese patient with severe pain in the finger tips and hypertrophy of the nail plate (plasma Se 1.13μg/ml).

Other trace elements

Several other elements are of indeterminate status or not proved to be of sufficient importance in human health and disease to receive more attention here (*Table 79*).

Table 79. Outline summary of some ultratrace elements.

Element	*Likely status*	*Major deficiency sign*	*Possible role*
Arsenic	E	Depressed growth	Methionine metabolism
Boron	E	Depressed growth	Bone mineralization
Chromium	E	Carbohydrate and lipid disorders	Insulin potentiation
Fluorine	NE*	Depressed growth	Calcified tissue structure
Lithium	PE	Depressed fertility	Endocrine regulation
Manganese	E	Various	Metalloenzymes
Molybdenum	E	Depressed growth	Xanthine, aldehyde and sulphite oxidases
Nickel	E	Depressed haemopoiesis	Iron absorption
Silicon	E	Depressed bone collagen	Cross-linking of connective tissue
Vanadium	PE	Various	Phosphoryl-transfer enzyme regulation

Key: E, essential; PE, probably essential; * Although fluorine is not known to be essential it has beneficial pharmacological properties (e.g. anticariogenic property).

7. Diet-Responsive Inherited Metabolic Diseases

One of the most important ways in which endogenous malnutrition (see Chapter 1) can arise is through a genetic defect that occurs at some stage in metabolism. Inborn errors of this kind are legion and their number is being added to constantly. Many of these conditions do not involve nutrients or do not respond to dietary manipulation and consequently are not considered here. Even so there is a considerable number that do and *Table 80* is a compilation of the principal ones.

Table 80. Principal diet- or nutrient-responsive inborn errors of metabolism (excluding vitamin dependency states – see **Table 81**).

Disorder	*Main clinical features*	*Management*
	Disorders of carbohydrate metabolism	
Glycogen storage diseases		
Glucose-6-phosphatase deficiency	Failure to thrive, hepatomegaly	High carbohydrate intake
Amylo-1, 6-glucosidase deficiency	Hepatomegaly	High carbohydrate intake
Muscle phosphorylase deficiency	Easy muscle fatigue	Oral glucose and fructose
Galactosaemia		
Galactose-1-phosphate transferase deficiency	Failure to thrive, cataract, liver failure, mental retardation	Galactose-free diet
Galactokinase deficiency	Cataract	Galactose-free diet
Disorders of fructose metabolism		
Fructose-1, 6-diphosphatase deficiency	Keto and lactic acidosis, hypoglycaemia	Fructose-free diet
Fructose-1-phosphate aldolase deficiency	Failure to thrive, hypoglycaemia, hepatic failure	Fructose-free diet
Disaccharide intolerance	Abdominal pain, diarrhoea	Disaccharide-free diet
	Disorders of amino acid metabolism	
Phenulketonuria (phenylalanine hydroxylase deficiency)	Mental retardation, growth failure	Phenylalanine restriction
Disorders of tyrosine metabolism		
Tyrosine aminotransferase deficiency	Mental retardation, skin and corneal changes	Diet low in tyrosine and phenylalanine
Fumarylacetoacetase deficiency	Liver failure, anaemia	Diet low in tyrosine and phenylalanine
Neonatal tyrosinaemia	Mild mental retardation	Diet low in protein and tyrosine
Histidase deficiency	Speech defects	Low histidine diet
Periodic hyperlysinaemia	Failure to thrive, dehydration	Restricted protein diet
Persistent hyperlysinaemia	Retardation	Restricted protein diet
Disorders of the urea cycle		
N-acetylglutamate synthetase deficiency	Hyperammonaemia syndrome	Low protein diet, arginine supplements

(Cont.)

Table 80. Continued:

Disorder	*Main clinical features*	*Management*
Argininosuccinate synthetase deficiency	Hyperammonaemia, orotic aciduria, neurologic changes	Low protein diet, arginine supplements
Isovaleric acidaemia	Failure to thrive, ketoacidosis	Protein restriction, glycine supplements
Cystinuria	Cystine stones	Low methionine diet
	Disorders of lipoprotein and lipid metabolism	
Lipoprotein lipase deficiency	Abdominal pain, pancreatitis, xanthomas	Low fat diet
Lecithin: cholesterol acyl transferase deficiency	Anaemia, corneal opacities, renal failure	Restricted fat diet
Phytanic acid storage disease (Refsum's disease)	Retinopathy, ataxia, peripheral neuropathy	Chlorophyll-free diet
	Disorders of porphyrin and haem metabolism	
Acute intermittent porphyria (porphobilinogen deaminase deficiency)	Nerve damage, abdominal pain	High carbohydrate diet
Erythropoietic protoporphyria (ferrochelatase deficiency)	Photosensitivity, anaemia, liver damage	Calorie restriction, B-carotene
Hereditary coproporphyria (coproporphyrinogen III oxidase deficiency)	Abdominal pain, photosensitivity	High carbohydrate diet
Variegate porphyria (protoporphyrinogen oxidase deficiency)	Photosensitivity, abdominal pain, neuropathy	High carbohydrate diet
Porphyria cutanea tarda (hepatic uroporphyrinogen decarboxylase deficiency)	Photosensitivity with skin lesions	Low alcohol
Congenital erythropoietic porphyria (uroporphyrinogen III cosynthetase deficiency)	Haemolysis, photosensitivity, skin scarring	B-carotene
	Other disorders	
Gout	Arthritis, tophi, hyperuricaemia	Protein, purine and alcohol restriction
Xanthine oxidase deficiency	Urinary tract stones	Low purine diet

It is useful to consider separately a group of disorders that respond to very large doses of certain vitamins – these are the vitamin dependency states (*Table 81*).

In all of these conditions, arising as they do soon after birth, there is as might be expected the common feature of growth retardation. It is probable that some defects are incompatible with intrauterine survival and all carry a guarded prognosis even when dietary treatment is quite effective. Some have distinctive clinical features and some of these are illustrated here.

Our understanding of the molecular basis of these diseases varies considerably. Most of them are due to absence or diminished production of an enzyme. In the vitamin dependencies there is some kind of defect in the binding of coenzyme to apoenzyme. Several conditions are due to a defect in the transport of amino acids across the intestinal mucosa and/or the renal tubule but its nature has not been discovered. In a few conditions nothing definite is known about the defect, for example cystic fibrosis and cystinosis. In some instances, as in familial hypercholesterolaemia, there is an abnormality in cell receptors, in this condition affecting those for LDL, which are either absent or defective.

Table 81. Principal inborn errors of metabolism responsive (some only partially) to large doses of vitamins.

Disorder	*Features*	*Vitamin*	*Dose (mg/day)*
Cystathionine synthase deficiency (classical homocystinuria)	Mental retardation, bony changes, lens dislocation, thromboembolism	Pyridoxine	5–500
Cystathioninuria	Usually none	Pyridoxine	5–500
Pyridoxine-responsive convulsions	Convulsions in infants	Pyridoxine	5–500
Pyridoxine-responsive anaemia	Normoblastic or sideroblastic anaemia	Pyridoxine	5–500
Familial xanthurenic aciduria	Urticaria	Pyridoxine	5–500
Primary hyperoxaluria	Oxalate kidney stones	Pyridoxine	5–500
Methylmalonic acidaemia	Metabolic acidosis	Vitamin B_{12}	1–2
Homocystinuria (one form)	Metabolic acidosis	Vitamin B_{12}	1–2
Biotinidase deficiency	Ketoacidosis, skin disorder, retardation, alopecia	Biotin	10
Holocarboxylase synthetase deficiency	Ketoacidosis, skin disorder, retardation, alopecia	Biotin	10
Glutaric aciduria (type I)	Metabolic acidosis, neurological damage	Riboflavin	250
Maple syrup urine disease	Retardation, ketoacidosis	Thiamin	10–100
Leigh's disease	Neurological damage	Thiamin	10–100
Dihydrofolate reductase deficiency	Anaemia, mental retardation	Folic acid	10–40
Homocystinuria (one form)	Anaemia, mental retardation	Folic acid	10–40
Hartnup disease	Dermatosis, cerebellar ataxia, amino aciduria	Nicotinamide	40–250
Type V hyperlipoproteinaemia	Xanthomas, recurrent pancreatitis, polyneuropathy	Nicotinamide	40–250
Familial hypercholesterolaemia	Xanthomas, atherosclerosis	Nicotinamide	40–250
Disorders of the glutamyl cycle	Acidosis, haemolysis, neurological damage	Vitamin E	100
Abetalipoproteinaemia	Ataxia, retinopathy, acanthocytosis, fat malabsorption	Vitamin E	100
Pseudohypoparathyroidism	Hypocalcaemia, skeletal deformities, cataracts, mental retardation	Vitamin D (in form of metabolite)	10–40 µg/day 1,25-$(OH)_2D_3$
Cystinosis	Rickets, renal failure	Vitamin D (in form of metabolite)	10–40 µg/day 1,25-$(OH)_2D_3$

Disorders of lipid metabolism

435 outlines the various aspects of lipid metabolism including absorption from the diet, transportation to the liver, fat depots and other tissues, and the various components that mediate these processes.

There are important differences in the composition of the various serum lipoproteins and these are shown in *Table 82*.

Disease results from both the total lack or deficiency of the various lipoproteins (*Table 83*) and also from excess levels (hyperlipaemia) (*Table 84*).

435

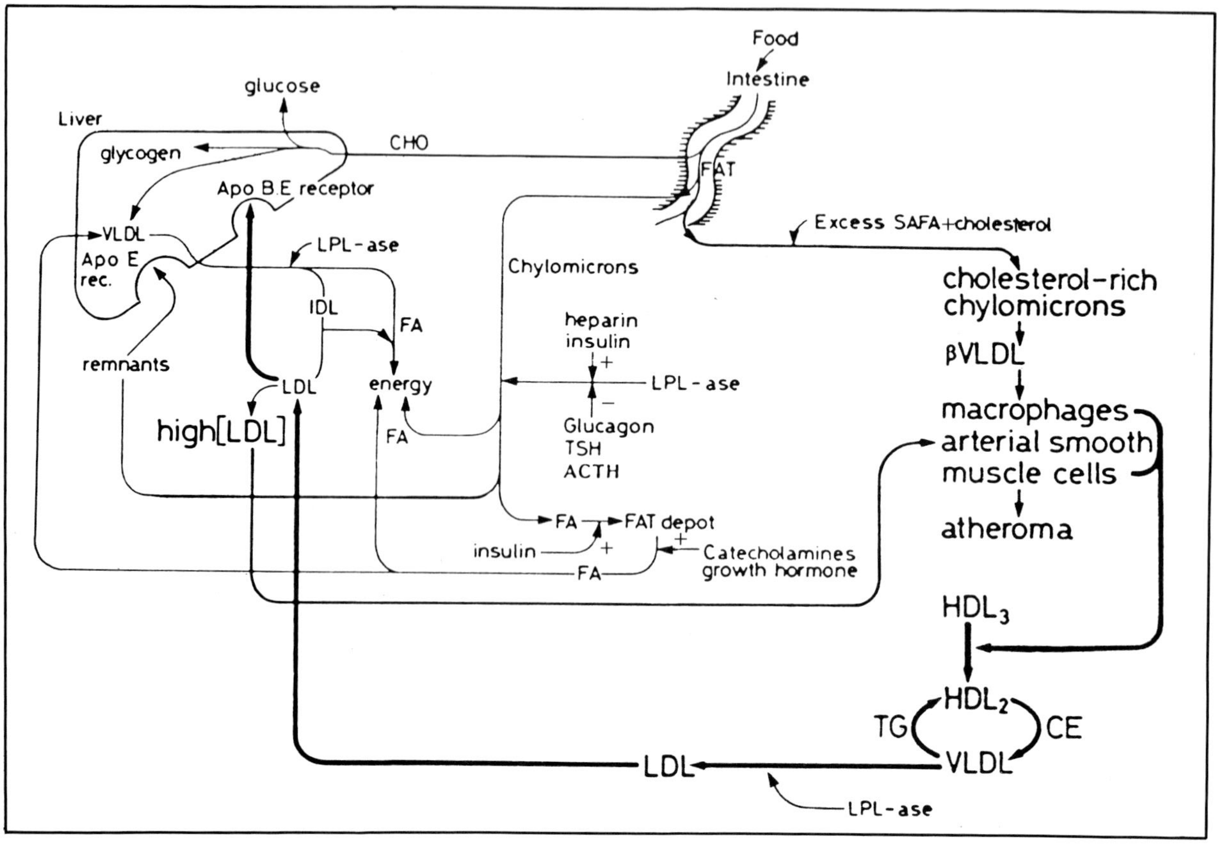

435 Disorders of lipid metabolism. Simplified scheme of the conversion of absorbed carbohydrates (CHO), fat and cholesterol to liver VLDL (with apo-B100), chylomicrons (with apo-B48) and B-VLDL. Lipoprotein lipase (LPL-ase) activity is stimulated by heparin and insulin and inhibited by glucagon, thyroid-stimulating hormone (TSH), and adrenocorticotrophic hormone (ACTH). Insulin stimulates triglyceride formation in fat depots, and catecholamines and growth hormone-stimulated adipose tissue lipase with fatty acid (FA) are released as a consequence. Excess VLDL formation in liver by excess dietary CHO or blood FA results in excess formation of LDL and atheroma. The same occurs at too high saturated fat (SAFA) and cholesterol consumption with the consequent formation of the atherogenic B-VLDL. HDL_3 is within certain limits capable of removing excess cholesterol from macrophages. The resulting HDL_2 particles transport the cholesterol to VLDL and are converted to LDL, which is taken up by liver and peripheral cells. The latter pathway is, however, contributing also to atheroma formation.

Table 82. Composition and some characteristics of serum lipoproteins.

Lipoprotein class	*Apolipoproteins*	*Percentage protein*	*Percentage cholesterol Free*	*Esthers*	*Percentage triglycerides*	*Percentage phospholipids*	*Main function*
Chylomicrons	A,B,C,E	2	1.5	2.5	83	8	Transport of triglycerides from small intestine to liver
(VLDL) Pre-betalipoprotein	B,C,E	7	10	5	52	18	Transport of triglycerides from liver to peripheral tissues
(LDL) Betalipoprotein	B	21	10	35	9	23	Transport and control of cholesterol
(HDL) Alphalipoprotein	A,C,E	46	5	15	8	27	Precise role not understood; some components probably involved in removing cholesterol from cells and inhibiting deposition in arteries

VLDL, very low density lipoproteins, LDL, low density lipoproteins, HDL, high density lipoproteins

Table 83. Classification and management of hypolipoproteinaemias.

Lipoprotein class involved	*Primary disorders*	*Complications*	*Treatment*
Chylomicrons	Abetalipoproteinaemia	Fat malabsorption	Low fat diet 5–20g/day, additional vitamins A,E,K
LDL	Abetalipoproteinaemia	Fat malabsorption	Low fat diet 5–20g/day, additional vitamins A,E,K
	Familial hypobetalipoproteinaemia (physiological in newborn)	Hyperthyroidism, hepatic failure, chronic anaemia	Not usually indicated
HDL	Familial alphalipoprotein deficiency (Tangier disease)	Hepatic failure	None
	Familial lecithin cholesterol-acyl-transferase (LCAT) deficiency	Non-specific	None

LDL, low density lipoproteins, HDL, high density lipoproteins

Table 84. The one-diet concept for prevention of atherosclerosis and treatment of hyperlipidaemia.

*Phase**	*Fat (percentage calories)*	*Saturated fat (percentage calories)*	*Cholesterol (mg/day)*	*Dietary measures*
I	30	10	300	Avoid foods rich in animal fats and cholesterol; use margarine, nonfat milk, and vegetable oils
II	25	8	200–250	Eat < 170–230g meat/day; use less fat and cheese, use more grains, fruit and vegetables
III	20	7	100–150	Eat mainly cereals, legumes, fruit and vegetables; eat meat as a condiment; use low cholesterol cheeses

* Phase I is appropriate for the population at large. Phase II is recommended for subjects with genetic forms of hyperlipidaemia, especially familial hypercholesterolaemia and familial combined hyperlipidaemia. Phase III may be required if there are other risk factors or strong family history of premature atherosclerotic complications.

Some of the characteristic clinical signs of these diseases are shown in **436–441.**

436

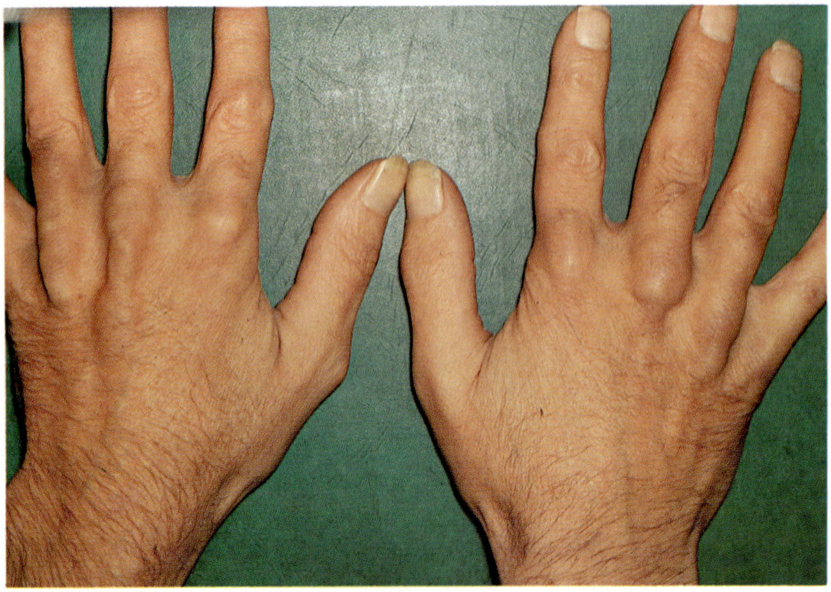

436 Tendon xanthomata. These consist of lipid accumulation in tissues in association with large foam cells. Type IIa familial hyperbetalipoproteinaemia or hypercholesterolaemia is usually present. In a rare familial condition with normal lipoproteins the upper part of the Achilles tendon is affected, followed by pulmonary insufficiency, dementia and spastic ataxia due to deposits of cholesterol and cholestanol. The metabolic defect has not been established.

437

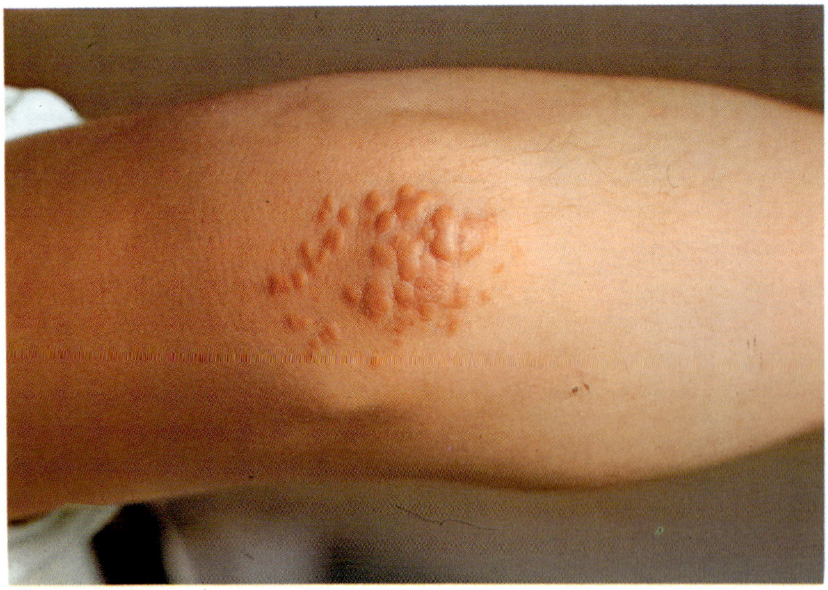

437 Cutaneous xanthomata (xanthoma tuberosum). Besides the elbows, the buttocks, palms and viscera are often affected. Type IIa, and less commonly Types IIb or III hyperlipoproteinaemia accompanies these lesions. In juveniles the plasma lipids may be normal.

438

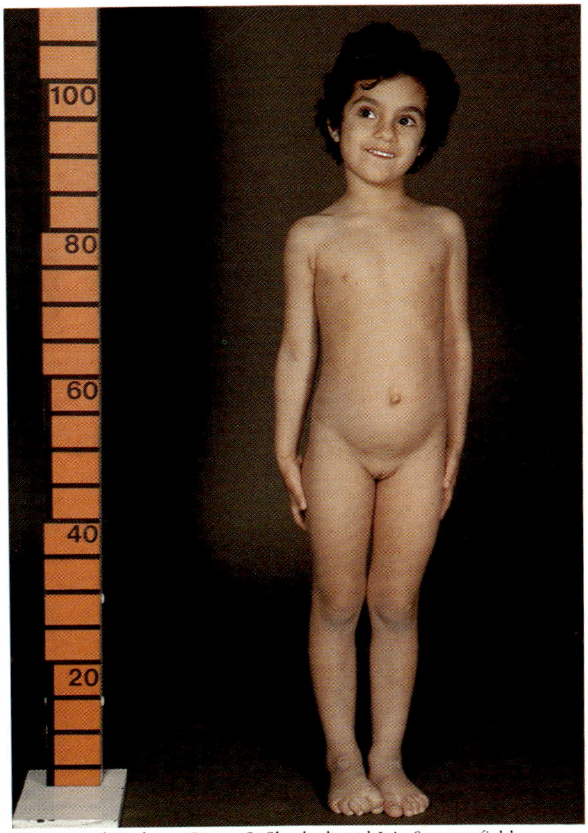

Courtesy of Professor Dame S. Sherlock and J.A. Summerfield.

439

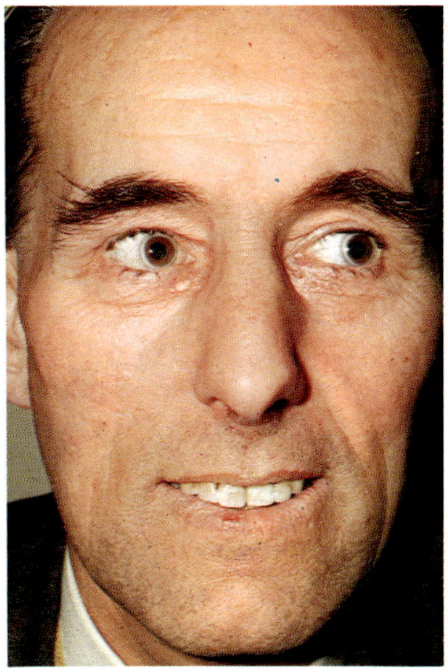

438 Familial hypercholesterolaemia. The heterozygote develops skin xanthomas and ischaemic heart disease in middle age. The homozygous state affects about 100,000 people in the U.K. and presents in childhood. The development of this 5-year-old homozygote girl was normal when she presented with skin xanthomas. Her serum cholesterol level was 420mg/100ml (10.92 mmol/l).

439 Corneal arcus. This is an infiltration of lipid forming a complete ring in the paralimbal periphery of the cornea. In young and middle aged subjects hyperlipoproteinaemia is often present, together with xanthoma or xanthelasma, and the term premature arcus and not arcus senilis should be used.

440

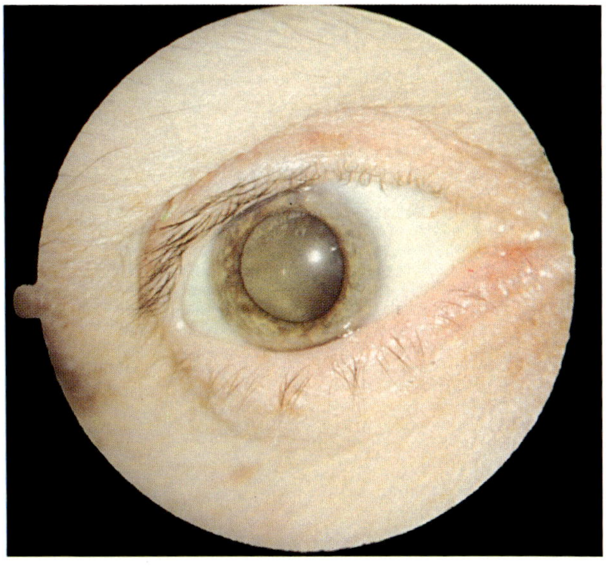

440 Arcus senilis (gerontoxon). In old age the plasma lipids are usually normal and other signs of disturbed lipid metabolism are absent.

441

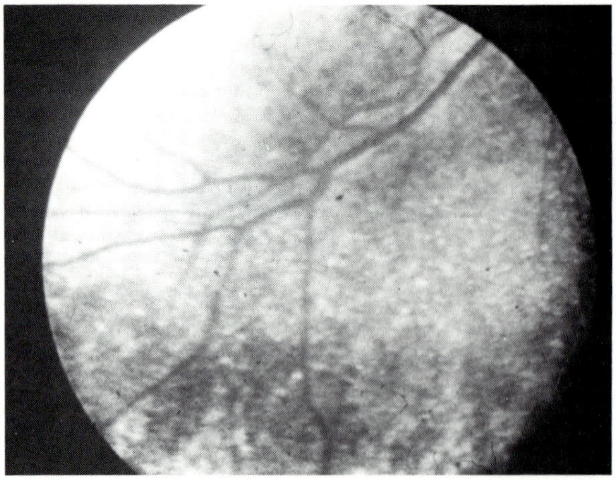

441 Retina in abetalipoproteinaemia. There is retinal pigmentary degeneration without evident narrowing and pigment clumping in the midperiphery. Some patients present a picture resembling retinitis punctata albescens, as does this one. Optic nerve pallor and posterior degeneration may occur. Nystagmus, strabismus and ptosis are common. A blue-yellow colour vision defect may be detected. Night blindness is common.

Refsum's disease results from damage caused by the accumulation of an abnormal fatty acid, phytanic acid, in tissues (**442, 443**).

442

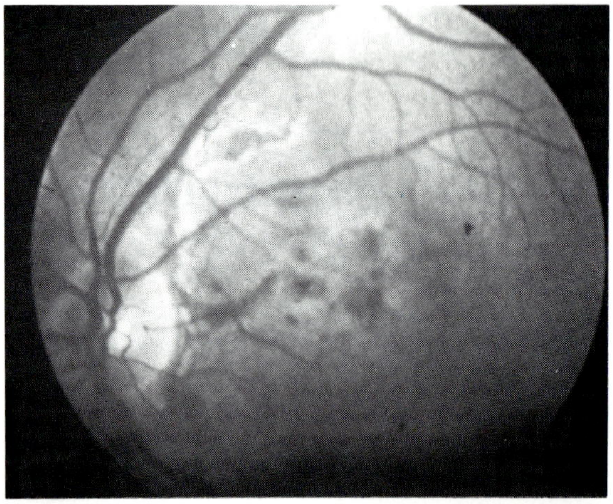

442 Retina in Refsum's disease. Night blindness is often the earliest abnormality. The electroretinogram (ERG) may be diminished or extinct. Visual field loss is common. Posterior cortical or subcapsular cataracts are present in about 35% of cases. This case shows pallor of the optic nerve head, arteriolar narrowing and retinal pigmentary disturbance.

443

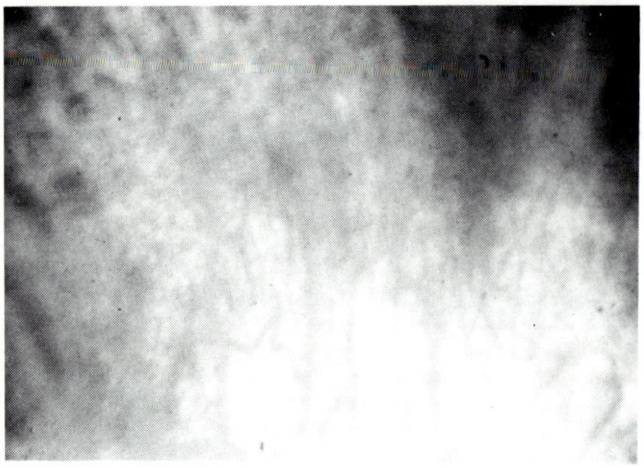

443 Retina in Refsum's disease. The peripheral retina shows mottling, 'salt and pepper' pattern, and 'bone spicule' pigmentary degeneration.

Disorders of carbohydrate metabolism

By far the most common disease in this group is diabetes mellitus. Although is has a polygenic component in its aetiology which has not yet been clearly identified it is also strongly determined by environmental factors among which diet and western life-style are important. It is discussed in Chapter 3.

There are several errors of glycogen storage, not all of which are amenable to dietary treatment (**444–447**).

444

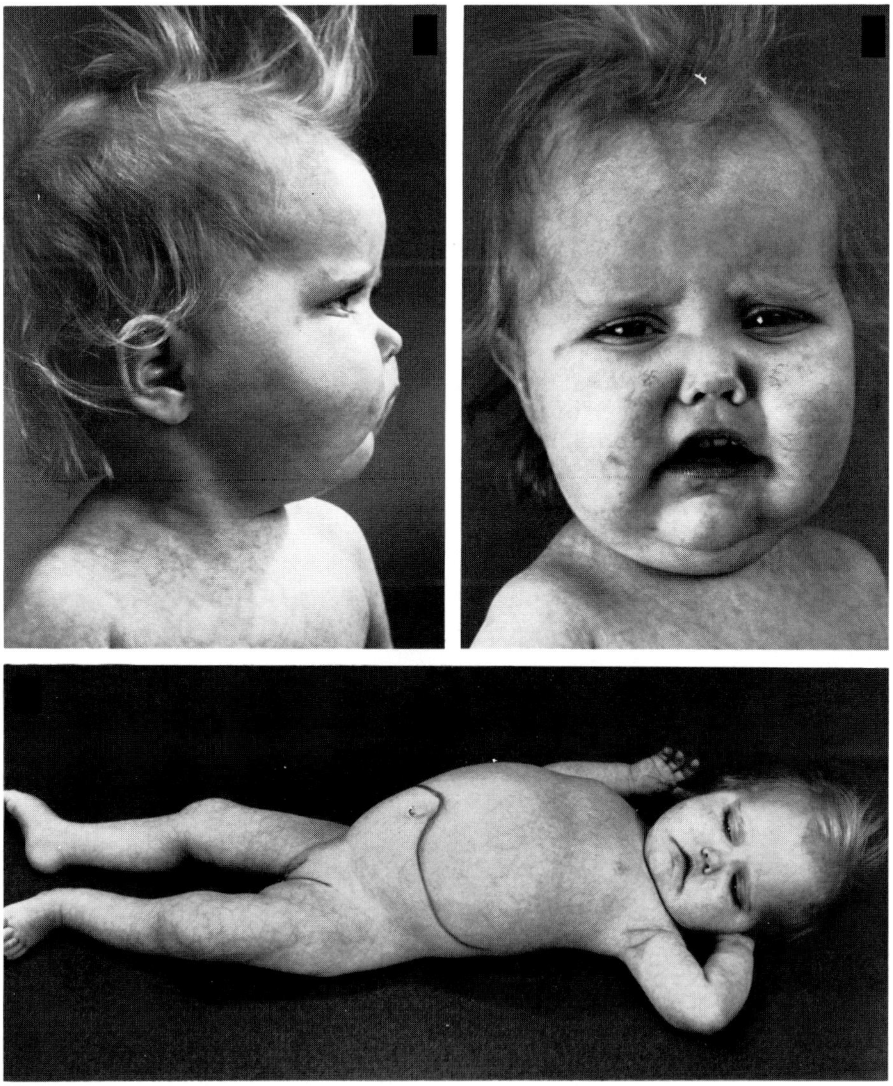

444 Von Gierke syndrome. Patient at age 1½ years. There is delayed development and a height deficit of 11 cm.

445

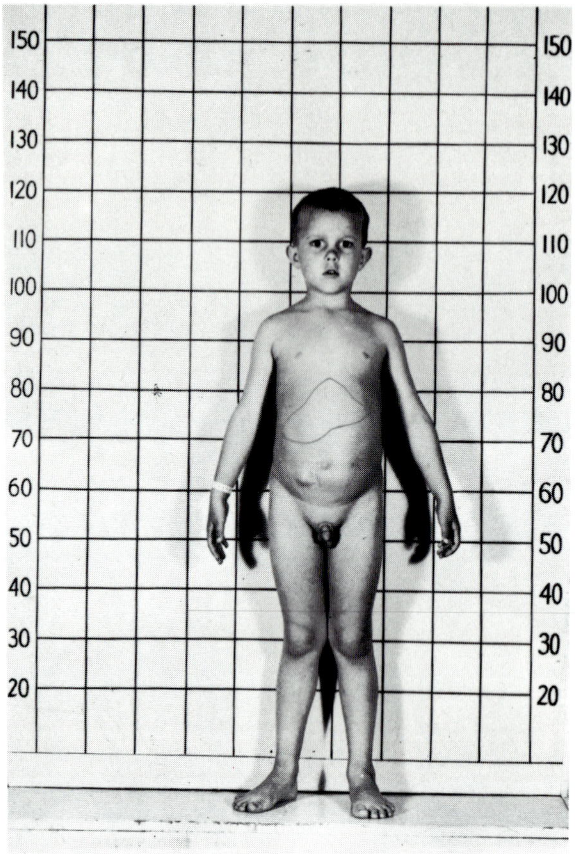

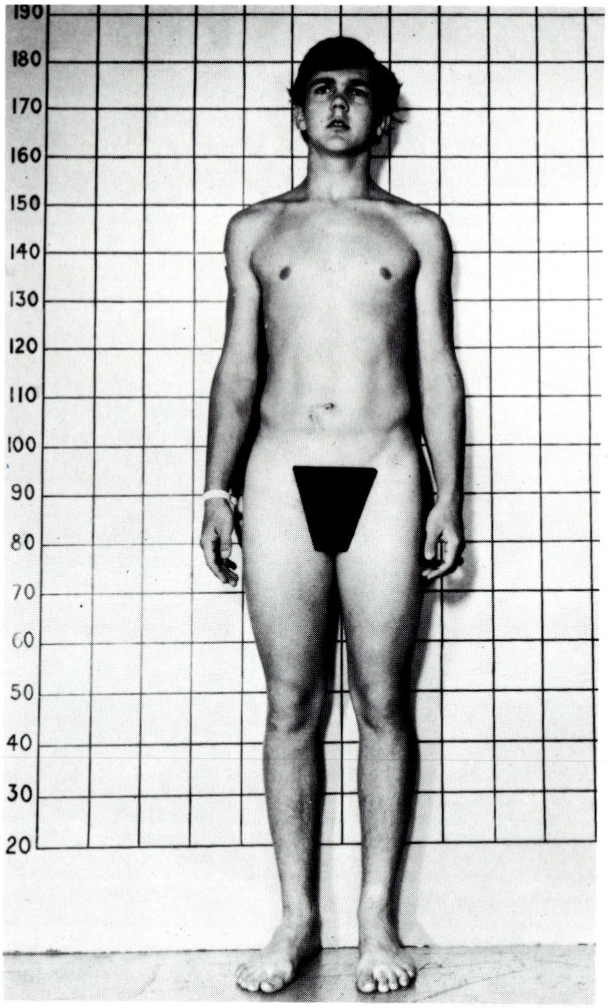

445 Glycogen storage disease. This picture shows hepatomegaly and stunting in a patient with Type III at 7 years of age.

446 Glycogen storage disease. This is the same patient at 17 years of age; growth and development are normal, the liver is not enlarged and there are no symptoms.

447

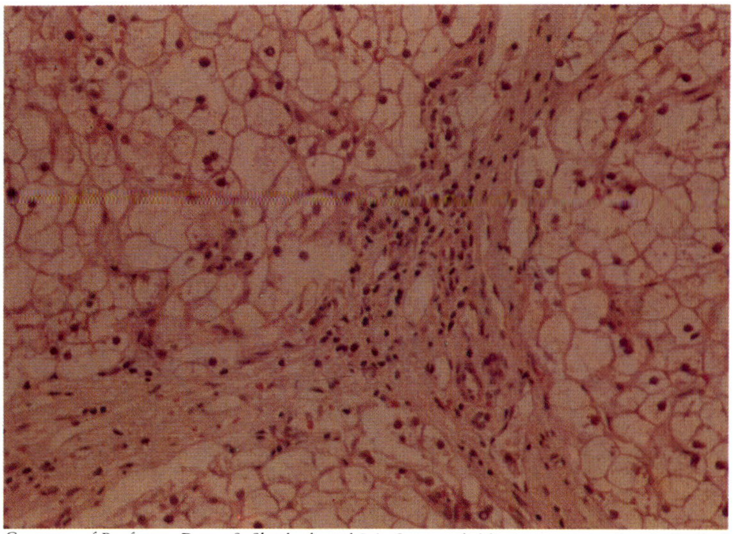

Courtesy of Professor Dame S. Sherlock and J.A. Summerfield.

447 Glycogen storage disease. In a liver biopsy processed in formol saline the glycogen is washed out of the cells. The liver cells then appear clear like plant cells. (*H&E*, × 40)

A deficiency or lack of the enzymes which take part in the metabolism of galactose (**448, 449**) and fructose (**450, 451**) causes disease which can be controlled by dietary modification.

448

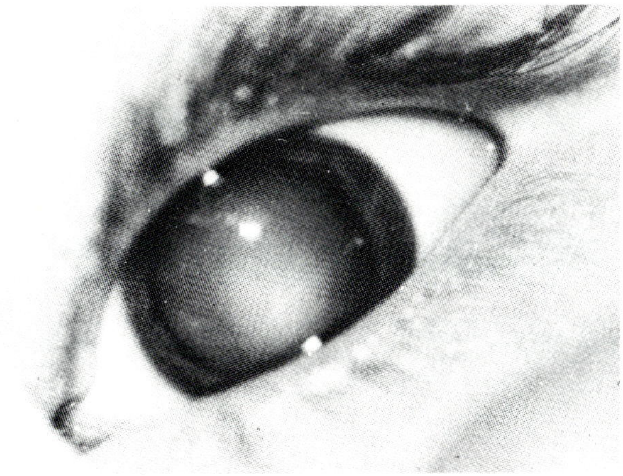

448 Galactosaemia. The first evidence may be cataract as in this infant.

449

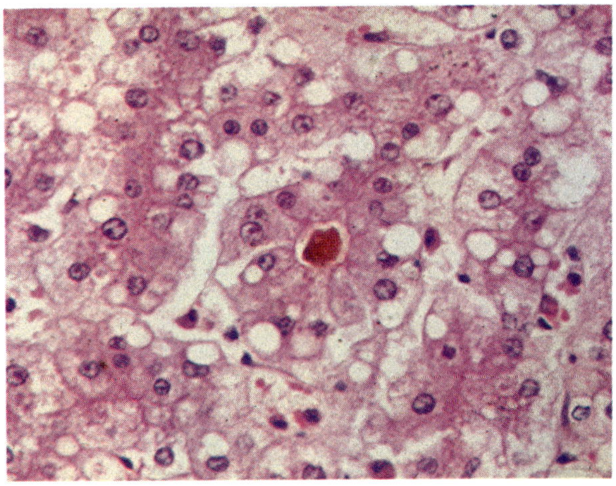

449 Liver in galactosaemia. Biopsy specimen from an infant showing pseudoacinus and fatty change in the parenchymal cells. (*H&E*, × 500)

450

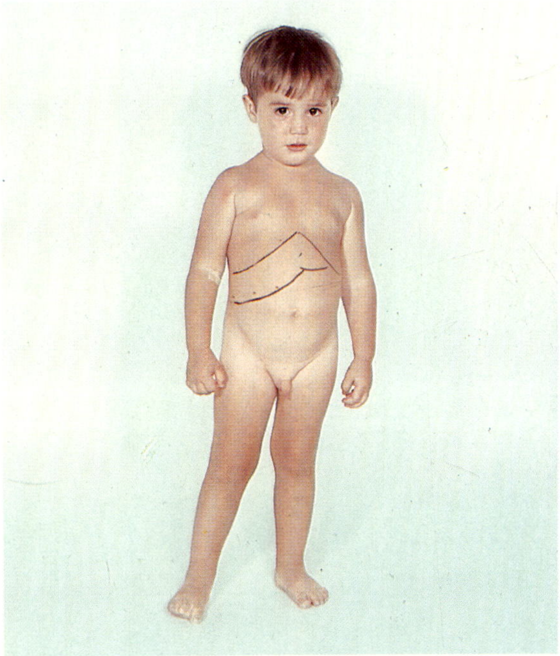

450 Hereditary fructose intolerance. This 2.5-year-old boy presented with nausea, vomiting and hepatomegaly. Hypoglycaemia, jaundice and aminoaciduria may also develop. Fructose intolerance resembles galactosaemia but the presentation is usually delayed until fruit and sucrose are introduced into the diet.

451 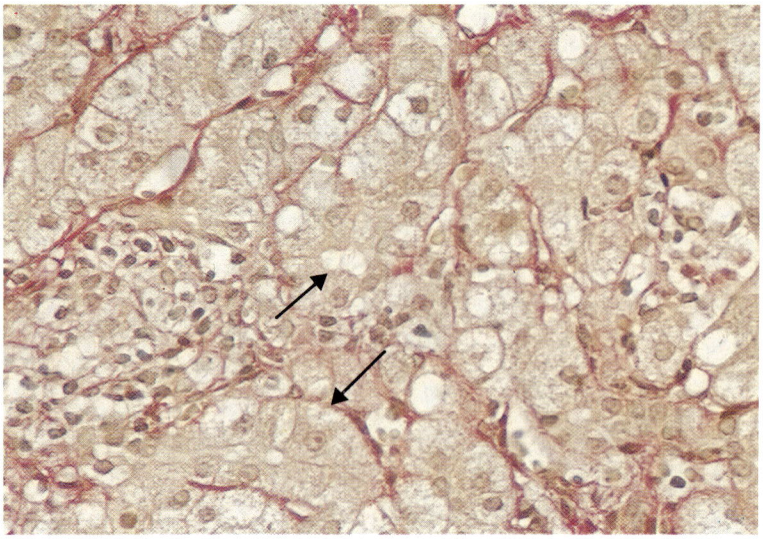

451 Hereditary fructose intolerance. Biopsy shows chronic inflammatory cell infiltration, fatty change and fibrosis. Groups of liver cells forming pseudo-acini (*arrowed*) are prominent. (× 100)

The congenital forms of disaccharide malabsorption may also be included in this category as well as the very rare forms involving the monosaccharides glucose and galactose. Symptoms consist of abdominal pain, flatulence and diarrhoea; lactose intolerance and sucrose–isomaltose intolerance have been described. Most cases are secondary to other diseases.

Disorders of amino acid and organic acid metabolism

A wide variety of symptoms and signs are produced by the aminoacidopathies (**452–462**).

452 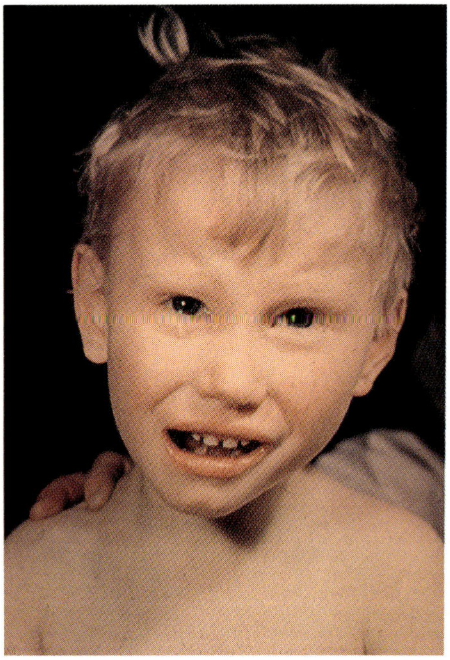

452 Phenylketonuria. This is one of the more common and most studied aminoacidopathies. Several forms have been described but most commonly there is deficiency of liver phenylalanine hydroxylase. Mental retardation is severe in the untreated case. A diet providing not more than between 200 and 500mg phenylalanine per day needs to be given at least for the first 6 years of life and probably longer to ensure full growth and development. Excessive restriction of phenylaline results in protein deficiency.

453 **Maple syrup urine disease.** This is a group of disorders involving metabolism of the branched-chain keto amino acids. Within a few days of birth feeding difficulties, hypertonicity and a shrill cry develop and unless these amino acids are restricted in the diet neurological damage and death will follow. This photomicrograph shows spongy degenerative changes in the globus pallidus.

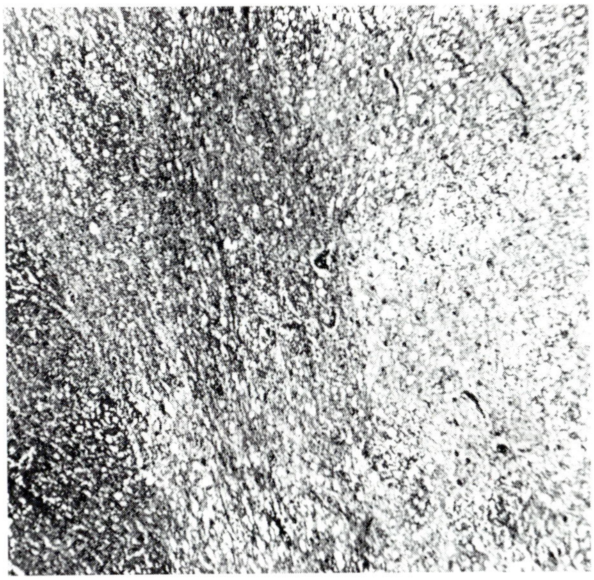

453

454 **Hartnup disease.** This appearance resembling Casal's necklace should suggest the possibility of Hartnup disease. In this aminoacidopathy there is an absorption defect of tryptophan. There is a dermatosis identical to that of pellagra, temporary cerebellar ataxia and a constant aminoaciduria. Nicotinamide (about 100mg daily) results in cure.

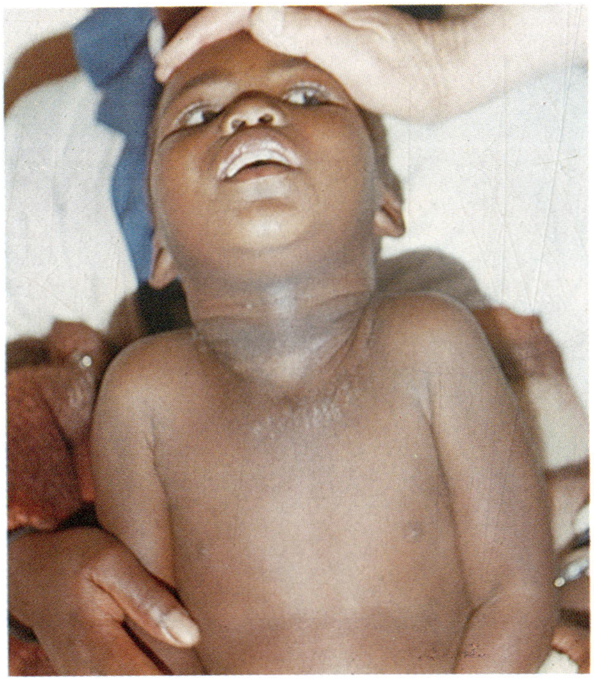

454

455

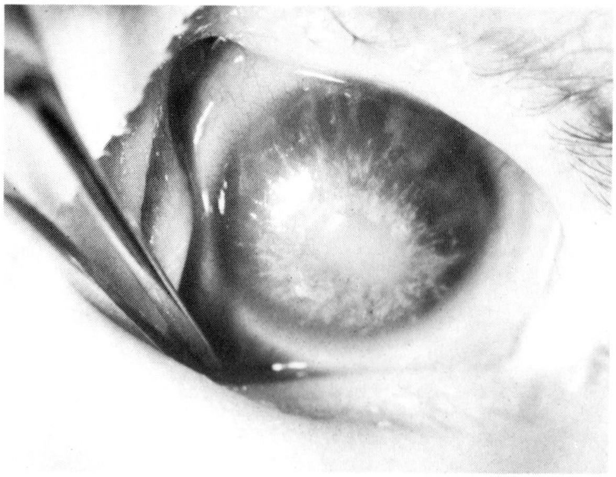

455 Tyrosinaemia (tyrosinosis). Bilateral corneal ulceration is common, together with liver and renal tubular dysfunction. A diet low in phenylalanine and tyrosine may permit normal growth and development.

456

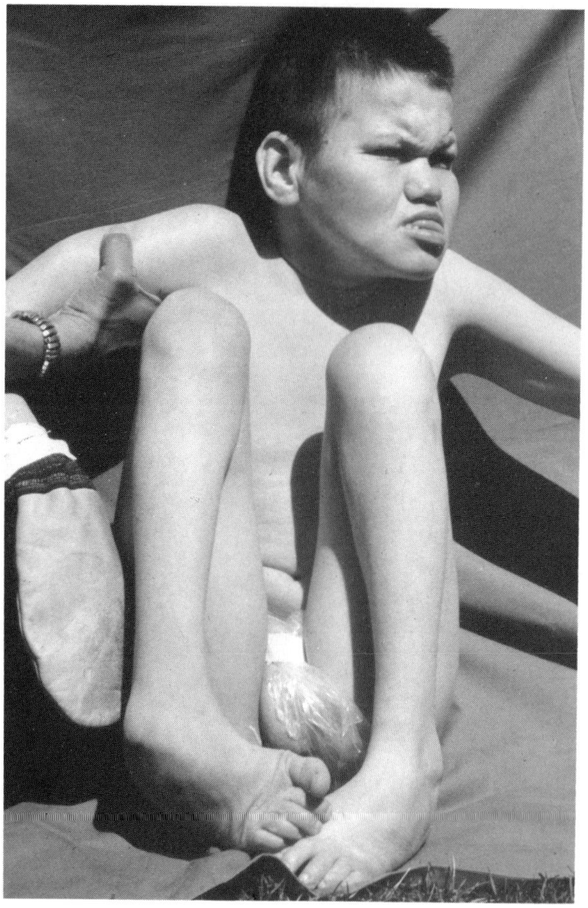

456 Hyperlysinaemia. This rare disorder of lysine metabolism may result in severe mental retardation and a variety of other clinical features. A diet low in lysine as soon as the diagnosis is made is advocated.

457

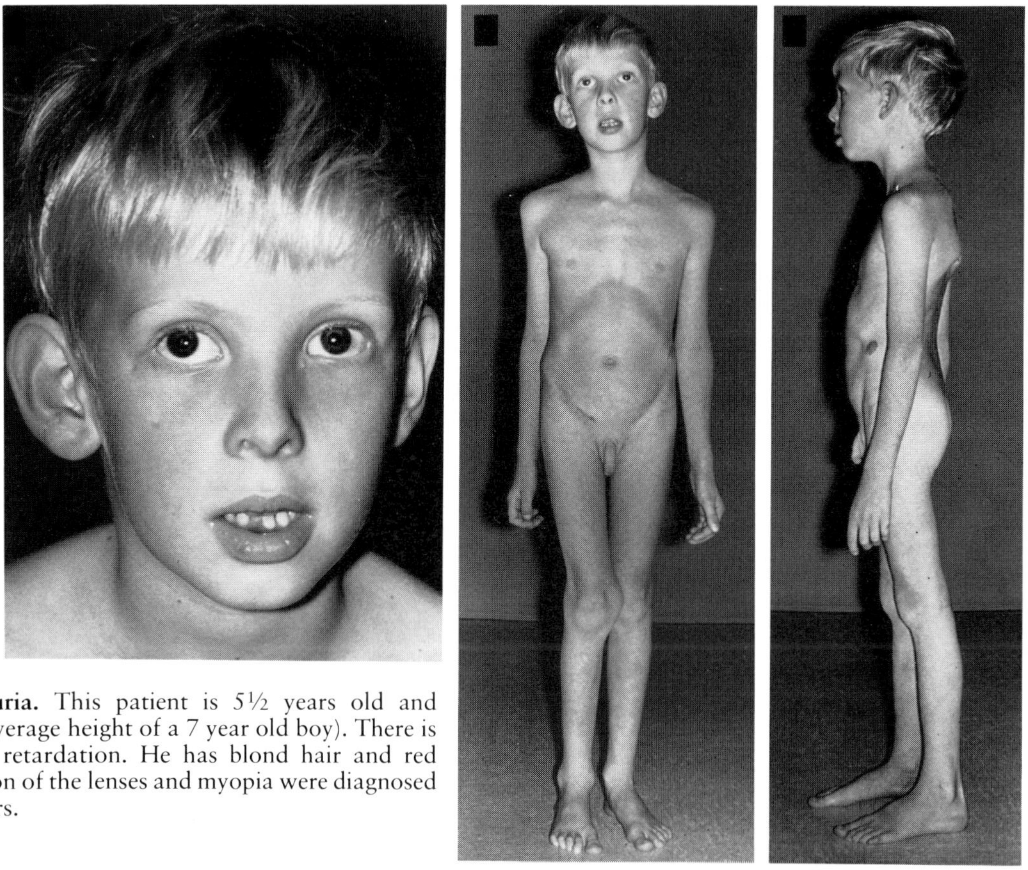

457 Homocystinuria. This patient is 5½ years old and 129 cm tall (the average height of a 7 year old boy). There is moderate mental retardation. He has blond hair and red cheeks. Subluxation of the lenses and myopia were diagnosed at an age of 2 years.

458

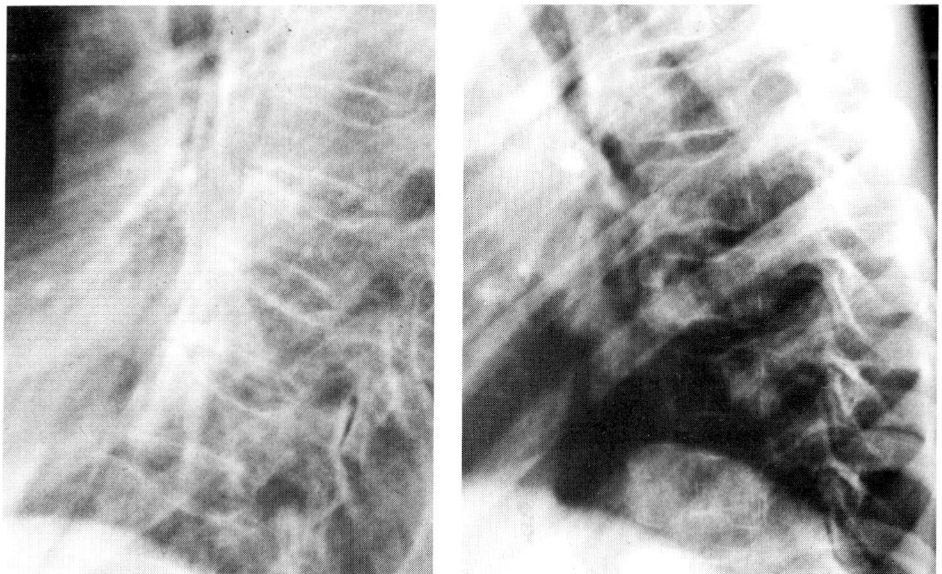

458 Homocystinuria. Cystothionine B-synthase, which facilitates the condensation of homocystine with serine to yield cystathionine, is lacking. Skeletal damage is prominent. Ocular, neurologic and premature atherosclerotic disease also occur. A low protein, low methionine diet is advocated and some patients respond to large doses of vitamin B_6. The X-ray (left) of an 18-year-old girl shows osteoporosis and characteristic biconcavity or 'cod fish' deformity of the vertebrae, seen more markedly in the X-ray (right) of an 11-year-old girl.

459

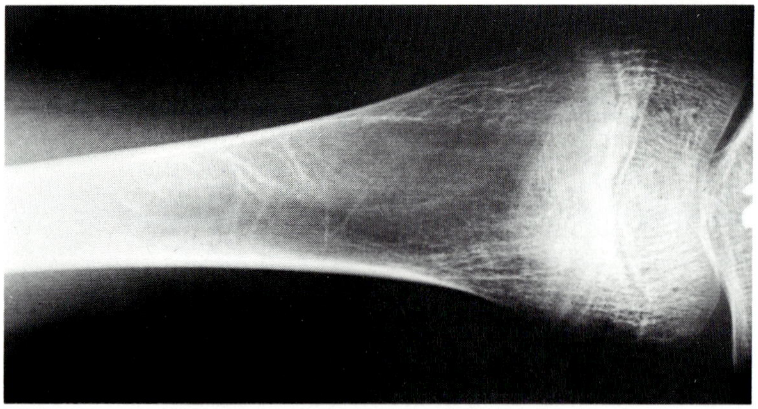

459 Homocystinuria. X-ray of the lower femur and knee shows osteoporosis and widening of the distal metaphysis and epiphysis of the femur.

460

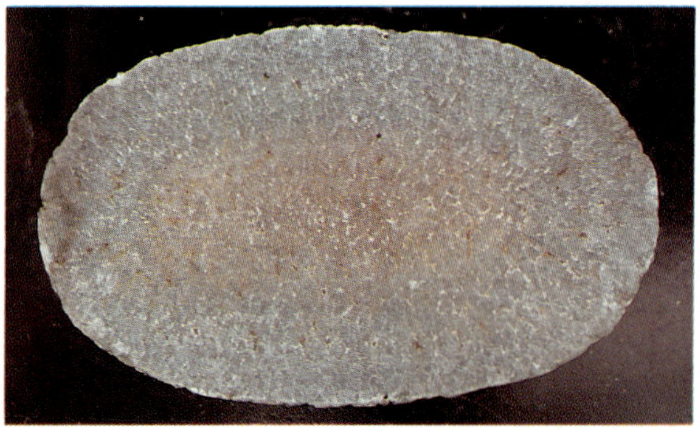

460 Cystine stone. This stone is blue in colour, interspaced with white areas caused by a combination of amino acids. The finding of cystine on the urine screening must always be followed up by an examination of a 24-hour specimem for all amino acids by amino acid chromatography in affected patients; the worst cases are in the homozygous group.

461

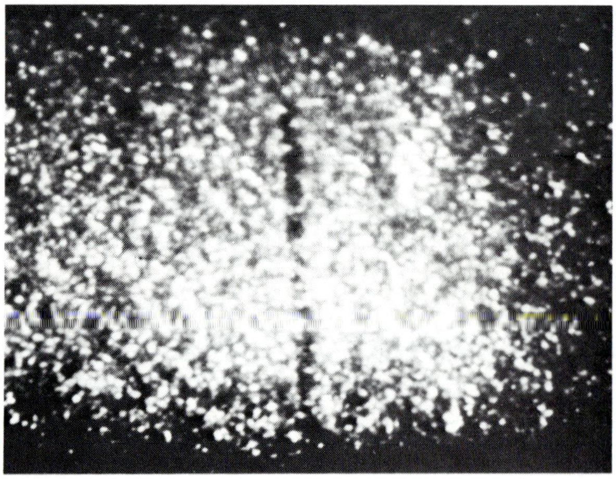

461 Cystinosis. Cystine is deposited in many tissues, shown here in the cornea, and especially as urinary calculi, in this relatively common autosomal recessive disorder. The diet should be relatively low in protein and methionine, but a high fluid intake and alkalinization of the urine are the most important measures.

462 Hyperornithinaemia. Ornithine transaminase is deficient in this rare disorder, and gyrate atrophy of the retina, shown here, is characteristic. Hyperammonaemia occurs, as it does in many disorders affecting urea cycle enzymes, with vomiting, somnolence and convulsions leading to coma and death, or mental retardation and neurological disorders in survivors. Treatment is difficult but dietary protein should be restricted to a minimum necessary to meet amino acid requirements.

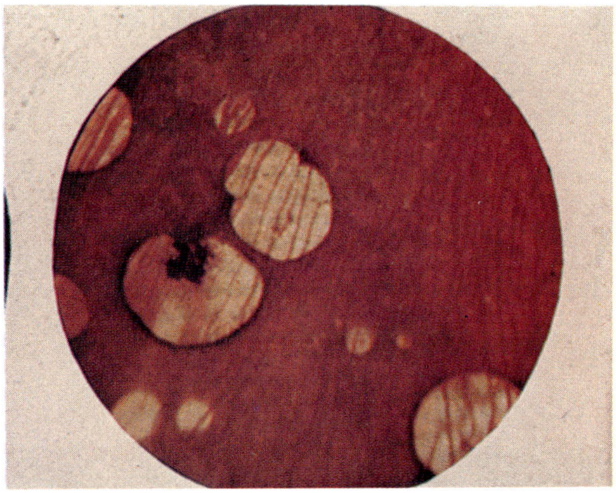

462

Biotin dependency (see *Table 81*) causes organic acidaemias (**463, 464**) which usually respond quite dramatically to large doses of the vitamin.

3

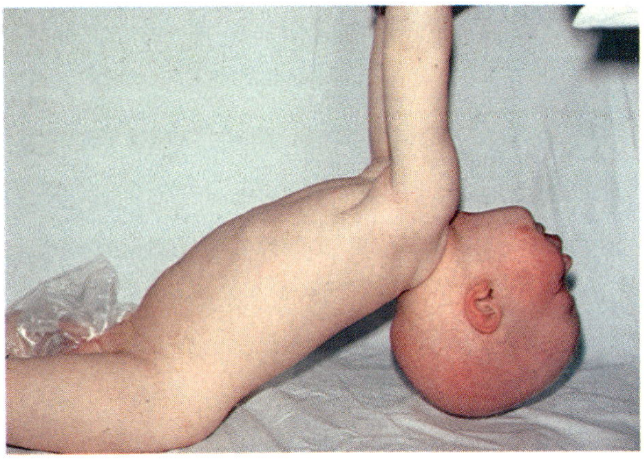

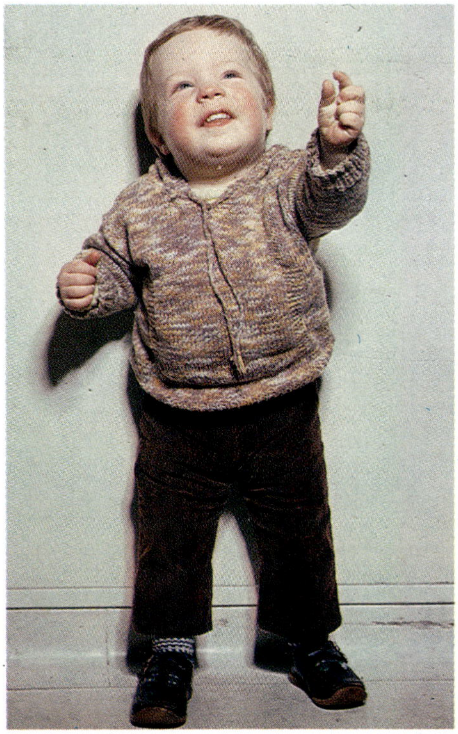

464

463, 464 Biotin dependency. A number of cases have been described in recent years of biotin-responsive disorders. Clinical features have included developmental regression and severe hypotonia, dermatitis, alopecia and defects in T-cell and B-cell immunity. Several cocarboxylase enzymes are affected and this results in increased urinary excretion of organic acids and lactic acidosis. Oral biotin, 5mg twice daily, has proved effective.

This child shows alopecia and lack of head control before treatment. The same child at 14 months of age, after 4 months of biotin therapy, has normal posture and hair growth.

Disorders of porphyrin and haem metabolism

The porphyrias

In this group of disorders the various genes which code for enzymes of haem biosynthesis are abnormal (see *Table 80*). Differential diagnosis depends upon variations in clinical presentation (**465–467**) and characteristic biochemical changes in blood and urine. Treatment differs considerably from disease to disease. The photosensitive skin changes of several of these conditions have been ameliorated by inducing hypercarotenosis (see page 120) with oral B-carotene 15-180mg/day.

In acute intermittent porphyria a high carbohydrate diet has been found to be helpful. Porphyria cutanea tarda responds to removal of iron.

465

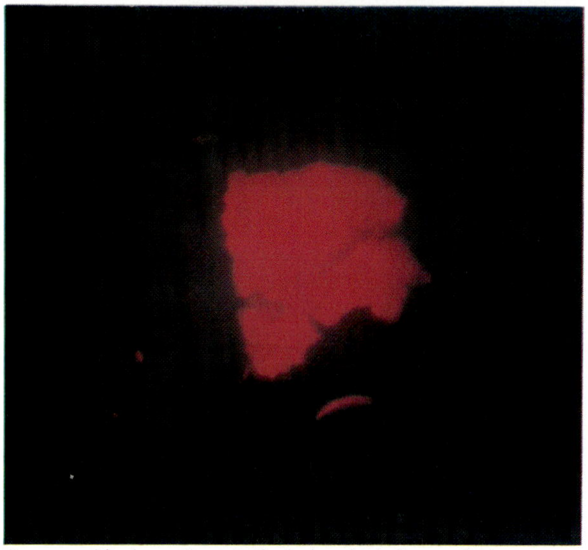

Courtesy of Professor Dame S. Sherlock and J.A. Summerfield.

465 Porphyria cutanea tarda (symptomatic cutaneous hepatic porphyria). Uroporphyrin in a fresh fragment of liver biopsy gives a red fluoresence in ultraviolet light. Light microscopy shows a hepatitis or cirrhosis and iron overload. Symptoms include photosensitivity with blistering and scarring of the skin. Alcoholism is a common association. Urinary uroporphyrin excretion is increased.

466 Porphyria cutanea tarda, face. Scarring and pigmentary changes are present. Hypertrichosis is also common. Suffused eyelids and conjunctivae are frequently seen.

467 Porphyria cutanea tarda, hand. There is often a history of increased skin fragility. Sometimes the only clinical sign of porphyria is the presence of brownish ill-defined macules with minimal atrophy on the backs of the hands. The brown marks are healed erosions or ulcers, produced by minor trauma. Similar lesions are seen in porphyria variegata. The patient may deny aggravation of lesions by exposure to sunlight.

466

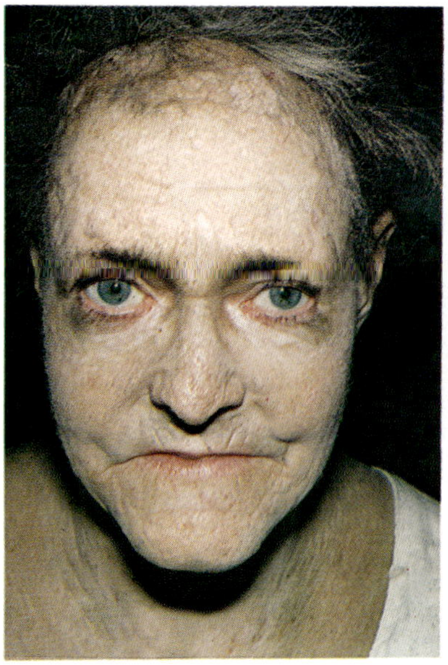

467

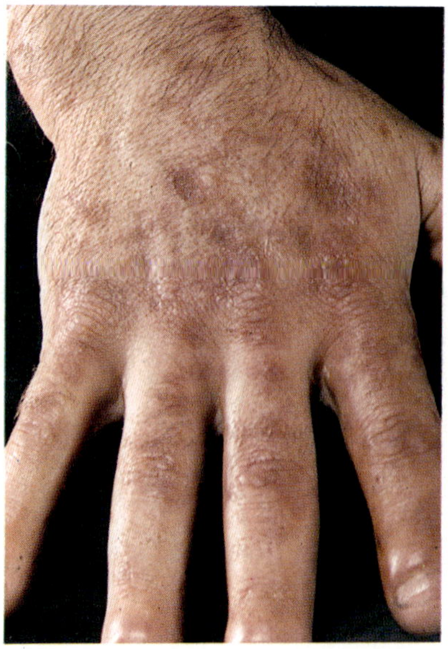

Disorders of purine metabolism

Gout

In some rare variants of the disease enzyme defects have been identified but in the usual form the cause is unknown. Raised blood uric acid is constant, but may be secondary to other diseases. Deposition of crystals of monosodium urate monohydrate in tissues, especially in certain joints, is responsible for the symptoms (**468–471**).

Supportive dietary management is helpful (*Table 85*).

468 Gouty tophus. This comprises a mass of urate crystals in the affected joint, surrounded by an inflammatory response composed of young fibroblasts intermingled with lymphocytes, plasma cells, macrophages and foreign body giant cells. (*H&E*, × 40)

468

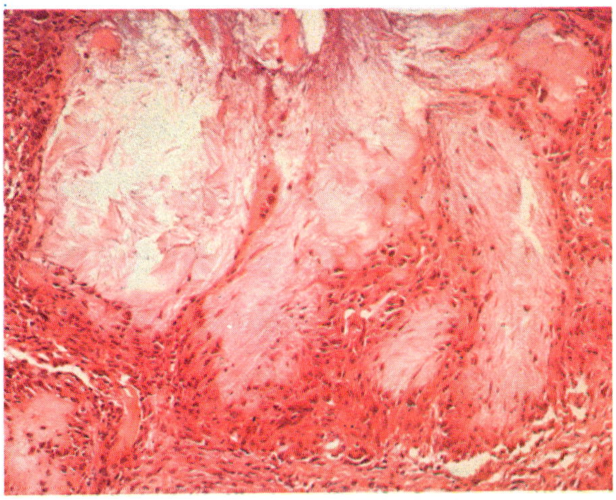

469

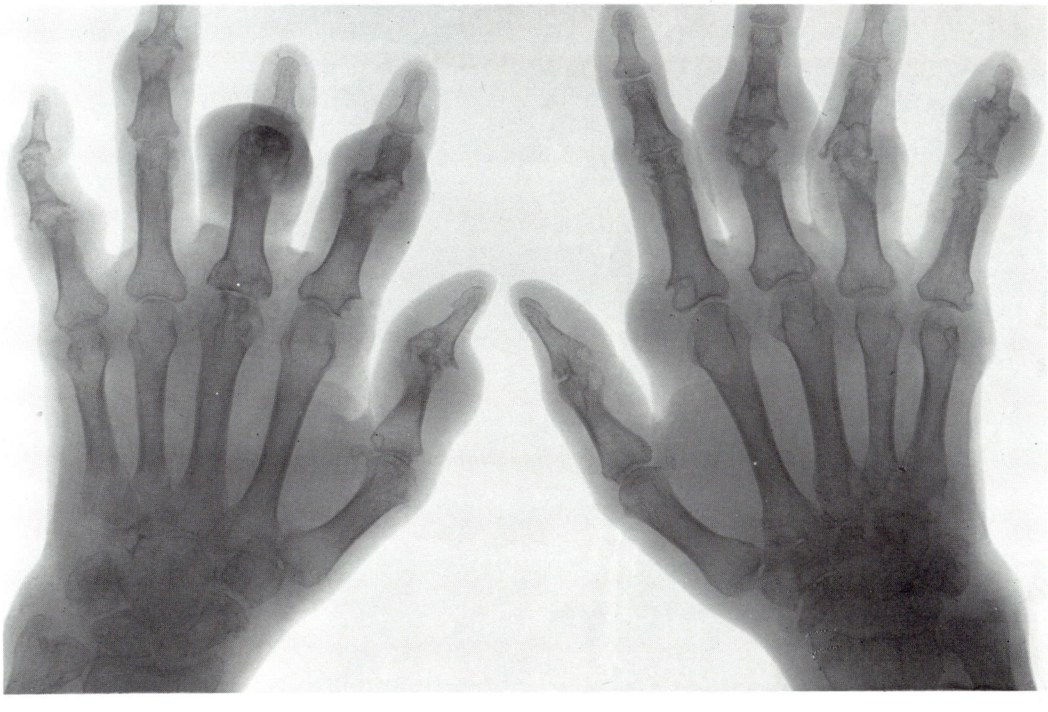

469 Chronic gouty arthritis of the hands. Note the extensive destruction of bone by urate deposits and the large soft tissue tophi.

470 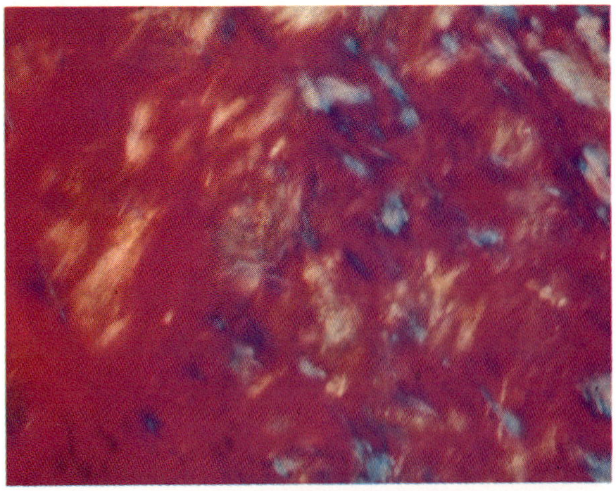

470 Urea crystals in gout. Taken with yellow parallel to the compensator and blue at 90° to the compensator.

471 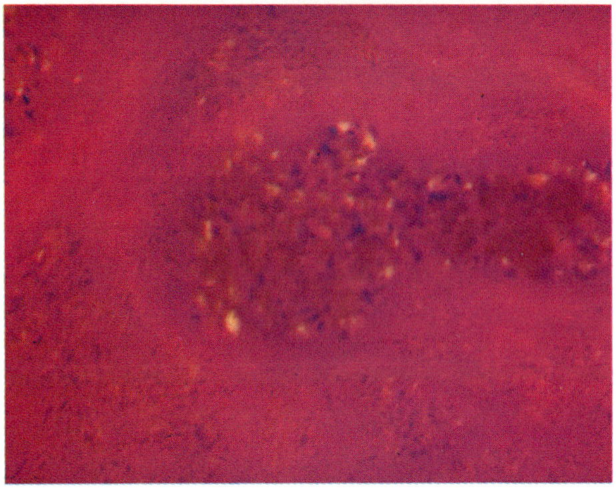

471 Chondrocalcinosis (pseudogout). Calcium pyrophosphate crystals to be distinguished from urate crystals in gout, with weak positive birefringence, taken with blue parallel to the compensator.

Table 85. Dietary management of hyperuricaemia and gout.

Gradual weight reduction towards ideal body weight
Avoidance of excessive alcohol consumption, especially beer
Reduction in intake of high-purine foods (liver, kidney, offal, sea food, peas and beans)
Consumption of a moderate amount of protein (approximately 1g/kg ideal body weight)
Consumption of a moderate amount of fat (< 40% of calories from fat); limitation of saturated fat
Reduction of simple sugars and increase of complex carbohydrate in the diet
Consumption of a liberal amount of non-alcoholic fluids

8. Food Idiosyncrasies

The word idiosyncrasy seems to be the most precise term available to describe the nature of the group of diseases covered in this chapter. It is used in the sense of one dictionary definition – 'a physical constitution peculiar to a person'. This implies that the vast majority of people will not react in this way to food, in strict contrast to the reactions to food toxins which form the subject of Chapter 9 and where the outcome is almost entirely dose-dependent.

To some extent some conditions overlap this chapter and one of the others in this book. For example, all of the diseases in Chapter 7 represent idiosyncratic behaviour to normal dietary items. The group of conditions called eating behaviour disorders could include, in addition to those that are discussed here, anorexia nervosa and bulimia; however, because of the resultant serious undernutrition they are discussed in Chapter 4.

The concept of diet-related diseases being either exogenous or endogenous in origin was developed in Chapter 1. Food idiosyncrasies are clearly endogenous and food toxicoses dealt with in Chapter 9 are exogenous. **472** shows the various categories in which each of these falls.

Food idiosyncrasies can be divided into three categories:

1. **Food allergy** – like other forms of allergy, for this diagnosis to be made there must be evidence of an abnormal immunological reaction to food; for example, increased IgE secretion.
2. **Non-allergic food idiosyncrasies** – there is no evidence of immunological reaction but symptoms and signs are similar to those seen in a true allergy.
3. **Disorders of eating behaviour** which relate to the process of eating, rather than ingredients of food as such, in a psychological rather than a chemical way.

472

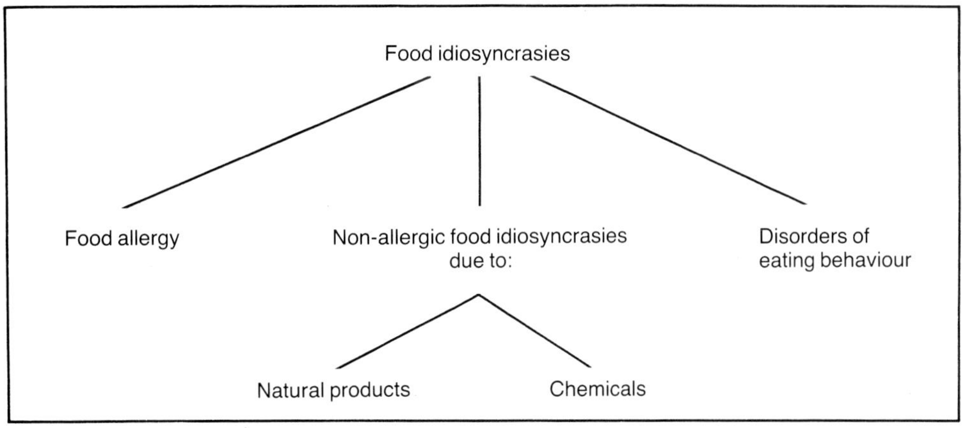

472 Categories of food idiosyncrasies.

Food allergy

Table 86 shows the symptoms and signs that have been commonly attributed to food allergy.

Table 87 lists foods that are most commonly responsible for these allergies. True allergy is much more commonly due to natural foods than to other substances such as food additives (**473–479**).

Table 86. Symptoms and signs associated with food allergy.

Skin
- Dermatitis
- Eczema
- Urticaria
- Angio-oedema

Gastrointestinal system
- Abdominal pain
- Abdominal distension
- Vomiting
- Diarrhoea
- Occult bleeding
- Malabsorption
- Protein-losing enteropathy

Haematological system
- Anaemia
- Eosinophilia
- Thrombocytopenia

Neurological system and behaviour
- Irritability
- Restlessness
- Fatigue
- Depression
- Hyperactivity
- Migraine

Respiratory system
- Sneezing
- Cough
- Rhinorrhoea
- Postnasal discharge
- Croup
- Bronchospasm
- Pneumonitis
- Serous otitis media

Other manifestations
- Anaphylaxis
- Arthritis
- Enuresis
- Sudden infant death syndrome(?)
- Nephrotic syndrome

Table 87. Foods commonly associated with allergic manifestations.

Urticaria, angio-oedema and anaphylaxis
- Egg ovalbumin
- Peanuts
- Cow's milk
- Fish

Gastrointestinal allergy
- Cow's milk
- Egg ovalbumin
- Nuts
- Seafood
- Some fruits
- Soya bean products

Rhinitis and asthma
- Egg
- Nuts
- Fish
- Chocolate
- Tartrazine, benzoates

Eczema
- Egg
- Cow's milk
- Wheat
- Colourings, preservatives

Migraine
- Cheese
- Tomatoes
- Chocolate
- Cow's milk
- Egg
- Orange
- Wheat
- Tartrazine, benzoates

473

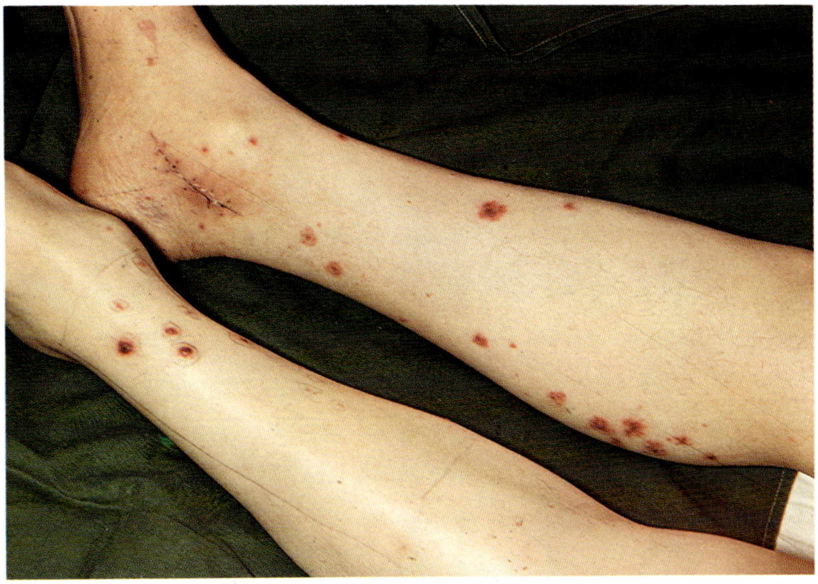

473 Purpura, cutaneous vasculitis, legs. There is damage to superficial blood vessels with small infarcts of the skin. Lesions come usually in crops, which may be recurrent, mostly on the legs and feet. Acute vasculitis associated with gut, renal, joint and other lesions is called 'Henoch–Schönlein purpura'. It is often associated with infections or drugs and occasionally due to food allergy.

474

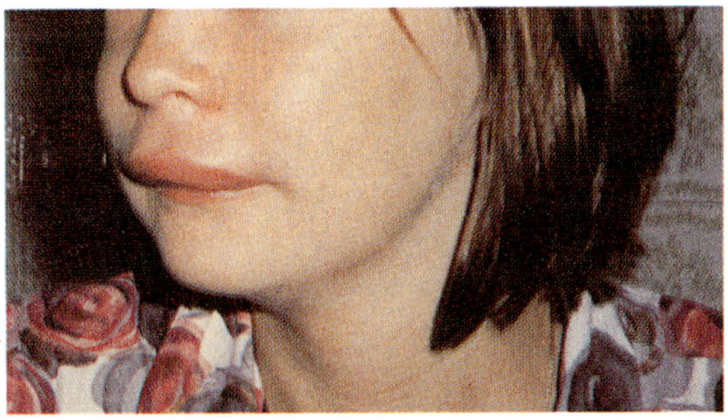

474 Angio-oedema resulting from tartrazine sensitivity. This girl had recurrent, severe angio-oedema and urticaria, with episodes of life-threatening laryngeal oedema. An exclusion diet showed tartrazine (E102) to be the cause of her symptoms. The food colouring is widely used in many processed foods and drinks, so a rigorous maintenance exclusion diet is required to prevent symptoms. The mechanism of tartrazine sensitivity is unclear, and it may not have an allergic basis. Cross sensitivity with other azo dyes and with aspirin is common.

475

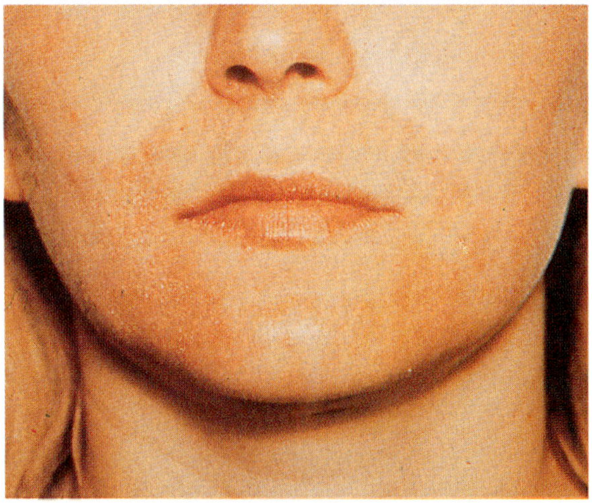

475 Eczema resulting from orange drink. The patient suspected the cause, and the perioral distribution of the lesions suggested a contact or ingested cause. An exclusion diet showed the cause to be the food-colouring azo dyes tartrazine (E102) and sunset yellow (E110), and not the orange juice itself (but note that citrus fruits are among the commoner causes of food-related symptoms).

476

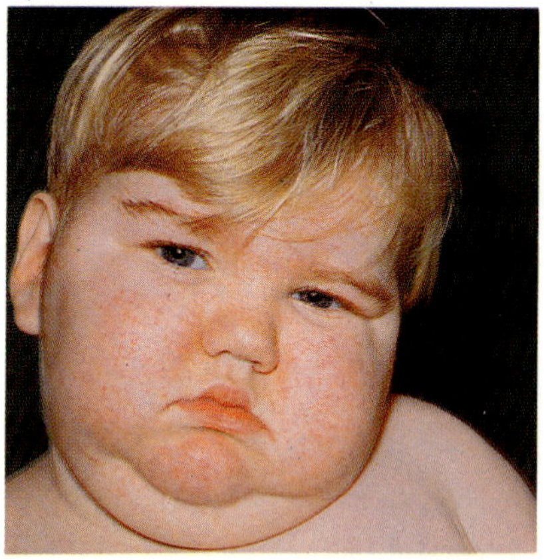

477

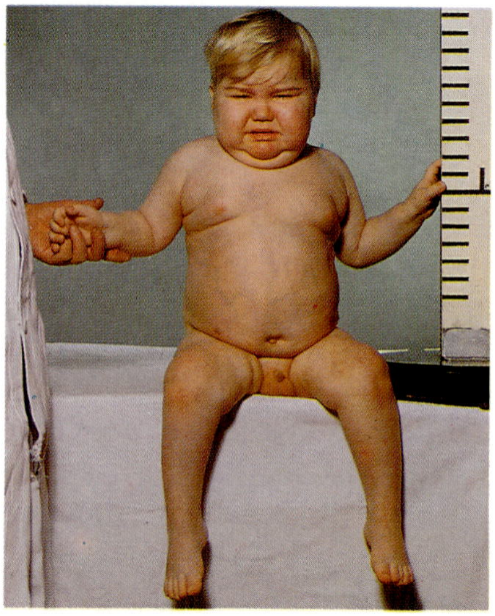

476, 477 Nephrotic syndrome in a 2.5-year-old boy. His severe facial and body oedema resulted from his gross proteinuria and hypoproteinaemia. Renal biopsy showed minimal change glomerulonephritis and he was treated with steroids to good effect, ultimately going into complete remission. Occasionally food allergy is responsible, especially cow's milk or eggs.

478

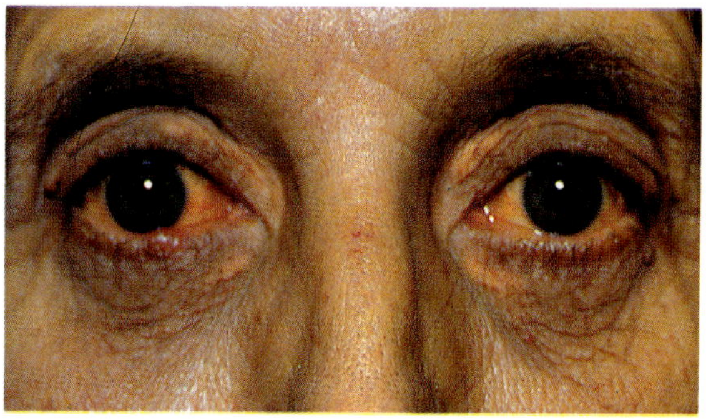

479

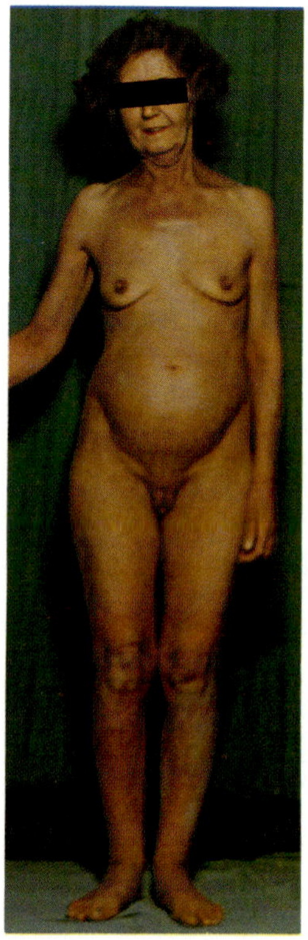

478, 479 Primary biliary cirrhosis. This 55-year-old woman presented originally with severe pruritus, and jaundice developed slowly over the next 3 years. The cause is unknown, allergy is a possible factor.

Non-allergic food idiosyncrasies

The symptomatology does not differ from that of true allergy. *Table 88* gives a selection of some of the most commonly implicated natural products and chemicals involved.

In either of these states the nutrition of the young child may be adversely affected through one or more of the mechanisms shown in *Table 89*.

Table 88. Well-documented examples of substances responsible for non-allergic food idiosyncrasies.

Natural products	*Chemicals*
Lactose	Sulphites
Sucrose	Nitrites
Galactose	Nitrates
Gluten	Monosodium glutamate
Broad beans (favism)	Tartrazine dyes
Lathyrus peas (lathyrism)	Benzoic acid
Caffeine	Oxalates
Theobromine	Heavy metals:
Histamine	mercury, lead
Tyramine	arsenic, copper
Tryptamine	Aspartame
Serotonin	Butylated hydroxytoluene
Phenylethylamine	Butylated hydroxyanisole
Solamine	

Table 89. Factors contributing to poor growth in children with allergic diseases.

Reduced dietary intake:	due to anorexia and vomiting with severe wheezing
Increased losses:	severe exudative eczema
Impaired utilization:	hypoxia in severe asthma; inflammation with eczema
Increased requirements:	extra respiratory work in asthma; increased cell turnover in eczema and continuous scratching

Coeliac disease (gluten-induced enteropathy)

This is due to an idiosyncrasy to the gliadin fraction of gluten, a cereal protein found in wheat and rye and to a lesser extent in barley and oats. Total exclusion of gluten from the diet results in cure. The disease is familial but there is no single genetic marker.

Clinical manifestations vary to some extent, depending upon the time of presentation (*Table 90*).

The untreated case can develop severe malnutrition from which recovery is rapid once the diagnosis has been made. The similarity to the marasmic form of PEM (see **119, 120**) should be noted. This illustrates the fact that endogenous and exogenous malnutrition do not differ in clinical presentation (**480, 481**).

Table 90. Clinical manifestations of coeliac disease.

Usual presentation	*Early presentation*	*Later presentations*
(9–18 months)	(1–2 months)	(i) (About 2–8 years)
Weight loss	Vomiting	Short stature
Poor appetite	Fluid diarrhoea	Iron-resistant anaemia
Stools – soft, pale, offensive, frequent	Acute weight loss	Rickets
Irritability	Abdominal distention	Behavioural problems
Abdominal distension	Irritability	(ii) (In adult at any age)
Muscle wasting		Earlier in women due to heightened clinical suspicion with anaemia in pregnancy and amenorrhoea in young women.
Hypotonia		Permanent-tooth enamel defects in all four sections of dentition; due to gluten
Retarded motor development		
Hypochromic anaemia		
Occasional constipation		
Occasional excessive vomits		

480

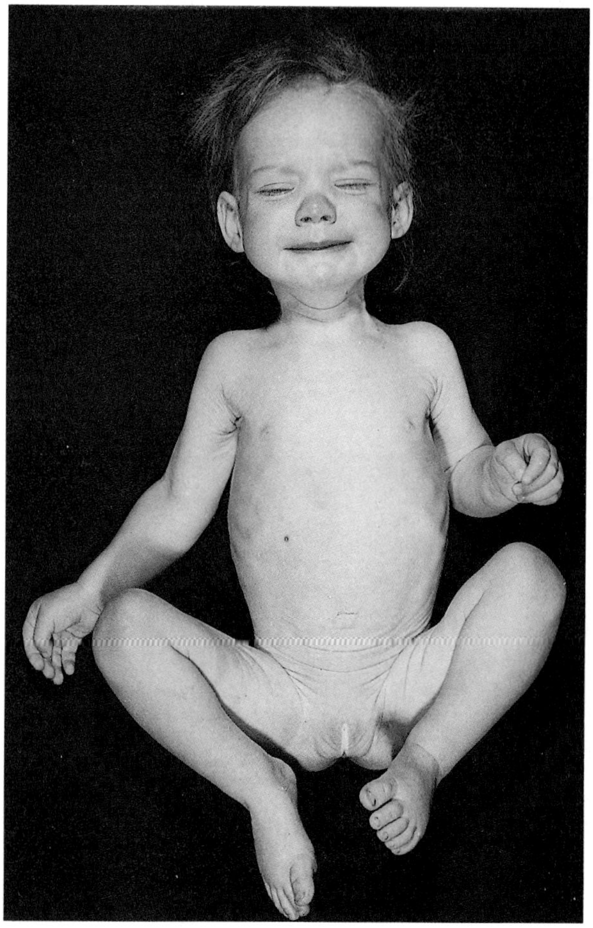

4

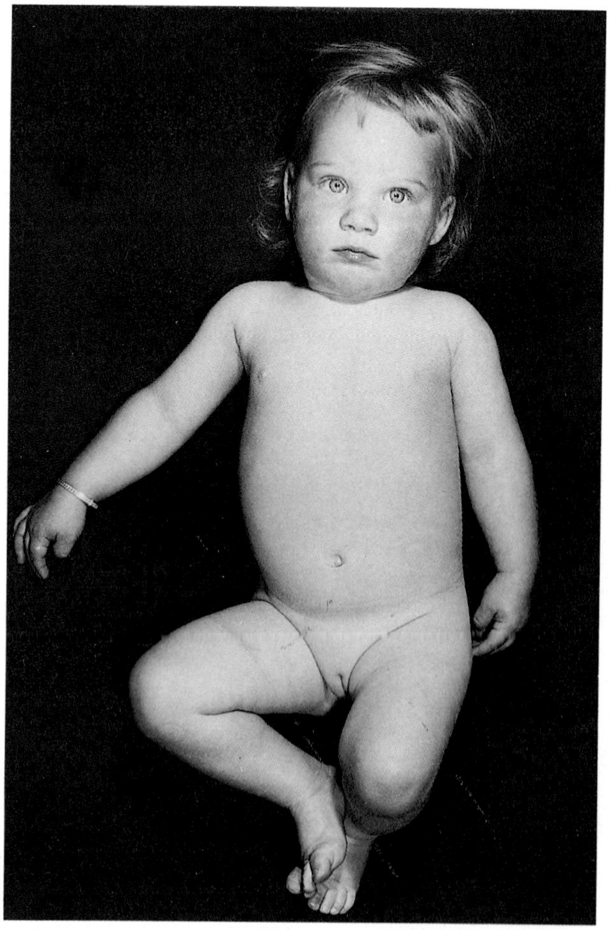

480 Patient with coeliac disease.

481 Same patient after a gluten-free diet for 3 months.

The changes revealed by intestinal biopsy (**482**) are not pathognomonic but the rapid return to normal on withdrawal of gluten is. Less importance is now given to the need for gluten challenge.

Eczema (**483**) and dermatitis herpetiformis (**484–486**) frequently accompany the bowel changes and also respond to treatment.

482 Coeliac disease. The jejunal biopsy of this adult case shows virtual absence of villi, long hyperplastic crypts of Lieberkuhn, abnormal cuboidal epithelial cells with an excess of lymphoid cells in the lamina propria; predominantly plasma cells, but lymphocytes, macrophages, eosinophils and mast cells are also present. (*H&E*, × 25)

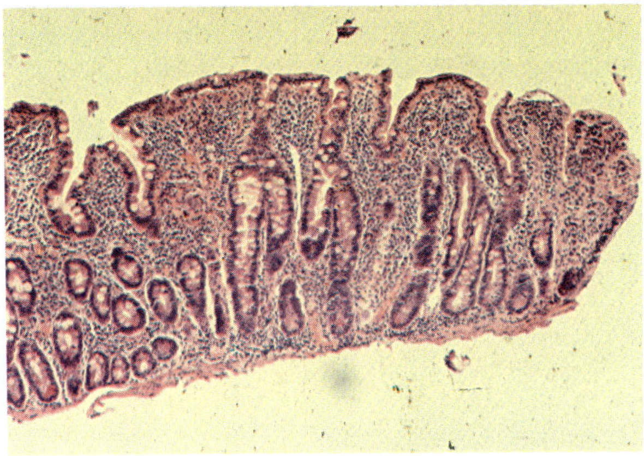

482

483 Eczema due to malabsorption. The patient had patchy eczema and hyperpigmentation associated with steatorrhoea. Lesions show no specific features and the association with malabsorption is not common. The eruption cleared after the patient started a gluten-free diet.

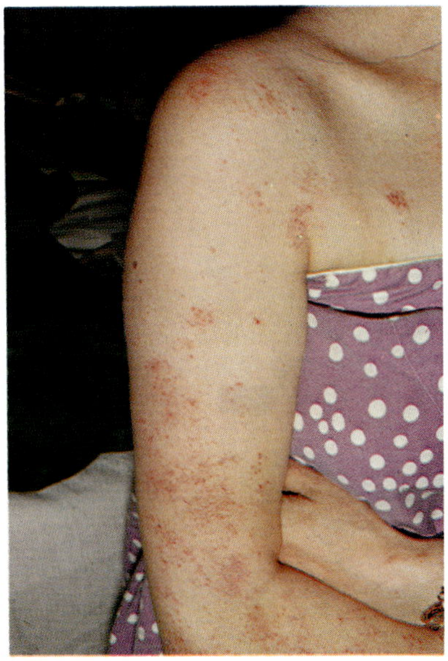

483

484

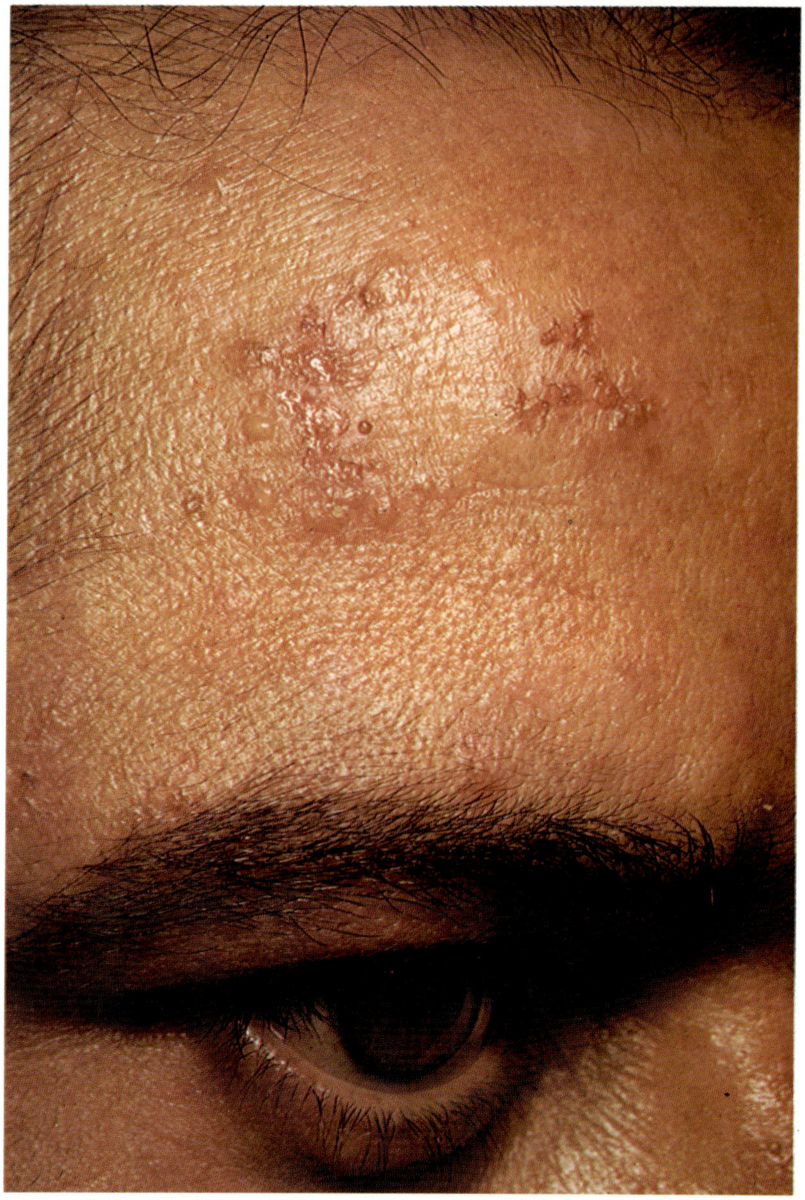

484 Dermatitis herpetiformis, forehead. Clusters of small, intensely pruritic blisters occur on the scalp, face, shoulders, lumbosacral area, the points of the elbows and the fronts of the knees. The disease may start as a 'toxic' erythema which can persist for weeks or months before blisters are seen. About two-thirds of cases have small bowel changes resembling gluten enteropathy and in these a malabsorption syndrome may be present.

485

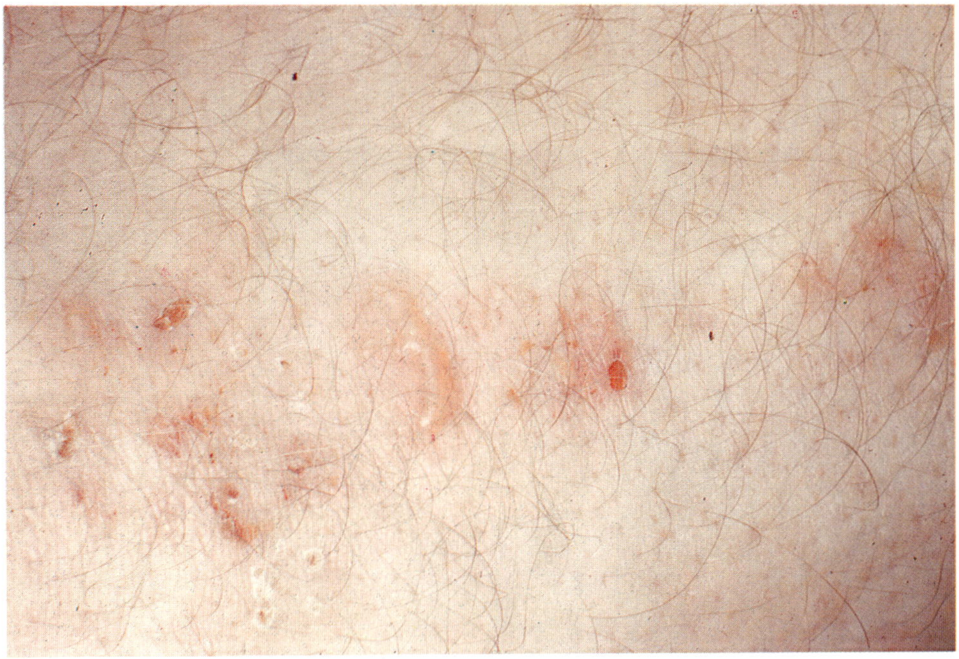

485 Dermatitis herpetiformis. This skin eruption is characterized by intensely itchy papular or vesicular lesions that lie on an urticarial or erythematous base. The elbows, knees, sacrum and shoulders are the most commonly affected sites. About 20% of patients with dermatitis herpetiformis have coeliac disease. The presence of both disorders in the same patient is linked genetically with the presence of human leucocyte antigens B8 and DR3. Sometimes patients with dermatitis herpetiformis have no symptoms to suggest coeliac disease, but are found to have mild or moderate jejunal mucosal abnormalities. Treatment with a gluten-free diet may ameliorate the skin condition.

486

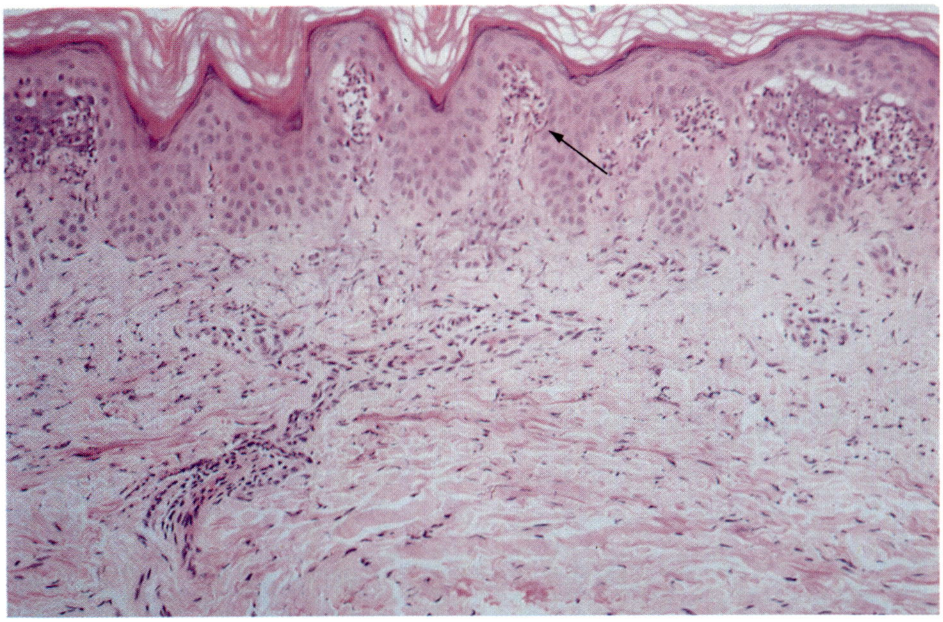

486 Dermatitis herpetiformis. Photomicrograph of a section of skin from a patient with dermatitis herpetiformis in association with coeliac disease. This is an early lesion with four separate micro-abscesses located at the tips of the dermal papillae (*arrowed*). In later lesions the micro-abscesses coalesce so that a bulla is formed with a plane of separation at the dermo-epidermal junction.

Adult coeliac disease, or non-tropical sprue (**487–489**) may elude diagnosis for years.

487

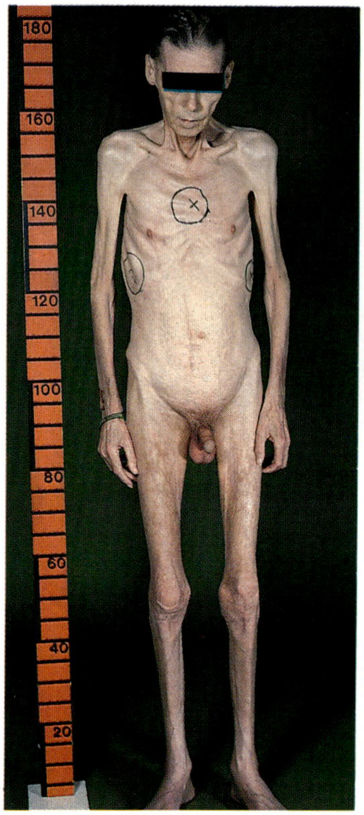

488

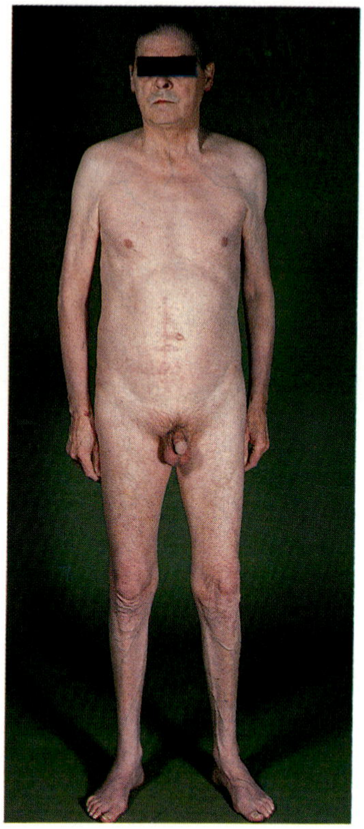

487, 488 Coeliac disease. This disease is the most common and most important cause of malabsorption in the West. It is characterized by partial or subtotal jejunal villous atrophy which improves morphologically when treated with a gluten-free diet, and which deteriorates again on reintroduction of gluten. This patient presented with combined iron and folic acid deficiency and severe emaciation. After 4 months' treatment with a gluten-free diet he had gained 23 kg in weight and his anaemia had resolved.

489

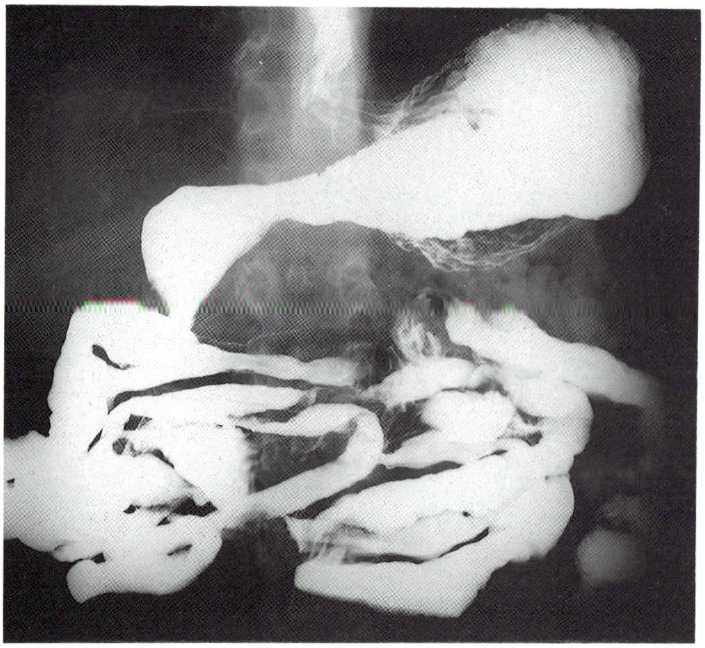

489 Coeliac disease. The small bowel meal X-ray is usually abnormal in coeliac disease. The mucosa becomes featureless and tubular, and the normal fine feathery appearance of the mucosa is lost. There may be flocculation of barium. These small bowel meal appearances are entirely non-specific, but they may suggest or confirm a clinical suspicion of malabsorption.

Disaccharide intolerance

This is a group of food idiosyncrasies in which intestinal enzymes for splitting disaccharide sugars to monosaccharides are either congenitally, or secondarily to disease. *Table 91* lists the main syndromes with their treatment.

Disaccharide intolerance secondary to other diseases (*Table 92*) recovers slowly once the underlying condition responds to treatment.

Table 93 shows the major and minor criteria for making a diagnosis.

Table 91. Sugar malabsorption syndromes and their treatment.

Malabsorption syndrome	*Cause*	*Dietary treatment*
Disaccharides		
Sucrose isomaltose	Congenital	Sucrose-free
Lactose	Congenital, Acquired, Secondary	Lactose-free
All disaccharides	Secondary	Starch, sucrose, and lactose-free
Monosaccharides		
Glucose, galactose	Congenital	Fructose only
All monosaccharides	Secondary	Parenteral feeding

Table 92. Causes of secondary disaccharide intolerance.

Low birthweight
Phototherapy
PEM
Immunologic deficiencies
Intestinal operations in infants
Intestinal infections and infestations, especially in infants
Infective hepatitis
Non-specific diarrhoea
Cystic fibrosis
Coeliac disease
Inflammatory bowel disease
Neomycin and other poorly absorbed antibiotics

Table 93. Criteria for the diagnosis of disaccharidase deficiency.

Major criteria
Symptoms produced by offending disaccharide (by history or during tolerance test)
Symptoms improved by removal of disaccharide
Abnormal disaccharide tolerance test
Low level of enzyme in mucosal biopsy
Minor criteria
Low faecal pH
Increased lactic acid in faeces
Small bowel X-ray (barium plus offending disaccharide) – malabsorption pattern

Disorders of eating behaviour

In recent years several periodic disorders of this nature have been identified.[89] They share a number of features but differ mainly in relation to the length of their periodicity. They are: seasonal affective disorder (SAD); carbohydrate craving obesity (CCO); and premenstrual syndrome (PMS). The shared symptoms include: depression, lethargy, inability to concentrate, episodic bouts of overeating and excessive weight gain.

CCO comes on in the late afternoon or early evening; PMS is monthly; and SAD occurs on an annual basis in the autumn or winter. Biochemical disturbances have been detected in two systems, both of which are known to be involved in photoperiodism: melatonin which affects mood and subjective energy levels, and serotonin, involved in the regulation of appetite for carbohydrate-rich foods.

9. Food Toxicoses

A classification scheme of food toxicoses is shown in **490**. This division is based on the source of the toxicant concerned. Natural foodborne toxicoses are caused by toxins that are normally present in the food but which reach toxic levels because something has gone wrong during processing. The chemical contaminants are substances that are not normally present in the food but also may reach toxic levels as the result of some breakdown in food processing. Food additives have been added to food intentionally and while in the vast majority of cases this appears to be fully justified and the results are beneficial there have been instances of harm resulting and permission for the additive to be used has been withdrawn. Occasionally additives may be responsible for allergic or other idiosyncratic reactions (see Chapter 8).

490

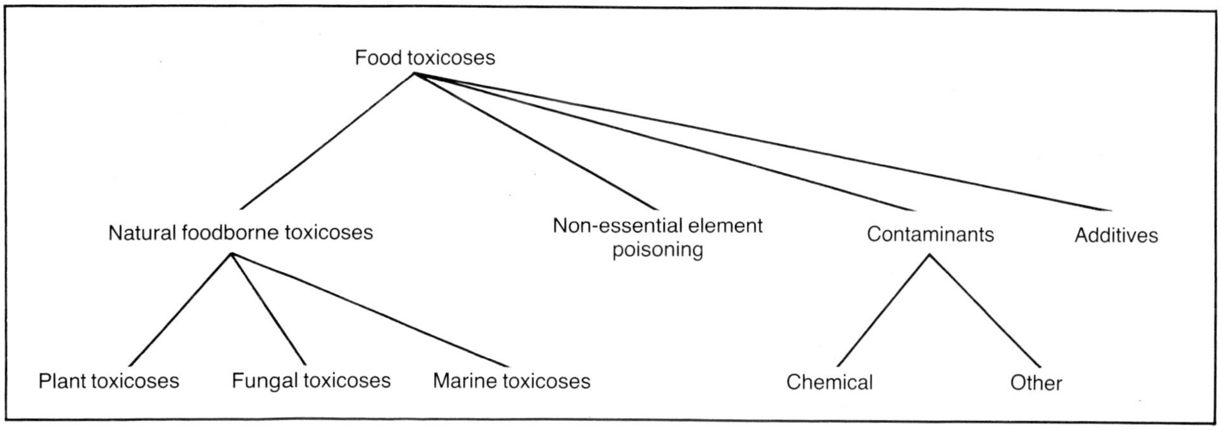

490 Classification of food toxicoses.

Plant toxicoses

The toxic effects of ethanol, both acute and chronic, can be considered under this heading as conveniently as anywhere as all forms of alcohol are plant derived. It does differ from all other forms of toxicosis in that it has a nutrient component, providing 7 kcal/g. When consumed chronically in excessive amounts this may contribute to thiamin deficiency (page 140) and also to obesity (page 90).

Chronic alcoholism causes damage to many systems in the body (*Table 94*).

Table 94. Systemic involvement in chronic alcoholism.

System	*Manifestations*
Gastrointestinal	Anorexia leading to weight loss Liver – hepatitis, fatty infiltration, cirrhosis, haemochromatosis, failure Pancreatitis and insufficiency, impaired glucose tolerance, malabsorption, especially of fat
Haemopoietic	Folate deficiency anaemia, macrocytosis (independent of folic acid)
Cardiovascular	Cardiomyopathy, dysrhythmias, hypertension, heart failure (wet beriberi)
Nervous	Wernicke's encephalopathy, Korsakoff psychosis, peripheral neuropathy (all thiamin deficiency-related), dementia
Fetus	Deformities of fetal alcohol syndrome

Fatty infiltration of the liver (**491, 492**) and later micronodular cirrhosis (**493**) are commonly seen.

A close association is seen to exist between the number of deaths due to cirrhosis of the liver per 100,000 people in a country and the number of litres of alcohol consumed per head per year.

491

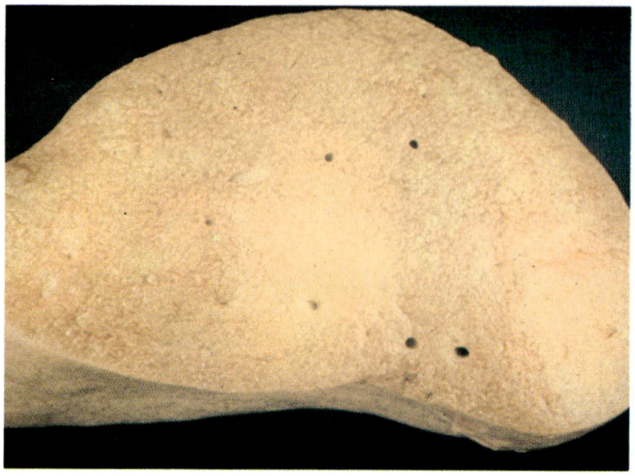

491 Alcoholic fatty liver. The liver is enlarged, smooth, yellowish in colour and obviously fatty. The hepatocytes around the central vein become filled with small vacuoles of triglyceride and appear paler than the surrounding hepatic parenchyma. Inflammatory cells surround the area of fatty deposition. The weight of evidence suggests that ethanol is a direct hepatotoxin, although in many patients chronic nutritional deficiency probably contributes.

492

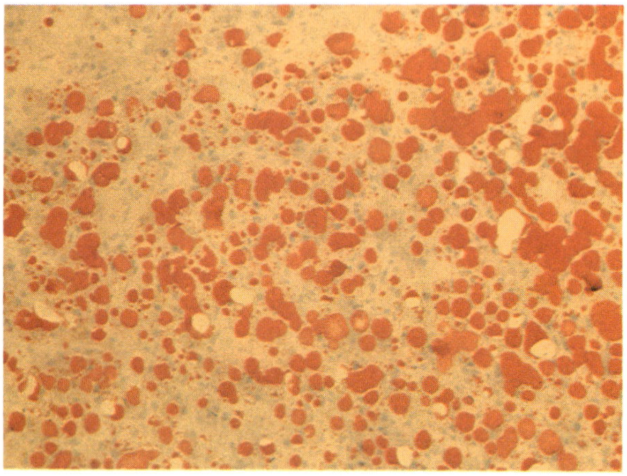

492 Fatty infiltration of the liver. In this section from an alcoholic patient the fat is stained by Sudan red.

493

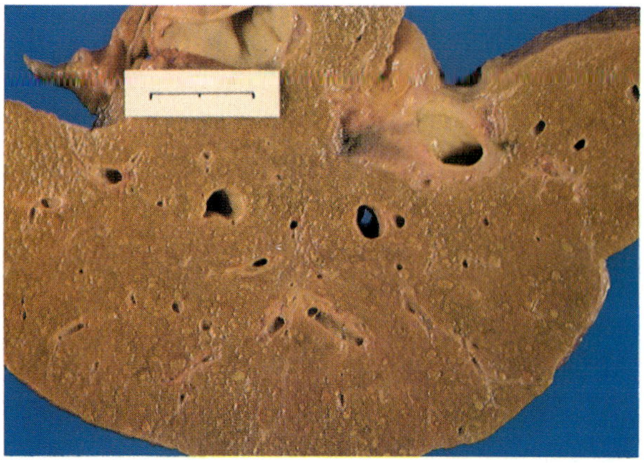

493 Alcoholic micronodular cirrhosis. This is the form of cirrhosis most characteristic of alcoholism. As the lesion evolves the liver decreases in size and becomes progressively nodular to produce a 'hob nail' pattern. It is yellow-orange in colour and diffusely scarred, beginning about the portal areas and eventually extending to interconnect adjacent portal triads.

In recent years there has been increased reporting of damage to the fetus resulting from heavy consumption of alcohol during pregnancy by the mother. This rise is related to the increase in the proportion of women drinking (**494–496**).

494

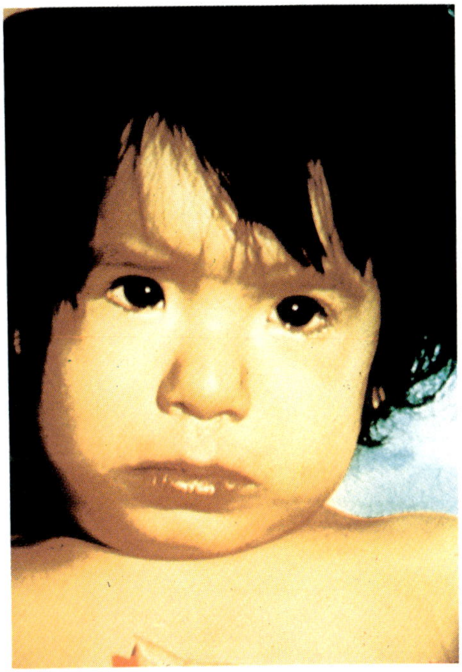

494 Fetal alcohol sydrome. Abnormality of the palpebral fissures, shown here, is characteristic of this syndrome first described in 1973 in the offspring of chronic alcoholic mothers.

In addition cranio-facial, limb and cardiovascular defects have been reported and there is prenatal-onset growth deficiency and developmental delay.

495

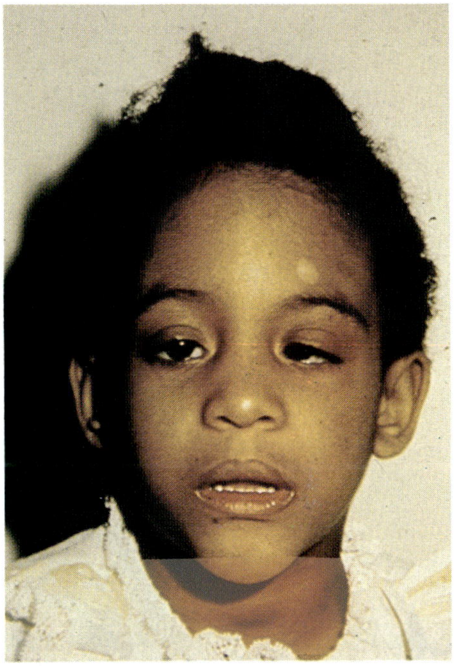

495 Fetal alcohol syndrome. A child 3 years and 9 months old with strabismus and asymmetric ptosis.

496

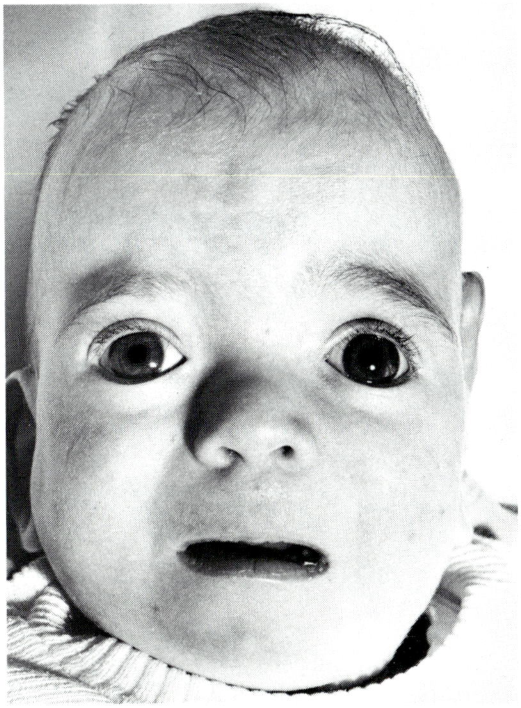

496 Fetal alcohol syndrome. This 6-month-old female shows several characteristic signs: hypertelorism, strabismus, small nose, long upper lip with narrow vermilion border.

Peripheral neuropathy especially affecting the lower limbs is not uncommon in undernourished alcoholics (**497**).

Cerebellar cortical degeneration and pontine myelinolysis (**498, 499**) cause a dementia which is largely due to chronic alcoholism *per se* but an element of nutritional deficiency is usually also present.

497

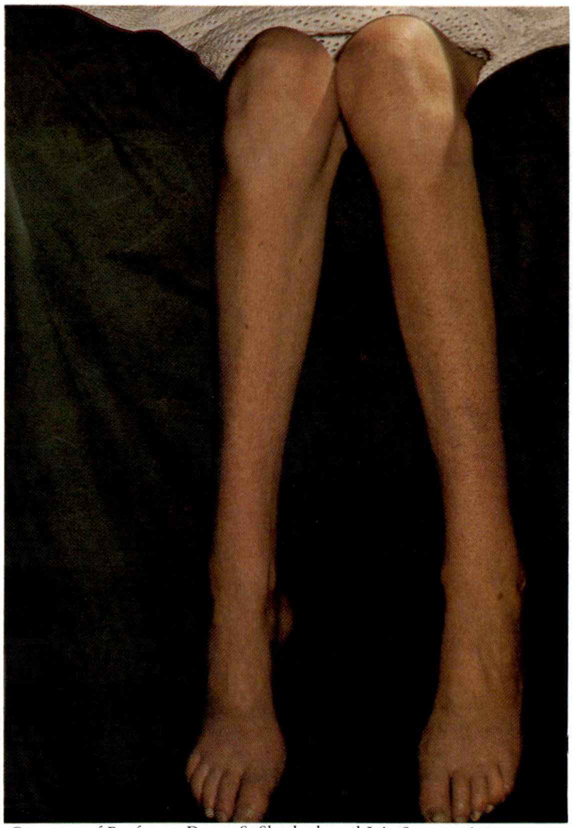

Courtesy of Professor Dame S. Sherlock and J.A. Summerfield.

497 Alcoholic neuropathy occasionally develops in poorly nourished alcoholics. Paraesthesiae, impaired pin prick and light touch sensation and absent ankle jerks are early signs of this peripheral neuropathy. In severe cases, such as this woman, gross muscle wasting results. The calf muscles are especially wasted.

498

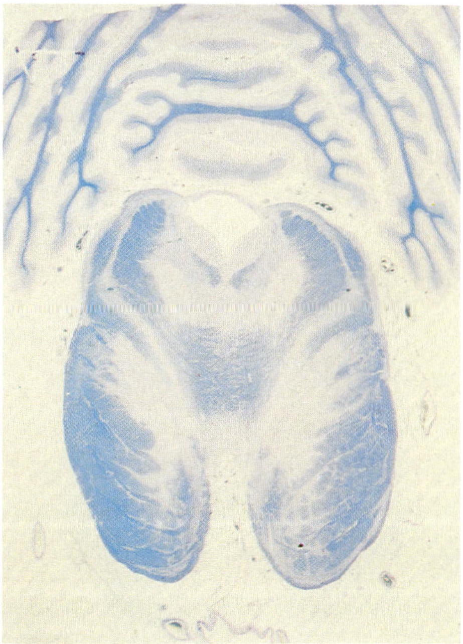

49

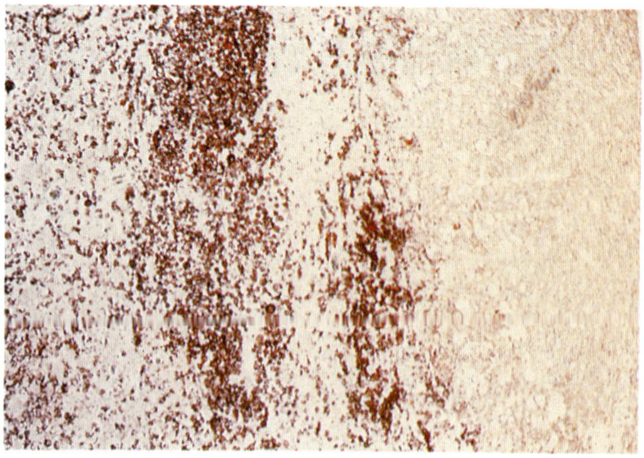

498 Central pontine myelinoclasis; degenerative changes in posterior midbrain. (*Luxol fast blue*, × 2).

499 Central pontine myelinoclasis. Sudanophilic myelin breakdown products (esterified cholesterol) within macrophages in an active case of CPM. (*Oil Red O*, × 80).

Jamaican vomiting sickness is due to poisoning with the ackee fruit (**500**). Herbal teas have been responsible for *Datura* poisoning (**501**). Comfrey herb and comfrey herbal tea are consumed by the public, in the false belief that because they are 'natural' they are safe to use for a host of conditions. They contain hepatoxic pyrrolizidine alkaloids and prolonged use has caused veno-occlusive disease (Budd–Chiari syndrome) (**502**).

500 **Jamaican vomiting sickness.** Consumption of ackee nut produces a severe, often fatal, form of hpoglycaemia. Although the fruit is widely distributed in the tropics, most cases have been reported from the Caribbean. The toxic compound is a breakdown product of hypoglycin in the nut. It blocks the access of long chain fatty acids to carnitine, necessary to, their transport into mitochondria for oxidation. It also blocks the participation of pyruvate in gluconeogenesis. As these two sources of energy are blocked glycogen stores are rapidly depleted, and severe hypoglycaemia ensues.

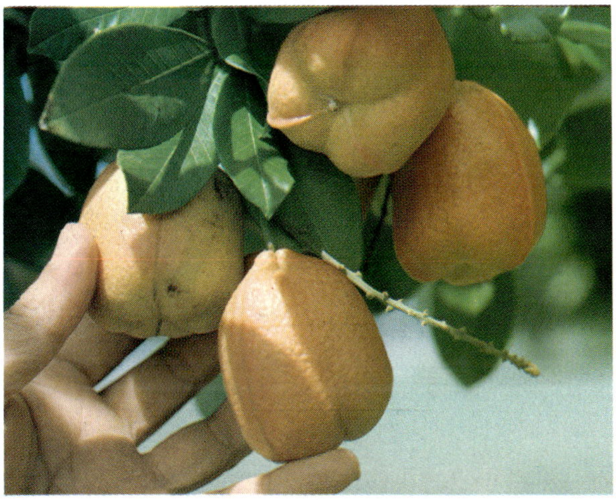

500

501 **The tonga plant, *Datura sanginea*.** Six cases were reported from Cornwall recently from eating the leaves or brewing a tea. The principle alkaloids are hyoscine, atropine and hyoscyamine. Visual hallucinations occur. Gastric lavage and sedation lead to recovery.

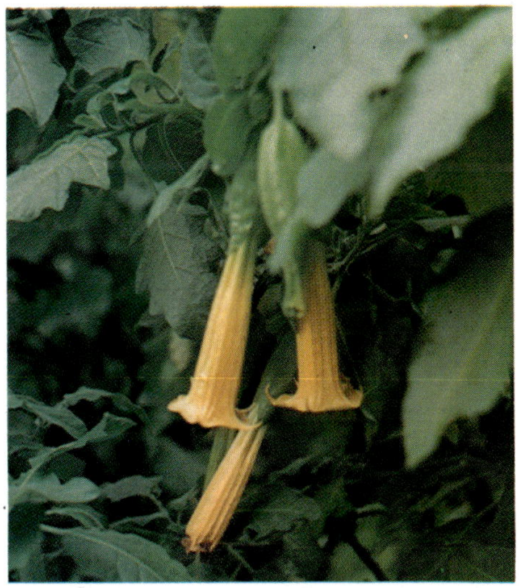

501

502

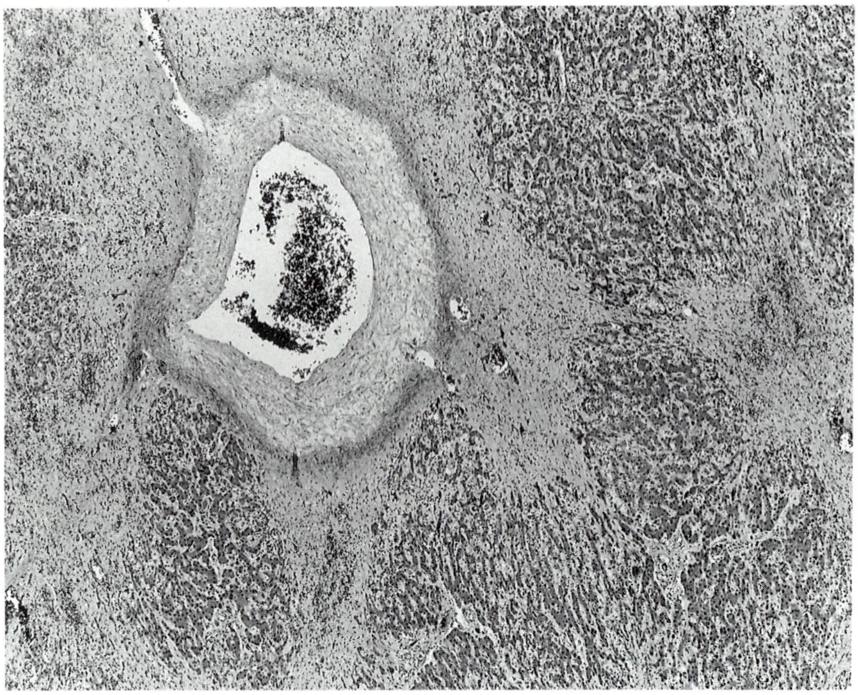

502 **Veno-occlusive disease** is a non-thrombotic obliterative process with narrowing of the small intrahepatic branches of the hepatic vein.

Cyanogenic glycosides

For millions of people in the third world cassava is the staple food and because it thrives in dry conditions and requires little attention it is being promoted in sub-Saharan Africa. However, without careful preparation cassava flour is very hazardous (**503**, **504**). Occasional reports suggest that cyanogenic glycosides may also be goitrogenic (**505**) (see pages 18 and 189). Detoxification of cyanide relates to the conversion to less toxic thiocyanate and in undernourished people low sulphur intake may impair this process and possibly explain the occurrence of spastic paralysis in some outbreaks[90].

503

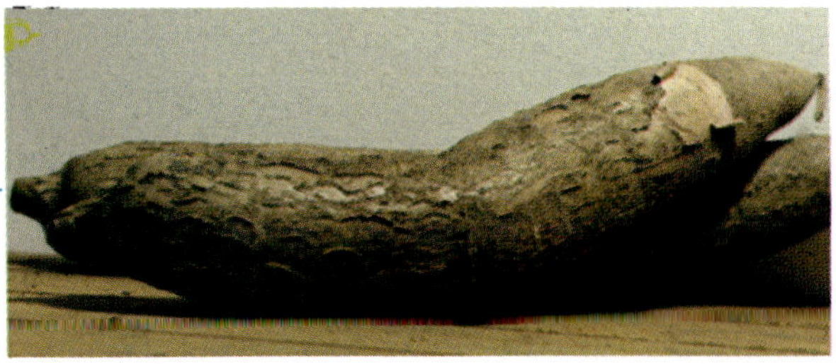

503 **Cyanogenic glycosides** occur in various plant tissues including cassava tubers from which they are usually leached out by prolonged soaking. Failure to do this is considered to be responsible for a syndrome consisting of ataxic polyneuropathy, amblyopia and tinnitus occurring in parts of Nigeria and other cassava-consuming regions. Highly toxic alkaloidal glycosides called solanines are produced by greening and sprouting potato tubers, consumption of which may be responsible for many mild episodes of gastroenteritis, and coma and convulsions have occasionally been reported.

504

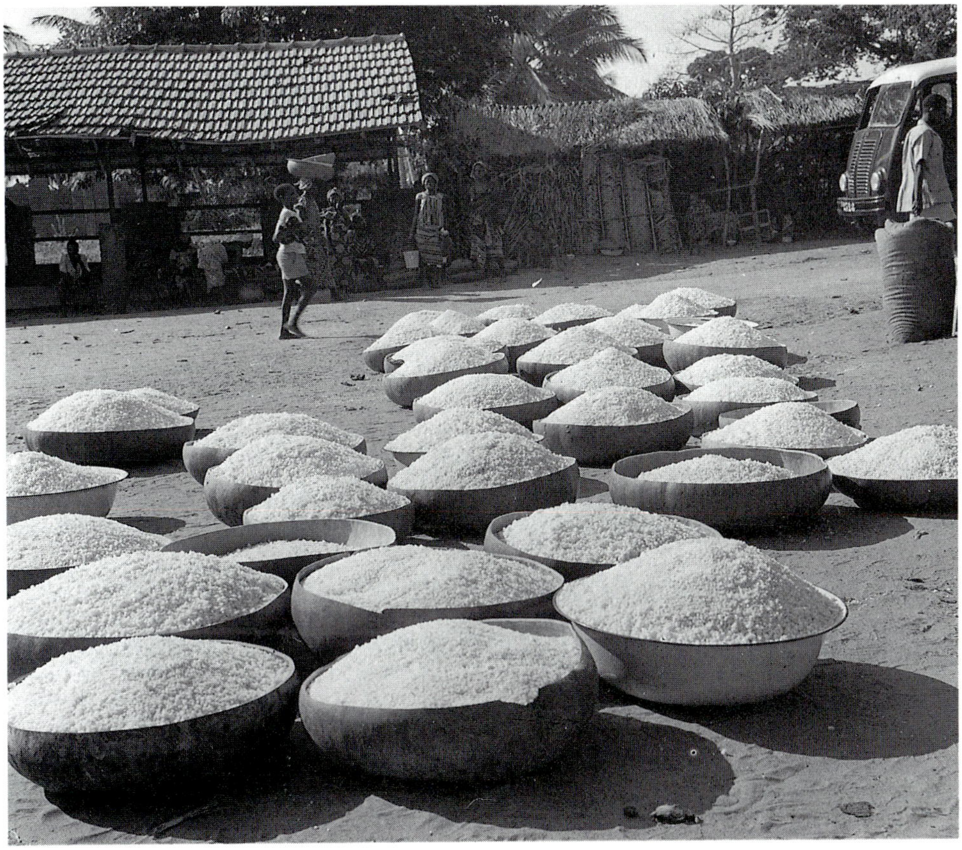

504 **Cassava flour** in Anfouin market, Togo, West Africa.

505 Goitrogens are an occasional cause of goitre with or without hypothyroidism. They differ from country to country. Cassava may be a goitrogen in areas of endemic iodine deficiency. Iodine from cough medicines, vitamin pills, X-ray contrast media or certain drugs such as amiodarone, may act as a goitrogen in the UK (see page 196).

505

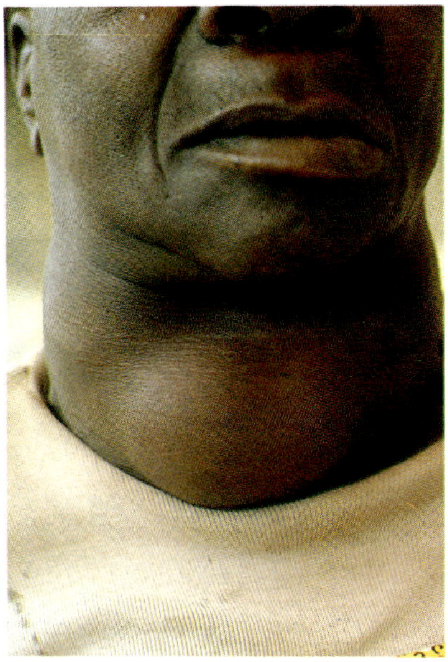

Fungal toxicoses

Amanita phalloides in the United Kingdom and *A. serua* in America are the commonest poisonous mushrooms, each having two types of toxin (506–508).

506
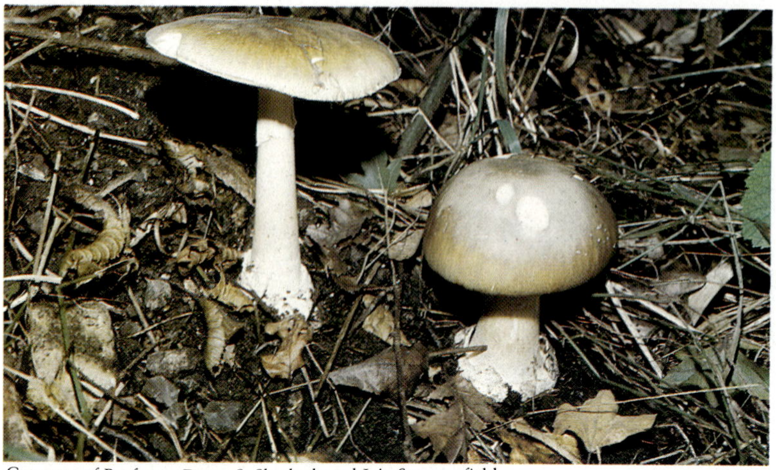

Courtesy of Professor Dame S. Sherlock and J.A. Summerfield.

506 ***Amanita phalloides*** is the only mushroom known to be hepatotoxic to man. Ingestion causes fulminant hepatic failure, usually in the autumn among holiday-makers who are unfamiliar with the recognition of edible fungi. *Amanita phalloides* is distinguished by a pale yellow to olive green cap and crowded white gills. The stipe (stem) has a bulbous base and is white, but may have a greenish tinge. Symptoms are delayed for 6–15 hours after poisoning with *Amanita phalloides*. Nausea, vomiting, abdominal cramps and diarrhoea are followed by signs of dehydration and vasomotor collapse. Jaundice and hepatic coma appear after 3 days. Signs of renal and central nervous system damage are also prominent.

507
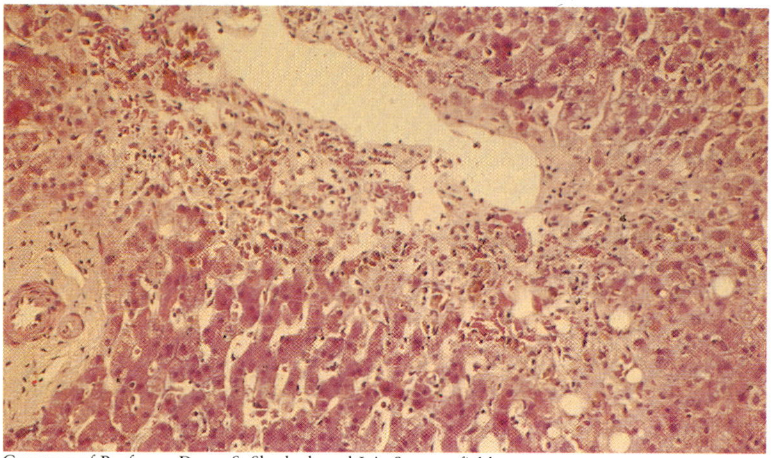

Courtesy of Professor Dame S. Sherlock and J.A. Summerfield.

507 ***Amanita phalloides.*** The liver biopsy shows massive centrilobular liver cell necrosis, infiltration with acute inflammatory cells and haemorrhage. Many liver cells contain fat droplets. (*H&E*, × 40)

508
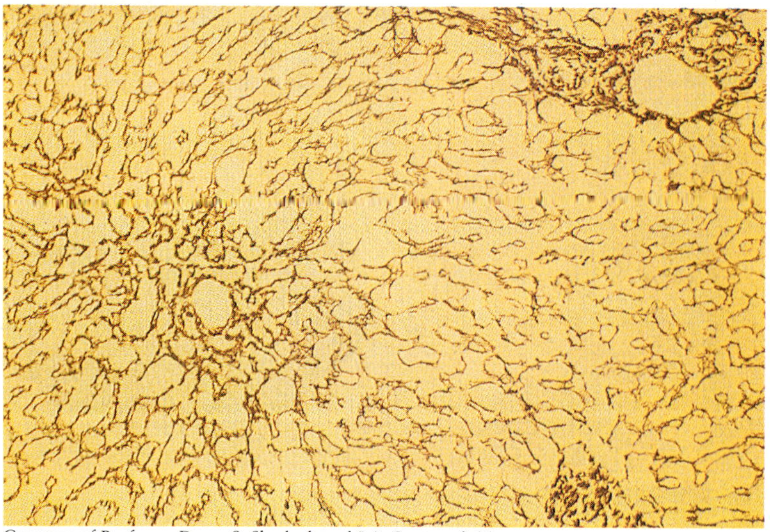

Courtesy of Professor Dame S. Sherlock and J.A. Summerfield.

508 ***Amanita phalloides.*** The reticulin stain of the liver biopsy shows more clearly the collapse of the reticulin framework around the central veins. (× 40)

Aflatoxins came into prominence after large numbers of young turkeys died with acute enteritis and hepatitis after being fed a ration containing imported groundnut meal contaminated with aflatoxin (**509**, **510**). Hepatoma has been produced experimentally in several animal species and the reported occurrence of this form of cancer in man (see **62**) lends some support to the suggestion that contaminated groundnut may be a factor in man also, although chronic hepatitis B virus infection and underlying cirrhosis are strongly associated.

There is evidence that undernourished individuals succumb to liver damage more readily than the well-nourished, but the suggestion that kwashiorkor is caused by aflatoxins has not received general support.

509

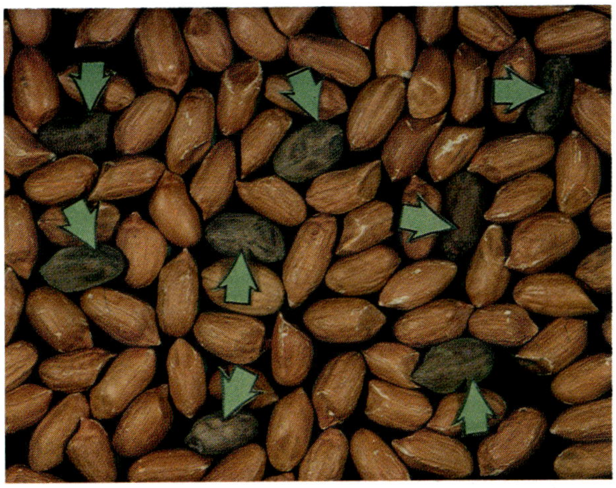

509 Aflatoxins are produced by the fungus *Aspergillis flavus*, a frequent contaminant of improperly stored groundnuts, as shown here, and some other foodstuffs. Liver cancer results from feeding contaminated groundnut to several animal species experimentally. There is some evidence for an association with hepatoma in man in parts of Africa and Asia where this is a common form of cancer (see **65**).

510

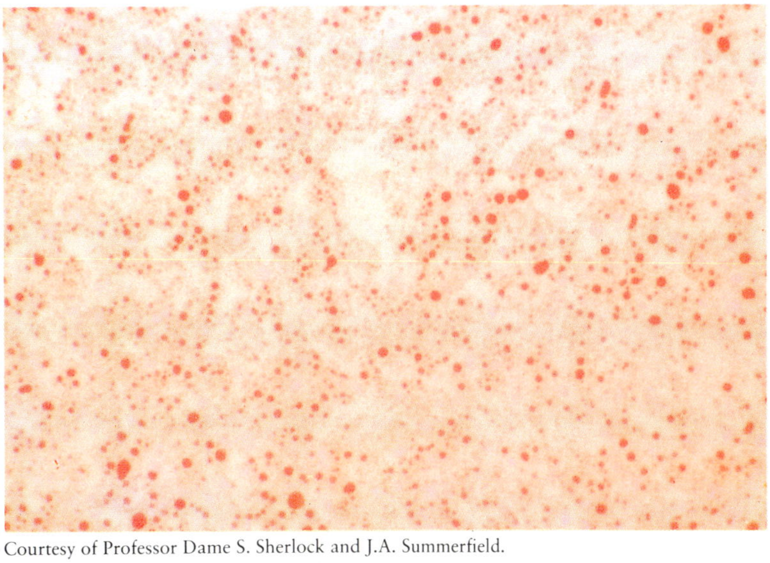

Courtesy of Professor Dame S. Sherlock and J.A. Summerfield.

510 Reye's syndrome. This is a highly fatal disease of uncertain aetiology in young children, with massive fatty infiltration of the liver, as shown here, and encephalopathy. In northern Thailand epidemics of this condition have been attributed to the consumption of glutinous rice contaminated with aspergillus fungus.

Ergotism (**511**) is largely of historical interest, but small outbreaks in recent years have been reported from Ethiopia from eating wild oats and from India associated with millet. Contaminated crops are only consumed in times of food shortage but with this situation endemic in much of sub-Saharan Africa the threat of new outbreaks cannot be ignored.

511

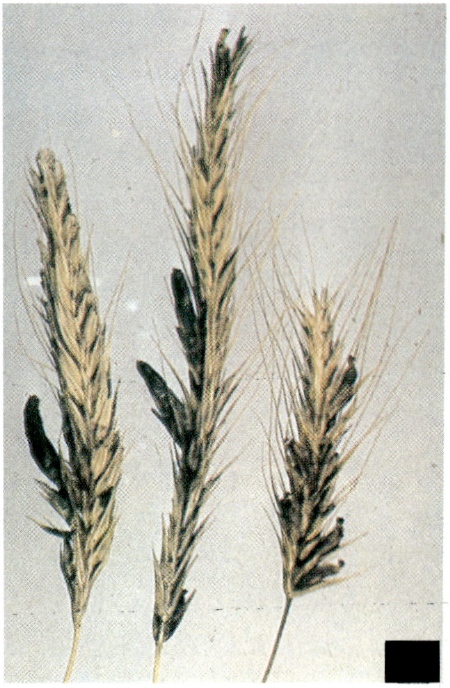

511 The fungus *Claviceps purpurea* commonly infects rye, as shown here, and less often wheat, barley and oats. Two distinct forms of ergotism occur, the gangrenous and convulsive, depending upon the combination of active *laevo* ergotamine compounds.

Vast epidemics of 'Saint Anthony's fire' from consuming contaminated crops in time of food shortage occurred in the past, and small outbreaks continue to be reported.

Marine toxicoses

According to Mills and Passmore[91] three main groups of seafood poisoning – puffer fish poisoning (**512**), ciguatera (**513**), and paralytic shellfish poisoning (**514**) – although caused by different poisons, have a common symptomatology, which they term pelagic paralysis, resulting from blockage of voltage-gated sodium channels in myelinated and non-myelinated nerve fibres.

512

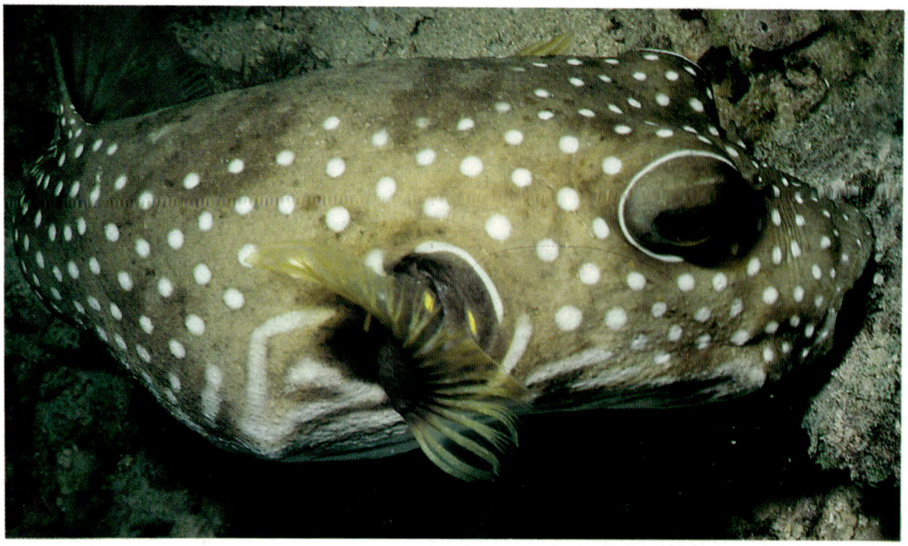

512 Arothron hispidus (Linnaeus). Also known as Maki-maki or deadly death puffer, it has a length of 50cm and is found in the Panama Canal, throughout the tropical Pacific to South America, Japan and the Red Sea.

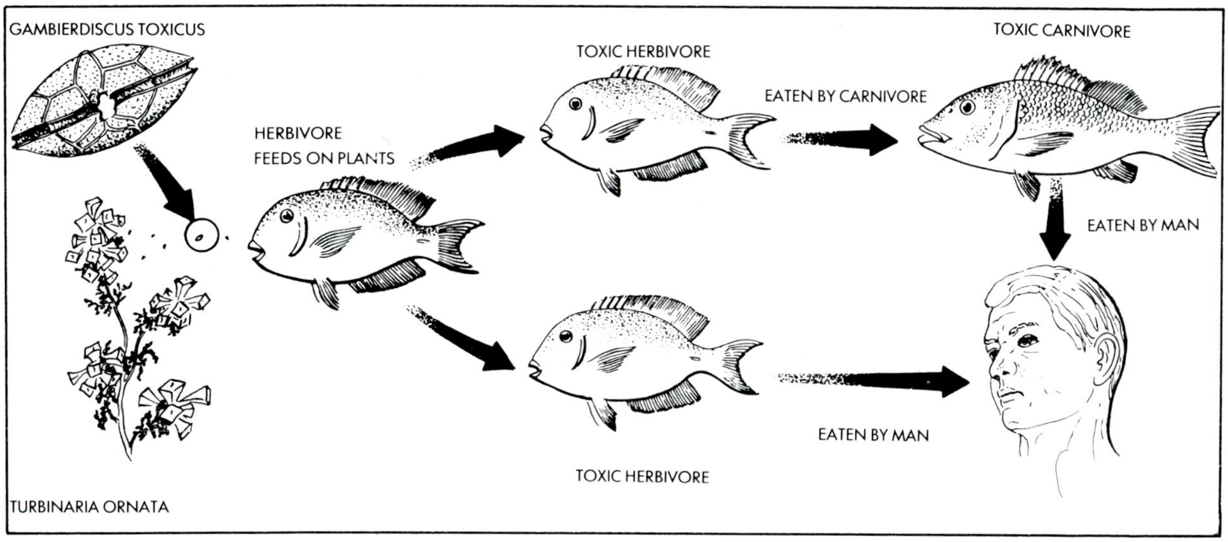

513

513 Ciguatera. Diagram showing the ways in which ciguatoxin enters the food chain.

514 Red tide in Lake Macquarie, New South Wales, Australia. Blooms of dangerous dinoflagellates often result in inshore waters becoming reddish-brown and are referred to as 'red tides'.

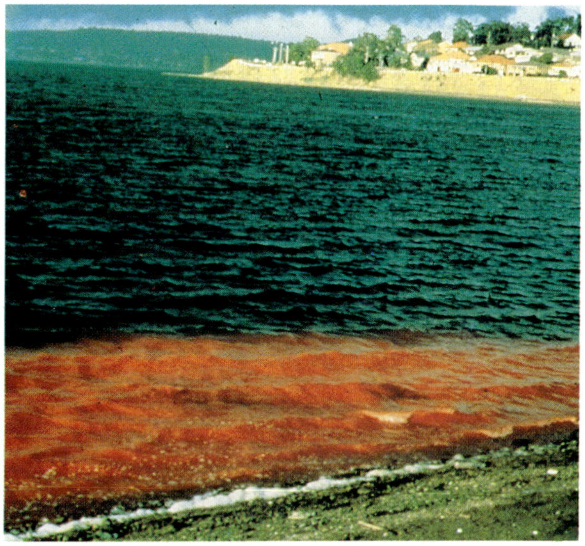

514

A different clinical picture, consisting of headache, palpitation, flushing and diarrhoea results a short time after ingestion of tunny, mackerel and related fish suffering bacterial spoilage. This is known as scombroid or scombrotoxic poisoning (**515**); it is prevented by cooking and is due to massive release of histamine.[92]

515 Euthynnus pelamis (Linnaeus). Also known as Oceanic bonito, it has a length of 50cm and is found in tropical areas around the world.

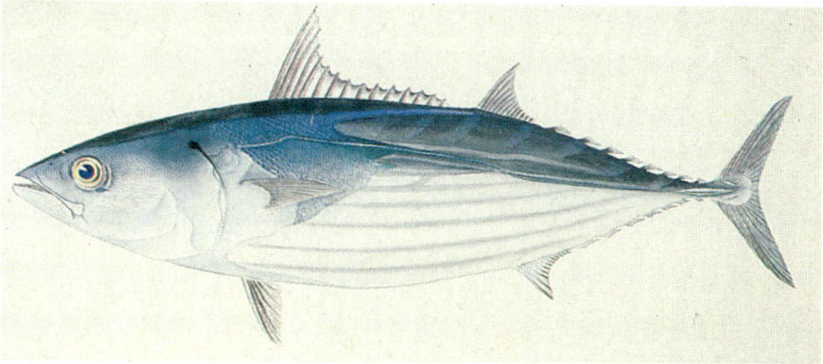

515

Non-essential element poisoning

Most of the essential elements are toxic in excessive amounts and are considered in Chapter 6. Poisoning from mercury, lead and aluminium (non-essential elements) is of special concern in relation to food as the source. Neurological damage has resulted from ingestion of mercury-contaminated fish from industrial effluents or of seed grains dressed with a fungicide. Excessive intake of lead mainly results from industrial exposure and atmospheric pollution; even in cities intake from food does not exceed about 400μg/day, 90% of which in unabsorbed and most of the rest excreted in urine. Bone has a high affinity for lead (**516**) and other evidence of poisoning includes hypertension and renal, bone marrow or nervous system damage. It has been found recently that decanters and crystal glasses are another source of

516

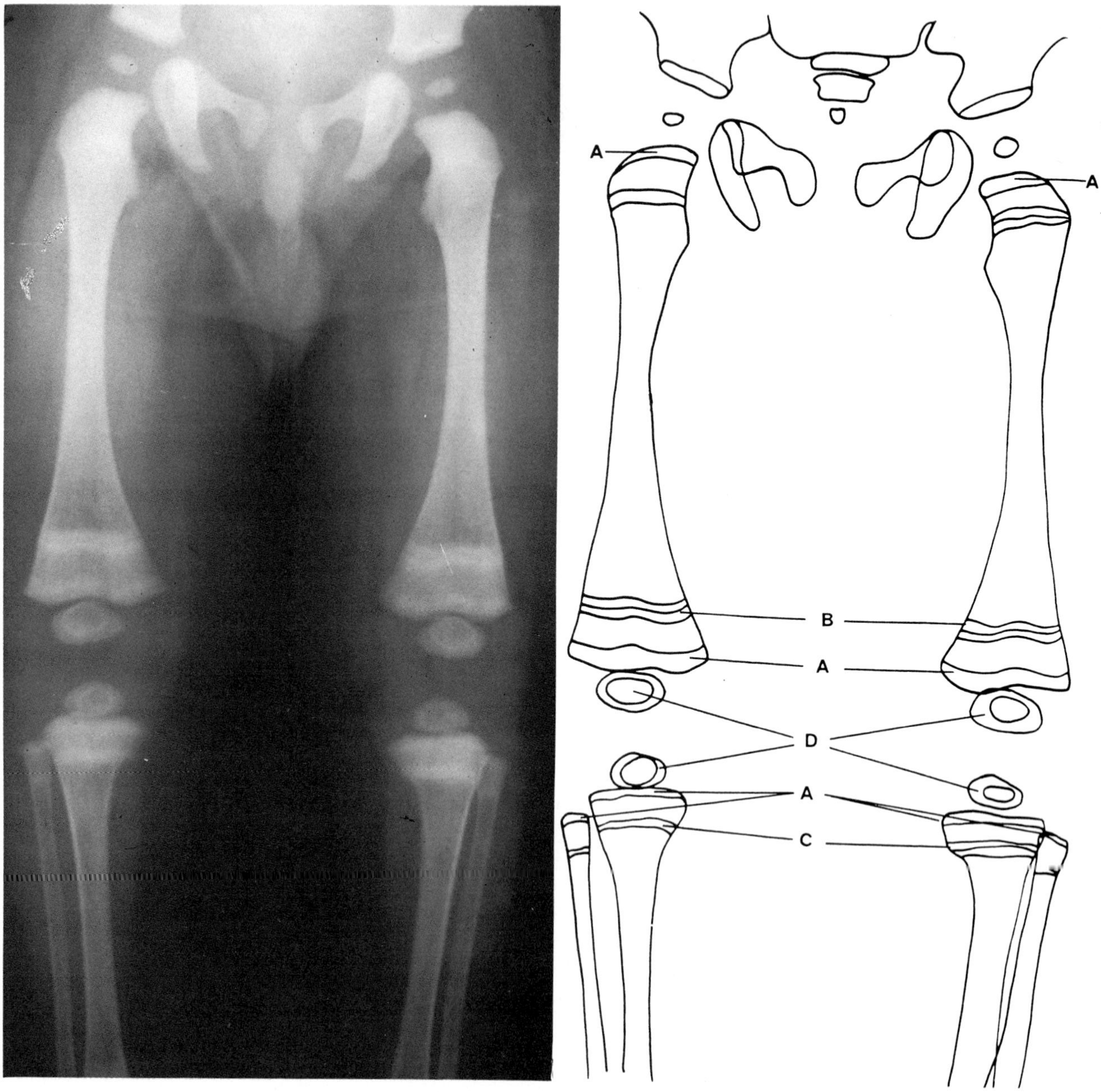

516 Lead poisoning. Lead deposition in growing bone causes a dense metaphyseal band (A). In this case, the presence of further submetaphyseal bands, particularly in the distal femora (B) and proximal tibiae (C), indicated that the poisoning was intermittent. The presence of dense circles (D) within the epiphyses has the same meaning.

poisoning due to lead dissolving into the liquid being drunk.[93] Aluminium presents a health hazard mainly to patients with chronic renal failure and especially those receiving haemodialysis. The hyperphosphataemia (see page 212) that commonly develops has customarily been counteracted by aluminium-containing antacids to bind phosphate in the intestines. Another possible source of aluminium is tap water used in very large amounts for dialysis. Two major syndromes have been provisionally attributed to aluminium toxicity under these circumstances – aluminium-related osteomalacia and so-called 'dialysis dementia' with progressive dementia, dyspraxia, facial grimaces, myoclonic seizures, and a characteristic EEG pattern.

Evidence for a role for aluminium toxicity in Alzheimer's disease is inconclusive (Chapter 11).

Other contaminants

In industrialized societies most foods are now packaged in some way and concern is now being expressed[94] concerning the possibility that harm may result from the penetration of food by chemicals in the package material, such as plasticizers in cling film.

The eosinophilia myalgia syndrome erupted in epidemic proportions in the United States and some European countries in 1989. In just over 12 months about 5000 people were affected and 27 died. The outbreak was soon traced to a dietary supplement containing tryptophan, advertized in health shops as relieving depression, insomnia and the premenstrual syndrome. The features included muscle pains, fever, oedema, rash and eosinophilia. All cases were eventually traced to a single Japanese company where tryptophan was genetically engineered. Whether it was this process or a contaminant that was responsible is not clear.

Since the recall of over-the-counter tryptophan preparations in November 1989 there has been a dramatic fall in the number of cases reported.[95]

Food additives

Most industrialized countries strictly control the use of chemical substances that may be added to food for various purposes by the food industry (517).[96]

The occurrence of idiosyncratic reaction to food additives is rare and has been exaggerated in the public mind. From time to time additives have been

517 Types of food additives used commercially in the United States.

517

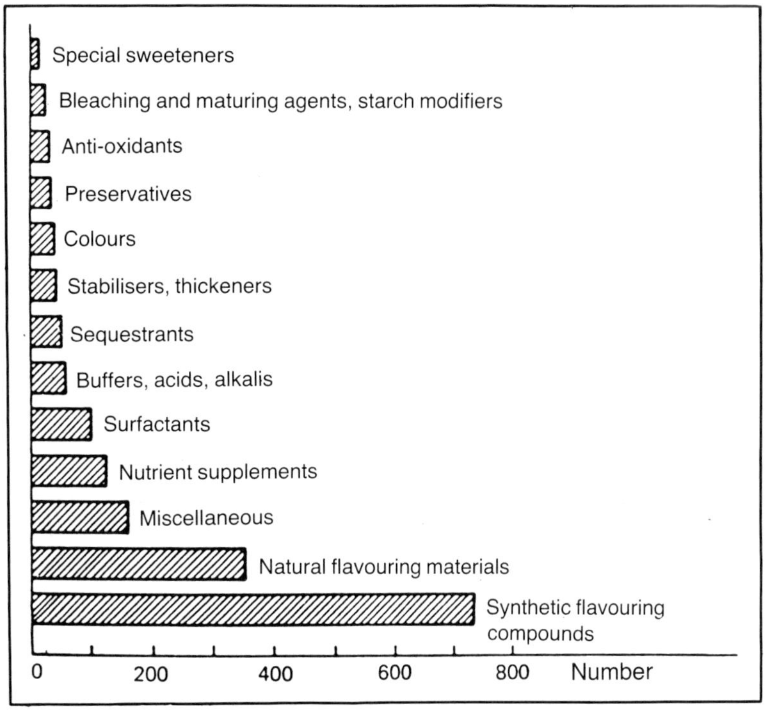

banned as the result of new evidence, usually either experimental or epidemiological, implicating them in predisposition to disease. Regulations increasingly become more stringent and new additives have to pass through very rigorous testing and evaluation.

10. Conditions Benefiting from Nutritional Support

There is a considerable number of conditions that are neither nutritional nor diet-related in origin but which benefit to a varying extent from nutritional support. In the past two decades increasing attention has been paid to the nutritional status of the hospitalized patient (see Chapter 4) and to the development of methods for improving that status. As a result Nutritional support has become an important medical speciality (518–522).

18

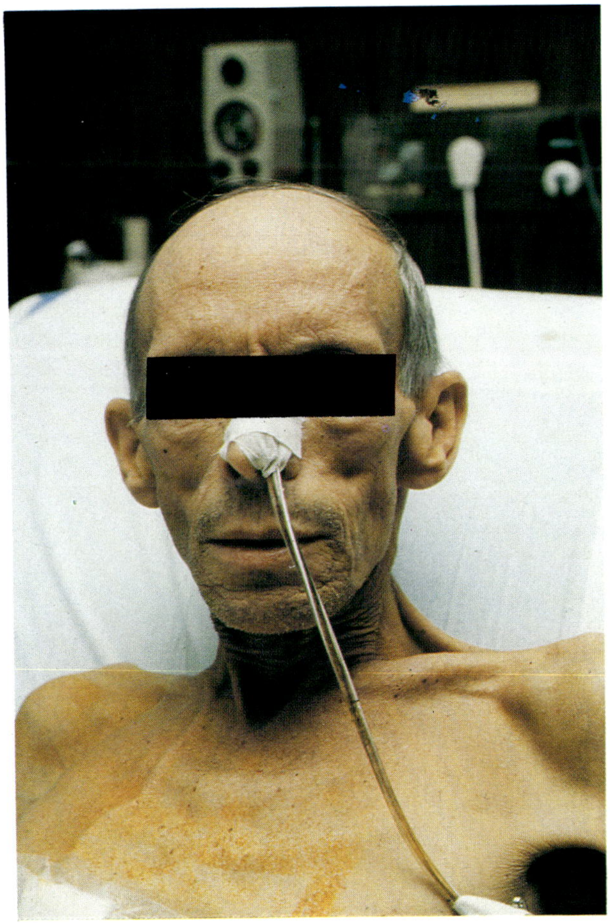

518 A patient receiving enteral nutrition through a nasogastric tube.

519

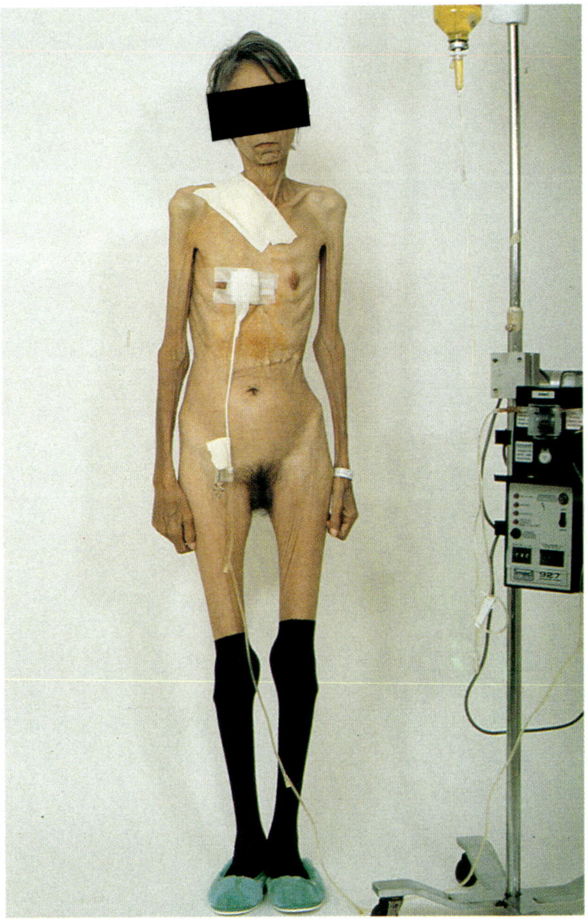

519 A patient being fed a complete nutritional formula by total parenteral nutrition through a catheter in a deep vein.

520

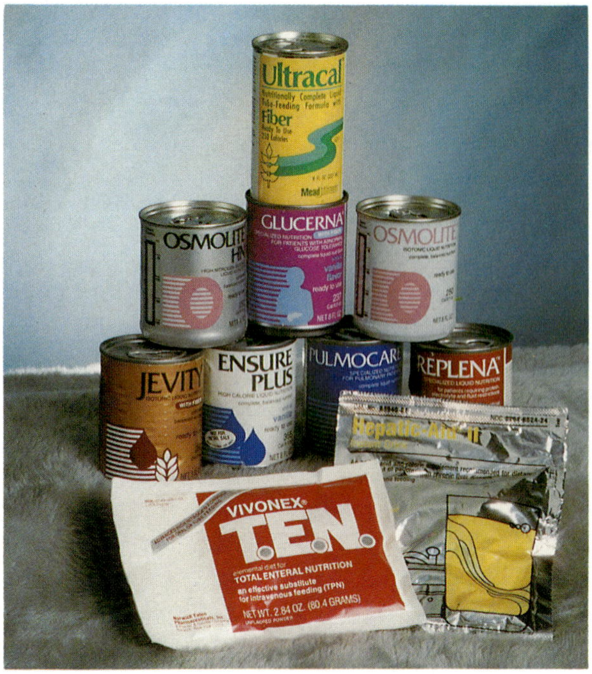

520 A selection of enteral feeds: Ultracal (with extra fibre in the form of wheat); Osmolite (high in nitrogen); Glucerna (for diabetics and patients with abnormal glucose tolerance); Osmolite (regular maintenance); Jevity (contains fibre from soya beans); Ensure plus (high energy); Pulmocare (high fat, low carbohydrate for patients with respiratory impairment); Replena (for renal patients); Vivonex (elemental diet); Hepatic aid (for acute liver failure; rich in brached-chain and no aromatic amino acids)

521

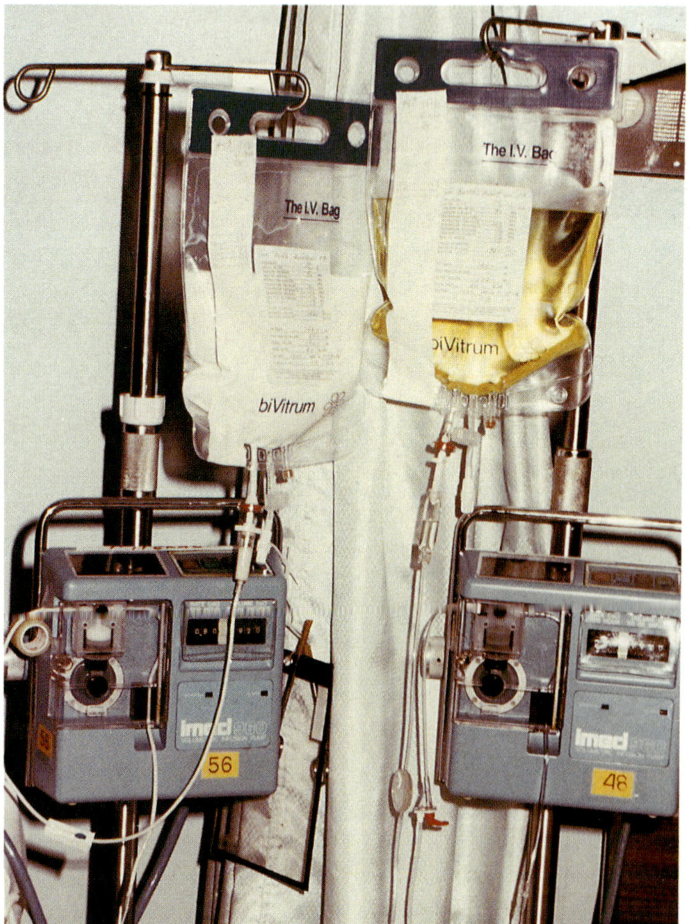

521 Parenteral feeds: on left – 'three-in-one' type system with an Imed diffusion pump delivering glucose (50%), fat (30%), and amino acids (20%) of total energy: on right – glucose (80%) and amino acids (20%) of total energy.

522 A variety of infusions for different patients: left to right – 20% fat (Intralipid); Osmolite (for nasogastric feeding); 5% dextrose (by peripheral vein); glucose–amino acid mixture; normal saline and fat.

522

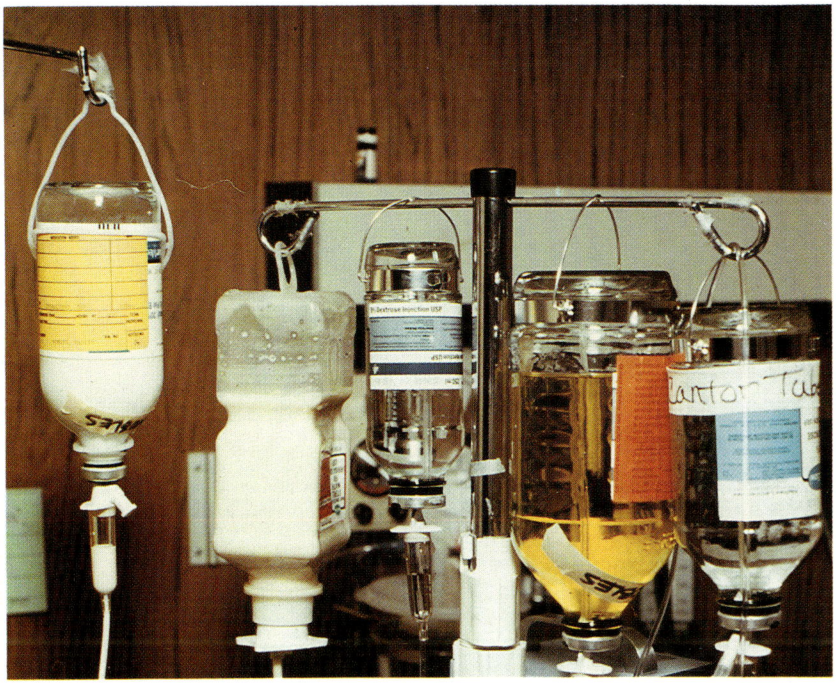

The decision tree in **523** indicates how choice of appropriate support can be made.

523

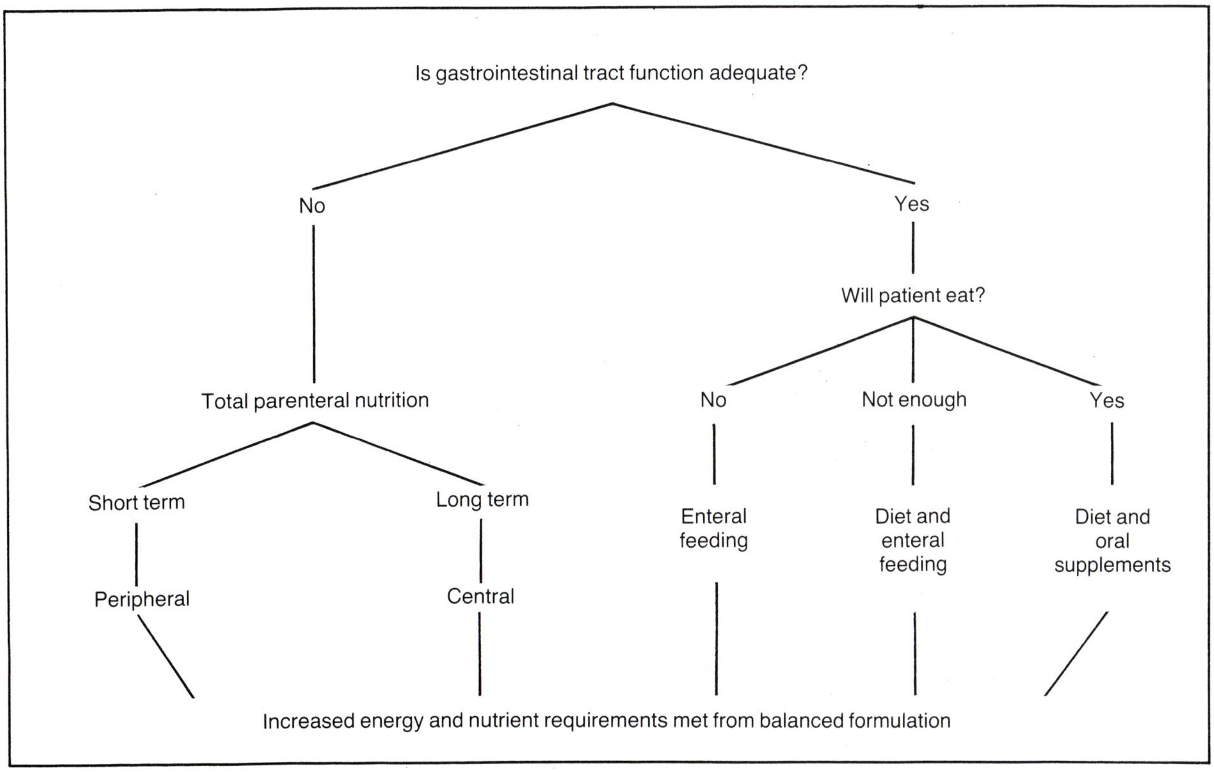

523 Decision tree for selecting mode of nutritional support.

Table 95 shows indications for parenteral nutrition.

Tube feeding is preferable as complications are less. It may be used for the conditions shown in *Table 95* in the absence of obstruction or severe loss of bowel surface, and when problems are less severe.

Some of the special features of the conditions considered here are discussed below.

Table 95. Indications for parenteral nutritional support.

Gastrointestinal tract obstruction
Prolonged ileus, pseudo-obstruction, adhesions, strictures, neoplasia, congenital atresia syndrome, gastroschisis or wound dehiscence

Severe loss of bowel surface
Necrotizing enterocolitis, radiation enteritis, inflammatory bowel disease, intractable diarrhoeal disease of infancy and failure to thrive, short bowel syndrome, high-output intestinal fistulas

Conditions associated with persistent vomiting or anorexia
Anorexia nervosa, cancer chemotherapy, severe depression, chronic renal failure, chronic liver failure

Increased nutrient requirements
Major trauma, burns, sepsis, cancer

Other occasional indications
Very low birthweight infants, intensive care/ventilatory support/coma

Trauma and infection

The metabolic and nutritional upset in trauma may be profound (*Table 96*). In burns, both complicating sepsis and fluid loss through exudates and heat loss add to the problem of management.

524 indicates the timing of onset of the many nutritional responses that follow upon a febrile illness. In recent years there has been increasing appreciation of the central role that the non-essential amino acid glutamine plays in the recovery of injured tissues.[97]

The marked undernutrition that accompanies the later stages of AIDS is of concern especially in young children and in third world countries (**525**).

Table 96. Some major metabolic responses following injury.

	Acute phase	*Chronic phase*
Duration in days (proportional to injury)	1–5	6–10+
Metabolic rate	High	Reducing
Core temperature	Below normal	Raised, lowering
Cardiac output	Below normal	Raised, lowering
Blood glucose	Raised	Reducing toward normal
Glucose production	Normal	Increased
Plasma insulin	Low	Normal or elevated
Plasma glucagon	Raised	Raised
Plasma catecholamines	Raised	Slightly raised
Blood lactate	Raised	Normal
Plasma fatty acids	Raised	Lowered
Oxygen consumption	Lowered	Raised
Nitrogen balance	Negative	Becoming positive

524

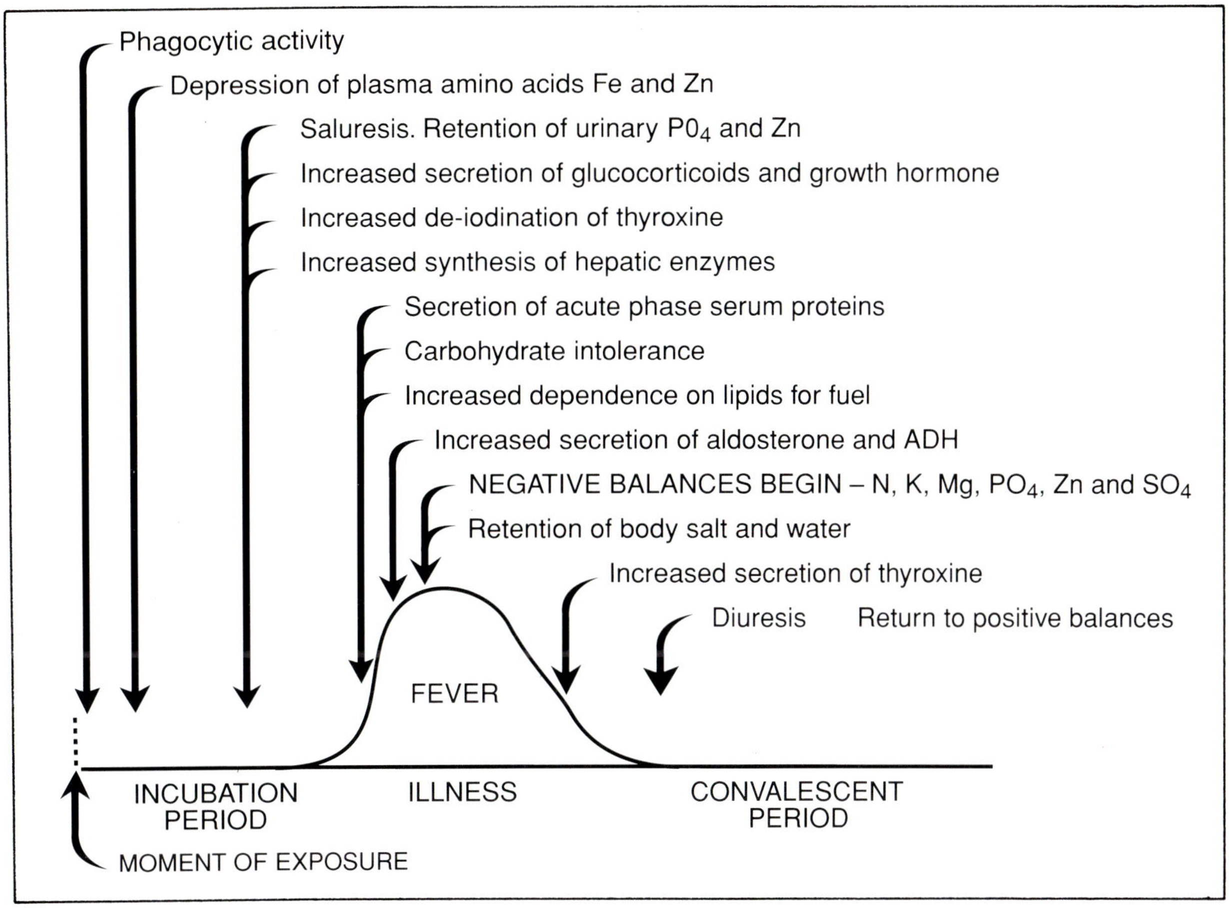

524 Metabolic response to pyrexia. Schematic representation of the sequence of nutritional responses that evolves during the course of a 'typical' generalized febrile infectious illness.

525

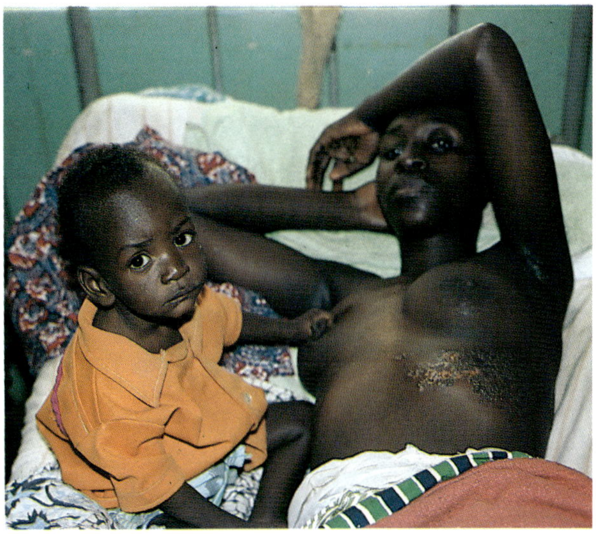

525 Perinatal transmission of AIDS. The virus in African communities is transmitted mainly by heterosexual contact, perinatally from infected mothers and by parenteral infection from contaminated blood in transfusions or dirty syringes. This woman with advanced AIDS has severe herpes zoster lesions. Her infant was also HIV positive.

Cancer

The possible aetiological role of dietary factors in cancer was considered in Chapter 3. Other aspects of nutrition and diet in relation to cancer include the impairment of nutritional status by various means in established malignant disease (*Table 97*).

Nutritional support can considerably improve prognosis by permitting the patient to undergo procedures that might otherwise not be possible. Sometimes malignant disease necessitates surgical, radiation or drug therapy that interferes with nutrition (*Table 98*).

Table 97. Nutritional implications of malignant disease.

Anorexia with progressive weight loss and undernutrition
Impaired food intake and malnutrition secondary to bowel obstruction at any level
Hypermetabolism in some cancers
Malabsorption associated with deficiency of pancreatic enzymes or bile salts; fistulous bypass of small bowel; infiltration of bowel, lymphatics or mesentry by malignant cells; blind loop syndrome with partial upper bowel obstruction leading to bacterial overgrowth; and malnutrition-induced villous hypoplasia
Protein-losing enteropathy with some malignancies
Hormonal abnormalities, e.g. hypercalcaemia induced by increased serum calcitriol and other hormones or by osteoclastic processes; osteomalacia with hypophosphataemia associated with depressed serum calcitriol; hypoglycaemia of insulin-secreting tumours; and hyperglycaemia with islet glucagonoma or somatostatinoma
Chronic blood loss and anaemia
Electrolyte and fluid problems with :– persistent vomiting with intestinal obstruction or intracranial tumours; intestinal fluid losses through fistulae or diarrhoea; intestinal secretory abnormalities with hormone-secreting tumours (e.g. carcinoid syndrome, Zollinger-Ellison syndrome (gastrinoma)); inappropriate antidiuretic hormone secretion (e.g. lung carcinoma); hyperadrenalism with tumours producing corticotropin or corticosteroid
Miscellaneous disorders, e.g. intractable gastric ulcers with gastrinomas; Fanconi syndrome with light-chain disease; coma with brain tumours

Table 98. Nutritional problems consequent upon cancer treatment.

Surgical treatment

Radical resection of oropharyngeal area:– chewing and swallowing difficulties

Oesophagectomy:– gastric stasis and hypochlorhydria, steatorrhoea, and diarrhoea secondary to vagotomy; early satiety, regurgitation

Gastrectomy (high subtotal or total):– dumping syndrome, malabsorption, achlorhydria and lack of intrinsic factor, hypoglycaemia, early satiety

Intestinal resection:– jejunum – decreased efficiency of absorption of many nutrients
ileum – vitamin B_{12} deficiency, bile salt loss with diarrhoea or steatorrhoea, hyperoxaluria and renal stone, calcium and magnesium depletion, fat and fat-soluble vitamin malabsorption
massive bowel resection:– life-threatening malabsorption, malnutrition, metabolic acidosis, dehydration
ileostomy and colostomy:– salt and water imbalance

Blind loop syndrome:– vitamin B_{12} malabsorption

Pancreatectomy:– malabsorption, diabetes mellitus

Radiation treatment

Oropharyngeal area:– destruction of sense of taste, xerostomia, loss of teeth

Lower neck and mediastinum:– oesophagitis and dysphagia, fibrosis with oesophageal stricture

Abdomen and pelvis:– diarrhoea, malabsorption, stenosis, obstruction, fistulization

Drug treatment

Corticosteroids:– fluid and electrolyte imbalance, nitrogen and calcium losses, hyperglycaemia

Sex hormone analogues:– nausea and vomiting

Immunotherapy:– interleukin-2 -azotaemia, hypotension, fluid retention

Cancer chemotherapy agents:– anorexia, nausea, diarrhoea, pain, ulceration

Cystic fibrosis (mucoviscidosis)

This is an autosomal recessively inherited disorder of exocrine glands primarily affecting the gastrointestinal and respiratory systems. Chromosome 7 is abnormal. It is the most common fatal genetic disease in white populations, but is much less common in blacks.

The effects of the disease are widespread throughout the gut and lungs and some other systems (*Table 99*). As a consequence in young children failure to thrive is frequent (*Table 100*).

Some major clinical changes are illustrated in **526, 527**.

Table 99. Cystic fibrosis: symptoms, signs and associated conditions.

General
Slow weight gain from birth
Large appetite
Recurrent or persistent harsh repetitive cough
Vomiting with cough
Salty taste when kissed

Respiratory tract
Upper
Sinusitis
Nasal polyps
Conductive hearing loss

Lower
Chronic respiratory infection: *staphylococci, Pseudomonas*
Progressive lung damage
Chronic respiratory failure
Cor pulmonale

Gastrointestinal system
Meconium ileus from birth
Pancreatic malabsorption
Fat-soluble vitamin deficiency
Biliary cholestasis in the newborn
Biliary cirrhosis
Gallstones
Rectal prolapse
Meconium ileus equivalent

Associated conditions
Diabetes mellitus
Delayed puberty
Spinocerebellar degeneration responsive to vitamin E
Polyarthropathy
Heatstroke
Psychosocial problems

Table 100. Factors contributing to failure to thrive in cystic fibrosis.

Diminished intake:	poor appetite
Energy loss:	glycosuria in diabetes
Reduced absorption:	pancreatic malabsorption biliary cirrhosis binding of nutrients to food residues in gut
Failure of utilization:	effects of chronic infection trace element deficiencies
Increased requirements:	effects of chronic respiratory disease possible cellular defect causing inefficient cellular metabolism

526 Cystic fibrosis. The chronic malabsorption of fat usually results in severe secondary undernutrition. This section of the pancreas shows the typical appearance of dilated ducts, containing inspissated secretion, fibrosis and disappearance of acini.

526

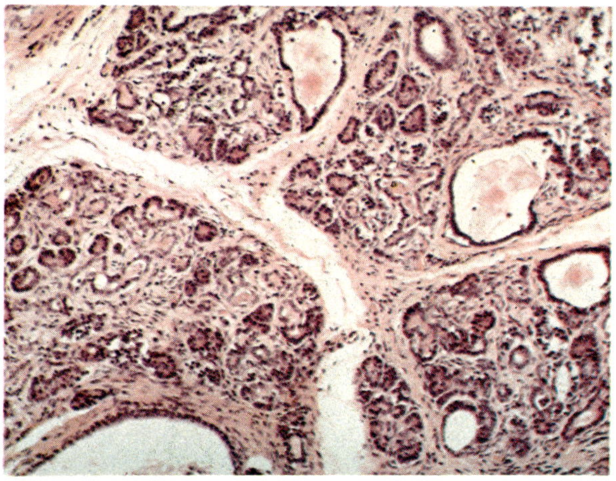

527 Cystic fibrosis. The lungs show emphysema, general and focal, thickened peribronchial markings and coarse nodular opacities throughout, denoting patchy bronchopneumonia in bronchiectatic lungs. The nutritional state usually correlates with that of the lungs rather than that of the pancreas.

527

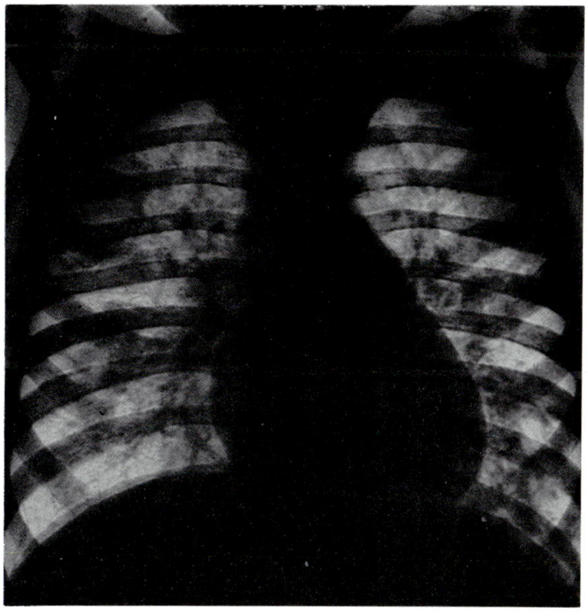

Gastrointestinal disease

Serious interference with absorption of the products of digestion, either from extensive disease or major resection of the gut, frequently necessitates nutritional support. In these circumstances this support is usually by the parenteral route.

528 outlines the absorption sites of the major nutrients; from this figure the likely effects on nutrition from different diseases may be deduced.

This process is seen clearly in relation to small bowel resection (529).

528

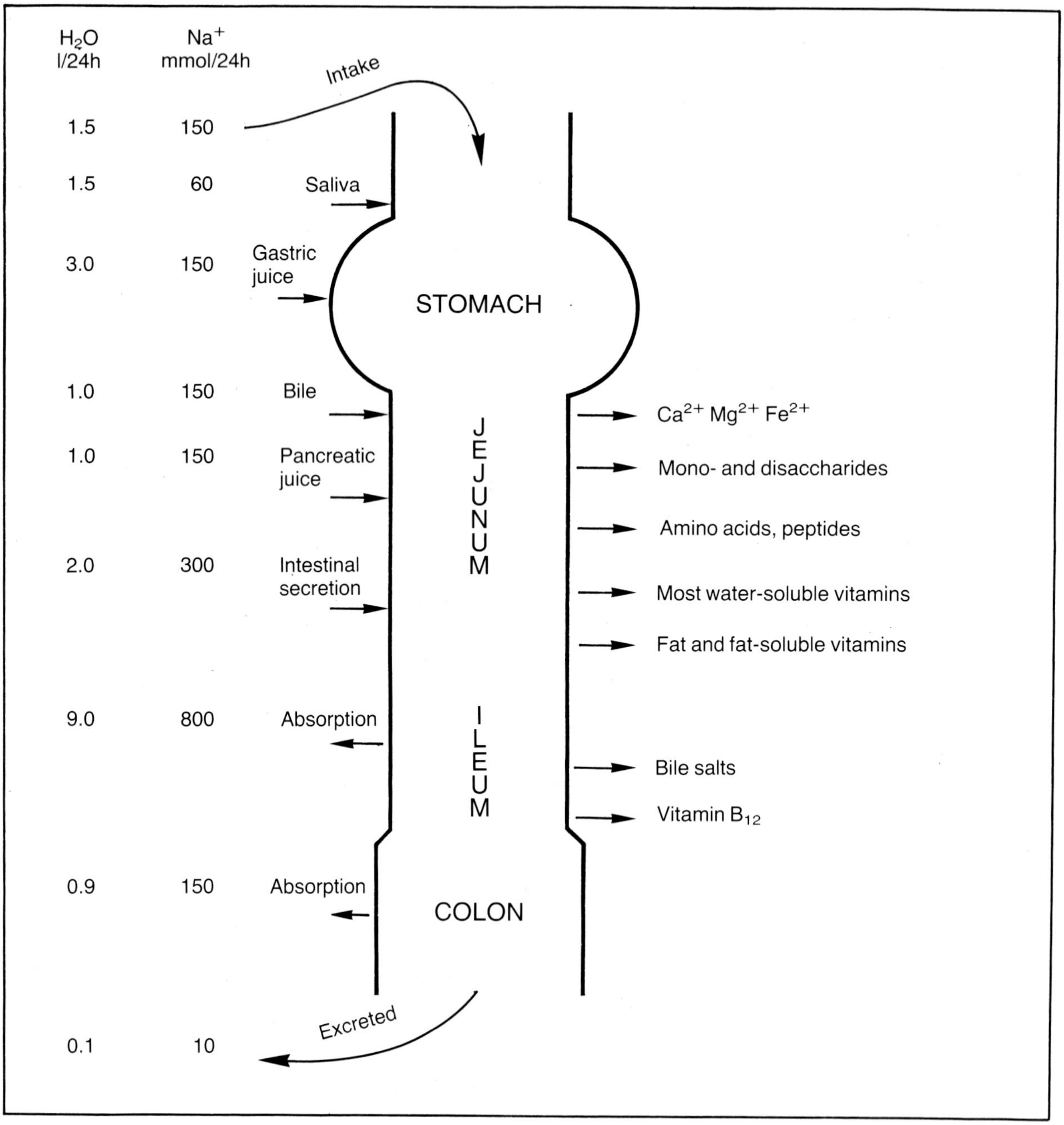

528 Gastrointestinal tract nutritional physiology. Some basic features of the localization in the gastrointestinal tract of absorption and secretion of water and sodium (left side) and absorption of nutrients (right side). The figures given for water and sodium are approximate for the average adult and with the information on nutrient absorption provide an indication of required replacement in the advent of surgical procedures and localized disease.

529 The effects of small intestinal resection.

529

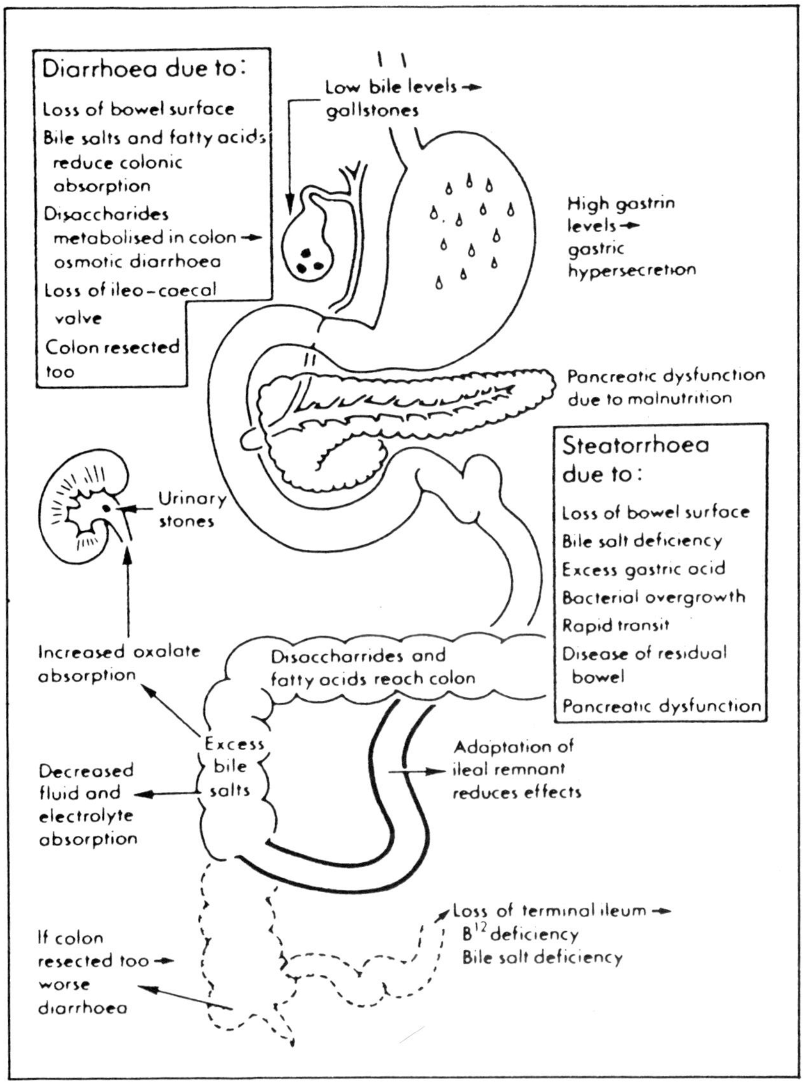

The short bowel syndrome

This is seen in a number of disease states (*Table 101*).

Table 101. Causes of short-bowel syndrome.

Crohn's disease	
Mesenteric embolism/thrombosis	
Radiation enteritis	
Intussusception	
Internal hernias	
Neonatal causes:	multiple atresias, malrotation with volvulus, meconium ileus, omphalocele/gastroschisis with volvulus, duplications, congenital short bowel

Inflammatory bowel disease

Nutritional problems arise from a number of causes as shown in *Table 102*, frequently necessitating nutritional support. Diet may be aetiologically involved in these diseases and they are considered further in Chapter 11.

Table 102. Nutritional problems in inflammatory bowel disease.

Factor	*Consequences*
Decreased dietary intake	As a consequence of abdominal pain: anorexia, nausea, vomiting, diarrhoea, iatrogenicity
Decreased absorption	Decreased absorptive surface due to: disease or resection, bile salt deficiency, bacterial overgrowth
Increased secretion	From protein-losing enteropathy, loss of elements, electrolytes in diarrhoea, gastrointestinal blood loss
Increased requirements	Inflammation and infection
Drug interference	Corticosteroids and calcium absorption or protein metabolism Sulphasalazine and folate absorption Cholestyramine and fat-soluble vitamin absorption

Irritable bowel syndrome

Other labels used in the past have included mucous colitis, spastic colon, spastic constipation and nervous diarrhoea. Abdominal pain accompanies constipation and/or diarrhoea. The syndrome is recognized to be due to functional disturbance of the colon as a result of abnormal responses to stress of some kind (**530, 531**). Adequate fibre intake should be encouraged and a normal diet is recommended.

530 'Spastic colon' or irritable bowel syndrome. A particularly bizarre stool, from a young woman with the irritable bowel syndrome, can be seen in the figure. Irritable bowel syndrome is a very common disorder accounting for abdominal symptoms in up to 50% of new referrals to gastroenterology outpatients in the UK. The pathophysiology of this syndrome is poorly understood. The pain has been correlated with colonic spasm and abdominal distension. Alternating constipation and diarrhoea may be associated with abnormalities in small and large bowel transit.

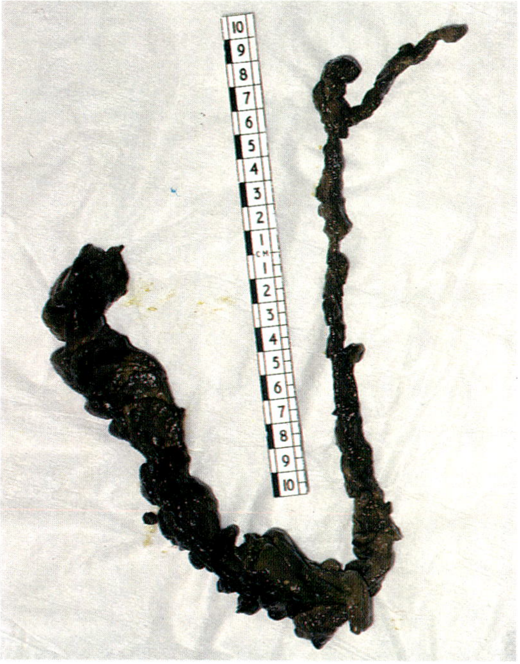

530

531 Irritable bowel syndrome. The investigation of patients with alteration in bowel habit should include sigmoidoscopy and barium enema. An example of an enema in a patient with irritable bowel syndrome and early diverticular disease is shown here. There are increased haustral markings and spasm, particularly in the transverse colon.

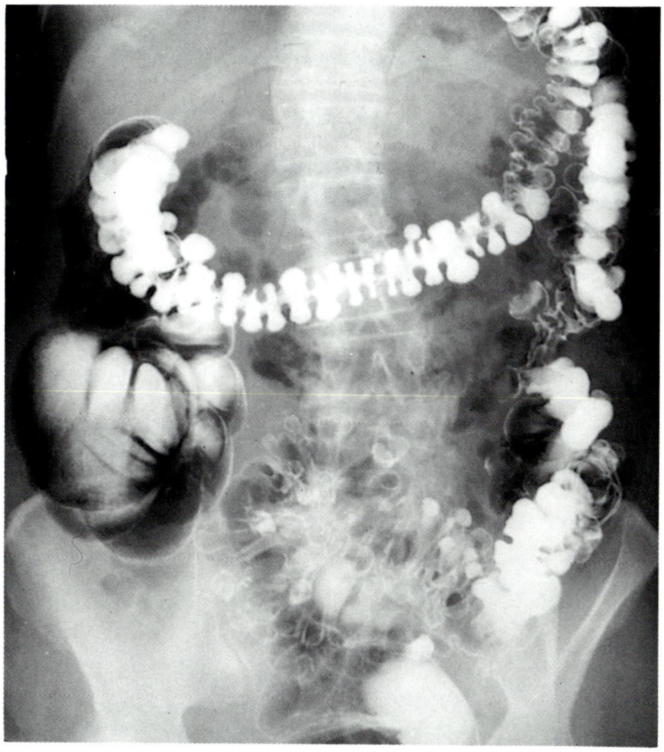

531

Acute diarrhoea and vomiting have many causes (*Table 103*) but with correct diagnosis and prompt treatment they rarely require nutritional support, apart from fluid and electrolyte replacement.

Table 103. Categories of acute diarrhoea and vomiting.

Gastroenteritis	
Viral	Most common is human rotavirus, which is responsible for 40–50% of acute diarrhoea in children
Bacterial	Usually various strains of *Escherichia coli, Shigella, Salmonella, Campylobacter jejuni,* and *Yersinia enterocolitica* and *Vibrio cholerae* in some developing countries
Parasitic	*Giardia lamblia, Entamoeba histolytica*
Inflammatory	Inflammatory bowel disease, Hirschsprung's enterocolitis, pseudomembranous colitis, necrotizing enterocolitis, radiation enteritis, eosinophilic gastroenteritis
Surgical	Acute appendicitis, intussusception, pyloric stenosis
Non-enteric disease	Urinary infection, meningitis, septicaemia, respiratory disease
Drugs	Laxatives, antibiotics, poisoning, cytotoxic agents
Metabolic disease	Diabetic ketoacidosis, haemolytic uraemic syndrome, congenital adrenal insufficiency
Food intolerance	Coeliac disease, acute food intolerance

If *protracted diarrhoea* supervenes, support is often indicated (*Table 104*). One of the causes of protracted diarrhoea in children, Schwachman–Diamond syndrome has a complex symptomatology and is especially likely to impair growth and development (*Table 105*).

Table 104. Categories of protracted diarrhoea.

Infectious	
Enteral	*Salmonella, Shigella,* enteropathogenic *E. coli, Giardia lamblia, Entamoeba histolytica,* measles
Parenteral	Chronic otitis and mastoiditis
Immune disorders	Severe combined immunodeficiency, autoimmune enteropathy
Food intolerance	Cow's milk and soya protein intolerances, coeliac disease
Enzyme deficiencies	Lactase, sucrase, isomaltase, enterokinase deficiencies
Drugs	Laxatives, cytotoxics, antibiotics
Other conditions	Inflammatory bowel disease, cystic fibrosis, Schwachman's syndrome, abetalipoproteinaemia, acrodermatitis enteropathica, primary bile acid malabsorption, Hirschsprung's disease, short gut syndrome

Table 105. Features of Schwachman–Diamond syndrome.

Familial incidence
Growth retardation especially in height, developmental retardation, poor feeding, diarrhoea
Recurrent infections (in 85%) – lungs, osteomyelitis, skin abscesses, otitis media; immune deficiency (especially IgA)
Non-specific enteropathy, occasionally Hirschsprung's disease, exocrine pancreatic insufficiency (steatorrhoea); mild cirrhosis of the liver
Haematological features: chronic neutropenia (95%), anaemia, mild thrombocytopenia
Dyschondroplasia of metaphyses and delayed maturation: rib abnormalities, long bone bowing, spinal abnormality, clinodactyly
Dental abnormalities
Ichthyotic skin and rashes

Acute and chronic pancreatitis and *pancreatic exocrine failure* (*Tables 106, 107*) tend to have intractable causes and malabsorption usually necessitates long-term nutritional support.

Table 106. Major causes of pancreatitis.

Alcoholism Biliary tract disease	account for about 80% of acute and chronic pancreatitis
Hereditary pancreatitis	
Hyperlipidaemia (especially Types I and IV)	
Hyperparathyroidism and hypercalcaemia	
Blunt and penetrating trauma	
Drugs (azathioprine, sulphasalazine, furosemide, valproic acid)	
Structural abnormalities of biliary system, pancreatic duct	
Calcific pancreatitis in the tropics (children and young adults)	

Table 107. Causes of pancreatic exocrine failure.

Cystic fibrosis
Schwachman–Diamond syndrome
PEM (occasionally in kwashiorkor)
Calcific pancreatitis of the tropics
In association with rare syndromes: with multiple congenital abnormalities in cartilage–hair hypoplasia
Surgical resection
Some specific enzyme deficiencies: lipase, amylase, trypsinogen

Renal disease

Acute renal failure has a number of causes that may or may not relate directly to the kidney itself (*Table 108*). Maintenance of nutrition is usually possible by oral feeding with dietary restrictions of protein, occasionally use of ketoacid analogues of some essential amino acids, and energy supplements.

Table 108. Major causes of acute renal failure.

Pre-renal	Fluid and electrolyte depletion, haemorrhage, septicaemia, cardiac failure, liver failure, burns, heatstroke
Post-renal	Calculi, prostatism, tumours of bladder, etc.
Renal	Acute glomerulonephritis, disseminated intravascular coagulation (DIC), vascular obstruction, intrarenal precipitation, acute tubulointerstitial nephritis (drug reaction, pyelonephritis, papillary necrosis), acute tubular injury (ischaemia, toxins, haemoglobinuria, myoglobinuria)

In the *nephrotic syndrome* massive proteinuria results in hypoalbuminaemia and oedema. Causes may be primary or secondary (*Table 109*).

Table 109. Major causes of the nephrotic syndrome.

Primary renal disease (90% in children, 75% in adults)
- Minimal change disease (MCD)
- Focal glomerulosclerosis (FGS)
- Membranous glomerulonephritis (MGN)
- Membranoproliferative glomerulonephritis (MPGN)
- Others: mesangial proliferative glomerulonephritis, IgA nephropathy, rapidly progressive glomerulonephritis (RPGN), focal glomerulonephritis (focal GN)

Secondary disease
- Metabolic: diabetes, amyloidosis
- Immunogenic: SLE, Henoch–Schönlein purpura, polyarteritis nodosa
- Neoplasia: leukaemias, lymphomas, Hodgkin's lymphoma, multiple myeloma, carcinoma (bronchus, breast, colon, stomach)
- Nephrotoxins
- Allergens
- Infections: bacterial, viral, protozoal, helminthic
- Miscellaneous: toxaemia of pregnancy, malignant hypertension

Replacement of lost protein has to be balanced against impairment of renal capacity to excrete nitrogenous waste products. Dialysis or renal transplant are eventually indicated.

Chronic renal failure (*Table 110*) usually passes through a phase where nutritional support is beneficial. Failure to thrive in children results from several mechanisms (*Table 111*).

Protein requirements are usually met by ordinary food of high biological value with energy supplements. Sodium may need to be restricted. Renal osteodystrophy (**532**) may be due either to rickets (1,25 $(OH_2)D_3$ is normally formed in the proximal tubule of the kidney, see page 123), secondary hyperparathyroidism, or metabolic acidosis. In the dialysis patient aluminium toxicity may cause bone disease (see page 269).

Table 110. Some main causes of chronic renal failure.

Glomerulonephritis
Reflux nephropathy
Hereditary diseases
Alport's syndrome
Nephronophthisis
Cystinosis
Polycystic disease
Dysplasia (with or without obstruction)
Haemolytic uraemic syndrome

Table 111. Causes of growth failure in children with chronic renal failure.

Inadequate dietary intake
Renal osteodystrophy
hyperparathyroidism
rickets
Acidosis
Salt wasting
Impaired energy utilization
Endocrine disturbances
'Uraemic toxicity'

532

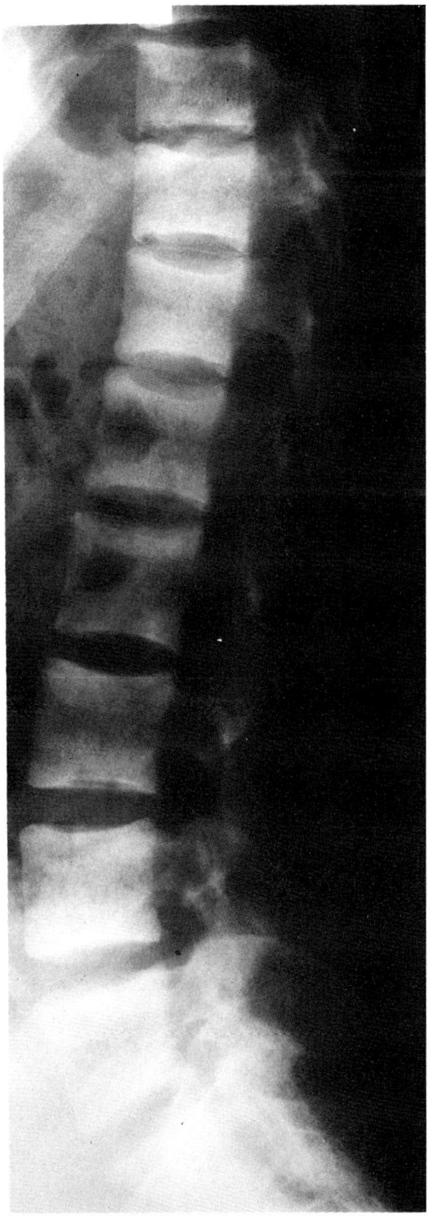

532 Renal osteodystrophy. Lateral spine X-ray: this lesion produces a 'rugger jersey' spine in patients with chronic renal failure. The appearance is due to alternating bands of sclerosis and rarefaction of the vertebrae.

Liver disease

The nutritional and dietary aspects of liver and gall-bladder diseases have been considered in several other parts of this book (cholelithiasis, Chapter 3; inborn errors, Chapter 7; toxins including ethanol, Chapter 9). Nutritional support is especially indicated in liver failure, usually resulting from cirrhosis (**533, 534**). The diet or feed should be high in energy, with normal protein and added vitamins. Sodium is restricted in the presence of ascites. If portalsystemic encephalopathy supervenes protein should be discontinued and slowly reintroduced with psychometric monitoring.

533

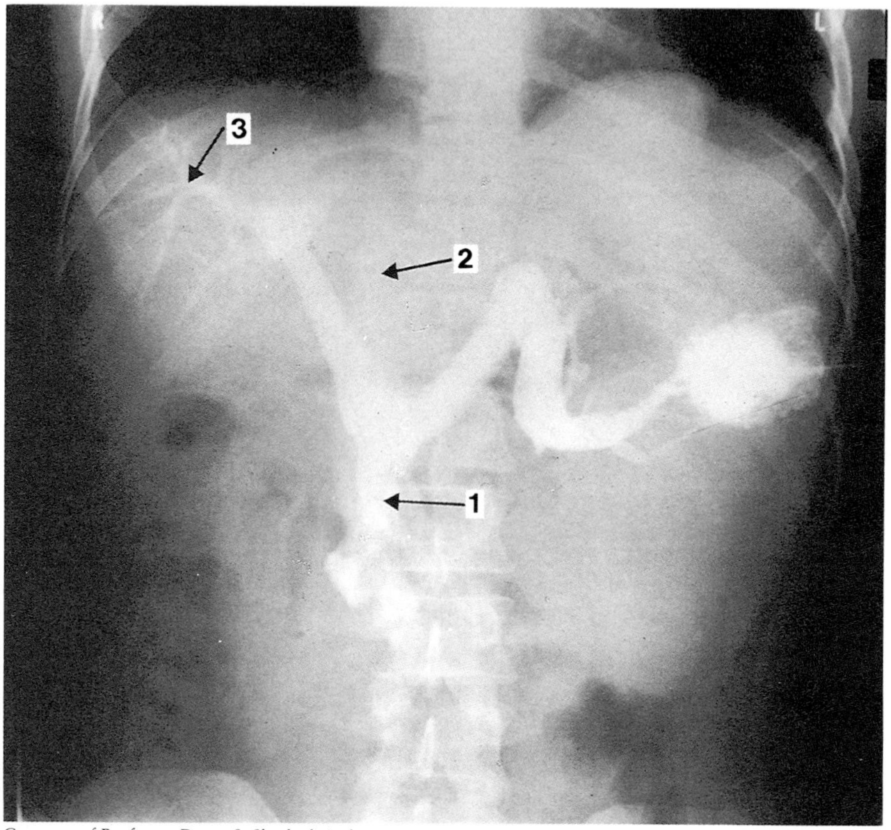

Courtesy of Professor Dame S. Sherlock and J.A. Summerfield.

533 **Liver failure.** A shunt between the superior mesenteric vein and the inferior vena cava (a meso-caval shunt) was performed in this patient. A splenic venogram showed much of the blood diverted down the superior mesenteric vein (1) which is draining into the inferior vena cava (2). Note that the portal blood supply to the liver (3) is reduced and that the oesophageal varices no longer fill.

534 Portal-systemic encephalopathy is an important complication of porto-caval shunts. This cirrhotic patient underwent a porto-caval shunt for recurrent variceal haemorrhage. Subsequently he became drowsy with a fetor and a coarse flapping tremor.

534

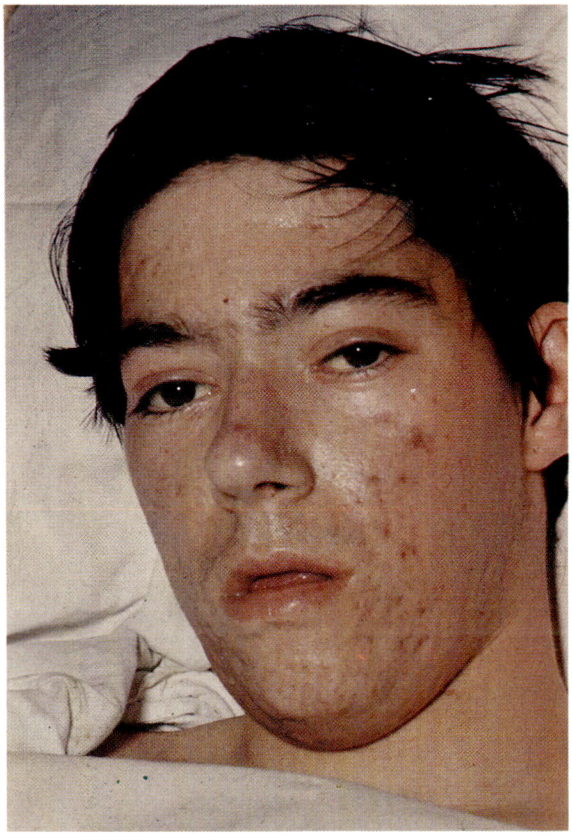

Courtesy of Professor Dame S. Sherlock and J.A. Summerfield.

11. Diseases Possibly Diet-related

In the first edition published over ten years ago seven diseases were included in this chapter. Five of these remain and have been joined by a further dozen or so. Diverticular disease is now clearly related to lack of dietary fibre and appears in Chapter 3. Cystic fibrosis has now been more precisely defined in genetic terms, but in the present context the need for nutritional support is emphasized in Chapter 10.

Osteoporosis

A great deal of research into the causes of osteoporosis has been undertaken in the past decade. It is clear that diet, especially low calcium (see Chapter 6), is only one of many risk factors (*Table 112, 535–537*).

Table 112. Risk factors for osteoporosis.

Well established evidence	**Less well established evidence**
Age (+)	Alcohol (+)
Black race (−)	Cigarette smoking (+)
Premenopausal	Exercise (−)
Oophorectomy (+)	Low dietary calcium (+)
Oestrogen use (−)	
Corticosteroid use (+)	
Marked immobility (+)	

(+) increased risk
(−) decreased risk

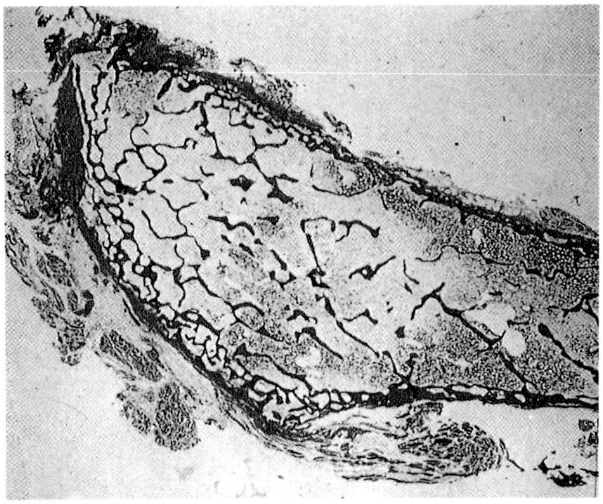
535

535 Osteoporosis. Almost the entire skeleton is usually affected but changes are most marked in the spine and pelvis. There is loss of bone mass, with thinning of the cortical bone, reabsorption of cancellous bone spicules and enlargement of the medullary cavity. Microscopically there is no evidence of new bone formation, the bone cortex is thinned and the trabeculae are narrow and delicate.

536

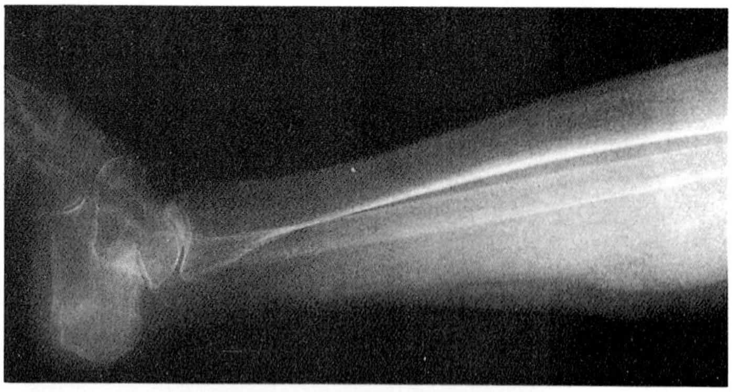

536 **Osteoporosis.** X-ray appearance of the lower leg with marked loss of density of the shafts of the tibia and fibula, and characteristic sharpening of the outlines of the small bones of the foot.

537

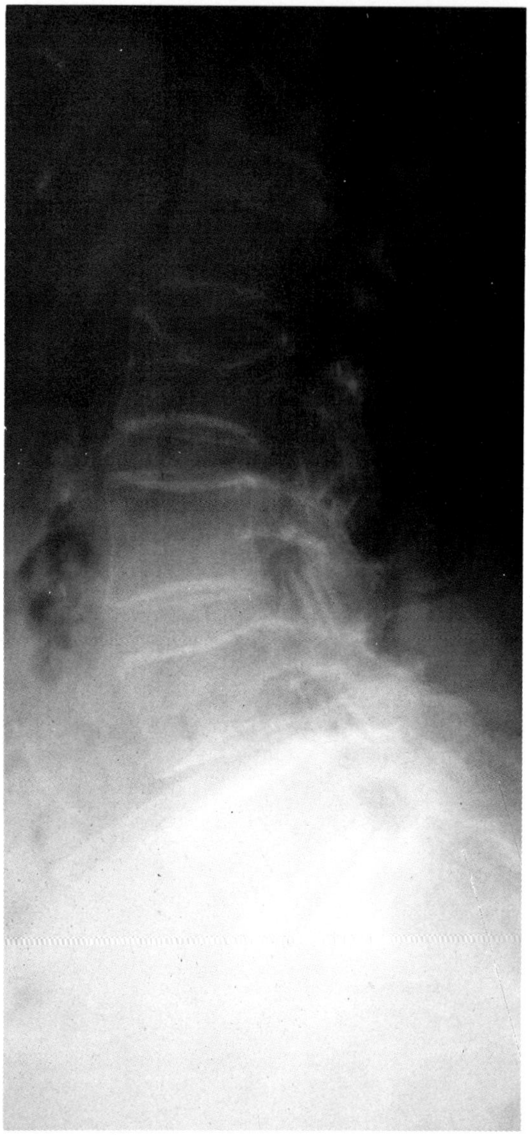

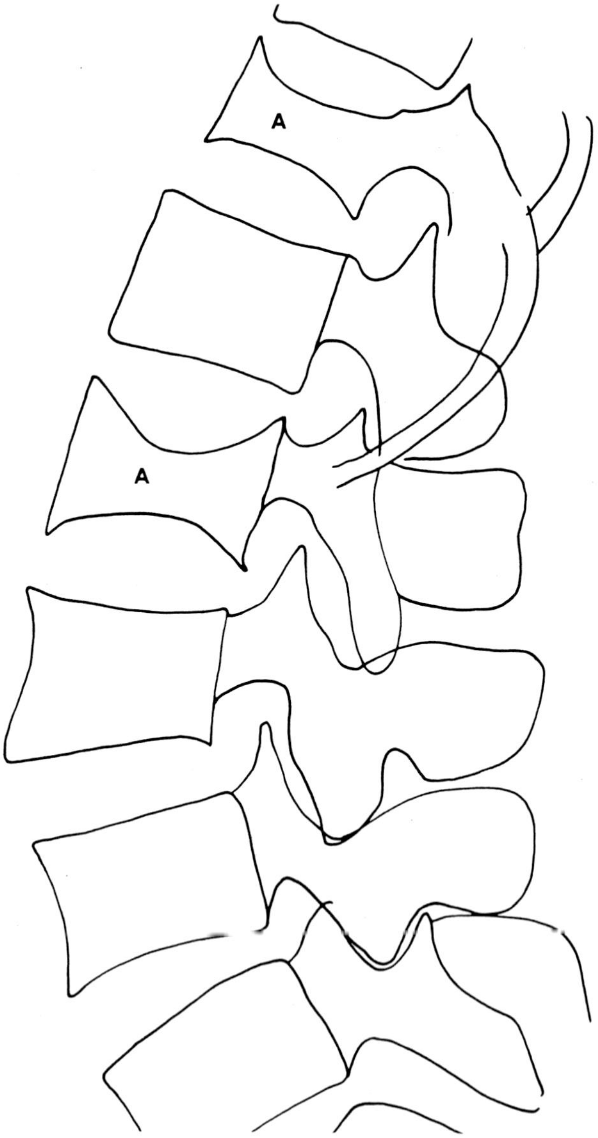

537 **Osteoporosis.** Whereas osteomalacia is due to deficient mineralization of osteoid, osteoporosis is due to deficient bone formation. In the early stages, loss of bone density is common to both disorders and differentiation may be difficult. Osteoporosis is much more common than osteomalacia and is present to some extent in most of the ageing population, particularly female. This lateral view of the lumbar spine shows loss of bone density and partial loss of height of two vertebrae (A), due to compression fractures.

Osteoporosis may be either primary in which certain factors appear to play a major part or secondary to other diseases (*Table 113*).

Osteomalacia (see Chapter 5) and osteoporosis may coexist, especially in the elderly, but the two disease states contrast markedly in many ways (*Table 114*).

Table 113. Classification of osteoporosis.

Primary (idiopathic) disease	
Decreased calcium intake	
Oestrogen deficiency	
High phosphate intake	
Immobilization	
PEM	
Secondary disease	
Hormonal	– Cushing's syndrome, steroid therapy
Genetic	– Osteogenesis imperfecta, Turner's syndrome, hypogonadism, hyperthyroidism, homocystinuria, hyperparathyroidism

Table 114. Comparison of osteoporosis with osteomalacia.

	Osteoporosis	*Osteomalacia*
Symptoms and signs		
Bone pain	Usually associated with fracture	Poorly localized, with bone tenderness
Muscle weakness	Often present	Present
Fractures	Common presenting feature	Uncommon
Skeletal deformity	Only with fracture	Common, especially kyphosis
Biochemical tests		
Plasma calcium	Normal	Low or normal
alkaline phosphatase	Normal	High
phosphate	Normal	Low
vitamin D metabolites	Normal	Very low
Urinary calcium	Normal or high	Often low
X-ray appearances		
Loss of density of bone	Irregular, mostly spine	Widespread
Loss of bone detail	None	Characteristic
Looser's zones	Absent	Diagnostic
Bone biopsy		
Histological changes	Bone mass diminished, normally mineralized	Demineralization with excess osteoid tissue

Bone mass increases during childhood and adolescence such that 97% of peak bone mass is achieved by the end of linear growth. Over the next 10–15 years it slowly reaches 100%; thereafter there is progressive loss with the rate increasing after the menopause in the female.

Peak bone mass is influenced by race (greater in black than white), sex (greater in male than female), heredity, hormones, pregnancy and the contraceptive pill. Calcium influences peak bone mass only during bone growth. Bone loss is influenced by the menopause, low body weight, smoking, alcohol, physical activity and decreased calcium absorption. The effect of calcium on fractures appears mainly to be on peak bone mass, i.e. in early life. Calcium reduces cortical bone loss, not trabecular; hormone replacement therapy (HRT) does both.[98] Calcium supplements are therefore especially recommended for children and adolescents, although a recent trial[99] with 800mg/day reduced bone loss in healthy older premenopausal women with a previous intake that was less than 400 mg. Calcium citrate malate was found to be more effective than calcium carbonate. Another study[100] suggests that axial (spine) rather than appendicular (limbs) skeleton is benefited (538).

538

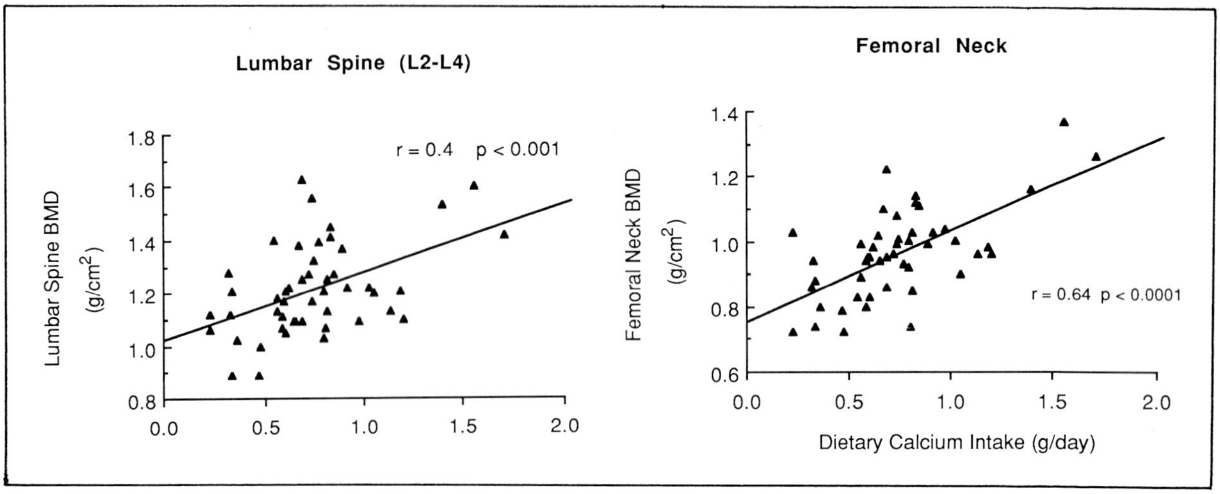

538 Relation between dietary calcium and bone mineral density (BMD) at lumbar spine and femoral neck in normal men.

Inflammatory bowel disease (IBD)

Crohn's disease (regional enteritis) (**539, 540**) and ulcerative colitis (**541, 542**) are included under this heading which covers a spectrum of disease of no known aetiology. Certain differences in disease patterns and known risk factors justify the distinction.

A recent review[101] estimates that there are between 250,000–500,000 cases in Europe with a north to south gradient. In Crohn's disease silica has been proposed as a dietary antigen causing the granulomatous reaction. Several studies have found a high sugar consumption and this is independent of smoking, which itself gives a four-fold increased risk. Patients are at increased risk of developing gastrointestinal cancer.

539 Crohn's disease. A small bowel meal demonstrating a long stricture of the terminal ileum (*arrowed*). About 30% of patients with Crohn's disease have exclusively small bowel involvement, 30% have colonic involvement alone, and 40% have combined small and large bowel disease.

539

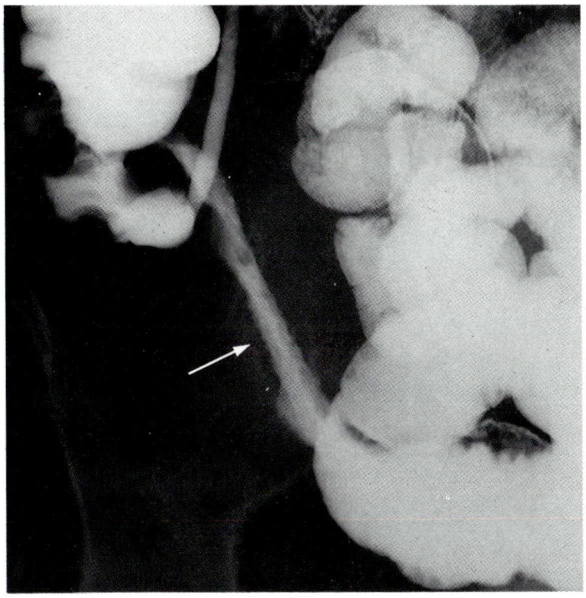

540 Crohn's disease. A surgical resection specimen from a young woman with Crohn's disease and subacute intestinal obstruction. The terminal ileum (on the right of the photograph) joins the caecum on the left. The terminal ileum is grossly thickened and inflamed (*arrowed*), and the mucosa has a cobblestone appearance except in the few centimetres proximal to the ileocaecal valve.

540

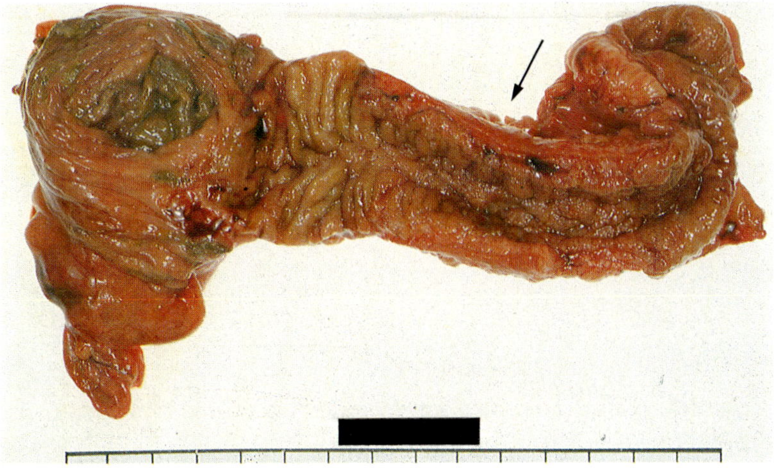

541

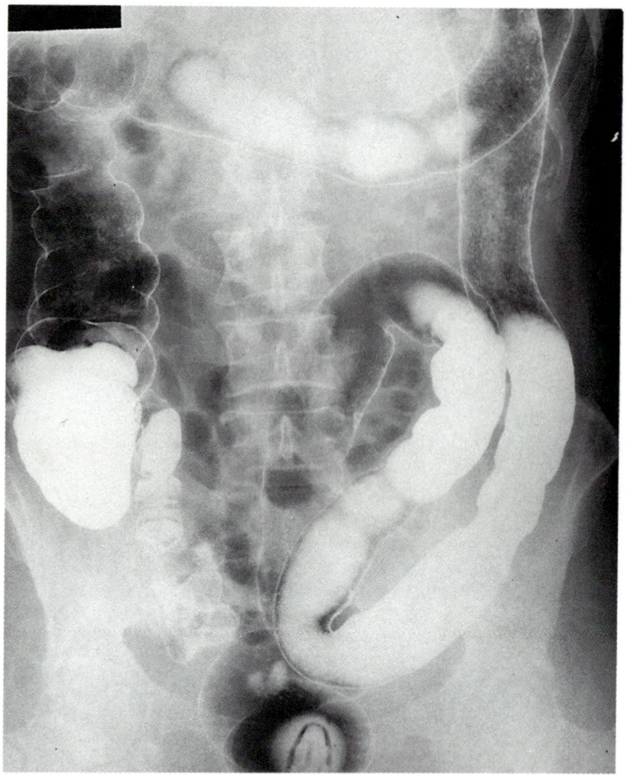

541 Ulcerative colitis. A barium enema showing a tubular colon with loss of haustral pattern. The disease extends as far as the proximal transverse colon. The rest of the colon appears spared. Barium has refluxed into the terminal ileum.

542

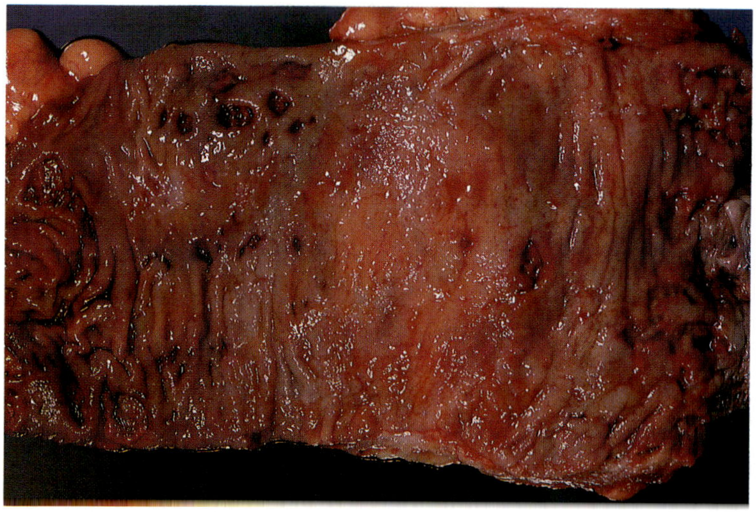

542 Ulcerative colitis. Most of the mucosa has been preserved, but punched-out ulcers are seen. Ulcers such as these may penetrate the muscle and serosa, resulting in colonic perforation.

In ulcerative colitis milk exacerbates symptoms. Many patients were either not breastfed or weaned very early, suggesting that early exposure to foreign milk protein might play a part. Smoking including nicotine may be protective as the disease has repeatedly been found to be much commoner in non-smokers.

Sprue

Steatorrhoea (**543, 544**) is a prominent feature of this tropical disease that affects expatriates more than indigenous peoples (**545–548**).

The aetiology has never been determined and a pathogen has not been isolated. Response is usually good to folic acid and a balanced diet but there is little evidence that nutritional deficiency is responsible.

543 Tropical sprue. The usual presenting complaint is persistent diarrhoea after an acute gastrointestinal infection. The figure is a dissecting micrograph of a jejunal biopsy in a patient with tropical sprue. There is partial villous atrophy, and villous fusion resulting in broad 'leaf-like' forms.

543

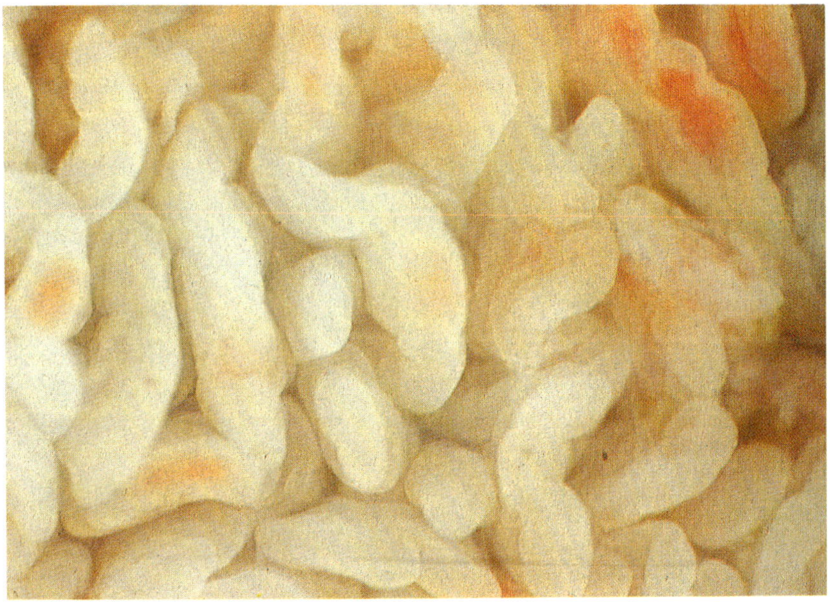

544 Tropical sprue. This jejunal biopsy section displays an increase in chronic inflammatory cells in the lamina propria and an excess of small lymphocytes within the epithelium. The villi are short and broad. These are the features of partial villous atrophy (crypt hyperplastic type).

544

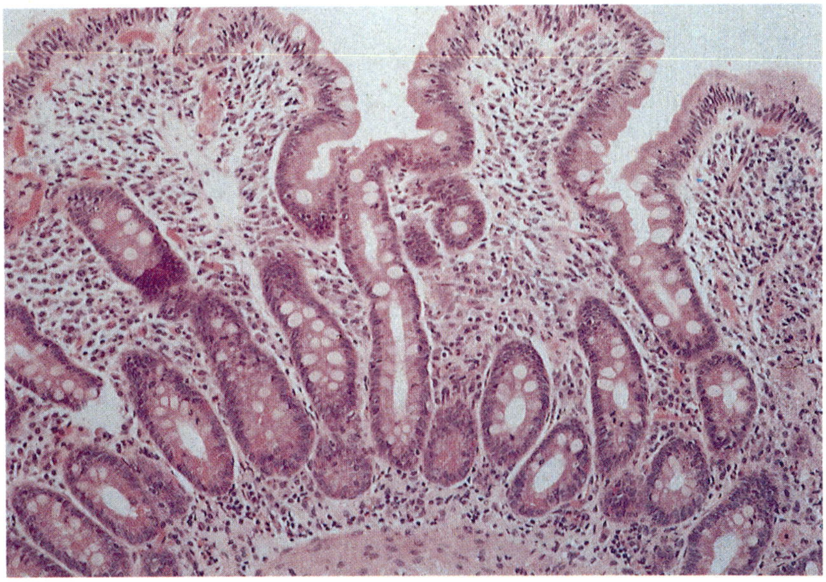

545

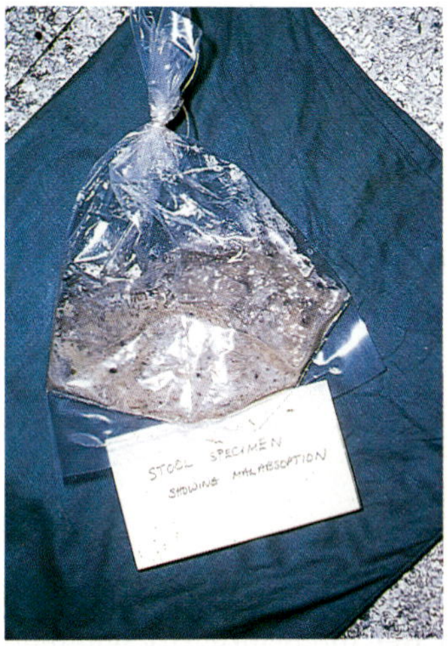

546

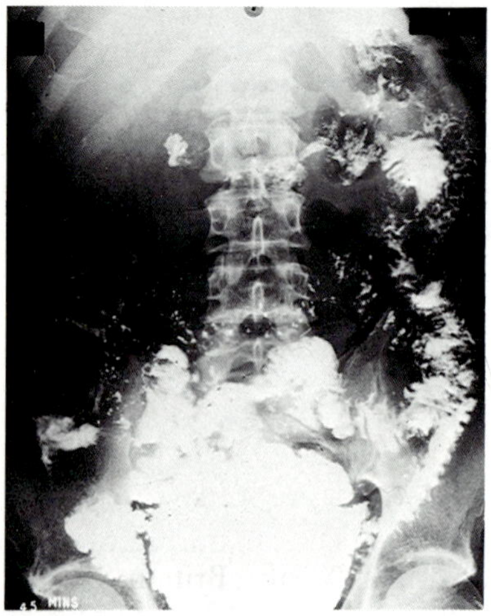

547

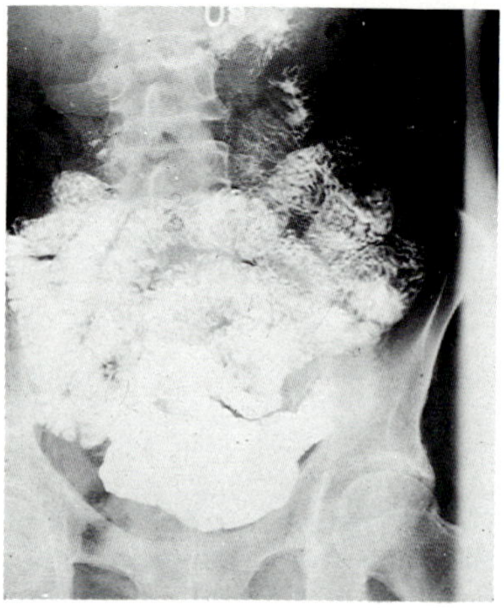

545 Sprue. Faeces from a patient with sprue. Sprue is characterized by chronic steatorrhoea with associated abdominal symptoms, glossitis and anaemia.

546, 547 Sprue. The X-rays show loss of normal intestinal pattern before (546) and recovery after 3 months of treatment (547).

548

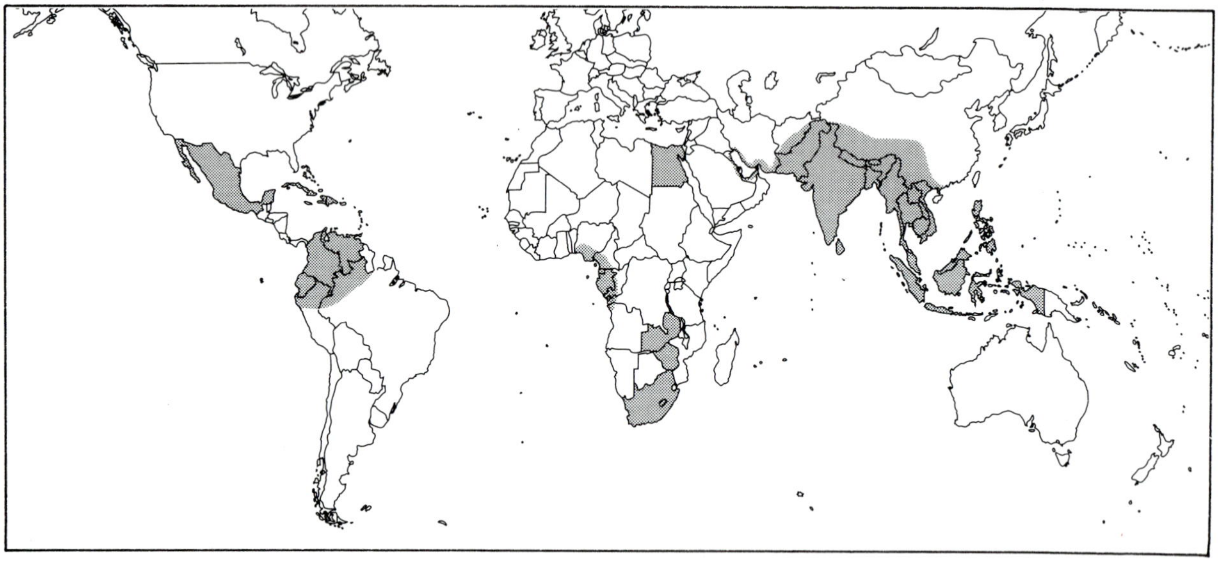

548 Sprue and sprue-like malabsorption in the tropics.

Acute appendicitis

Low dietary fibre has been favoured as the cause of the much greater prevalence of this disease in western societies. However, this does not explain the marked reduction in recent years, as fibre intake has not tended to rise over the same period. Green vegetables and tomatoes appear to provide some protection and the same group has suggested that improvements in hygiene decrease the likelihood of infections including appendicitis.[102]

Urolithiasis

There are many causes of stone formation in the urinary tract but only two types are considered here.

Endemic bladder stones affect males in 90% of cases (usually boys 2–4 years of age) and are nearly always solitary and rarely recur (**549**).

Endemic areas are southern China, Laos, northern Thailand, northern India, parts of the Middle East, Egypt, Turkey and South Africa (**550**).[103]

In some other places the disease has disappeared during this century – New York State, Norfolk in Britain, Beirut, Lebanon.[104] The stones are usually rich in urate, and a low pH and osmolarity will tend to cause saturation with calcium oxalate and a low pH will reduce the solubility of uric acid.[105] A role for diet has not been satisfactorily demonstrated.

549

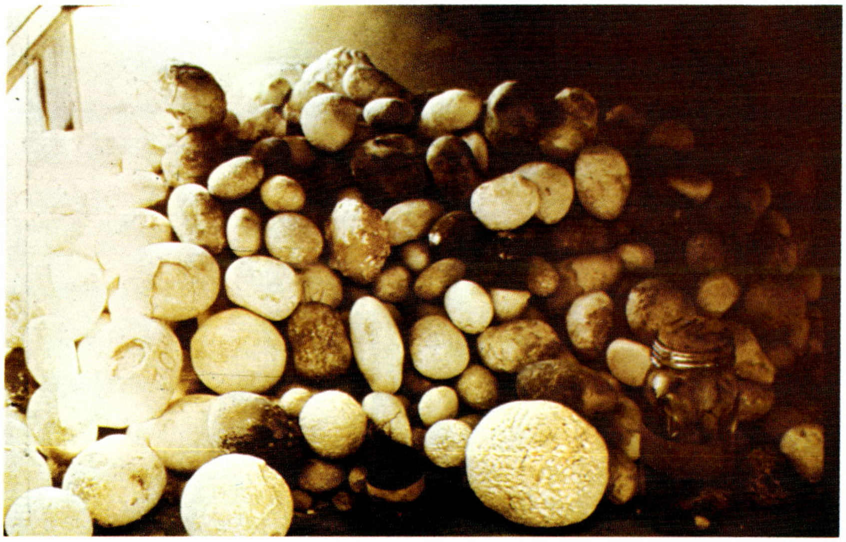

549 Endemic bladder stones. Unlike calculus formation elsewhere in the urinary tract they occur with high frequency only in certain parts of the world (see **550**). They are common in Northern Thailand where this collection was made in one hospital. There is oxalate crystaluria and this has been reduced and episodes made less frequent by increasing dietary phosphate intake. It has been suggested that phytate in a high cereal diet may chelate phosphate.

550

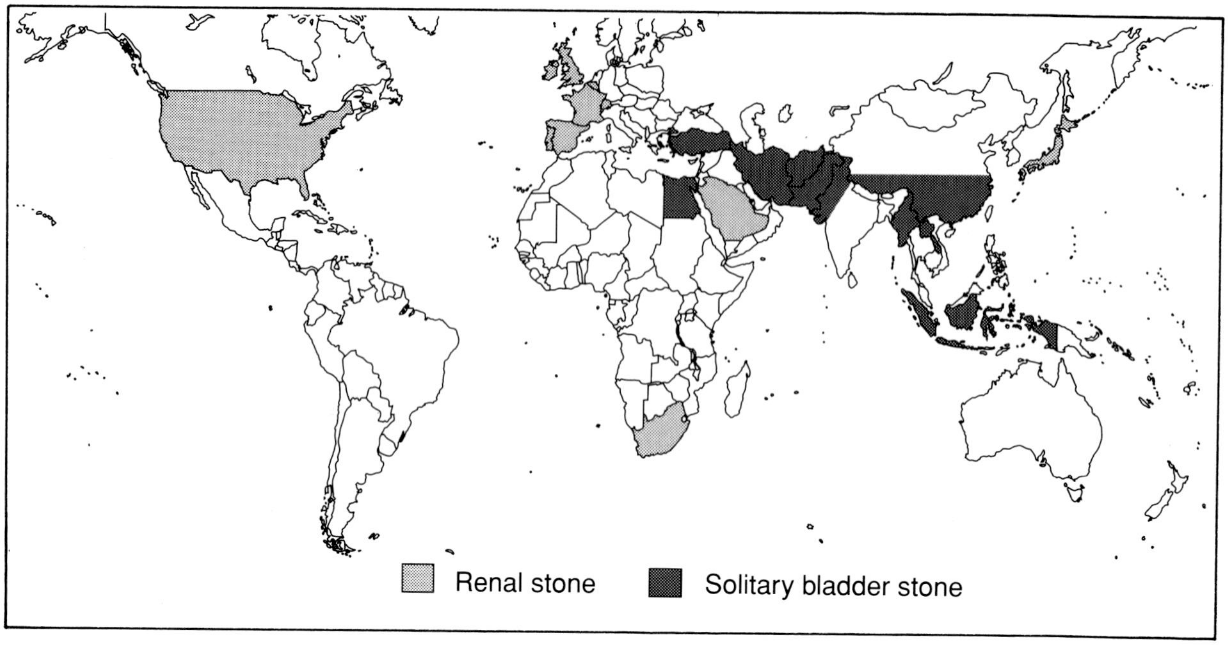

550 Global distribution of urinary tract stones.

Renal calculi are most common in Europe, North America and Japan.[106] In South Africa whites and Asians have the same high rates as in Europe but the rate is low in Bantus. In the United States the rate in blacks is increasing to become similar to that in whites.

The absolute amount of dietary calcium and the composition of the diet are important factors in influencing urinary calcium excretion. Hypercalciuria can result from a very high dietary calcium intake of more than 30mmol/day. In idiopathic calcium stone disease hypercalciuria is usually absorptive in nature; the mechanism is unknown. It has never been shown that stone formers have a higher dietary calcium intake than non-stone formers or that the diets differ in any way.

Psoriasis

Over the years many diets have been devised but no lasting benefit has been demonstrated. This scaling, papular disease (**551**) affects about 2–4% of white people and is much less common among blacks. The increased epidermal cell proliferation has led to the use of retinoids (see Chapter 5) with some success. A dose of etretinate 1mg/kg/day with meals is reduced to 0.25–0.50mg for maintenance.

551

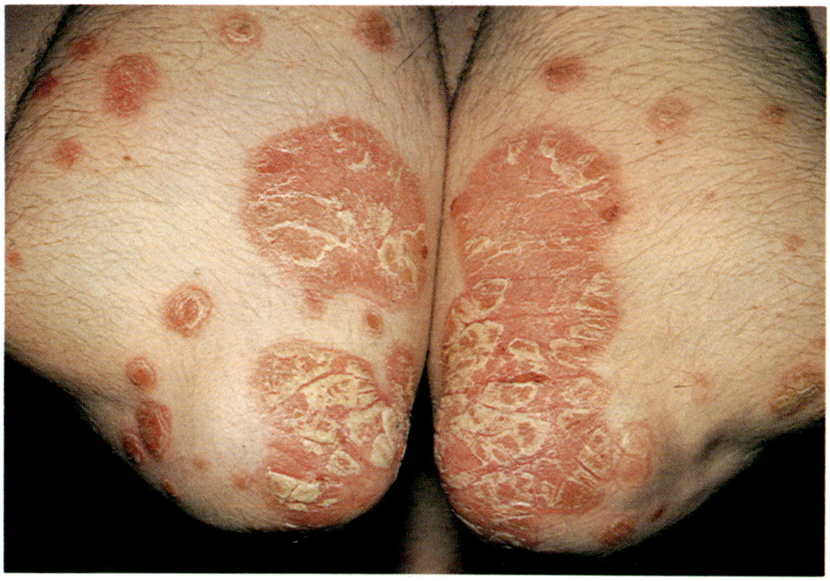

551 Psoriasis, elbows. Lesions are sharply circumscribed bright red plaques covered with coarse silvery scales. The elbows and knees are commonly involved and lesions are usually symmetrically distributed. The cause of psoriasis is unknown.

Endomyocardial fibrosis

It is now generally accepted that this disease is the same as Löffler's endocarditis seen in temperate climates (**552**).[107] In developing countries most reports have come from Uganda, Rwanda (especially in children), Nigeria, India, Sri Lanka, Brazil and Colombia. No evidence has been found for a specific nutrient deficiency.

552

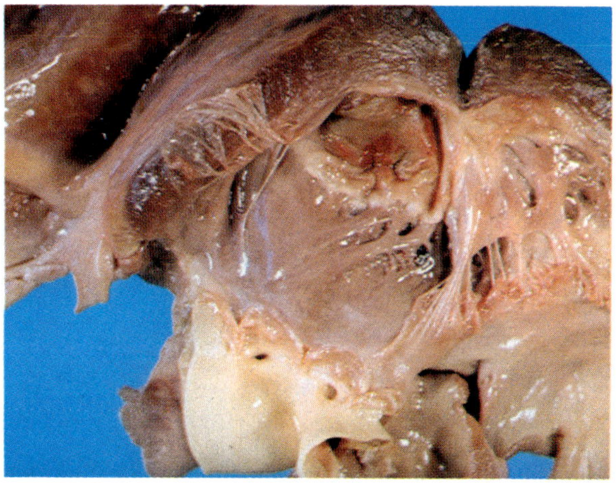

552 Endomyocardial fibrosis. The process affects the endocardium of the apices of the ventricles, extending into the cusps of the atrioventricular valves as shown here. It presents in three clinical forms: mainly left sided as mitral incompetence; right sided with features suggestive of constrictive pericarditis; and involving both sides of the heart presenting as congestive heart failure.

Cancrum oris (noma, infective gangrene of the mouth)

This grossly destructive lesion of uncertain aetiology is an occasional accompaniment of PEM of the kwashiorkor or marasmic type. Reports have come from most parts of Africa, some areas in southeast Asia and tropical America, especially in relation to famine. In the nineteenth century it occurred in Europe in association with measles, typhus, or typhoid fever (**553, 554**).

553

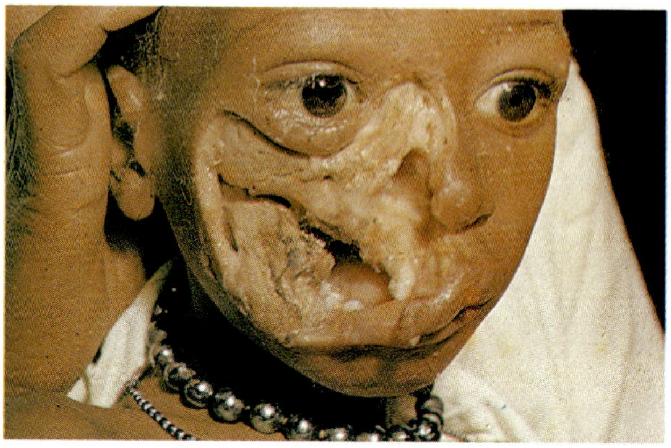

553 Cancrum oris. Undernourished subjects, especially young children, tend to show unusual patterns of infection such as generalized herpes simplex infection, severe reaction to measles (**104**), anergic and afebrile reactions to infection and, as in this condition, gangrene rather than suppuration. Impairment of the immune response is thought to be responsible. Vincent's organisms, *Borrelia vincenti* and fusiform bacteria are invariably present in cancrum oris. The lesion usually starts as an area of ulcerating stomatitis with a tender, firm swelling of the upper gum and underlying maxilla and some swelling of the overlying part of the face. The teeth become loose, and inflammation spreads into underlying bone with osteitis and a sequestrum. The cheek usually ulcerates, producing a cavity leading directly into the mouth. Good diet and antibiotics result in eventual healing but usually with gross disfigurement. Occasionally the process starts in the nose, vulva or elsewhere.

554

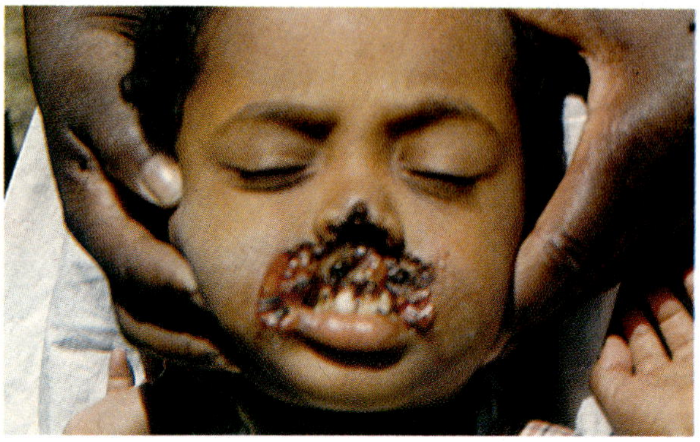

554 Cancrum oris. A healed case with less deformity than frequently seen.

Multiple sclerosis

The aetiology of multiple sclerosis (**555**) remains elusive after decades of research into all aspects.[108] This is partly due to the difficulty of making a diagnosis early in the course of the disease and also because this course is characterized by frequent remissions and relapses. Response to any modality of treatment is consequently difficult to substantiate and claims abound. These circumstances have probably conspired to permit a single investigator[109,110] over a period of more than forty years to maintain the theory that high animal fat intake is causative and that a diet high in polyunsaturated fat is beneficial. Others have been unable to confirm these claims.

555 **Multiple sclerosis.** A very common appearance. Multiple subcortical, periventricular and central white matter plaques. Note grey translucency of chronic lesions (× 0.5).

555

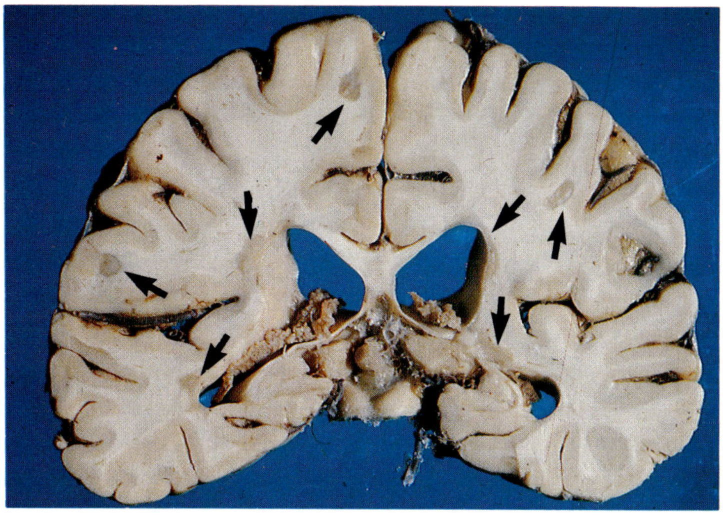

Alzheimer's disease (senile dementia)

A similar state of dementia in dialysis patients has been attributed to aluminium toxicity (see page 269). One group of workers[111] has put forward evidence to support the theory that both aluminium and silica may be involved in Alzheimer's disease in the form of amorphous aluminosilicates which they have demonstrated at the core of senile plaques in the brains of patients dying with the disease (556).

556

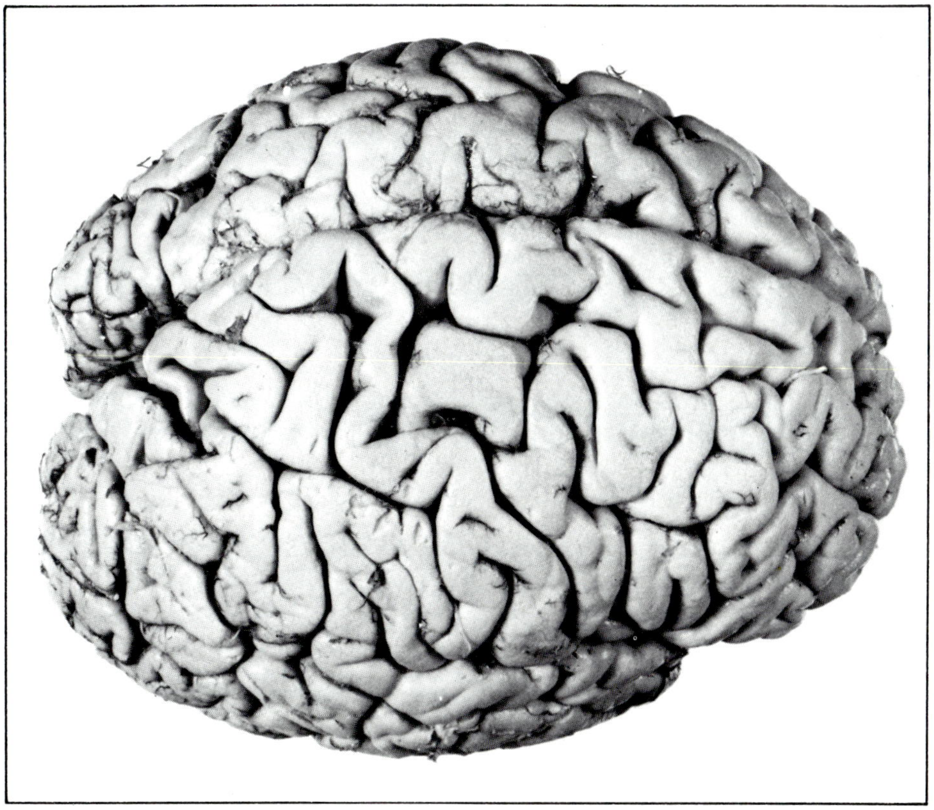

556 **Alzheimer's disease.** Generalized cerebral cortical atrophy has resulted in narrowing of gyri and widening of sulci, particularly in the parietal region. (× 0.7)

Chronic fatigue syndrome (myalgic encephalomyelitis)

Failure to recover normal energy and persistence of muscle pains after trivial febrile illness has attracted much attention recently. There is no obvious aetiology and some doubt the existence of such an entity. In a recent clinical trial[112] the red blood cell content of magnesium was found to be low, and magnesium supplementation restored levels to normal accompanied by symptomatic improvement and return of energy. Confirmation is awaited.

Discrete colliquative keratopathy (DCK)

This term was applied to a painless, non-inflammatory localized perforation of a small area of the cornea, frequently with a small prolapsed knuckle of iris by the writer from his experience with a number of cases in East Africa in the early 1960s. It had previously been described in South Africa as 'malnutrition keratitis' although there is no definite evidence that nutritional deficiency plays a part. Young children are usually affected. The condition spontaneously heals, unlike keratomalacia (see 207–209) leaving a small leucoma and vitamin A is not effective (557, 558).

557

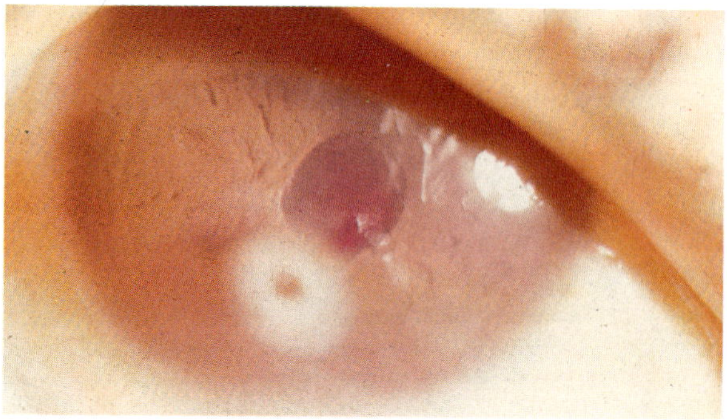

557 **Discrete colliquative keratopathy** (DCK). This is an active lesion.

558

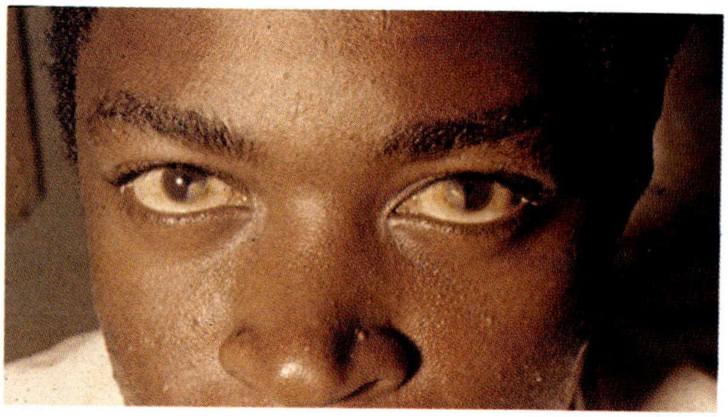

558 **Discrete colliquative keratopathy** (DCK). Typical healed lesions.

Refractive errors

During fetal life the retina takes over the function of 'organizer' of emmetropia (normal refraction). Studies of twins have shown that heredity plays a dominant role normally in determining refraction.[113] However, under adverse circumstances environmental factors might come into play. The possible effects of famine in pre- and early postnatal life on refraction were investigated in Tanzania by the author in the 1960s.[114] 559 shows the marked differences in the incidence of refractive errors between a famine area (Mvumi) and a non-famine area (Mwanza).

In Japan myopia has been reported to have declined by 50–70% in recent years and this has occurred in step with marked improvement in nutrition although a causal relationship is not proved.

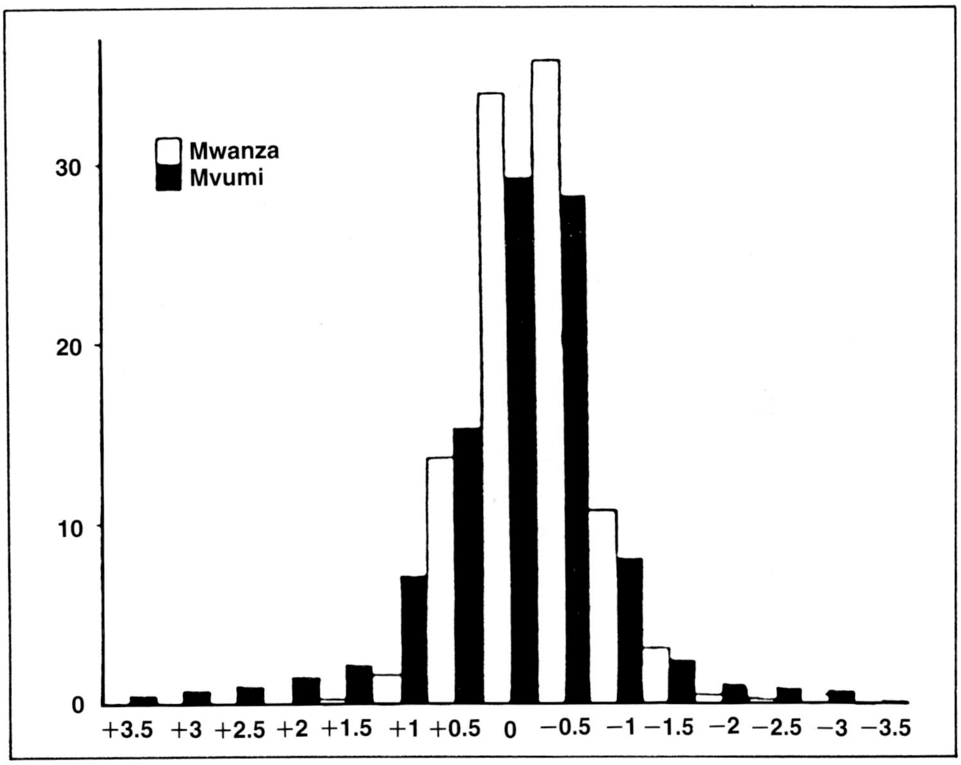

559 Refractive errors and undernutrition. Percentage distribution of mean refraction within the limits ±4.0D. Beyond these limits the differences were even more marked: 23 high myopes and 5 high hypermetropes at Mvumi compared with 1 high hypermetrope at Mwanza.

Age-related macular degeneration

Over the age of 75 almost 30% of the population in western societies are affected and the condition has become the leading cause of visual loss among the elderly (see **413**). There is a high proportion of polyunsaturated fatty acids in the photoreceptors of the macula and it has the highest oxygen consumption of any tissue in the body. These fatty acids are very susceptible to oxidative degredation and it has been postulated that natural dietary antioxidants such as vitamin E, vitamin C and B-carotene may be protective.[115] Other work has suggested that zinc, which is normally in high concentration in the retinal pigment epithelium and in which the elderly are often deficient (see Chapter 6), may be involved. Improvement has been claimed with zinc supplementation.[116]

Rheumatoid arthritis

Many diets have been devised for this prevalent disease without true benefit (**560**). Arthritic patients are often undernourished but this is most likely to be secondary to the disease from anorexia, interference with chewing and swallowing if the temporomandibular joint is involved, pain, fever, and discomfort. On the basis that the disease is considered to be rare among Eskimos (see page 25) supplementing patients' diets with fish oils has been tested. In one well-designed study supplementation of the diet with fatty fish such as mackerel and cod which are rich in the oils eicosapentaenoic acid (EPA) and docosahexaenoic acid (DHA) brought about a significant improvement in the time of onset of fatigue and tenderness of joints.[117] The effect was proportional to the decrease in production of neutrophil leukotriene B_4, possibly involved in the inflammatory process.

560

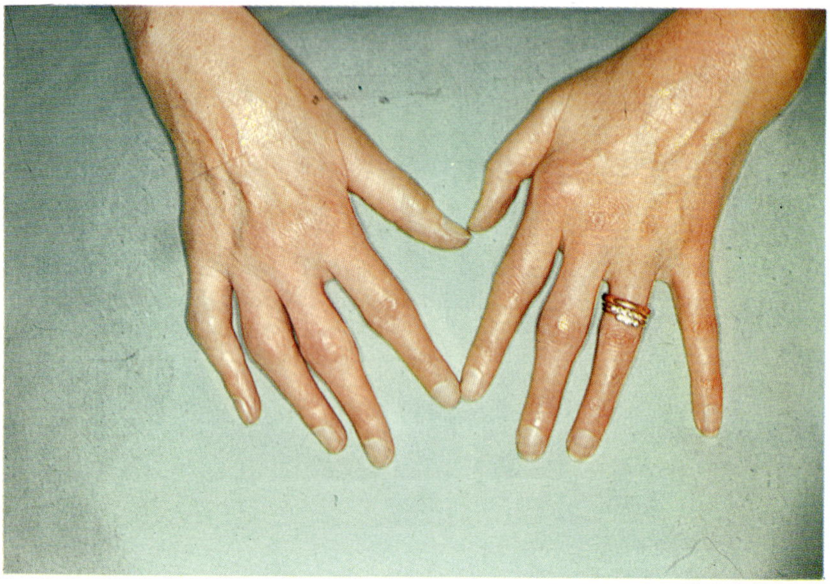

560 **Early rheumatoid arthritis of the hands.** Although sometimes starting as a monarthritis, this disease usually begins as a symmetrical polyarthritis, the finger joints commonly presenting the earliest manifestations of pain, swelling and stiffness most marked in the early morning.

Systemic lupus erythematosus

This common inflammatory connective tissue disorder is of unknown aetiology but the presence of antinuclear antibodies in the serum suggests that it is autoimmune in origin. Many systems are affected and the serious form is life threatening, requiring steroid therapy. Until recently there has been no specific form of treatment but the results of a double-blind cross-over study suggest that a good clinical response occurs with a diet low in fat but containing 20g of marine oil (Maxepa, see Chapter 2) daily for many weeks (**561**).[118]

561 An erythematous 'butterfly' rash on the face is a classic sign in systemic lupus erythematosus.

561

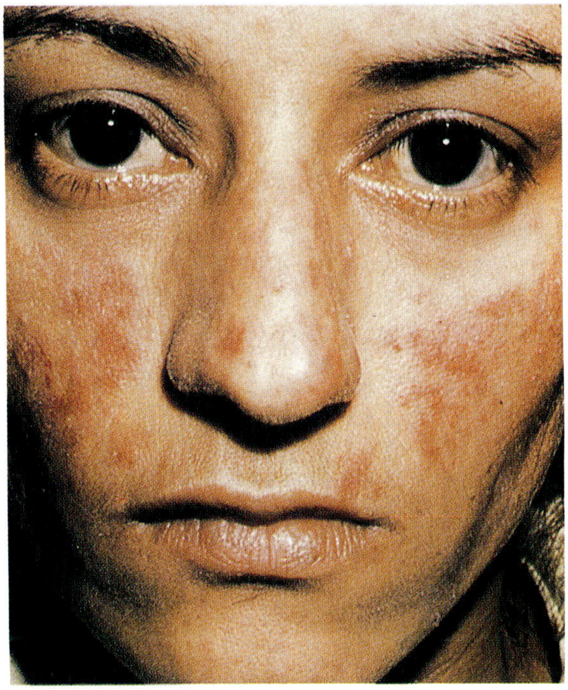

Appendix I

Table 1. Estimated Average Requirements (EARs) for energy.

Ages	*EARs MJ/day (kcal/day)*	
	Males	**Females**
0–3 months	2.28 (545)	2.16 (515)
4–6 months	2.89 (690)	2.69 (645)
7–9 months	3.44 (825)	3.20 (765)
10–12 months	3.85 (920)	3.61 (865)
1–3 years	5.15 (1,230)	4.86 (1,165)
4–6 years	7.16 (1,715)	6.46 (1,545)
7–10 years	8.24 (1,970)	7.28 (1,740)
11–14 years	9.27 (2,220)	7.92 (1,845)
15–18 years	11.51 (2,755)	8.83 (2,110)
19–50 years	10.60 (2,550)	8.10 (1,940)
51–59 years	10.60 (2,550)	8.00 (1,900)
60–64 years	9.93 (2,380)	7.99 (1,900)
65–74 years	9.71 (2,330)	7.96 (1,900)
75 + years	8.77 (2,100)	7.61 (1,810)
Pregnancy		+ 0.80* (200)
Lactation:		
1 month		+ 1.90 (450)
2 months		+ 2.20 (530)
3 months		+ 2.40 (570)
4–6 months (Group 1)		+ 2.00 (480)
4–6 months (Group 2)		+ 2.40 (570)
> 6 months (Group 1)		+ 1.00 (240)
> 6 months (Group 2)		+ 2.30 (550)

* Last trimester only

Table 2. Dietary Reference Values for fat and carbohydrate for adults as a percentage of daily total energy intake (percentage of food energy).

	Individual minimum		*Population average*	*Individual maximum*
Saturated fatty acids			10 (11)	
Cis-polyunsaturated fatty acids			6 (6.5)	10
	n–3	0.2		
	n–6	1.0		
Cis-monounsaturated fatty acids			12 (13)	
Trans fatty acids			2 (2)	
Total fatty acids			30 (32.5)	
Total fat			33 (35)	
Non-milk extrinsic sugars		0	10 (11)	
Intrinsic and milk sugars and starch			37 (39)	
Total carbohydrate			47 (50)	
Non-starch polysaccharide (g/day)		12	18	24

The average percentage contribution to total energy does not total 100% because figures for protein and alcohol are excluded. Protein intakes average 15% of total energy which is above the RNI. It is recognized that many individuals will derive some energy from alcohol, and this has been assumed to average 5% approximating to current intakes. However, the Panel allowed that some groups might not drink alcohol and that for some purposes nutrient intakes as a proportion of food energy (without alcohol) might be useful. Therefore average figures are given as percentages both of total energy and, in parentheses, of food energy.

Table 3. Reference Nutrient Intakes for protein.

Age	*Reference Nutrient Intake* (g/day)*
0–3 months	12.5**
4–6 months	12.7
7–9 months	13.7
10–12 months	14.9
1–3 years	14.5
4–6 years	19.7
7–10 years	28.3
Males	
11–14 years	42.1
15–18 years	55.2
19–50 years	55.5
50+ years	53.3
Females	
11–14 years	41.2
15–18 years	45.0
19–50 years	45.0
50+ years	46.5
*Pregnancy****	+6
*Lactation****	
0–4 months	+11
4+ months	+8

* These figures, based on egg and milk protein, assume complete digestibility.
** No values for infants 0–3 months are given by WHO.
*** To be added to adult requirement through all stages of pregnancy and lactation.

Table 4. Reference Nutrient Intakes for vitamins.

Age	*Thiamin*	*Riboflavin*	*Niacin (nicotinic acid equivalent)*	*Vitamin B_6*	*Vitamin B_{12}*	*Folate*	*Vitamin C*	*Vitamin A*	*Vitamin D*
	mg/day	*mg/day*	*mg/day*	*mg/day†*	*µg/day*	*µg/day*	*mg/day*	*µg/day*	*µg/day*
0–3 months	0.2	0.4	3	0.2	0.3	50	25	350	8.5
4–6 months	0.2	0.4	3	0.2	0.3	50	25	350	8.5
7–9 months	0.2	0.4	4	0.3	0.4	50	25	350	7
10–12 months	0.3	0.4	5	0.4	0.4	50	25	350	7
1–3 years	0.5	0.6	8	0.7	0.5	70	30	400	7
4–6 years	0.7	0.8	11	0.9	0.8	100	30	500	—
7–10 years	0.7	1.0	12	1.0	1.0	150	30	500	—
Males									
11–14 years	0.9	1.2	15	1.2	1.2	200	35	600	—
15–18 years	1.1	1.3	18	1.5	1.5	200	40	700	—
19–50 years	1.0	1.3	17	1.4	1.5	200	40	700	—
50+ years	0.9	1.3	16	1.4	1.5	200	40	700	**
Females									
11–14 years	0.7	1.1	12	1.0	1.2	200	35	600	—
15–18 years	0.8	1.1	14	1.2	1.5	200	40	600	—
19–50 years	0.8	1.1	13	1.2	1.5	200	40	600	—
50+ years	0.8	1.1	12	1.2	1.5	200	40	600	**
Pregnancy	+0.1***	+0.3	*	*	*	+100	+10	+100	10
Lactation:									
0–4 months	+0.2	+0.5	+2	*	+0.5	+ 60	>0	>50	10
4+ months	+0.2	+0.5	+2	*	+0.5	+ 60	+30	+350	10

* No increment
** After age 65 the RNI is 10µg/day for men and women
*** For last trimester only
† Based on protein providing 14.7% of EAR for energy

Table 5. Reference Nutrient Intakes for minerals (SI units).

Age	*Calcium*	*Phos-phorus***	*Magne-sium*	*Sodium****	*Potassium*†	*Chloride*††	*Iron*	*Zinc*	*Copper*	*Selenium*	*Iodine*
	mmol/day	*mmol/day*	*mmol/day*	*mmol/day*	*mmol/day*	*mmol/day*	*μmol/day*	*μmol/day*	*μmol/day*	*μmol/day*	*μmol/day*
0–3 months	13.1	13.1	2.2	9	20	9	30	60	5	0.1	0.4
4–6 months	13.1	13.1	2.5	12	22	12	80	60	5	0.2	0.5
7–9 months	13.1	13.1	3.2	14	18	14	140	75	5	0.1	0.5
10–12 months	13.1	13.1	3.3	15	18	15	140	75	5	0.1	0.5
1–3 years	8.8	8.8	3.5	22	20	22	120	75	6	0.2	0.6
4–6 years	11.3	11.3	4.8	30	28	30	110	100	9	0.3	0.8
7–10 years	13.8	13.8	8.0	50	50	50	160	110	11	0.4	0.9
Males											
11–14 years	25.0	25.0	11.5	70	80	70	200	140	13	0.6	1.0
15–18 years	25.0	25.0	12.3	70	90	70	200	145	16	0.9	1.0
19–50 years	17.5	17.5	12.3	70	90	70	160	145	19	0.9	1.0
50+ years	17.5	17.5	12.3	70	90	70	160	145	19	0.9	1.0
Females											
11–14 years	20.0	10.0	11.5	70	80	70	260†††	140	13	0.6	1.0
15–18 years	20.0	20.0	12.3	70	90	70	260†††	110	16	0.8	1.1
19–50 years	17.5	17.5	10.9	70	90	70	260†††	110	19	0.8	1.1
50+ years	17.5	17.5	10.9	70	90	70	160	110	19	0.8	1.1
Pregnancy	*	*	*	*	*	*	*	*	*	*	*
Lactation:											
0–4 months	+14.3	+14.3	+2.1	*	*	*	*	+90	+5	+0.2	*
4+ months	+14.3	+14.3	+2.1	*	*	*	*	+40	+5	+0.2	*

* No increment
** Phosphorus RNI is set equal to calcium in molar terms
*** 1 mmol sodium = 23 mg
† 1 mmol potassium = 39 mg
†† Corresponds to sodium 1 mmol = 35.5 mg
††† Insufficient for women with high menstrual losses where the most practical way of meeting iron requirements is to take iron supplements.

Table 6. Reference Nutrient Intakes for minerals (metric units).

Age	*Calcium*	*Phos-phorus***	*Magne-sium*	*Sodium****	*Potassium†*	*Chlo-ride††*	*Iron*	*Zinc*	*Copper*	*Selenium*	*Iodine*
	mg/day	*mg/day*	*mg/day*	*mg/day*	*mg/day*	*mg/day*	*mg/day*	*mg/day*	*mg/day*	*μg/day*	*μg/day*
0–3 months	525	400	55	210	800	320	1.7	4.0	0.2	10	50
4–6 months	525	400	60	280	850	400	4.3	4.0	0.3	13	60
7–9 months	525	400	75	320	700	500	7.8	5.0	0.3	10	60
10–12 months	525	400	80	350	700	500	7.8	5.0	0.3	10	60
1–3 years	350	270	85	500	800	800	6.9	5.0	0.4	15	70
4–6 years	450	350	120	700	1100	1100	6.1	6.5	0.6	20	100
7–10 years	550	450	200	1200	2000	1800	8.7	7.0	0.7	30	110
Males											
11–14 years	1000	775	280	1600	3100	2500	11.3	9.0	0.8	45	130
15–18 years	1000	775	300	1600	3500	2500	11.3	9.5	1.0	70	140
19–50 years	700	550	300	1600	3500	2500	8.7	9.5	1.2	75	140
50+ years	700	550	300	1600	3500	2500	8.7	9.5	1.2	75	140
Females											
11–14 years	800	625	280	1600	3100	2500	14.8†††	9.0	0.8	45	130
15–18 years	800	625	300	1600	3500	2500	14.8†††	7.0	1.0	60	140
19–50 years	700	550	270	1600	3500	2500	14.8†††	7.0	1.2	60	140
50+ years	700	550	270	1600	3500	2500	8.7	7.0	1.2	60	140
Pregnancy	*	*	*	*	*	*	*	*	*	*	*
Lactation:											
0–4 months	+550	+440	+ 50	*	*	*	*	+6.0	+0.3	+15	*
4+ months	+550	+440	+ 50	*	*	*	*	+2.5	+0.3	+15	*

* No increment
** Phosphorus RNI is set equal to calcium in molar terms
*** 1 mmol sodium = 23 mg
† 1 mmol potassium = 39 mg
†† Corresponds to sodium 1 mmol = 35.5 mg
††† Insufficient for women with high menstrual losses where the most practical way of meeting iron requirements is to take iron supplements.

Table 7. Safe intakes

Nutrient	*Safe intake*
Vitamins	
Pantothenic acid	
adults	3–7 mg/day
infants	1.7 mg/day
Biotin	10–200 μg/day
Vitamin E	
men	above 4 mg/day
women	above 3 mg/day
infants	0.4 mg/g polyunsaturated fatty acids
Vitamin K	
adults	1 μg/kg/day
infants	10 μg/day
Minerals	
Manganese	
adults	1.4 mg (26 μmol)/day
infants and children	16 μg (0.3 μmol)/day
Molybdenum	
adults	50–400 μg/day
infants, children and adolescents	0.5–1.5 μg/kg/day
Chromium	
adults	25 μg (0.5 μmol)/day
children and adolescents	0.1–1.0 μg (2–20 μmol)/kg/day
Fluoride (for infants only)	0.05 mg (3 μmol)/kg/day

Appendix II

Table 1. Estimated requirements of indispensable amino acids (mg/kg/day).

Amino acid	*Infants*	*Children (10–12 years)*	*Adults*
Isoleucine	111	30	10
Leucine	153	49	13
Lysine	96	59	10
Methionine + cystine	50	27	13
Phenylalanine + tyrosine	90	27	13
Threonine	66	34	7
Tryptophan	19	4	3
Valine	95	33	11
Histidine	28	–	–

Table 2. Indispensability of amino acids.

Classical indispensable	
	Lysine, threonine, isoleucine, leucine, valine, methionine, phenylalanine, tryptophan (the first two are totally indispensable; for the others the ketoacid or hydroxyacid analogue can be converted in the body to the corresponding amino acid)
Now considered indispensable for all age groups	
	Histidine
Conditionally indispensable	
	Taurine (especially in low birthweight infants and long-term parenteral nutrition)
	Cysteine (term and pre-term infants, older children with inborn errors e.g. homocystinuria, liver damage)
	Tyrosine (pre-term and some full-term infants, liver damage)
	Arginine, citrulline, ornithine (in some genetic disorders and liver failure; arginine has strong antitumour activity and improves the immune response after trauma and sepsis)

Appendix III

Table 1. Biochemical assessment of vitamin nutritional status.

Vitamin	*Laboratory test(s)*	*Normal value or range*
Vitamin A (retinol)	Serum retinol	0.7–1.7 μmol/l
Vitamin D (cholecalciferol)	Serum level	
25-OHD		23.8–111 nmol/l
$24,25(OH)_2D_3$		12.5–125 nmol/l
$1,25(OH)_2D_3$		1.25–7.5 nmol/l 50–100 pmol/l
Vitamin E (tocopherol)	Serum tocopherol Haemolysis test with H_2O_2	0.5 mg/dl > 20%
Vitamin K (phylloquinone)	Plasma prothrombin PIVKA II test	20% reduction is deficient > 4 AU/ml is deficient
Essential fatty acids	Ratio in plasma of 20:3w9/20:4	ratio ≥ 0.4
Thiamin (vitamin B_1)	Red cell transketolase	40–90 i.u./l activation coefficient 1.25
Niacin (nicotinic acid)	Urinary N^1-methyl nicotinamide	1.5 mmol/l
Riboflavin	Plasma Red cell glutathione reductase	21.3 nmol/l activation coefficient 1.30
Pyridoxine (vitamin B_6)	Plasma	178 nmol/l
Folic acid	Serum folate Red cell folate	6.8 nmol/l 0.23 μmol/l
Vitamin B_{12} (cobalamin)	Serum vitamin B_{12}	110 pmol/l
Vitamin C (ascorbic acid)	Serum ascorbate Buffy coat ascorbate	11 μmol/l 40 nmol/10^8WBC

Table 2. Biochemical assessment of essential element nutritional status.

Essential element	*Laboratory test(s)*	*Normal value or range*
Iron	Serum total iron binding capacity Serum ferritin	54–75 μmol/l male: 14–31 μmol/l female: 11–30 μmol/l
Iodine	Urinary iodine Serum protein-bound iodine	50 μg/g creatinine 276–550 nmol/l
Sodium	Plasma sodium	135–145 mmol/l
Chloride	Plasma chloride	95–105 mmol/l
Potassium	Plasma potassium	3.3–4.7 mmol/l
Magnesium	Plasma magnesium	0.75–1.05 mmol/l
Calcium	Plasma calcium (ionized) (total)	1.0–1.25 mmol/l 2.12–2.65 mmol/l
Phosphate (inorganic)	Plasma phosphate	0.9–1.38 mmol/l
Zinc	Plasma	6–25 μmol/l
Copper	Plasma	12–26 mmol/l
Selenium	Plasma Plasma glutathione peroxidase	1–2 μmol/l –
Cobalt	Plasma	8 nmol/l
Manganese	Plasma	0.15 μmol/l

Appendix IV

Table 1. Clinical signs of nutritional deficiency and their interpretation.

Signs	*Associated disorder or nutrient*
Hair	
Lack of lustre	
Thinness and sparseness	
Straightness	Protein energy malnutrition
Dyspigmentation	(kwashiorkor more commonly than marasmus)
Flag sign	
Easy pluckability	
'Swan neck' deformity	Scurvy
Face	
Nasolabial dyssebacia	Riboflavin
Moon-face	Kwashiorkor
Eyes	
Pale conjunctiva	Anaemia (iron etc.)
Bitot's spot	
Conjunctival xerosis	Vitamin A
Corneal xerosis	
Keratomalacia	
Angular palpebritis	Riboflavin, pyridoxine
Lips	
Angular stomatitis	Riboflavin
Angular scars (rhagades)	Riboflavin
Cheilosis	Riboflavin
Tongue	
Scarlet and raw tongue	Niacin
Magenta tongue	Riboflavin
Glossitis	Vitamin B_{12}, folate, iron, vitamin B_6
Teeth	
Mottled enamel	Fluorosis
Pitted enamel	More severe fluorosis
Caries	Associated with low fluorine intake
Gums	
Spongy, bleeding	Scurvy
Hypertrophied interdental papillae	Scurvy
Glands	
Thyroid enlargement, goitre	Iodine
Parotid enlargement (painless)	Starvation

Table 1. Continued.

Signs	*Associated disorder or nutrient*
Nails	
Brittle, ridged	Protein-energy malnutrition, zinc
Spoon-shaped (koilonychia)	Iron
White nail beds	Selenium
Skin	
Perifollicular hyperkeratosis	Vitamin A and other factors
Dry, scaling	Essential fatty acids, zinc and other factors
Petechiae	Scurvy and other causes
Ecchymoses	Scurvy and other causes
Symmetrical dermatosis, photosensitive	Pellagra
Flaky paint and 'crazy paving' dermatosis	Kwashiorkor
Scrotal and vulval dermatosis	Riboflavin
Subcutaneous tissue	
Oedema	Kwashiorkor
Fat decreased	Starvation, marasmus
Muscular and skeletal systems	
Muscle wasting	Starvation, PEM
Craniotabes	
Frontal and parietal bossing	
Epiphyseal enlargement	
Persistently open anterior fontanelle	Rickets
Knock knees, bow legs	also fluorosis
Thoracic rosary	also scurvy
Musculoskeletal haemorrhages	Scurvy
Other systems	
Hepatomegaly	Kwashiorkor
Psychomotor changes	Kwashiorkor
Mental confusion	Beriberi, pellagra
Sensory loss	
Motor weakness	
Motor weakness	
Loss of position sense	
Loss of vibration sense	Beriberi
Loss of ankle and knee jerks	
Calf tenderness	
Ophthalmoplegia	
Cardiac enlargement	
Cardiomyopathy	Selenium

Appendix V

Table 1. Recommendations of the Report on Nutrition and Health.[22]

Issues for Most People:

- *Fats and cholesterol:* Reduce consumption of fat (especially saturated fat) and cholesterol. Choose foods relatively low in these substances, such as vegetables, fruits, whole grain foods, fish, poultry, lean meats, and low-fat dairy products. Use food preparation methods that add little or no fat.

- *Energy and weight control:* Achieve and maintain a desirable body weight. To do so, choose a dietary pattern in which energy (caloric) intake is consistent with energy expenditure. To reduce energy intake, limit consumption of foods relatively high in calories, fats, and sugars, and minimize alcohol consumption. Increase energy expenditure through regular and sustained physical activity.

- *Complex carbohydrates and fibre:* Increase consumption of whole grain foods and cereal products, vegetables (including dried beans and peas), and fruits.

- *Sodium:* Reduce intake of sodium by choosing foods relatively low in sodium and limiting amount of salt added in food preparation and at the table.

- *Alcohol:* To reduce the risk for chronic disease, take alcohol only in moderation (no more than two drinks a day), if at all. Avoid drinking any alcohol before or while driving, operating machinery, taking medications, or engaging in any other activity requiring judgment. Avoid drinking alcohol while pregnant.

Other Issues for Some People:

- *Fluoride:* Community water systems should contain fluoride at optimal levels for prevention of tooth decay. If such water is not available, use other appropriate sources of fluoride.

- *Sugars:* Those who are particularly vulnerable to dental caries (cavities), especially children, should limit their consumption and frequency of use of foods high in sugars.

- *Calcium:* Adolescent girls and adult women should increase consumption of foods high in calcium, including low-fat dairy products.

- *Iron:* Children, adolescents, and women of childbearing age should be sure to consume foods that are good sources of iron, such as lean meats, fish, certain beans, and iron-enriched cereals and whole grain products. This issue is of special concern for low-income families.

References

[1] Sheldon, W.H., Stevens, S.S., and Tucker, W.B. (1940). *The Varieties of Human Physique,* Harper, New York.

[2] Hartl, E.M., Mornelly, E.P., and Elderkin, R.D. (1982). *Physique and Delinquent Behaviour: a Thiry-year Follow-up of William H. Sheldon's Varieties of Delinquent Youth,* Academic Press, New York.

[3] Vague, J. (1956). The degree of masculine differentiation of obesities: a factor determining predisposition to diabetes, atherosclerosis, gout and uric calculous disease, *American Journal of Clinical Nutrition,* **4**, 20–34.

[4] Solomons, N.W. and Allen, L.H. (1983). The functional assessment of nutritional status: principles, practice and potential, *Nutrition Reviews,* **41**, 33–50.

[5] Eaton, S.B. and Konner, M. (1985). Paleolithic nutrition: a consideration of its nature and current implications. *New England Journal of Medicine,* **312**, 283–289.

[6] O'Keefe, S.J.D. and Lavender, R. (1989). The plight of modern bushmen. *Lancet,* **ii**, 255–258.

[7] Perissé, J. Sizaret, F., and François, P. (1969). The effect of income on the structure of diet. *FAO Nutrition Newsletter,* 7, 1–9.

[8] Keys, A. (1980). *Seven Countries: A Multivariate Analysis of Death and Coronary Heart Disease,* Harvard University Press, Cambridge, Mass.

[9] Munro, H.N. (1982). Interaction of liver and muscle in the regulation of metabolism in response to nutritional and other factors. In *The Liver: Biology and Pathobiology.* Editors Arias, I., Popper, H., Schachter, D. and Schafritz, D.A., pp 677–691. Raven Press, New York.

[10] Panel on Dietary Sugars (1989). *Dietary Sugars and Human Disease. Reports on Health and Social Subjects,* no **37**, HMSO, London.

[11] Zmora, E., Gorodischer, R., Bar-Ziv, J. (1979). Multiple nutritional deficiencies in infants from a strict vegetarian community. *American Journal of Diseases of Children,* **133**, 141–144.

[12] Henderson, J.B., Dunnigan, M.G., McIntosh, W.B. *et al.* (1990). Asian osteomalacia is determined by dietary factors when exposure to ultraviolet radiation is restricted: a risk factor model. *Quarterly Journal of Medicine,* **76**, 923–933.

[13] Bang, H.O., Dyerberg, J. and Sinclair, H.M., (1980). The composition of the Eskimo food in north western Greenland. *American Journal of Clinical Nutrition,* **33**, 2657–2661.

[14] Dyerberg, J., Bang, H.O., Stoffersen, E., *et al.* (1978). Eicosapentaenoic acid and prevention of thrombosis and atherosclerosis? *Lancet,* **ii**, 117–119.

[15] Kinsella, J.E., Lokesh, R., and Stone, R.A. (1990). Dietary n-3 polyunsaturated fatty acids and amelioration of cardiovascular disease: possible mechanisms. *American Journal of Clinical Nutrition*, **52**, 1–28.

[16] Munger, R.G., Prineas, R.J., Crow, R.S. et al. (1991). Prolonged QT interval and risk of sudden death in South-East Asian men. *Lancet*, **338**, 280–281.

[17] National Center for Health Statistics (1988). *Monthly Vital Statistics Report*, vol **37**, no 1 April 25.

[18] Brown, M.S., Kovanen, P.T. and Goldstein, J.L. (1981). Regulation of plasma cholesterol by lipoprotein receptors. *Science*, **212**, 628–635.

[19] Steinberg, D. and Witzum, J.L. (1990). Lipoproteins and atherogenesis. *Journal of the American Medical Association*, **264**, 3047–3052.

[20] Dawber, T.R. (1980). *The Framingham Study: the Epidemiology of Atherosclerotic Disease*, Harvard University Press, Cambridge, Mass.

[21] Grundy, S.M. (1986). Cholesterol and coronary heart disease: a new era. *Journal of the American Medical Association*, **256**, 2849–2858.

[22] The Surgeon General, (1988). *Report on Nutrition and Health*. DHHS (PHS) Publication No. 88–50210, p 110, U.S. Department of Health and Human Services, Washington, D.C.

[23] Glueck, C.J., and Connor, W.E. (1978). Diet–coronary heart disease relationships reconnoitred. *American Journal of Clinical Nutrition*, **31**, 727–737.

[24] Meade, T.W., Brozovic, M., Chakrabarti, R.R., *et al.*, (1986). Haemostatic function and ischaemic heart disease: principal results of the Northwick Park Heart Study. *Lancet*, **ii**, 533–537.

[25] The Surgeon General (1988). *Report on Nutrition and Health*. DHHS (PHS) Publication No. 88–50210, pp 95–106, U.S. Department of Health and Human Services, Washington, D.C.

[26] Medical Research Council Working Party (1977). Randomized controlled trial of treatment for mild hypertension: design and pilot trial. *British Medical Journal*, **i**, 1437–1440.

[27] Law, M.R., Frost, C.D., and Wald, N.J. (1991). By how much does dietary salt restriction lower blood pressure? I. Analysis of observational data among populations. *British Medical Journal*, **302**, 811–815.

[28] McCarron, D.A. (1982). Low serum concentration of ionized calcium in patients with hypertension. *New England Journal of Medicine*, **307**, 226–228

[29] Liu, K., Cooper, R., McKeever, J. *et al.* (1979). Assessment of the association between habitual salt intake and blood pressure: methodological problems. *American Journal of Epidemiology*, **110**, 219–226.

[30] MacMahon, S., Cutler, J., Brittain, E. *et al.* (1987). Obesity and hypertension: epidemiological and clinical issues. *European Heart Journal* **8**, (Suppl B), 57–70.

[31] Salomaa, V.V., Standberg, T.E., Vanhanen, H. *et al.* (1991). Glucose tolerance and blood pressure: long term follow up in middle aged men. *British Medical Journal*, **302**, 493–496.

[32] Saad, M.F., Lillioja, S., Nyomba, B.L. *et al.* (1991). Racial differences in the relation between blood pressure and insulin resistance. *New England Journal of Medicine,* **324**, 733–739.

[33] Jenkins, D.J.A., Wolever, T.M.S., and Jenkins, A.L. (1988). Starchy foods and glycaemic index. *Diabetes Care,* **11**, 149–159.

[34] The Surgeon General. (1988). *Report on Nutrition and Health.* DHHS (PHS) Publication No. 88–50210, p 257, U.S. Department of Health and Human Services, Washington, D.C.

[35] Jenkins, D.J.A., Leeds, A.R., Gassull, M.A. *et al.* (1977). Decrease in postprandial insulin and glucose concentrations by guar and pectin. *Annals of Internal Medicine,* **86**, 20–23.

[36] Sherlock, S. (1989). *Disease of the Liver and Biliary System,* 8th edition. Blackwell, Oxford.

[37] Small, D.M. (1968). Gallstones. *New England Journal of Medicine,* **279**, 588–593.

[38] Montgomery, R., Dryer, R.L., Conway, T.W. *et al.* (1983). *Biochemistry, a Case Orientated Approach,* 4th edition, p 453, CV Mosby, St Louis, 1983.

[39] Doll, R. and Peto, R. (1981). The causes of cancer: quantitative estimates of avoidable risks of cancer in the United States today. *Journal of the National Cancer Institute,* **66**, 1191–1308.

[40] The Surgeon General (1988). *Report on Nutrition and Health.* DHHS (PHS) Publication No. 88–50210, Chapter 4, Cancer, pp 177–247, U.S. Department of Health and Human Services, Washington, D.C.

[41] American Cancer Society (1991). *Cancer Facts and Figures,* p 3.

[42] Carroll, K.K. and Khor, H.T. (1975). Dietary fat in relation to tumorigenesis. *Progress in Biochemical Pharmacology,* **10**, 308–353.

[43] The Surgeon General (1988). *Report on Nutrition and Health.* DHHS (PHS) Publication No. 88–50210, pp 651–652, U.S. Department of Health and Human Services, Washington, D.C.

[44] Pilch, S.M., Editor (1987). *Physiological Effects and Health Consequences of Dietary Fiber.* Bethesda MD, Federation of American Societies for Experimental Biology.

[45] Murray, M.J., Murray, M.B., Murray, A.B. *et al.* (1976). Somali food shelters in the Ogaden famine and their impact on health. *Lancet,* **i**, 1283–1285.

[46] Moore, F.D. (1959). *The Metabolic Care of the Surgical Patient.* Saunders, Philadelphia.

[47] Cuthbertson, D.P. (1932). Observations on the disturbance of metabolism produced by injury to the limbs. *Quarterly Journal of Medicine,* **1**, 233–246.

[48] Bistrian, B.R. (1977). Interaction of nutrition and infection in the hospital setting. *American Journal of Clinical Nutrition,* **30**, 1228–1235.

[49] Buzby, G.L., Mullen, J.L., Matthews, D.C. *et al.* (1980). Prognostic nutritional index in gastrointestinal surgery. *American Journal of Surgery,* **139**, 160–167.

[50] McLaren, D.S. (1987). A fresh look at some perinatal growth and nutritional standards. *World Review of Nutrition and Dietetics*, **49**, 87–120.

[51] Barker, D.J.P. (1990). The fetal and infant origins of adult disease. *British Medical Journal*, **301**, 1111.

[52] Seidman, D.S., Last, A., Gale, R. *et al.* (1991). Birth weight, current body weight, and blood pressure in late adolescence. *British Medical Journal*, **302**, 1235–1237.

[53] Widdowson, E.M. (1951). Mental contentment and human growth. *Lancet*, **260**, 1316–1318.

[54] Jelliffe, D.B. (1959). Protein-calorie malnutrition in tropical pre-school children: a review of recent knowledge. *Journal of Pediatrics*, **54**, 227–250.

[55] McLaren, D.S. (1966). A fresh look at protein-calorie malnutrition. *Lancet*, **2**, 485–488.

[56] McLaren, D.S. (1988). A fresh look at protein-energy malnutrition in the hospitalized patient. *Nutrition*, **4**, 1–6.

[57] de Garine, I. and Koppert, G.J.A. (1991). Guru-fattening sessions among the Massa. *Ecology of Food and Nutrition*, **25**, 1–28.

[58] Jung, R.T. (1990). *A Colour Atlas of Obesity*. Wolfe Medical Publications, London.

[59] Bray, G. (1985). Obesity: definition, diagnosis and disadvantages. *Medical Journal of Australia*, **142**, S2–8.

[60] Stunkard, A.J., Sorensen, T.I.A., Hanis, C. *et al.* (1988). An adoption study of human obesity. *New England Journal of Medicine*, **314**, 193–198.

[61] Larsson, B., Svardsudd, K., Welin, L. *et al.* (1984). Abdominal adipose tissue distribution, obesity, and risk of cardiovascular disease and death: 13 year follow up of participants in the study of men born in 1913. *British Medical Journal*, **288**, 1401–1404.

[62] Krotkiewski, M. (1988). Can body fat be changed? *Acta Medica Scandinavica*, Suppl **723**, 213–223.

[63] Bouchard, C. (1988). Inheritance of human fat distribution. In *Fat Distribution During Growth and Later Health Outcomes.* Editors Bouchard, C. and Johnston, F.E., pp 103–125. Alan R. Liss, New York.

[64] Blomhoff, R., Green, M.H., Berg, T. *et al.* (1990). Transport and storage of vitamin A. *Science*, **250**, 399–404.

[65] Natadisastra, G., Wittpenn, J.R., West, K.P. Jr., *et al.* (1987). Impression cytology for detection of vitamin A deficiency. *Archives of Ophthalmology*, **105**, 1224–1228.

[66] Sommer, A., Tarwotjo, I., Djunaedi, E. *et al.* (1986). Impact of vitamin A supplementation on childhood mortality: a randomised controlled community trial. *Lancet*, **i**, 1169–1173.

[67] World Health Organization. (1982). *Control of Vitamin A Deficiency and Xerophthalmia. Technical Report Series*, no **672**, WHO, Geneva.

[68] McLaren, D.S. and Zekian, B. (1971). Failure of enzyme cleavage of beta-carotene: the cause of vitamin A deficiency in a child. *American Journal of Diseases of Children*, **121**, 278–280.

[69] Ahmed, F., Ellis, J., Murphy, J. *et al.* (1990). Excessive faecal loss of vitamin A (retinol) in cystic fibrosis. *Archives of Disease in Childhood*, **65**, 589–593.

[70] Matsuo, T., Matsuo, N., Shiraga, F. et al. (1988). Keratomalacia in a child with familial hypo-retinol-binding proteinaemia. *Japanese Journal of Ophthalmology*, **32**, 249–254.

[71] Harnois, C., Samson, J., Malenfant, M. *et al.* (1989). Canthaxanthin retinopathy: anatomic and functional reversibility. *Archives of Ophthalmology*, **107**, 538–540.

[72] McLaren, D.S. (1991). The fat soluble vitamins. In *Textbook of Paediatric Nutrition*, 4th edition, pp 391–403. Editors McLaren, D.S., Burman, D., Belton, N.R. and Williams, A.F. Churchill Livingstone, Edinburgh.

[73] Victor, M., Adams, R.D., and Collins, G.H. (1971). *The Wernicke-Korsakoff Syndrome*. Davis, Philadelphia.

[74] Anon. (1990). Korsakoff's syndrome. *Lancet*, **336**, 912–913.

[75] Campbell, C.H. (1984). The severe lactic acidosis of thiamine deficiency: acute pernicious or fulminating beriberi. *Lancet*, **ii**, 446–449.

[76] Schaumberg, H., Kaplan, J., Windebank, A. *et al.* (1983). Sensory neuropathy from pyridoxine abuse. A new megavitamin syndrome. *New England Journal of Medicine*, **309**, 445–448.

[77] MRC Vitamin Study Research Group. (1991). Prevention of neural tube defects: results of the Medical Research Council vitamin study. *Lancet*, **338**, 131–137.

[78] Herbert, V.D. and Colman, N. (1988). Folic acid and vitamin B_{12}. In *Modern Nutrition in Health and Disease*, 7th edition, pp 388–416. Editors Shils, M. and Young, V.R. Lea and Febiger, Philadelphia.

[79] Danford, D.E., and Munro, H.N. (1982). The liver in relation to the B vitamins, pp 367–384. In *The Liver: Biology and Pathobiology*. Editors Arias, I., Popper, H., Schechter, D. and Shafritz, D.A. Raven Press, New York.

[80] Hetzel, B.S. (1989). The iodine deficiency disorders: their nature and prevention. *Annual Review of Nutrition*,**9**, 21–38.

[81] Mu, L., Chengyi, Q., Qidong, Q. *et al.* (1987). Endemic goitre in central China caused by excessive iodine intake. *Lancet*, **ii**, 257–259.

[82] Hall, R. and Lazarus, J.H. (1987). Changing iodine intake and the effect on thyroid disease. *British Medical Journal*, **294**, 721.

[83] Jenkins, G.N. (1985) Recent changes in dental caries. *British Medical Journal*, **291**, 1297–1298.

[84] The Surgeon General (1988). *Report on Nutrition and Health*. DHHS(PHS) Publication No. 88–50210, pp 330–331, U.S. Department of Health and Human Resources, Washington, D.C.

[85] Passmore, R. Meiklejohn, A.P., Dewar, A.D. *et al.* (1955). Energy utilization in overfed thin young men. *British Journal of Nutrition,* **9**, 20–27.

[86] Fine, K.D., Santa Ana, C.A. and Fordtran, J.S. (1991). Diagnosis of magnesium-induced diarrhea. *New England Journal of Medicine,* **304**, 1012–1017.

[87] Dormandy, T.L. (1986). Trace element analysis of hair. *British Medical Journal,* **293**, 975–976.

[88] Broun, E.R., Greist, A., Tricot, G. *et al.* (1990) Excessive zinc ingestion: a reversible cause of sideroblastic anemia and bone marrow depression. *Journal of the American Medical Association,* **264**, 1441–1443.

[89] Wurtman, J.J. and Wurtman, R.J. (1983). Studies on the appetite for carbohydrates in rats and humans. *Journal of Psychiatric Research,* **13**, 213–221.

[90] Cliff, J., Lundqvist, P., Martensson, J. *et al.* (1985). Association of high cyanide and low sulphur intake in cassava-induced spastic paralysis. *Lancet,* **ii**, 1211–1213.

[91] Mills, A.A. and Passmore, R. (1988). Pelagic paralysis. *Lancet,* **i**, 161–164.

[92] Morrow, J.D., Margolies, G.R. and Rowland, J. (1991). Evidence that histamine is the causative toxin of scombroid-fish poisoning. *New England Journal of Medicine,* **324**, 716–720.

[93] Graziano, J.H. and Blum, C. (1991). Lead exposure from lead crystal. *Lancet,* **337**, 141–142.

[94] Walker, A. (1990). Warnings over cling film. *British Medical Journal,* **301**, 1179.

[95] Belongia, E.A., Hedberg, C.W., Gleich, G.J. *et al.* (1990). An investigation of the cause of the eosinophilia-myalgia syndrome associated with tryptophan use. *New England Journal of Medicine,* **323**, 357–365.

[96] Senti, F.R. (1988). Food additives and contaminants. In *Modern Nutrition in Health and Disease,* 7th edition, pp 698–711. Editors Shils, M. and Young, V.R., Lea and Febiger, Philadelphia.

[97] Anon. (1989). Nutritonal and metabolic response to injury. *Lancet,* **i**, 995–997.

[98] Francis, R.M. (1990). The calcium controversy. In *Osteoporosis,* pp 125–133. Editor Smith, R., Royal College of Physicians, London.

[99] Dawson-Hughes, B. Dallal, G.E., Krall, E.A. *et al.* (1990). A controlled trial of the effect of calcium supplementation on bone density in postmenopausal women. *New England Journal of Medicine,* **323**, 878–883.

[100] Kelly, P.J., Peacock, N.A., Sambrook, P.N. *et al.* (1990). Dietary calcium, sex hormones, and bone mineral density in man. *British Medical Journal,* **300**, 1361–1364.

[101] Jayanthi, V., Probert, C.S.J. and Mayberry, J.F. (1991). Epidemiology of inflammatory bowel disease. *Quarterly Journal of Medicine,* **78**, 5–12.

[102] Barker, D.J.P. and Morris, J. (1988). Acute appendicitis, bathrooms, and diet in Britain and Ireland. *British Medical Journal,* **296**, 953–955.

[103] Ashworth, M. (1990). Endemic bladder stones. *British Medical Journal,* **301**, 826–827.

[104] McLaren, D.S. (1963). Nutritional factors in urinary lithiasis. *East African Medical Journal,* **40**, 178–185.

[105] Valyasevi, A., Halstead, S.B. and Dhanamitta, S. (1967). Studies in bladder stone disease in Thailand. 6. Urinary studies in children, 2–10 years old, resident in a hypo- and hyperendemic area. *American Journal of Clinical Nutrition,* **20**, 1362–1368.

[106] Wickham, J.E.A. Editor (1979). *Urinary Calculous Disease.* Churchill Livingstone, Edinburgh.

[107] Braunwald, E. Editor (1988). *Heart Disease: a Textbook of Cardiovascular Medicine.* vol **2** p 1436, WB Saunders, Philadelphia.

[108] Matthews, W.B., Acheson, E.D. Batchelor, J.B. and Weller, R.O. (1985). *McAlpine's Multiple Sclerosis.* Churchill Livingstone, Edinburgh.

[109] Swank, R.L. (1950). Multiple sclerosis: a correlation of its incidence with dietary fat. *American Journal of the Medical Sciences,* **220**, 421–430.

[110] Swank, R.L. and Dugan, B.B. (1990). Effect of low saturated fat diet in early and late cases of multiple sclerosis. *Lancet,* **336**, 37–39.

[111] Birchall, J.D. and Chappell, J.S. (1988). The chemistry of aluminium and silicon in relation to Alzheimer disease. *Clinical Chemistry,* **34**, 265–267.

[112] Cox, I.M., Campbell, M.J. and Dowson, D. (1991). Red blood cell magnesium and chronic fatigue syndrome. *Lancet,* **337**, 757–760.

[113] Sorsby, A., Benjamin, B., Sheridan, M. *et al.* (1957). *Emmetropia and its aberrations: a study in the correlation of the optical components of the eye. Special Report Series Medical Research Council,* no **293**, HMSO, London.

[114] McLaren, D.S. (1980). *Nutritional Ophthalmology,* pp 318–322. Academic Press, London.

[115] Gerster, H. (1991). Review: antioxidant protection of the ageing macula. *Age and Ageing,* **20**, 60–69.

[116] Anon. (1990). Zinc and macular degeneration. *Nutrition Reviews,* **48**, 285–287.

[117] Kremer, J.M., Jubiz, W., Michalek, A. *et al.* (1987). Fish-oil fatty acid supplementation in active rheumatoid arthritis. A double-blinded, controlled, crossover study. *Annals of Internal Medicine,* **106**, 497–503.

[118] Walton, A.J.E., Snaith, M.L., Locniskar, M. *et al.* (1991). Dietary fish oil and the severity of symptoms in patients with systemic lupus erythematosus. *Annals of the Rheumatic Diseases,* **50**, 463–466.

Index

Numbers in bold type refer to figure captions.